VOLUME **2**

DISEASE CONTROL PRIORITIES • FOURTH EDITION

# Investing in Pandemic Prevention, Preparedness, and Response

Scan to see all titles in this series.

# DISEASE CONTROL PRIORITIES • FOURTH EDITION

## SERIES EDITORS

Ole F. Norheim
David A. Watkins
Kalipso Chalkidou
Victoria Y. Fan
Muhammad Ali Pate
Dean T. Jamison

## VOLUMES IN THE SERIES

Country-Led Priority-Setting for Health
**Investing in Pandemic Prevention, Preparedness, and Response**
Interventions Outside the Health Care System
Universal Health Coverage: Priorities and Value for Money

## VOLUME EDITORS

Siddhanth Sharma
Stefano M. Bertozzi
Victoria Y. Fan
Dean T. Jamison
Ole F. Norheim
Hitoshi Oshitani
Muhammad Ali Pate

# Disease Control Priorities

This fourth edition of *Disease Control Priorities* (*DCP4*) builds on the first three editions, all published by the World Bank. Through collaboration and capacity strengthening in a select number of low- and middle-income countries, *DCP4* summarizes, produces, and helps translate economic evidence into better priority setting for universal health coverage, public health functions, pandemic preparedness and response, and intersectoral and international action for health. *DCP4* aims to be relevant for countries committed to increasing public financing of universal health coverage and other health-improving policies, recognizing the need to set priorities on those countries' path to achieving the Sustainable Development Goals and beyond. The project is a collaboration between the World Bank and the University of Bergen, Norway, to develop and co-publish *DCP4* in four volumes with broad inputs from individuals and institutions around the world. These plans will likely evolve in the course of the work.

More people live longer and have better lives today compared to any other time in history. The world's population is aging at a dramatic speed. Improved living standards and new technologies are driving this change. However, we live in times of increased risks. No country can afford all technologies that are effective at improving health and well-being—and progress is unequal. The COVID-19 (coronavirus) pandemic has emphasized the vulnerability of countries when a threatening new infection affects life, the health system, work, and the economy. Climate change is another major challenge. Those already worse off are especially affected, by both direct and indirect effects on the health system, the economy, and the environment. During times of crisis, health care providers and policy makers must decide whom to prioritize and which programs to protect, expand, contract, or terminate.

These challenges are not unique to pandemics and climate change. Resource allocation decisions under scarcity are always being made, creating winners and losers when compared to the status quo. Such decisions may exacerbate or ameliorate existing inequities, which are often substantial. These risks are not the only reminders of the importance and urgency of priority setting in global health; in many low-income countries, the unfinished agenda with respect to infections and maternal and child mortality competes with increasing needs to prevent and treat chronic conditions such as cardiovascular diseases, cancer, and mental health. How should countries prioritize among infectious diseases, maternal and child health programs, and prevention of noncommunicable diseases? How should a health ministry define essential health benefit packages to be financed under universal health coverage reforms? Priority setting is key, and we now have the experience and the tools needed to improve and implement decision support for more efficient and fair resource allocation on the path to better health and well-being for all.

*Disease Control Priorities* provides a periodic review of the most up-to-date evidence on cost-effective and equitable interventions to address the burden of disease in low-resource settings. The third edition (*DCP3*), published by the World Bank Group, included nine volumes laying out a total of 21 essential universal health coverage packages and 71 intersectoral policies. Each essential package addressed the concerns of a major professional community and contained a mix of intersectoral policies and health sector interventions. Since then, several countries have used this evidence and translated it into revised health system priorities. In many countries, experts from the World Health Organization and the World Bank have been substantially involved. Key results have been published in a series of high-impact journal articles. *DCP3* relied primarily on cost-effectiveness analysis to evaluate interventions, using benefit-cost analysis in some cases to address the overall impacts on social welfare. It also introduced a new extended cost-effectiveness analysis method to account for the equity and financial protection impacts of extending coverage of proven effective interventions. *DCP4* builds on these methods but differs substantially from its predecessors by adopting a country-led approach to priority setting.

*Ole F. Norheim*
*David A. Watkins*
*Kalipso Chalkidou*
*Victoria Y. Fan*
*Muhammad Ali Pate*
*Dean T. Jamison*

VOLUME 2

DISEASE CONTROL PRIORITIES • FOURTH EDITION

# Investing in Pandemic Prevention, Preparedness, and Response

**Editors**

Siddhanth Sharma

Stefano M. Bertozzi

Victoria Y. Fan

Dean T. Jamison

Ole F. Norheim

Hitoshi Oshitani

Muhammad Ali Pate

WORLD BANK GROUP

# Contents

# Foreword by The Right Honourable Helen Clark

When public notification was provided for a pneumonia of unknown origin in the last days of 2019, some governments took notice and action, but life continued as usual in most countries. The World Health Organization's (WHO) declaration of a public health emergency of international concern (PHEIC) on January 30, 2020—the highest level of global public health alert at the time—failed to prompt meaningful action in many national capitals.

It was not until March 11, when the WHO Director-General characterized COVID-19 as a pandemic, that the gravity of the situation began to penetrate the halls of power. Apathy gave way to fear and panic. As the virus spread across borders with alarming speed, people began to ask: How could COVID-19 cause so much destruction so quickly?

At The Independent Panel for Pandemic Preparedness & Response—which I co-chair with President Ellen Johnson Sirleaf—we were determined to help answer that question. Our task, requested by the World Health Assembly, was clear: to examine the global response to COVID-19; identify the strengths, gaps, and failures; and provide actionable recommendations for the future. In May 2021, we presented our evidence-based package of proposals to the World Health Assembly. Our goal was to ensure that COVID-19 would be the last pandemic of such devastation. Our recommendations were urgent, ambitious, and practical.

We called for transformative change in several areas: highest-level political leadership; financing for pandemic prevention, preparedness, and response (PPPR) as a global common good; a strong and independent WHO; a modern and rapid system for surveillance and alert; equitable access to medical countermeasures; and accountability.

Since 2021, there have been areas of progress. WHO Member States have adopted amendments to the International Health Regulations. In May 2025, the World Health Assembly adopted a landmark Pandemic Agreement that provides a new framework for collective international action. The Pandemic Fund, launched in 2021, has raised much-needed financing for preparedness for low- and middle-income countries. An innovative mRNA technology transfer programme—engaging 15 middle-income countries—is helping to build scientific capacity and a geo-diversified research and development ecosystem.

Although these are important steps, we must be clear: progress has been neither fast enough nor far-reaching enough. If a novel pathogen were to emerge today, it would still find dangerous gaps in our systems that could allow an outbreak to escalate into a pandemic and prevent a rapid, equitable response if the worst were to occur.

Preparedness and response financing remains vastly insufficient and overly reliant on development assistance, which is itself now in grave jeopardy. Many countries and communities still lack access to the tools, systems, and resources they need to detect outbreaks early and respond effectively. Gaps in risk and readiness monitoring leave the world blind to emerging threats.

The recent responses to outbreaks of mpox and avian influenza A (H5N1) serve as sobering reminders of these shortcomings. The H5N1 response has exposed tensions between human and animal health sectors. The mpox response has seen reactive and delayed funding and a continued reliance on charitable models that leave low- and middle-income countries dependent on the goodwill of others. The development and stockpiling of medical countermeasures remains largely concentrated in high-income countries, and One Health approaches—essential to tackling zoonotic threats—are still not meaningfully integrated across sectors.

Despite these challenges, I remain optimistic. Of all the complex global problems that we face today, preventing a new pandemic is one we know how to address.

This important new collection brings together evidence and lessons from COVID-19 that can support policy makers in preparing better and in taking effective measures against new threats. The evidence-based discussion of a range of issues in these pages—including future mortality estimates, Always On systems, outbreak detection, public health measures, acute care, and financing—provides evidence upon which we can act.

The question is not whether we can do it, but whether we choose to do it. It is a matter of political will and collective action. Leaders must see pandemic prevention, preparedness, and response as core elements of a resilient, secure, and just world.

COVID-19 showed, in the starkest possible terms, that pandemic preparedness is not a theoretical or technocratic exercise. It is about lives, livelihoods, and the bonds of trust that hold societies together.

A new pandemic threat will emerge, and it will test us all again. Presidents, Prime Ministers, Ministers of Health and Finance—all leaders at every level—must recognize the responsibility they share. They have the lessons and the evidence to act now to prepare and respond. Not to learn from those lessons and act on that evidence puts us all at great risk. A virtue of this volume is that it provides options for any government with the foresight to address that risk.

*Helen Clark*
Co-Chair of The Independent Panel for Pandemic
Preparedness & Response;
Former Prime Minister of New Zealand;
Former Administrator of the United Nations
Development Programme

# Foreword by Gabriel M. Leung

The vocative title of this latest volume of the Disease Control Priorities project is spot-on: resourcing pandemic prevention, preparedness, and response is very much an "investment"—or at least insurance—as opposed to an expense. It yields one of the best health and economic impact returns, not least to reduce potential attributable lives (and livelihoods) lost, as chapter 2 attests. Every post hoc evaluation of past pandemics or consensus report to better prepare the world for the next global outbreak presents reinforcing empirical evidence. The case is indisputable.

Despite decades of recent experience—from influenza to severe acute respiratory syndrome (SARS), Ebola to mpox, and most recently COVID-19—gaps remain, particularly in implementing difficult but vital changes in the way governments prepare and respond. Some of these lacunae have remained unaddressed from epidemic to epidemic, whereas others arise from dynamic new developments in external circumstances. Chapter 3 on One Health presents an example of the former. Effective realization of this concept requires a whole-of-society approach, across all countries, to fundamentally redress frailties in animal husbandry and environmental degradation, reflecting recognition of their causative role in the generation and recrudescence of the zoonotic origins of many public health emergencies of international concern. The authors of chapter 1, echoing the 78th World Health Assembly that adopted the Pandemic Agreement by consensus, put the primary responsibility for this work squarely on the shoulders of countries and local authorities, albeit with external assistance as appropriate.

On how broader external changes can improve outbreak control, chapters 6 through 8 describe anti-epidemic measures that trace their first deployment to the fourteenth century. The very term "quarantine" descends from "quarantino" ("40 days" in old Italian)—the duration of holding incoming ships anchored off the Adriatic port of Ragusa to keep the bubonic plague at bay. These chapters illustrate how modern innovations have revolutionized what is now possible, for instance, the effectiveness of total lockdown of societal functions until vaccines became available during

COVID-19. In China, the powerful combination of "neighborhood committees" on the ground enforcing home quarantine, the conversion of community halls and sports stadiums to Fangcang shelter hospitals for isolation, and the ubiquitous use of the "super app" WeChat enabled the longest and most robust cordon sanitaire in history. Although sickness records of English boarding schools and the rotating term times of French schools by region have long established closures as an effective transmission-limiting measure, the prolonged nature of such closures during the COVID-19 pandemic tested the optimality between disease control and child development to the limit.

Chapters 9 and 10 remind us of the transformative role of vaccination, accelerated and empowered by the latest scientific breakthroughs on a timescale hitherto unseen, but increasingly threatened by populist "infodemics" and still made inaccessible to the most socially and medically needy through perpetuation of preexisting inequities. Unless and until satisfactory agreement is reached on the vexed annex of the Pandemic Agreement—the so-called product access and benefit sharing system—this Achilles' heel of global health security will remain so.

Whereas Chapter 11 gives us a reassuring glimpse of a future of Always On surveillance and early warning, the subsequent three chapters offer a sobering reminder of the critical turnkey of just-in-time and judicious financing. That financing must be guided by a nonpartisan and compassionate ethical compass to a world better protected from infectious perils is discussed in chapter 15.

Finally, hard science and rational policy often cannot overcome the realpolitik between and within countries. The recent upswing in nationalist populism across multiple countries and the corollary of wholesale diversion of overseas development aid to buttress defense budgets have shaken the global health architecture to its core. Ironically, those that built this system are particularly responsible for the demise of global health 1.0. Whether and how a 2.0 version will pan out—perhaps via a shifting and more transactional coupling of regional or otherwise like-minded sets of sovereign and philanthropic actors—remains uncertain.

That is precisely why the present volume is such a timely and valuable contribution of reasoned thinking to guide us through these interesting times. When making decisions, those in positions of authority who are entrusted to rebuild and reinforce our prevention, preparedness, and response system would do well to reflect on the chapters herein.

*Gabriel M. Leung*
Executive Director,
Hong Kong Jockey Club Charities Trust;
Honorary Professor, The University of Hong Kong,
Tsinghua University, and Peking Union Medical College Hospital
Hong Kong SAR, China

# Abbreviations

| | |
|---|---|
| AAL | average annual loss |
| ACER | average cost-effectiveness ratio |
| ADB | Asian Development Bank |
| AfDB | African Development Bank |
| AI | artificial intelligence |
| AMC | advance market commitment |
| AMR | antimicrobial resistance |
| ARDS | acute respiratory distress syndrome |
| AVMA | African Vaccine Manufacturing Accelerator |
| BCEPS | Bergen Centre for Ethics and Priority Setting in Health |
| BRICS | Brazil, Russian Federation, India, China, and South Africa |
| BSE | bovine spongiform encephalitis |
| BSL1 | biosafety level 1 |
| BSL2 | biosafety level 2 |
| BSL3 | biosafety level 3 |
| BSL3+ | biosafety level 3+ |
| BSL4 | biosafety level 4 |
| C19RM | COVID-19 Response Mechanism |
| CAT DDO | Catastrophic Deferred Drawdown Option |
| CCRT | Catastrophe Containment and Relief Trust |
| CEP | cumulative exceedance probability |
| CEPI | Coalition for Epidemic Preparedness Innovations |
| CERC | Contingency Emergency Response Component |
| CERF | Central Emergency Response Fund |
| CFE | Contingency Fund for Emergencies |
| CFR | case fatality ratio |
| CHI | controlled human infection |

| | |
|---|---|
| CHR | case hospitalization ratio |
| CI | confidence interval |
| C-MHI-MFI | combined mandatory home- and facility-based isolation |
| COPD | chronic obstructive pulmonary disease |
| COVAX | COVID-19 Vaccines Global Access |
| COVID-19 | coronavirus disease 2019 |
| CPRO | COVID-19 Pandemic Response Option |
| CRW | Crisis Response Window |
| CSF | Countercyclical Support Facility |
| CT | computed tomography |
| C-VHI-VFI | combined voluntary home- and facility-based isolation |
| DALY | disability-adjusted life year |
| DCP | Disease Control Priorities |
| DCP3 | *Disease Control Priorities, Third Edition* |
| DCP4 | *Disease Control Priorities, Fourth Edition* |
| DPL | Development Policy Loan |
| DURC | dual-use research of concern |
| EBRD | European Bank for Reconstruction and Development |
| ECF | Extended Fund & Credit Facility |
| ECMO | extracorporeal membrane oxygenation |
| ECSC | emergency, critical, and surgical care |
| EDCTP2 | European & Developing Countries Clinical Trials Partnership, Second Programme (2014–24) |
| EKG | electrocardiogram |
| EP | exceedance probability |
| EPF | exceedance probability function |
| EPI | Expanded Programme on Immunization |
| EVD | Ebola virus disease |
| FAO | Food and Agricultural Organization of the United Nations |
| FMD | foot and mouth disease |
| FOI | force of infection |
| Gavi | Gavi, the Vaccine Alliance |
| GDP | gross domestic product |
| GFATM | Global Fund to Fight AIDS, Tuberculosis and Malaria |
| GHI | global health initiative |
| GHSI | Global Health Security Index |
| GNI | gross national income |
| H1N1 | swine flu |
| HEPR | health emergency prevention, preparedness, response, and resilience |
| HIC | high-income country |

| | |
|---|---|
| HIV | human immunodeficiency virus |
| HIV/AIDS | human immunodeficiency virus and acquired immune deficiency syndrome |
| IBRD | International Bank for Reconstruction and Development |
| ICER | incremental cost-effectiveness ratio |
| ICU | intensive care unit |
| IDA | International Development Association |
| IDB | Inter-American Development Bank |
| IDSR | Integrated Disease Surveillance and Response |
| IFFIm | International Finance Facility for Immunisation |
| IHR | International Health Regulations |
| IM | intramuscular |
| IMF | International Monetary Fund |
| IP | intellectual property |
| IPF | Investment Project Financing |
| IRM | Immediate Response Mechanism |
| IsDB | Islamic Development Bank |
| ISO | International Organization for Standardization |
| IV | intravenous |
| JEE | Joint External Evaluation |
| LAI | laboratory-acquired infection |
| LIC | low-income country |
| LMICs | low- and middle-income countries |
| MCER | marginal cost-effectiveness ratio |
| MDB | multilateral development bank |
| MERS | Middle East respiratory syndrome |
| MFI | mandatory facility-based isolation |
| MHI | mandatory home-based isolation |
| MIC | middle-income country |
| ML | machine learning |
| MPA | Multiphase Programmatic Approach |
| MRI | magnetic resonance imaging |
| Norad | Norwegian Agency for Development Cooperation |
| OCR | Ordinary Capital Resources |
| ODA | official development assistance |
| ODF | official development finance |
| OIE | Office International des Epizooties |
| OOF | other official flows |
| OT | occupational therapy |
| P&P | prevention and preparedness |
| PAHO | Pan American Health Organization |

| | |
|---|---|
| PEF | Pandemic Emergency Financing Facility |
| PEP | post-exposure prophylaxis |
| PforR | Program-for-Results |
| PHEIC | public health emergency of international concern |
| PHSM | public health and social measures |
| PISA | Programme for International Student Assessment |
| POC | point of care |
| PPE | personal protective equipment |
| PPP | purchasing power parity |
| PT | physical therapy |
| QALY | quality-adjusted life year |
| R | South African rand |
| R&D | research and development |
| RR | reporting ratio |
| RSF | Resilience and Sustainability Facility |
| SARI | severe acute respiratory infection |
| SARS | severe acute respiratory syndrome |
| SEIHR | Susceptible–Exposed–Infectious–Hospitalized–Recovered |
| SLP | speech language pathology |
| SMC | School Meals Coalition |
| TB | tuberculosis |
| TRIPS | Agreement on Trade-Related Aspects of Intellectual Property Rights |
| UHC | Universal Health Coverage |
| UN | United Nations |
| UNAIDS | Joint United Nations Programme on HIV/AIDS |
| UNEP | United Nations Environment Programme |
| UNFPA | United Nations Population Fund |
| UNICEF | United Nations Children's Fund |
| UNOCHA | United Nations Office for the Coordination of Humanitarian Affairs |
| UV | ultraviolet |
| VFI | voluntary facility-based isolation |
| VHF | viral hemorrhagic fever |
| VHI | voluntary home-based isolation |
| VOC | variant of concern |
| VSL | value per statistical life |
| VxRate | vaccination rate |
| VxEff | vaccination efficacy |
| WB_IBRD | World Bank, International Bank for Reconstruction and Development |

| | |
|---|---|
| WB_IDA | World Bank, International Development Association |
| WHO | World Health Organization |
| WOAH | World Organisation for Animal Health (founded in 1924 as Office International des Epizooties [OIE]) |
| WPV3 | wild poliovirus type 3 |

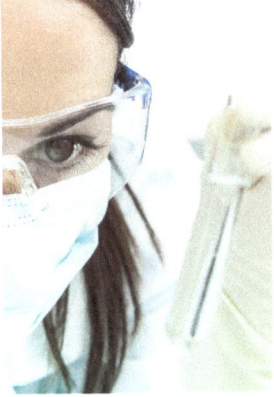

# Introduction: Lessons for Pandemic Policy

Stefano M. Bertozzi, Victoria Y. Fan, Dean T. Jamison, Ole F. Norheim,
Hitoshi Oshitani, Muhammad Ali Pate, and Siddhanth Sharma

This second volume in the World Bank's *Disease Control Priorities* series, *fourth edition* (*DCP4*), deals with pandemic prevention, preparedness, and response. A distinguished group of authors has reviewed the available evidence and experience to draw conclusions for policy. The volume's chapter 1 provides an overview of the main findings in the volume. In this Introduction, the editors present their own conclusions for policy by drawing on but stepping back from the specifics of the volume to convey the lessons we have drawn from working with each other and the authors over a number of years, including during our mutual experience of COVID-19 (coronavirus).

The Introduction focuses on lessons for policy, which raises the question of "whose policy?" Lessons tend to be general and potentially serve multiple policy communities. That said, previous editions of *Disease Control Priorities* focused principally on a global audience of interested academic institutions, international organizations, and major bilateral donors to health. This volume, in contrast, addresses what we view as the policy options of those individual countries whose governments actively seek to be prepared. It shares widespread concerns that some governments show little commitment to preparation—the United States in the years subsequent to the pandemic phase of COVID-19 is but one example. Communication directed to these governments (until well into the next pandemic) is likely of little value. Thus, this volume addresses the narrower audience of concerned policy makers, including those in government.

We start with the conclusion that policy matters. The *Lancet* Commission on Investing in Health found that, among the 30 most populous countries, the poorest-performing against mortality from COVID-19 (Bangladesh, Mexico, and the Russian Federation) experienced over five times the level of excess mortality as did well-performing countries (for example, China, France, and Japan) (Jamison et al. 2024). Even the best-performing countries, however, experienced severe losses of life, as well as economic and social disruption. The specific causal chains leading from policy to success or failure remain to be determined, will differ from pandemic to pandemic, and may never be definitively known. Even success will likely be incomplete. Policy plausibly makes an important difference, though, in separating merely bad outcomes from terrible ones.

The magnitude of pandemic risk provides the context for considering the significance of policy. Mortality risk remains high. In 2021, 2.6 million people died from AIDS, tuberculosis, or malaria (WHO 2024). In a particular year, it is unlikely that anyone will die in a pandemic; however, on average over time, and at current levels of risk, the analyses reported in this volume conclude that about 1.6 million people per year can be expected to die from an influenza pandemic and another 0.9 million from a coronavirus pandemic. These numbers should be viewed as only approximate, as known unknowns. In addition, unknown unknown sources of pandemic risk exist. Despite the unknown unknowns, the main dimensions of risk prove well enough understood to prepare for, and preventive measures to reduce risk are at least partially understood.

Our main conclusions for policy fall under five headings, which we will deal with in turn:

1. National policy makers would be mistaken to count on operating in a "good" environment.
2. Effective public health and social measures (PHSM) exist to slow transmission.
3. Effective medical countermeasures will likely be key to mitigating mortality.
4. Taking full advantage of vaccines, when and if they become available, will entail maximizing ease of access for those at high risk and with high motivation to be vaccinated.
5. Science is critically important, and much science will or can be local.

## 1. DIMENSIONS OF A GOOD ENVIRONMENT

Several dimensions of a "good" environment for pandemic prevention and response have been persuasively delineated in recent major reviews (Clark and Sirleaf 2025; Fisher 2025; Horton 2021; Osterholm and Olshaker 2025; Patrick, Larnder, and Ruck 2025; Sachs et al. 2022; Sridhar 2022; Yamey et al. 2024). They include the following:

- National governments and international organizations should support efforts at early detection of emergence of new pathogens, closely monitor gain-of-function research, and regulate activities involving high risk of animal-to-human transmission.
- Major international organizations should be well financed to respond quickly to global and country needs. International collaborations should invest in vaccine development and manufacturing capacity, increasing the probability of a quickly available vaccine with intellectual property that is widely shared.
- National populations should be induced to respond to national leadership in a cooperative spirit to contain the pandemic.

- Both mainstream and social media should be educated to provide an honest picture of the current state of the science and the trade-offs that science poses for individual and collective choice.
- National governments should prepare seriously for the next pandemic.

We join these other analysts in advocating for the creation of such a favorable environment, but little in the evolution of national and international politics in the past decade offers much hope. Although a final pandemic agreement (treaty) was agreed on in 2025, and reflects progress, reaching closure required so many compromises that little optimism is warranted. We feel that prudent national policy makers cannot realistically assume that an effective strain-specific vaccine will be available in their country any time early in a pandemic, that other governments will be prepared, that international cooperation will result in financial support, or that, for many countries, important segments of their own populations and media will be cooperative. Despite this bleak policy environment, much can still be done.

## 2. PUBLIC HEALTH AND SOCIAL MEASURES

Rapid implementation underpins attenuation of a pandemic's impact. Quick scientific assessment and publication on COVID-19 enabled the rapid responses actually implemented in many countries of the Western Pacific as early as mid-January 2020 (Wang et al. 2020). In addition to the Wang et al. warning of pandemic risk, *The Lancet* also published in January 2020 a prescient projection of the global spread of COVID-19 (Wu, Leung, and Leung 2020) and, in early March 2020, an assessment of the probable impact (or lack thereof) of mitigation measures that also proved prescient (Anderson et al. 2020).

Domains of early action include isolating known sources of infection (individual and community), isolating susceptible individuals from infection, and introducing measures to slow the spread of what will, with high probability, be an aerosol-transmitted virus. These measures will typically include masks, ventilation and air filtration, and social distancing including venue closures.

Isolating known sources of infection may involve unpopular measures like closing national borders or quarantining cities. Identifying (including through testing) and isolating infectious individuals is a lesson from public health 101, but remarkably many countries in the COVID-19 pandemic made essentially no effort to do so. At the same time many countries of the Western Pacific did create means for infectious individuals to isolate and effective incentives for that isolation. Arguably, these efforts contributed importantly to their success.

Rapid action involves not only rapid implementation of measures expected to slow transmission but also rapid relaxation of those measures when they are no longer needed (or when learning from experience has shown them to be ineffective). School closures provide an important example. Early in the course of COVID-19, epidemiologists learned that schools were not an important venue of transmission and that school-aged children were at minimal risk of death. Nevertheless, school closures remained in place in far too many countries for far too long. As frightened populations will undertake efforts to isolate themselves, public policy's role may well importantly lie in convincing individuals to return to normal life.

## 3. MEDICAL COUNTERMEASURES

In the early days of COVID-19, the case fatality ratios in Wuhan, China, were very high. Clinicians in Wuhan quickly developed approaches to supportive care that significantly improved survival prospects—and their findings were published in *The Lancet* less than two months after the pandemic began (Huang et al. 2020). Case management matters.

It is correct to say that each pandemic will differ from its predecessors. It is also true that, in all likelihood, aerosol transmission and respiratory distress will characterize the next pandemic. Thus, assuring good supplies of oxygen and appropriate isolation rooms will prove valuable not only for pandemic preparation but also more generally for health system strengthening. Ensuring that clinical staff are as protected as possible will also be key to ethically strengthening clinical response.

Rapid trial and error learning offers the promise of relatively quickly generating the clinical tools to enhance survival, and we return to this point in our discussion of the importance for governments to facilitate and encourage scientific understanding for responses to an unfolding pandemic. Rapid initiation of clinical learning, including identification and evaluation of effective medicines (and of which potentially promising medicines are ineffective), will be important.

## 4. VACCINES

Vaccines can provide protection against severe disease and death. Relatively early in COVID-19, strong government incentives and support resulted in German and US mRNA vaccines that provided such protection. Also apparently successful against mortality were more traditionally developed vaccines such as a vaccine from Oxford/AstraZeneca and another from Sinovac in China.

To the (possibly substantial) extent that vaccines primarily will confer individual protection, government policies to vigorously encourage or even coerce vaccine uptake are likely to prove counterproductive. Particularly early in a pandemic, vaccines are likely to remain in short supply and there will be high payoff to making available supplies easily accessible to individuals who wish to be immunized—prioritizing among them the most at risk like health care and other essential workers.

Unless it turns out that already-existing vaccines have some effectiveness against a new pandemic pathogen—and there is some evidence for this possibility—vaccines will, as we have stressed, become available only late into a pandemic if at all. PHSM combined with medical countermeasures thus will remain of primary importance even if, as with COVID-19, vaccines ultimately prove of significant value. Investing in vaccine development also provides insurance against the evolution of the pathogen into highly transmissible forms relatively invulnerable to PHSM. The much less good relative performance of China and Japan late in COVID-19 resulted, in all likelihood, from the evolution (elsewhere) of the Omicron variant, which was so transmissible that PHSM were less effective.

An implication of the potential to adapt relatively standard vaccines to deal with a new pathogen is that many individual countries will find it within their scientific capacity to develop and manufacture a potentially successful vaccine.

## 5. THE CRITICAL ROLE OF EVER-EVOLVING SCIENCE

Science underpins development of the understanding of pandemic characteristics, medical countermeasures, effective PHSM, diagnostics, and vaccines. Countries will, of course, differ in the extents to which they can mobilize effective scientific responses, but rapid mobilization of available resources will, at a minimum, facilitate rapid uptake of advances from elsewhere and systematic learning about what is working locally.

The effectiveness of masks, hand hygiene, and air filtration—to take a few examples—will depend on transmission characteristics of the virus and is thus knowledge that can be acquired locally while simultaneously learning from efforts elsewhere. At the same time much is known, or could be known, from the COVID-19 experience and accumulated experience with airborne transmission of respiratory viruses. It is thus puzzling that distillation of this experience into information of direct use to policy makers, clinicians, and the public remains so limited. There likewise appeared to be no up-to-date distillation that this volume could turn to of the best available evidence on the protectiveness of the major COVID-19 vaccines against infection, against severe disease, and against onward transmission. Distilling such information now would help pre-position a country's scientific community for action against a new outbreak. It would likewise help guide decisions about investing in stockpiles and reserve manufacturing and clinical capacity. Chapters in this volume provide valuable starting points on the evidence base, but much remains to be done.

Policy makers and the public will be well advised to listen carefully to science as it adds to existing knowledge. But listening carefully in no way implies "following the science." Scientists will (rightly) have their own views about trade-offs between vaccine safety and efficacy. Or between acting quickly on weak evidence or waiting for the evidence base to improve. Or about how to balance risks of quickly reopening schools against the social costs of prolonged closure. Their role as scientists, however, lies in providing policy makers and the public with the best available evidence on the trade-offs. Policy makers and the public should retain responsibility for making their own determinations—informed by science but not dictated by scientists. Governments that choose to take this perspective may find that they need to resist pressure from regulatory agencies and medical or public health establishments that would prefer to keep these trade-off judgments for themselves.

We judge that rapid mobilization of the scientific community, and committing substantial resources to it, will have high payoffs in national pandemic control. The scientific role is no less essential for being circumscribed.

*****

Collective striving for a better global environment for pandemic preparedness may well have some success, and that is to be hoped for—hoped for, but not planned for. We have in this volume attempted to elucidate the multiple pathways that a committed national government could follow for effective response despite an unsupportive international environment.

## REFERENCES

Anderson, R. M., H. Heesterbeek, D. Klinkenberg, and T. D. Hollingsworth. 2020. "How Will Country-Based Mitigation Measures Influence the Course of the COVID-19 Epidemic?" *The Lancet* 395 (10228): 931–34.

Clark, H., and E J. Sirleaf. 2025. "The Pandemic Agreement Is a Milestone: Now It Is Time for Action in National Capitals." *The Lancet* 405 (10495): 2109–11.

Fisher, D., ed. 2025. *Infectious Disease Emergencies: Preparedness and Response.* National University of Singapore Press.

Horton, R. 2021. *The COVID Catastrophe: What's Gone Wrong and How to Stop It Happening Again, 2nd Edition.* London: Wiley.

Huang, C., Y. Wang, X. Li, L. Ren, J. Zhao, Y. Hu, L. Zhang, et al. 2020. "Clinical Features of Patients Infected with 2019 Novel Coronavirus in Wuhan, China." *The Lancet* 395 (10223): 497–506.

Jamison, D. T., L. H. Summers, A. Y. Chang, O. Karlsson, W. Mao, O. F. Norheim, O. Ogbuoji, et al. 2024. "Global Health 2050: The Path To Halving Premature Death by Mid-Century." *The Lancet* 404 (10462): 1561–1614.

Osterholm, M. T., and M. Olshaker. 2025. *The Big One: How We Must Prepare for Future Deadly Pandemics.* New York: Hachette Book Group.

Patrick, D., A. Larnder, and C. Ruck, eds. 2025. *Understanding and Controlling Pandemics: Lessons Learned from COVID-19.* Volume 1 of *Effective Pandemic Response: Linking Evidence, Intervention, Politics, Organization, and Governance*, edited by P. Berman. Singapore: World Scientific.

Sachs, J. D., S. S. Abdool Karim, L. Aknin, J. Allen, K. Brosbøl, F. Colombo, G. Cuevas Berron, et al. 2022. "The *Lancet* Commission on Lessons for the Future from the COVID-19 Pandemic." *The Lancet* 400 (10359): 1224–80.

Sridhar, D. 2022. *Preventable: How a Pandemic Changed the World & How to Stop the Next One.* London: Viking.

Wang, C., P. W. Horby, F. G. Hayden, and G. F. Gao. 2020. "A Novel Coronavirus Outbreak of Global Health Concern." *The Lancet* 395: (10223): 470–73.

WHO (World Health Organization). 2024. "WHO Methods and Data Sources for Country-Level Causes of Death 2000–2021." Global Health Estimates Technical Paper WHO/DDI/DNA/GHE/2024.2, WHO, Geneva.

Wu, J. T., K. Leung, and G. M. Leung. 2020. "Nowcasting and Forecasting the Potential Domestic and International Spread of the 2019-nCoV Outbreak Originating in Wuhan, China: A Modelling Study. *The Lancet* 395 (10225): 689–97.

Yamey, G., A. V. Diez Roux, J. Clark, and K. Abbasi. 2024. "Pandemic Lessons for the 2024 US Presidential Election." *BMJ* 384: q150.

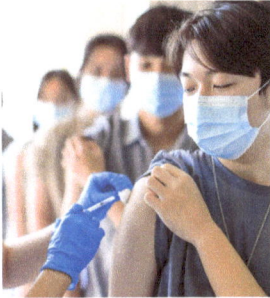

# 1

# Responding to Pandemic Risk: What Countries and Regions Can Do within the Constraints of Limited Global Cooperation and Solidarity

Siddhanth Sharma, Stefano M. Bertozzi, Victoria Y. Fan, Dean T. Jamison, Ole F. Norheim, Hitoshi Oshitani, Brett N. Archer, Till Bärnighausen, David E. Bloom, Donald A. P. Bundy, Simiao Chen, Maddalena Ferranna, Rachel Glennerster, Julian Jamison, Sun Kim, Nita K. Madhav, Jonna Mazet, Ben Oppenheim, Govind Persad, John Rose, Linda Schultz, Gabriel Seidman, David A. Watkins, Bridget Williams, and Muhammad Ali Pate

## ABSTRACT

The global response to pandemic threats remains inadequate, failing to translate the lessons of COVID-19 (coronavirus) into sustained investment and preparedness. The "panic and neglect" cycle persists, amplified by pandemic fatigue, denialism, misinformation, resistance to public health measures, and limited international cooperation. Against this backdrop, volume 2 of the fourth edition of *Disease Control Priorities* (*DCP4*) synthesizes scientific literature and expert knowledge to establish priorities for preventing, preparing for, and responding to future pandemics. This chapter synthesizes key insights from volume 2. It identifies priority actions based on the available evidence, while acknowledging that economic evaluations remain limited. Substantial reductions in pandemic risk can be achievable through targeted national and regional efforts, including the following:

- Recognizing the high ongoing pandemic risk (especially from influenza) and building adaptable, threat-agnostic frameworks rather than focusing solely on past experiences
- Implementing measures to minimize pathogen introduction from natural and human-made sources, and developing robust, layered early warning surveillance systems

- Rapidly characterizing novel pathogens to assess transmission and severity risks, and initiating timely containment actions based on available evidence, even if incomplete
- Investing in core public health functions (for example, surveillance and contact tracing), interlinked with resilient health care systems (for example, laboratory networks, oxygen supply, and emergency care) with adaptable surge capacity
- Tailoring public health and social measures to the specific pathogen, timing, and local socioeconomic context, moving beyond rigid preexisting pandemic plans
- Making critical investments in both rapid medical countermeasure development and regional manufacturing capacity, alongside streamlined regulatory pathways and robust delivery systems
- Establishing prearranged financing with swift disbursement based on clear, effectively designed triggers; prioritizing investments in dual-purpose infrastructure (for example, ventilation); and differentiating financial instruments for early (collective) versus late (domestic) needs.

*DCP4* underscores that pandemic preparedness can be markedly improved through national and regional efforts. The annex to this chapter offers an initial prioritization framework synthesized from expert opinion. Although the evidence base for many interventions continues to evolve, this framework provides a structured starting point for context-specific adaptation and helps identify priority areas for future research and evaluation. Breaking the cycle of panic and neglect requires action now—not after the next pandemic begins.

---

## INTRODUCTION

The fourth edition of *Disease Control Priorities* (*DCP4*) expands upon the foundation laid by previous DCP editions, translating health and economic evidence to help countries navigate a fair pathway to achieving universal health coverage. For the first time, an entire volume (volume 2) focuses on pandemics—a decision catalyzed by COVID-19 (coronavirus). Even before the pandemic, *DCP3* demonstrated foresight by dedicating two chapters to pandemic preparedness (Fan, Jamison, and Summers 2017; Madhav et al. 2017). The first chapter highlighted the magnitude of the economic risk posed by influenza pandemics, arguing that they received insufficient attention compared to other health priorities (Fan, Jamison, and Summers 2017). The second presented estimates of the probability of influenza pandemics, assessed the evidence on pandemic impacts (health, economic, social, and political), and synthesized the limited evidence on pandemic response measures and cost-effectiveness (Madhav et al. 2017). Like others (Hoffman and Silverberg 2018; International Working Group on Financing Preparedness 2017), this work highlighted the persistent "panic and neglect" cycle driven by multiple barriers: systematic underestimation of pandemic risk, constrained budgets, disincentives for investing in global public goods, and challenges in preparing for hypothetical threats.

The work of curating *DCP4*, volume 2, has shown that these challenges have only intensified. Widespread fatigue and disillusionment with pandemic response measures and public health interventions after COVD-19 have further complicated preparedness efforts. Despite numerous high-level reports outlining necessary improvements for pandemic preparedness (Horton 2021; Sachs et al. 2022; The Independent Panel 2021), momentum for change remains weak. As Helen Clark and Ellen Johnson Sirleaf noted in June 2024, the enormous political challenges to negotiating and ratifying a pandemic treaty, along with international mistrust, have left critical vulnerabilities, allowing "pathogens to spill over, slip through, and spread fast" (Clark and Sirleaf 2024, 9).

This chapter synthesizes key insights from volume 2 of *DCP4*. The volume addresses the full pandemic cycle framework (figure 1.1): prevention (actions to reduce spillover risk and pathogen emergence before outbreaks occur), preparedness (building capabilities to respond effectively when threats emerge), response (containing outbreaks and mitigating pandemic impacts), and recovery (rebuilding systems and communities after a pandemic).

**Figure 1.1** Framework for the Phases of the Pandemic Cycle

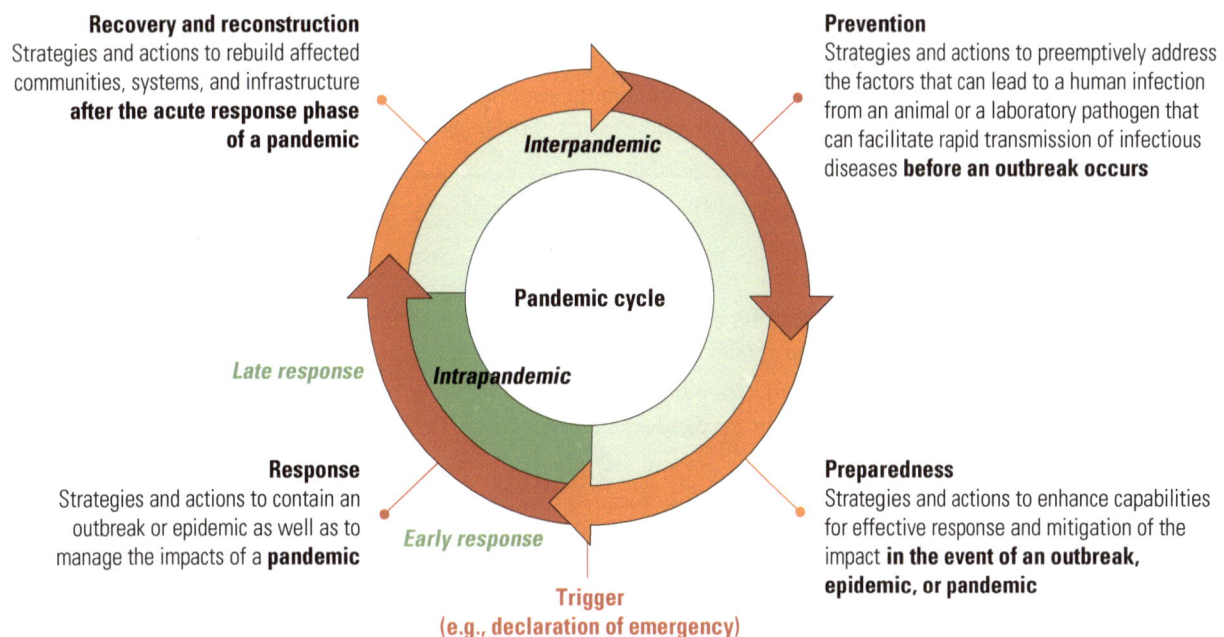

**Recovery and reconstruction**
Strategies and actions to rebuild affected communities, systems, and infrastructure **after the acute response phase of a pandemic**

**Prevention**
Strategies and actions to preemptively address the factors that can lead to a human infection from an animal or a laboratory pathogen that can facilitate rapid transmission of infectious diseases **before an outbreak occurs**

*Interpandemic*

Pandemic cycle

*Late response*

**Intrapandemic**

**Response**
Strategies and actions to contain an outbreak or epidemic as well as to manage the impacts of a **pandemic**

*Early response*

**Trigger**
(e.g., declaration of emergency)

**Preparedness**
Strategies and actions to enhance capabilities for effective response and mitigation of the impact **in the event of an outbreak, epidemic, or pandemic**

*Source:* Original figure created for this publication.

Given persistent global gridlock, the recommendations focus primarily on actions achievable at regional, national, and local levels. To support these recommendations, the annex to this chapter (comprising tables 1A.1–1A.6) presents a set of interventions prioritized through a synthesis of expert opinion. This chapter argues that targeted investments and reforms across all phases of the pandemic cycle can substantially reduce pandemic risks, even without global alignment and collective action. Despite a limited number of economic evaluations, the chapter identifies priority actions based on the available evidence and expert consensus. Although international reforms remain important, countries and regions need not wait for global consensus to strengthen their pandemic readiness.

## REASSESSING PANDEMIC RISK: OVERCOMING RESISTANCE AND COMPLACENCY

During COVID-19, a common narrative emerged that such catastrophic events occur only once per century (Gates 2020). This narrative fosters complacency and undermines efforts to invest in preparedness (International Working Group on Financing Preparedness 2017). Today, the challenges facing pandemic preparedness extend beyond mere complacency. The experience of COVID-19 has transformed public attitudes in many societies from indifference into active resistance against public health measures, creating substantial barriers to implementing even basic preparedness initiatives (Nicolo et al. 2023).

However, new modeling by Madhav et al. in chapter 2 of this volume challenges the assumption that pandemics on the scale of COVID-19 are a once-in-a-century phenomenon. Using historical outbreak data and probabilistic modeling (while acknowledging the inherent uncertainties in any attempt to model extreme events), those authors estimate that the likelihood of another respiratory pandemic with mortality on the scale of COVID-19 or worse is roughly 20 percent over the next decade. On average, this translates to about 2.5 million estimated deaths annually, implying that their expected harm ranks on par with the greatest global infectious disease challenges we face.

The modeling finds that pandemic influenza presents the greatest threat, with expected annual losses roughly double those from epidemic novel coronaviruses, and greatly exceeding expected losses from filoviruses. This finding carries implications for pandemic preparedness. Although we must learn from COVID-19 response strategies and their varying success across nations, we cannot allow these lessons to narrow our focus to coronavirus-like threats alone. Influenza pandemics typically affect younger populations more severely than COVID-19 did—a key consideration for health care planning, public health and social measures (PHSM), and financial risk protection. Even within influenza pandemics, however, there is enormous variation: historical pandemics have varied widely in terms of their severity, duration, health impacts across age and demographic groups, and broader economic and societal impacts. Our preparedness frameworks must therefore remain adaptable to diverse threat profiles, rather than becoming overly calibrated to historical experience (including our most recent experience).

## OPPORTUNITIES FOR PREVENTION: ADDRESSING SPILLOVERS, BIOSAFETY, AND BIOSECURITY

Most pandemics have originated from zoonotic pathogens that crossed from animals to humans. The frequency and severity of these spillover events continue to increase, largely because of changes in land use, agriculture, and wildlife trade (Meadows et al. 2023). In principle, preventing such spillovers at or near their source could avert a pandemic (Morse et al. 2012). Dobson et al. (2020) estimate that interventions to achieve this goal might cost about US$20 billion–US$30 billion per year. Despite uncertainty about the effectiveness of these measures, which makes optimal investment levels difficult to pinpoint, the potential cost of inaction is significant.

Chapter 3 explains how preventing spillovers requires first detecting and monitoring potential pandemic pathogens in animal populations before they reach humans. Strengthening integrated surveillance systems across wildlife, livestock, human, and environmental health sectors (a "One Health" approach) is a prudent step toward prevention. Early detection in animal populations allows authorities to implement preventive measures before widespread human cases occur, making such surveillance systems critical for pandemic prevention.

Detection alone, however, is insufficient. Effective containment—the capacity to control animal disease outbreaks once identified—is also required. The ongoing spread of highly pathogenic avian influenza A (H5N1) demonstrates both the value of surveillance and the immense challenge of containment (Peacock et al. 2025). This virus originally emerged in wild birds, later spread to poultry, and now infects dairy cattle (Peacock et al. 2025). It has shown concerning adaptations that could enable human-to-human transmission (Garg et al. 2024). Despite detection of the virus, insufficient livestock biosecurity has allowed for extensive spread in dairy herds. This containment failure not only threatens animal health but also creates more opportunities for viral adaptation through repeated spillovers (Simoneau, Hirshfield, and Speer 2024). Achieving better control also faces systemic barriers: farmers risk significant economic losses from livestock culling or trade bans, and authorities may fear political or reputational damage from acknowledging outbreaks. Policy solutions, including fair compensation for losses, may help overcome these barriers by building trust and encouraging transparency (Rushton et al. 2005).

Further upstream, preventing wildlife-to-human spillovers requires different approaches than controlling livestock outbreaks. Reducing wildlife-to-human transmission risk calls for careful monitoring and regulation of markets and trade (Vora et al. 2023). The origins of COVID-19, likely linked to the sale of wildlife in Wuhan's live animal markets (Crits-Christoph et al. 2024), illustrate both the catastrophic potential of wildlife trade and the speed with which policy can change once threats are taken seriously. China's 2020 wildlife trade ban demonstrates that rapid regulatory shifts are possible when political will aligns with public health imperatives (Koh, Li, and Lee 2021).

Chapter 4 illustrates how advancements in biotechnology present a separate source of pandemic risk beyond zoonotic spillovers. Although biological research is a cornerstone in reducing pandemic risks, as more facilities engage in high-level research, the potential for accidental pathogen release increases. Even minor laboratory mishaps can have major consequences, yet reporting of such incidents remains inconsistent. Unlike wildlife-human interfaces, the scale of which makes selective sampling necessary, laboratory biosafety requires universal surveillance. National and local authorities should, in line with the high-priority interventions outlined in table 1A.1, enforce mandatory lab biosafety standards, licensing, and incident reporting. Transparent reporting is essential for identifying common failure points, improving biosafety standards, and preventing unintentional outbreaks.

A parallel concern is the deliberate misuse of biotechnology, including the potential development of bioweapons. The accelerating capabilities of synthetic biology, automated laboratories, and artificial intelligence could enable smaller groups, or even individuals, to create or modify pathogens with pandemic potential (Pannu et al. 2024). This risk requires a dual approach to security. For legitimate research, governance frameworks must balance innovation with appropriate oversight of dual-use research (Wheeler 2025). However, malicious actors operating outside regulatory frameworks, like hostile states or criminal organizations, require different countermeasures. These countermeasures include robust intelligence capabilities, monitoring and regulation of equipment and material transfers (for example, DNA synthesis screening), and technical safeguards that limit a large language model's ability (like ChatGPT) to facilitate malicious acts. Addressing these interconnected threats requires coordination between scientific, security, and technology communities across borders (Lipsitch and Bloom 2012).

## EARLY DETECTION AND IDENTIFYING NOVEL THREATS

Once a pathogen has emerged in human populations, swift and accurate detection determines whether an outbreak is contained or escalates globally. Early identification provides a critical window for intervention, enabling timely resource allocation and response. Although understanding a pathogen's characteristics (for example, transmissibility and severity) is discussed in the next section, it bears emphasizing that timely and comprehensive detection lays the groundwork for these deeper assessments and the evidence-based decisions and actions they inform.

Frontline clinicians and diagnostic laboratories are often the first to raise the alarm (Hussein 2014; Lingappa et al. 2004; Mahase 2020; MMWR 1996, 2009; Pellejero-Sagastizábal et al., forthcoming). In December 2019, a cluster of atypical pneumonia flagged by Wuhan doctors signaled the earliest stage of the COVID-19 pandemic (The Independent Panel 2021). Relying solely on clinical vigilance can delay detection, however, because new pathogens are rarely top-of-mind for busy practitioners and often suspected only after excluding common causes, potentially weeks into hospital care (Chappell et al. 2021; Ecker 2020; Pellejero-Sagastizábal et al., forthcoming). To catch outbreaks earlier will require more systematic approaches. Chapters 5 and 11 illustrate how strengthening passive surveillance with genomic sequencing offers a promising strategy. For instance, targeted sequencing of a representative subset of influenza and COVID-19 polymerase chain reaction (PCR) detections can track pathogen evolution and diversity, whereas more novel approaches, such as respiratory viral metagenomics for severe acute respiratory infection (SARI) may enable the detection of entirely new pathogens.[1] By moving beyond predefined test panels, genomic methods reduce the risk of missing emergent threats and may avert weeks or months of undetected community transmission (Chappell et al. 2021).

Pathogen genomics, although powerful, presents challenges for low-resource settings because of its cost and complexity (Marais, Hardie, and Brink 2023; WHO 2021). Investing in sequencing infrastructure, specialized reagents, and trained staff may not seem locally cost-effective when the threat of a new pathogen appears low (Marais, Hardie, and Brink 2023; WHO 2021); however, this calculation changes dramatically when viewed from a global perspective. The localized expense of surveillance is orders of magnitude smaller than the societal and economic costs averted by stopping a pathogen at its source. For this reason, genomic surveillance and early warning systems should be treated as a global public good that merits external financing and coordinated support. Under such arrangements, countries with fewer resources can begin with simpler, tiered approaches: initially focusing on foundational laboratory and surveillance capacity and then establishing targeted sequencing of a small subset of influenza or COVID-19 samples, and referring more unusual or complex cases to regional reference laboratories for more advanced, untargeted sequencing. Over time, broader capacity to monitor febrile or respiratory illnesses can be expanded, enabling earlier detection and characterization of zoonotic threats that may spill over without yet transmitting from human to human.

Alongside clinical genomic sequencing, wastewater surveillance offers a complementary, relatively inexpensive approach (lower in cost per person than individual testing) for early detection (Sanjak et al. 2024). Municipal systems typically require substantial numbers of infected individuals to produce a detectable signal; however, targeted sampling in high-risk or high-traffic nodes (such as airports or hospitals) may yield earlier insights because such sampling requires fewer cases to produce a measurable signal (Morfino 2022). This approach can be particularly valuable in areas with limited clinical testing capacity or where health care access barriers exist.

## RAPID CHARACTERIZATION AND CONTAINMENT

When a novel pathogen is detected, rapid characterization of its epidemiological and molecular features is essential. That initial assessment determines the public health risk, guides immediate containment measures, and informs the development of countermeasures. A key early task, clarifying whether human-to-human transmission is occurring, is achieved through epidemiological investigation and genomic sequencing. If transmissibility is low, targeted measures like case isolation and controlling the zoonotic source may halt the spread. If an outbreak shows efficient person-to-person spread, however, governments face a narrow window to avert wider dissemination. The early response hinges on understanding key parameters including transmissibility, severity, and the extent of asymptomatic and presymptomatic spread.

Initially, determining these key parameters relies on intensive epidemiological work: detailed case finding, contact tracing, and analysis of early transmission chains. If a pathogen spreads rapidly, however, these traditional outbreak investigation methods can be quickly overwhelmed. The sheer volume of cases can make individual-level tracing unsustainable, leaving public health authorities with an incomplete picture of the outbreak's true scale and speed. In such scenarios, broader surveillance tools become valuable. Although expanding PCR testing capacity is critical, early-stage bottlenecks in laboratory infrastructure and supply chains are common. Developing and mass-producing point-of-care tests, particularly as a prepandemic goal supported by global research and development efforts (table 1A.5), may offer a more viable way to rapidly scale testing. Complementing individual diagnostics, wastewater surveillance can help track the extent of community spread. In several cities during the COVID-19 omicron wave, wastewater monitoring often predicted spikes 5–10 days before official case counts rose, providing valuable lead time for interventions (Cheng et al. 2023; Torabi et al. 2023).

Even with robust surveillance it may still be unclear whether the outbreak will evolve into a pandemic and cause significant harm. This uncertainty necessitates acting on incomplete information. Rapid risk assessment and decisive action, even with suggestive evidence, are more effective than waiting for certainty when the potential consequences are catastrophic. The COVID-19 timeline demonstrates this point: despite mounting evidence suggesting human-to-human transmission by mid-January 2020, many country, regional, and global health authorities waited for definitive proof before acting (The Independent Panel 2021). It took the World Health Organization (WHO) several weeks to gather sufficient evidence to confirm human transmission, and a full month to declare a public health emergency of international concern (The Independent Panel 2021). Major centers for disease control (for example, the European Centre for Disease Control and Prevention, and the US Centers for Disease Control and Prevention) showed similar hesitancy in their pathogen characterization and risk assessment, waiting for conclusive evidence before recommending important public health measures (ECDC 2020; Patel 2020).

Some Asia-Pacific economies moved faster. The Republic of Korea, Singapore, and Taiwan, China, quickly recognized presymptomatic and airborne transmission risks, enabling early deployment of large-scale testing, border closures, contact tracing, and mask recommendations—measures other countries adopted months later (Jamison et al. 2024; Jamison and Wu 2021). Their experience illustrates a key pandemic response principle, often described as a "no regrets" approach: decisions must be made using available evidence weighing the relatively low costs of early intervention against the potentially catastrophic consequences of delay (Smallwood et al. 2021). These economies achieved lower transmission rates and less economic disruption throughout 2020 precisely because they acted on incomplete but suggestive information. Accordingly, this chapter lists PHSM decision frameworks as a key priority (table 1A.2) to prepare before the next pandemic (Jamison et al. 2024; Jamison and Wu 2021). Early interventions can often be adjusted or scaled back if the threat proves less severe than initially feared, whereas opportunities for effective containment, once missed, may be impossible to recover.

Political and social barriers, however, often block early action. Leaders hesitate to implement substantial measures that might later appear unnecessary if successful—creating a paradox in which effective prevention appears in hindsight to be an overreaction. Pathogens with moderate severity but high transmissibility, as witnessed with COVID-19, create a distinctive risk perception challenge. Unlike diseases with high case fatality rates that immediately trigger alarm (such as Ebola), pathogens that cause more moderate levels of severe disease or death appear manageable when viewing individual cases. Their high transmissibility, however, means that they can rapidly infect millions, transforming a seemingly moderate threat into one with catastrophic aggregate impact that can overwhelm health care capacity. This combination is particularly challenging for decision-making because the window for effective early intervention often closes before the cumulative harm becomes evident enough to overcome political resistance to disruptive containment measures. Data-driven triggers—which chapter 14 argues should be simple, transparent, objective, verifiable, and preagreed—may help overcome these obstacles by making decisions more technical than political.

Infectious disease modeling can help guide the early response through understanding core parameters such as reproduction number, incubation period, and asymptomatic transmission rates (Davies et al. 2020; Ferguson et al. 2020). By simulating different scenarios, models can also help project future cases, anticipate hospital surges, and evaluate which interventions might best reduce transmission. Whereas single models provide useful insights, ensemble approaches like the US COVID-19 Forecast Hub better account for uncertainties and varying assumptions (Howerton et al. 2023). Modeling effectiveness, however, depends on data quality and transparent communication of results and limitations, highlighting the need for integrated surveillance systems and a clear description of model assumptions, uncertainties, and scenario analyses.

When effective pathogen characterization, risk assessment, and timely response align—backed by political commitment—containment becomes possible. If containment is deemed infeasible (Fraser et al. 2004), these same tools guide the shift to harm reduction and health care system resilience. Building these capabilities into preparedness plans enables faster mobilization during the critical containment window, or swift pivot to mitigation if that window closes (Craxì et al. 2020).

## STRENGTHENING CORE PUBLIC HEALTH AND HEALTH SYSTEM CAPABILITIES

Chapters 5, 6, 7, and 12 emphasize that a core lesson from COVID-19 is the need for strong public health and health system capacities. Basic functions such as surveillance, contact tracing, laboratory networks, and clear protocols for isolation were pivotal in controlling transmission. Foundational investments such as building disease notification and contact tracing systems are essential for enabling seamless use of these functions. Japan and Korea demonstrated how applying these measures effectively, particularly before vaccines became available, can slow outbreaks (Imamura, Saito, and Oshitani 2021; Issac et al. 2020). Japan's approach was especially instructive. Health authorities focused on the "three Cs" (closed spaces, crowded places, and close-contact settings) and prioritized backward contact tracing in these high-risk environments. This targeted strategy helped authorities identify infection sources, disrupt transmission chains, and use limited public health resources more efficiently (Imamura, Saito, and Oshitani 2021; Imamura et al. 2020).

Investing in foundational health care capabilities, especially oxygen systems, basic clinical care, and essential diagnostics (refer to the high priority health system interventions in table 1A.2), may be one of the highest-priority actions nations can take, as chapters 11 and 12 illustrate. These core capabilities serve dual purposes: they strengthen routine care for chronic conditions while providing surge capacity for outbreaks. The tragic oxygen shortages during India's Delta wave in 2021 highlighted this critical need: hospitals simply could not maintain adequate oxygen supplies as demand surged (Acosta et al. 2022; Sachs et al. 2022). Effective oxygen delivery requires reliable electricity, enabling facilities to generate oxygen on-site rather than relying on transported cylinders, thus providing greater scalability and lower long-term costs.

All core capabilities must include surge capacity. COVID-19 showed how rapidly demands can escalate across all aspects of response, from contact tracing teams to laboratory networks to hospital beds (Imamura, Saito, and Oshitani 2021; Sachs et al. 2022). Many countries struggled to expand these systems during the crisis, creating bottlenecks that undermined effective response. Building flexibility into routine systems, with clear escalation protocols and regular scenario exercises, enables more rapid and effective scale-up when needed. This approach helps health systems manage both the initial surge of cases and the sustained pressure of a full pandemic.

## PUBLIC HEALTH AND SOCIAL MEASURES: BALANCING EVIDENCE, TIMING, AND CONTEXT

COVID-19 prompted governments worldwide to implement a broad range of PHSM, from mask mandates to complete lockdowns. As chapters 6 and 8 explain, however, strong evidence on the effectiveness of each individual measure remains limited. Evaluating these interventions has been difficult because many countries (and jurisdictions within countries) introduced multiple measures simultaneously, with different degrees of strictness, in varying social and economic contexts (Talic et al. 2021). Still, comparing how different nations responded has offered useful insights on designing and implementing PHSM.

A key lesson is that PHSM deployment should be guided more by the specific epidemiological characteristics of the pathogen than by predefined pandemic plans (Huang et al. 2021). Decisions about stricter measures depend on factors such as how the pathogen spreads, its severity, and who is most at risk—all of which underscore the importance of gathering and analyzing evidence quickly in an emerging outbreak instead of simply applying strategies from past pandemics. Guided by preexisting influenza pandemic playbooks, many governments prioritized droplet- and fomite-based nonpharmaceutical interventions: physical distancing, hand hygiene, surface disinfection, and school closures (GIP 2019; Viner et al. 2020). Evidence from cluster investigations and an open letter by 239 scientists soon highlighted aerosol build-up in poorly ventilated venues as a dominant transmission route (Morawska and Milton 2020). Nevertheless, authoritative ventilation guidance and broad mask mandates often lagged by several months, especially in Europe and North America, compared with early adopters in East Asia.[2] Similarly, although pre-COVID-19 evidence suggested that travel restrictions would merely delay rather than prevent spread and would incur significant economic costs, during COVID-19 this delay proved important in buying time to prepare health systems and avoid overwhelming hospital capacity, especially before vaccines become available.

The timing of PHSM implementation strongly influences impact, particularly for highly restrictive measures such as stay-at-home orders (Zweig et al. 2021). Acting early when transmission is still low buys time to strengthen health systems, limit case numbers, and implement more targeted controls and shorter lockdowns; however, context matters significantly. India's nationwide lockdown in early 2020 demonstrated that strategies successful in wealthier countries can cause serious harm where social safety nets and financial support are weaker (Miguel and Mobarak 2022). This problem underscores the importance of tailoring public health responses to local conditions, with careful consideration of social and economic impacts, particularly in resource-limited settings.

## JUMPSTARTING MEDICAL COUNTERMEASURE PRODUCTION AND DELIVERY

COVID-19 exposed profound inequities in access to medical countermeasures. High-income countries, representing just 19 percent of the world's adult population, secured over half of all COVID-19 vaccine doses through advance purchase agreements, as illustrated in chapter 9. By mid-2022, only 16 percent of people in low-income countries had received a single vaccine dose, compared to 80 percent in high-income countries. The pandemic also demonstrated unprecedented acceleration in vaccine development. Traditional vaccine development typically takes a decade or more, but mRNA platforms, overlapping phase I–III trials, and substantial investments compressed this timeline to under a year (GAO 2021). This achievement showed how concentrated global effort and innovative technologies could dramatically speed up the development of medical countermeasures.

The economic case for investing in accelerated vaccine development and manufacturing capacity is compelling. Chapter 9 compares "100-day vaccines" to a one-year development timeline under two pandemic scenarios. In a moderate scenario with an estimated 38 million deaths, fast vaccine creation prevented 99 percent of deaths and saved a combined US$53.7 trillion in mortality and economic losses. Under a more severe scenario with 146 million potential deaths, 97 percent of deaths were averted and US$191.6 trillion saved. Although equitable distribution enhanced these benefits, the greatest gains came from speed of development and deployment. Achieving the full scale of these benefits depends critically on having sufficient manufacturing capacity in place before a pandemic strikes. After the first COVID-19 vaccines were authorized, supply constraints were the main bottleneck to increasing global coverage through most of 2021.[3] Chapter 10 estimates that, to build this capacity, investing approximately US$60 billion up front and US$5 billion annually to build worldwide production capacity could yield US$500 billion in net present value over 10 years.

Geographically distributed manufacturing capacity improves resilience by insulating supply from export controls and purchasing power imbalances. During COVID-19, nations with strong purchasing power dominated vaccine supply, and manufacturing countries occasionally restricted exports (Duke Global Health Institute 2020). Although regional production may incur higher peacetime costs, it provides protection against supply nationalism. Smaller economies can share the fixed costs by establishing joint manufacturing hubs, which in interpandemic periods can produce routine adult influenza and COVID-19 vaccines. In many low-income settings, however, demand for seasonal influenza vaccines remains low, partly because its moderate efficacy and uncertain cost-effectiveness weaken the case for large public procurement (Gharpure et al. 2022).

Regulatory frameworks and delivery systems require equal attention to ensure that innovations translate into impact. Swift rollout of vaccines, diagnostics, and treatments depends on streamlined regulatory approvals and robust clinical trial networks capable of rapidly evaluating new candidates (Mak et al. 2020; Wright et al. 2023). During COVID-19, WHO's Emergency-Use Listing and regional joint-review platforms such as the African Vaccine Regulatory Forum provided expedited pathways that dramatically shortened the usual regulatory timeline, allowing vaccines and other countermeasures to reach patients far sooner than would have been possible under routine procedures (Mak et al. 2020; Wright et al. 2023).

Meanwhile, last-mile delivery depends on resilient cold-chain logistics, well-trained health care workers, and proactive community engagement to foster trust and counter misinformation. Unlike typical mass vaccination campaigns for diseases like measles or polio that rely on substantial external support, pandemic vaccination efforts must often be scaled using local resources, because many countries simultaneously compete for scarce resources. COVID-19 highlighted how even abundant supplies can fail to achieve widespread coverage in a timely manner if public health systems do not receive sufficient resources or if misinformation erodes confidence. Strengthening these foundational elements (both upstream in regulatory processes and downstream in distribution) can accelerate equitable access and maximize the effectiveness of pandemic response efforts.

## REFORMING PANDEMIC FINANCING ACROSS THE PANDEMIC CYCLE

Chapter 13 explains how COVID-19 exposed critical weaknesses in global health financing. Reliance on multiple organizations and disparate funding mechanisms increased complexity and slowed the mobilization of resources. Most financing was negotiated during the outbreak rather than prearranged, leading to avoidable delays when rapid action was essential. These delays in securing and distributing resources hindered early containment efforts and later attempts to reduce morbidity and mortality. Wealthier countries secured supplies more swiftly, exacerbating global inequities. New initiatives like COVID-19 Vaccines Global Access (commonly known as COVAX), launched to promote equitable vaccine access, arrived late and were overshadowed by individual countries' bilateral purchasing. Although international coordination remains important to address these disparities, current geopolitical realities, such as the United States' withdrawal from WHO and significant cuts to its international aid, underscore the need for alternative approaches. Strengthening regional financing mechanisms (such as the African Union's African Vaccine Acquisition Trust and the Association of Southeast Asian Nations' COVID-19 response fund) could provide a more reliable and agile solution, allowing funds to be activated quickly and managed more efficiently than through global efforts alone.

Regional financing could support pandemic prevention and preparedness activities that function as global public goods—activities that safeguard every country by lowering both the chance that new pathogens emerge and the speed at which they spread. To ensure that regional or national investments genuinely boost these capacities, however, chapter 13 recommends the use of clear and independently verified metrics for readiness. Such indicators may be drawn from frameworks like WHO's International Health Regulations (or a comparable system) and tied to incentive-based funding, ensuring that resources directly strengthen prevention. Priority should go to building dual-purpose infrastructure (such as laboratory networks, surveillance systems, and clinical care and public health workforces) that both improve routine health care delivery and bolster outbreak response capacity. Countries with greater capacity can bear a larger share of these costs, whereas lower-income nations will require collective regional financing to address critical gaps. Whether funded domestically or through pooled mechanisms, these efforts contribute to global health security by strengthening frontline defenses against emerging threats.

Chapters 13 and 14 also draw attention to the need for clear, predefined release mechanisms to enable swift early outbreak response. The system should operate like a circuit breaker, releasing funds when key thresholds are met without requiring lengthy approval processes. A combination of contingency funds and pandemic insurance could provide this rapid funding, with preset agreements governing how and when money flows. Early regional collaboration carries strong incentives for all parties: swift, coordinated action at the outset of an outbreak serves collective interests, similar to how (as chapter 13 illustrates) containing a small fire protects an entire neighborhood from widespread damage.

In contrast, late response and reconstruction efforts primarily address domestic concerns. Although humanitarian considerations might justify external assistance, the incentive for collective self-interest is not there. Continuing the fire analogy made in chapter 13, although neighbors might help extinguish the blaze, responsibility for repairs and rebuilding generally falls on the homeowner. For this phase, prepurchased pandemic insurance, prearranged contingent loans, or grants act as essential financial safeguards. These mechanisms, tailored to a country's ability to pay, can provide a practical path to recovery.

## CONCLUSION

In summary, this second volume of *DCP4* confirms that the challenges highlighted in prior editions—neglected pandemic risks, weak preparedness, and political inertia—have only intensified. Nevertheless, this volume identifies clear opportunities for meaningful progress at national and regional levels. Among the top of these insights is that early decisive action based on incomplete information often achieved better outcomes than waiting for certainty. The COVID-19 pandemic also highlighted significant gaps across the preparedness and response spectrum—from surveillance and health system readiness to equitable access to countermeasures and the importance of context-specific public health measures. The expert analysis and evidence synthesized in this volume demonstrates that timely, evidence-based, and context-specific measures can save millions of lives and trillions in economic losses, even in today's era of fractured global cooperation.

## ANNEX 1A

Tables 1A.1–1A.6 present a set of interventions prioritized through a synthesis of expert opinion. The interventions specifically address pandemic prevention, preparedness, and response rather than broader global health priorities. This prioritization considered factors such as potential impact, feasibility, and cost, aiming to identify interventions offering significant value in pandemic prevention, preparedness, and response. The set of interventions is not exhaustive. Interventions are delineated for both national/local (tables 1A.1–1A.3) and global/regional (tables 1A.4–1A.6) contexts. Because of the currently limited evidence base for many interventions in diverse low- and middle-income country settings, the priorities should be considered tentative and are intended to stimulate context-specific analysis and guide future research to build a more robust evidence base. For global/regional contexts, tables focus on high-priority strategic interventions requiring international collaboration and coordination.

The national/local tables distinguish two key intervention categories: targeted measures refer to test, trace, isolate, and quarantine programs focused on identifying infectious individuals and their contacts; and PHSM encompass populationwide interventions such as gathering limits, mask mandates, ventilation improvements, and border controls. The tables use relative cost indicators ($, $$, $$$) for broad comparative prioritization of financial investment within a low- or middle-income country setting:

- $ **(low cost).** Modest financial resources (for example, policy, coordination, and leveraging existing resources)
- $$ **(medium cost).** Substantial investment (for example, comprehensive training, new protocols/equipment, and moderate infrastructure)
- $$$ **(high cost).** Significant financial outlay (for example, large-scale infrastructure, extensive technology, and broad multisectoral programs).

**Table 1A.1** Pandemic Prevention Prioritization, National/Local

| Priority | High | Medium | Low |
|---|---|---|---|
| One Health | • Implement livestock biosecurity. $$<br><br>• Establish intersectoral One Health coordination (risk assessment and data sharing). $<br><br>• Train frontline human/animal health staff within hot spots in zoonoses. $$ | • Conduct animal-human interface surveillance (sentinel surveillance with sampling and sequencing at hot spots). $$<br><br>• Implement wet market risk reduction (licensing and regulation). $$<br><br>• Implement livestock vaccination. $$ | • Reduce deforestation. $$$ |
| Biosafety/biosecurity | • Enforce mandatory lab biosafety standards, licensing, and incident reporting. $<br><br>• Implement biological research governance (review boards and risk-benefit assessments). $$ | • Invest in biorisk workforce (training, career paths, and certification). $$<br><br>• Tabletop exercises for accidental or deliberate threats. $$ | |

*Source:* Original table compiled for this report.

*Note:* $ = low cost; $$ = medium cost; $$$ = high cost.

**Table 1A.2** Pandemic Preparedness Prioritization, National/Local

| Priority | High | Medium | Low |
|---|---|---|---|
| Targeted measures | • Build local capacity for contact tracing. $$<br><br>• Plan repurposing of existing venues for isolation/quarantine facilities. $ | • Plan to support home isolation and quarantine. $<br><br>• Develop digital tools to support contact tracing. $$ | • Construct purpose-built isolation/quarantine facilities. $$$ |
| PHSM | • Establish PHSM evidence-based decision frameworks. $<br><br>• Develop and maintain essential service continuity plans. $<br><br>• Develop community engagement and risk communication plans. $<br><br>• Implement low-cost ventilation/filtration upgrades. $ | • Define context-specific border control protocols (closure, screening, testing, and quarantine). $<br><br>• Develop hybrid work/education infrastructure and policies. $$<br><br>• Expand ventilation/filtration upgrades. $ | • Support evidence generation to determine PHSM effectiveness. $$$ |
| Health systems | • Develop clinical care surge plans. $<br><br>• Invest in dual-purpose capacity (emergency care and infrastructure/workforce). $$<br><br>• Strengthen critical supply chains (for example, oxygen, PPE, and therapeutics). $$ | • Ensure universal basic/advanced life support training and equipment. $$<br><br>• Develop modules to rapidly expand critical care competencies during emergencies. $$ | • Strengthen advanced care capabilities (ECMO and renal replacement) at referral centers. $$$<br><br>• Develop adult immunization delivery platforms. $$$ |

*table continues next page*

| Priority | High | Medium | Low |
|---|---|---|---|
| Surveillance | • Strengthen disease notification systems. $$ <br><br>• Build essential public health lab capacity. $$ <br><br>• Strengthen syndromic and event-based surveillance capabilities. $$ | • Establish clinical-laboratory data link. $$ <br><br>• Build genomic surveillance. $$ <br><br>• Implement wastewater monitoring in targeted settings. $$ <br><br>• Build epidemological modeling capabilities. $$ | • Implement comprehensive genomic and wastewater surveillance. $$$ |
| Products and manufacturing | • Develop rapid procurement processes. $ <br><br>• Build and manage stockpiles. $$ <br><br>• Invest in cold chain infrastructure. $ <br><br>• Establish expedited regulatory review for emergencies. $ <br><br>• Establish lines of credit to finance at-risk capacity investments. $$ | • Develop local manufacturing capabilities for essential countermeasures. $$ | • Invest in full-scale countermeasure development. $$$ |

*Source:* Original table compiled for this report.

*Note:* ECMO = extracorporeal membrane oxygenation; PHSM = public health and social measures; PPE = personal protective equipment; $ = low cost; $$ = medium cost; $$$ = high cost.

**Table 1A.3** Pandemic Response Prioritization, National/Local

| Priority | High | Medium | Low |
|---|---|---|---|
| Targeted measures | • Implement contact tracing for high-risk contexts/settings. $ <br><br>• Provide guidance and support for self-isolation and quarantine. $ <br><br>• Test symptomatic contacts. $$ | • Expand contact tracing to low- to medium-risk contacts. $$ <br><br>• Establish/repurpose isolation facilities. $$ <br><br>• Deploy digital tools to support contact tracing. $ | • Attempt comprehensive contact tracing for all potential exposures. $$$ |
| PHSM | • Develop and activate emergency operations centers to coordinate surveillance, planning, and operational response. $ <br><br>• Deliver timely, transparent, and factual risk communication. $ <br><br>• Promote and enable core personal protective behaviors (for example, mask use and hand hygiene). $ <br><br>• Improve ventilation and air quality in high-traffic areas, prioritizing low-cost solutions. $$ <br><br>• Adopt school modifications that minimally disrupt education. $$ | • Implement policies to reduce workplace density. $$ <br><br>• Enforce capacity limits in public venues. $$$ <br><br>• Implement mask mandates, particularly for specific high-risk indoor settings (for example, health care, aged care, and public transportation). $ | • Implement broad restrictions on movement, nonessential business operations, or public access (lockdowns). $$$ <br><br>• Implement widespread domestic travel restrictions. $$$ <br><br>• Implement hotel quarantine and testing upon border entry. $$$ |

*table continues next page*

| Priority | High | Medium | Low |
|---|---|---|---|
| Health systems | • Activate national and subnational surge policies (as mentioned in table 1A.2). $$$<br><br>• Redirect resources to essential interventions:<br><br>– Health centers and clinics (triage and basic life support, including oxygen) $$<br><br>– First-level hospitals (basic diagnostics and supportive care for respiratory failure and shock, such as mechanical ventilation). $$<br><br>• Manage supplies of key commodities, especially oxygen. $$$ | • Maintain/protect essential nonpandemic services (including interventions in health benefits package). $$<br><br>• Expand rehabilitation services for patients following critical illness episodes and patients with postinfection disability syndromes. $$<br><br>• Expand supportive care for respiratory failure and shock to health centers. $$ | • Designate select referral hospitals for<br><br>– Advanced diagnostics and supportive care and $$$<br><br>– Advanced surgical and intensive care procedures. $$$ |
| Surveillance | • Monitor and openly report key indicators (for example, cases, hospitalizations, and deaths). $<br><br>• Ensure laboratory capacity for essential pandemic diagnostics (for example, PCR and culture). $$<br><br>• Conduct targeted genomic surveillance. $$<br><br>• Apply epidemiological analyses to inform response actions. $ | • Perform strategic wastewater monitoring. $$<br><br>• Deploy targeted asymptomatic testing in high-risk groups. $$<br><br>• Conduct epidemiological modeling to inform response planning. $$ | • Undertake populationwide asymptomatic testing. $$$ |
| Products and manufacturing | • Activate emergency procurement plans for diagnostics, therapeutics, oxygen, and basic PPE. $$$<br><br>• Streamline emergency regulatory pathways for pandemic products. $ | • Boost domestic production of essential generic medicines, basic medical supplies (for example, PPE and sanitizers), and relevant raw materials. $$<br><br>• Participate actively in international clinical trials for new pandemic countermeasures. $ | • Independently fund development of novel (early-stage) vaccine candidates. $$$<br><br>• Lead "moonshot" (high-risk, high-reward) biomedical R&D programs $$$ |

*Source:* Original table compiled for this report.

*Note:* PCR = polymerase chain reaction; PHSM = public health and social measures; PPE = personal protective equipment; R&D = research and development; $ = low cost; $$ = medium cost; $$$ = high cost.

**Table 1A.4** Pandemic Prevention High-Priority Interventions, Global/Regional

| Priority | High-priority interventions |
|---|---|
| One Health | • Develop coordinated animal-human interface surveillance networks (for example, testing humans at spillover hotspots and cross-border and intersectoral data sharing). |
| | • Implement harmonized wildlife trade regulation (coordinated monitoring, bans, and enforcement on the riskiest zoonotic species). |
| Biosafety/biosecurity | • Develop and implement international biosafety standards and peer-review audits. |
| | • Establish multilateral research governance norms and funding conditions (for example, mandatory risk reviews in donor requirements and journal policies). |
| | • Form a global DNA synthesis security consortium (access-controlled sequence databases, uniform screening protocols, and cross-border enforcement). |
| | • Establish a global registry of BSL3 and BSL4 labs, including both public and private. |

*Source:* Original table compiled for this report.

*Note:* BSL3 = biosafety level 3; BSL4 = biosafety level 4.

**Table 1A.5** Pandemic Preparedness High-Priority Interventions, Global/Regional

| Priority | High-priority interventions |
|---|---|
| PHSM | • Support evidence generation to determine effectiveness of PHSM. |
| | • Invest in R&D for improved environmental controls (ventilation, filtration, and germicidal ultraviolet light) and PPE. |
| Surveillance | • Strengthen global pathogen data-sharing platform (genetic sequences, test protocols, and validation data). |
| | • Strengthen global pathogen alert and rapid-response systems (rules for escalating high-risk signals and triggering regional/global support). |
| | • Implement strategic genomic surveillance at novel pathogen emergence hot spots. |
| | • Implement and strengthen strategic wastewater surveillance at high-risk areas (for example, major transportation hubs). |
| | • Drive R&D for broad-spectrum point-of-care diagnostics. |
| **Priority** | **High-priority interventions** |
| Products and manufacturing | • Invest in "warm" (rapidly repurposable) global manufacturing capacity. |
| | • Fund R&D for countermeasure platform technologies (vaccines, therapeutics, and diagnostics). |
| | • Prioritize R&D for high-priority pathogens (for example, universal vaccines and broad-spectrum antivirals). |
| | • Strengthen global clinical trial infrastructure (for example, recruit preselected cohorts who have given consent ex ante). |
| | • Strengthen oxygen supply chain and production capacity. |
| | • Multilateral development banks should establish credit mechanisms to help low- and middle-income countries finance at-risk capacity investments in the event of a pandemic |

*Source:* Original table compiled for this report.

*Note:* PHSM = public health and social measures; PPE = personal protective equipment; R&D = research and development.

**Table 1A.6** Pandemic Response High-Priority Interventions, Global/Regional

| Priority | High-priority interventions |
|---|---|
| PHSM | • Facilitate rapid evidence synthesis, and disseminate updated PHSM guidance for the current pathogen and its variants.<br>• Support systematic evidence generation to evaluate PHSM guidance. |
| Surveillance | • Standardize and facilitate global reporting of core epidemiological indicators (for example, cases, deaths, hospitalizations).<br>• Coordinate global surveillance (genomic, phenotypic), and enable rapid data sharing.<br>• Provide global/regional epidemiological modeling, forecasting, and technical support to countries.<br>• Conduct rapid risk assessments of transmission and disease potential to guide country responses.<br>• Support and coordinate international wastewater surveillance to monitor pathogen trends. |
| Products and manufacturing | • Mobilize and coordinate global manufacturing capacity for the rapid scale-up of needed countermeasures.<br>• Coordinate equitable global allocation and distribution of essential countermeasures (diagnostics, therapeutics, vaccines, and PPE).<br>• Support and expedite the rapid development, evaluation (including clinical trials), and adaptation of countermeasures.<br>• Coordinate global efforts to ensure access to medical oxygen and essential related clinical supplies.<br>• Incentivize vaccine manufacturing firms to build at-risk capacity.<br>• Use vaccine capacity efficiently (for example, "first doses first" policy).<br>• Invest in a diverse portfolio of vaccine candidates (across vaccine platforms). |

*Source:* Original table compiled for this report.

*Note:* PHSM = public health and social measures; PPE = personal protective equipment.

## NOTES

1. World Health Organization, "Surveillance Case Definitions for ILI and SARI" (accessed February 22, 2025), https://www.who.int/teams/global-influenza-programme/surveillance -and-monitoring/case-definitions-for-ili-and-sari.
2. Our World in Data, "Face Covering Policies during the COVID-19 Pandemic" (accessed April 19, 2025), https://ourworldindata.org/grapher/face-covering-policies-covid.
3. World Health Organization, "CoVDP Frequently Asked Questions" (accessed May 12, 2025), https://www.who.int/news-room/questions-and-answers/item/covdp-frequently -asked-questions.

## REFERENCES

Acosta, R. J., B. Patnaik, C. Buckee, M. V. Kiang, R. A. Irizarry, S. Balsari, and A. Mahmud 2022. "All-Cause Excess Mortality across 90 Municipalities in Gujarat, India, during the COVID-19 Pandemic (March 2020–April 2021)." *PLOS Global Public Health* 2 (8): e0000824.

Chappell, J. G., T. Tsoleridis, G. Clark, L. Berry, N. Holmes, C. Moore, M. Carlile, et al. 2021. "Retrospective Screening of Routine Respiratory Samples Revealed Undetected Community Transmission and Missed Intervention Opportunities for SARS-CoV-2 in the

United Kingdom." *Journal of General Virology* 102 (6). https://www.microbiologyresearch
.org/content/journal/jgv/10.1099/jgv.0.001595.

Cheng, L., H. A. Dhiyebi, M. Varia, K. Atanas, N. Srikanthan, S. Hayat, H. Ikert, et al. 2023.
"Omicron COVID-19 Case Estimates Based on Previous SARS-CoV-2 Wastewater Load,
Regional Municipality of Peel, Ontario, Canada." *Emerging Infectious Diseases* 29 (8).
https://wwwnc.cdc.gov/eid/article/29/8/22-1580_article.

Clark, H., and E. J. Sirleaf. 2024. "No Time to Gamble: Leaders Must Unite to Prevent
Pandemics." The Independent Panel for Pandemic Preparedness & Response.
https://theindependentpanel.org/wp-content/uploads/2024/06/The-Independent-Panel
_No-time-to-gamble.pdf.

Craxì, L., M. Vergano, J. Savulescu, and D. Wilkinson. 2020. "Rationing in a Pandemic:
Lessons from Italy." *Asian Bioethics Review* 12 (3): 325–30.

Crits-Christoph, A., J. I. Levy, J. E. Pekar, S. A. Goldstein, R. Singh, Z. Hensel,
K. Gangavarapu, et al. 2024. "Genetic Tracing of Market Wildlife and Viruses at
the Epicenter of the COVID-19 Pandemic." *Cell* 187 (19): 5468–82.

Davies, N. G., A. J. Kucharski, R. M. Eggo, A. Gimma, and W. J. Edmunds. 2020. "Effects
of Non-pharmaceutical Interventions on COVID-19 Cases, Deaths, and Demand for
Hospital Services in the UK: A Modelling Study." *The Lancet Public Health* 5 (7): e375–85.

Dobson, A. P., S. L. Pimm, L. Hannah, L. Kaufman, J. A. Ahumada, A. W. Ando, A. Bernstein,
et al. 2020. "Ecology and Economics for Pandemic Prevention." *Science* 369 (6502):
379–81.

Duke Global Health Institute. 2020. "Will Low-Income Countries Be Left Behind When
COVID-19 Vaccines Arrive?" *Research News*, November 9. https://globalhealth.duke.edu
/news/will-low-income-countries-be-left-behind-when-covid-19-vaccines-arrive.

ECDC (European Centre for Disease Prevention and Control). 2020. "Rapid Risk Assessment:
Cluster of Pneumonia Cases Caused by a Novel Coronavirus, Wuhan, China, 2020."
ECDC. https://www.ecdc.europa.eu/en/publications-data/rapid-risk-assessment-cluster
-pneumonia-cases-caused-novel-coronavirus-wuhan.

Ecker, D. J. 2020. "How to Snuff Out the Next Pandemic." *Scientific American*, May 18,
2020. https://www.scientificamerican.com/blog/observations/how-to-snuff-out-the-next
-pandemic/.

Fan, V. Y., D. T. Jamison, and L. H. Summers. 2017. "The Loss from Pandemic Influenza
Risk." In *Disease Control Priorities: Improving Health and Reducing Poverty* (third edition),
Volume 9, edited by D. T. Jamison, H. Gelband, S. Horton, P. Jha, R. Laxminarayan,
C. N. Mock, and R. Nugent. Washington, DC: World Bank. http://www.ncbi.nlm.nih.gov
/books/NBK525291/.

Ferguson, N. M., D. Laydon, G. Nedjati-Gilani, N. Imai, K. Ainslie, M. Baguelin,
S. Bhatia, et al. 2020. "Impact of Non-pharmaceutical Interventions (NPIs) to Reduce
COVID-19 Mortality and Healthcare Demand." Report No. 9, Imperial College
COVID-19 Response Team, Imperial College London. https://www.imperial.ac.uk/media
/imperial-college/medicine/sph/ide/gida-fellowships/Imperial-College-COVID19-NPI
-modelling-16-03-2020.pdf.

Fraser, C., S. Riley, R. M. Anderson, and N. M. Ferguson. 2004. "Factors That Make an
Infectious Disease Outbreak Controllable." *Proceedings of the National Academy of Sciences
of the United States of America* 101 (16): 6146–51.

GAO (United States Government Accountability Office). 2021. "Operation Warp
Speed: Accelerated COVID-19 Vaccine Development Status and Efforts to Address
Manufacturing Challenges." GAO-21-319, GAO, Washington, DC. https://www.gao.gov
/products/gao-21-319.

Garg, S., K. Reinhart, A. Couture, K. Kniss, C. T. Davis, M. K. Kirby, E. L. Murray, et al. 2024.
"Highly Pathogenic Avian Influenza A(H5N1) Virus Infections in Humans." *New England
Journal of Medicine* 392 (9): 843–54.

Gates B. 2020. "Responding to Covid-19—A Once-in-a-Century Pandemic?" *New England Journal of Medicine* 382 (18): 1677–79.

Gharpure, R., A. N. Chard, M. Cabrera Escobar, W. Zhou, M. M. Valleau, T. S. Yau, J. S. Bresee, et al. 2022. "Costs and Cost-Effectiveness of Influenza Illness and Vaccination in Low- and Middle-Income Countries: A Systematic Review from 2012 to 2022." *PLOS Medicine* 21 (1): e1004333.

GIP (Global Influenza Programme). 2019. "Non-pharmaceutical Public Health Measures for Mitigating the Risk and Impact of Epidemic and Pandemic Influenza." World Health Organization, Geneva. https://www.who.int/publications/i/item/non-pharmaceutical -public-health-measuresfor-mitigating-the-risk-and-impact-of-epidemic-and-pandemic -influenza.

Hoffman, S. J., and S. L. Silverberg. 2018. "Delays in Global Disease Outbreak Responses: Lessons from H1N1, Ebola, and Zika." *American Journal of Public Health* 108 (3): 329–33.

Horton, R. 2021. *The COVID-19 Catastrophe: What's Gone Wrong and How to Stop It Happening Again.* John Wiley & Sons.

Howerton, E., L. Contamin, L. C. Mullany, M. Qin, N. G. Reich, S. Bents, R. Borchering, et al. 2023. "Evaluation of the US COVID-19 Scenario Modeling Hub for Informing Pandemic Response under Uncertainty." *Nature Communications* 14 (1): 7260.

Huang, Q. S., T. Wood, L. Jelley, T. Jennings, S. Jefferies, K. Daniells, A. Nesdale, et al. 2021. "Impact of the COVID-19 Nonpharmaceutical Interventions on Influenza and Other Respiratory Viral Infections in New Zealand." *Nature Communications* 12: 1001.

Hussein, I. 2014. "The Story of the First MERS Patient." *Nature Middle East*, June 2, 2014. https://www.natureasia.com/en/nmiddleeast/article/10.1038/nmiddleeast.2014.134.

Imamura, T., T. Saito, and H. Oshitani. 2021. "Roles of Public Health Centers and Cluster-Based Approach for COVID-19 Response in Japan." *Health Security* 19 (2): 229–31.

Imamura, T., A. Watanabe, Y. Serizawa, M. Nakashita, M. Saito, M. Okada, A. Ogawa, et al. 2020. "Transmission of COVID-19 in Nightlife, Household, and Health Care Settings in Tokyo, Japan, in 2020." *JAMA Network Open* 6 (2): e230589.

International Working Group on Financing Preparedness. 2017. "From Panic and Neglect to Investing in Health Security." World Bank, Washington, DC. https://documents .worldbank.org/en/publication/documents-reports/documentdetail/979591495652724770 /from-panic-and-neglect-to-investing-in-health-security-financing-pandemic -preparedness-at-a-national-level.

Issac, A., S. Stephen, J. Jacob, V. Vr, R. V. Radhakrishnan, N. Krishnan, M. Dhandapani, et al. 2020. "The Pandemic League of COVID-19: Korea versus the United States, with Lessons for the Entire World." *Journal of Preventive Medicine and Public Health* 53 (4): 228–32.

Jamison, D. T., L. H. Summers, A. Y. Chang, O. Karlsson, W. Mao, O. F. Norheim, O. Ogbuoji, et al. 2024. "Global Health 2050: The Path to Halving Premature Death by Mid-century." *The Lancet* 404 (10462): 1561–614.

Jamison, D. T., and K. B. Wu. 2021. "The East–West Divide in Response to COVID-19." *Engineering* 7 (7): 936–47.

Koh, L. P., Y. Li, and J. S. H. Lee. 2021. "The Value of China's Ban on Wildlife Trade and Consumption." *Nature Sustainability* 4: 2–4. https://www.nature.com/articles/s41893-020 -00677-0.

Lingappa, J. R., L. C. McDonald, P. Simone, and U. D. Parashar. 2004. "Wresting SARS from Uncertainty." *Emerging Infectious Diseases* 10 (2). https://wwwnc.cdc.gov/eid /article/10/2/03-1032_article.

Lipsitch, M., and B. R. Bloom. 2012. "Rethinking Biosafety in Research on Potential Pandemic Pathogens." *mBio* 3 (5).

Madhav, N., B. Oppenheim, M. Gallivan, P. Mulembakani, E. Rubin, and N. Wolfe. 2017. "Pandemics: Risks, Impacts, and Mitigation." In *Disease Control Priorities: Improving Health and Reducing Poverty* (third edition), Volume 9, edited by D. T. Jamison,

H. Gelband, S. Horton, P. Jha, R. Laxminarayan, C. N. Mock, and R. Nugent. Washington, DC: World Bank. http://www.ncbi.nlm.nih.gov/books/NBK525302/.

Mahase, E. 2020. "Coronavirus: Doctor Who Faced Backlash from Police after Warning of Outbreak Dies." *BMJ* 368: m528. https://www.bmj.com/content/368/bmj.m528.

Mak, T. K., J. C. Lim, P. Thanaphollert, G. N. Mahlangu, E. Cooke, and M. M. Lumpkin. 2020. "Global Regulatory Agility during COVID-19 and Other Health Emergencies." *BMJ* 369: m1575. https://www.bmj.com/content/369/bmj.m1575.long.

Marais, G., D. Hardie, and A. Brink. 2023. "A Case for Investment in Clinical Metagenomics in Low-Income and Middle-Income Countries." *The Lancet Microbe* 4 (3): e192–9.

Meadows, A. J., N. Stephenson, N. K. Madhav, and B. Oppenheim. 2023. "Historical Trends Demonstrate a Pattern of Increasingly Frequent and Severe Spillover Events of High -Consequence Zoonotic Viruses." *BMJ Global Health* 8 (11): e012026.

Miguel, E., and A. M. Mobarak. 2022. "The Economics of the COVID-19 Pandemic in Poor Countries." *Annual Review of Economics* 14: 253–85. https://www.annualreviews.org/content/journals/10.1146/annurev-economics-051520-025412.

MMWR (Morbidity and Mortality Weekly Report). 1996. "Pneumocystis Pneumonia—Los Angeles." *MMWR* 1996 (45): 729–33. https://www.cdc.gov/mmwr/preview/mmwrhtml/lmrk077.htm.

MMWR (Morbidity and Mortality Weekly Report). 2009. "Outbreak of Swine-Origin Influenza A (H1N1) Virus Infection—Mexico, March–April 2009." *MMWR* 2009 (58–Dispatch): 1–3. https://www.cdc.gov/mmwr/preview/mmwrhtml/mm58d0430a2.htm.

Morawska, L., and D. K. Milton. 2020. "It Is Time to Address Airborne Transmission of Coronavirus Disease 2019 (COVID-19)." *Clinical Infectious Diseases* 71 (9): 2311–13.

Morfino, R. C. 2022. "Notes from the Field: Aircraft Wastewater Surveillance for Early Detection of SARS-CoV-2 Variants—John F. Kennedy International Airport, New York City, August–September 2022." *Morbidity and Mortality Weekly Report* 72 (8): 210–11. https://www.cdc.gov/mmwr/volumes/72/wr/mm7208a3.htm.

Morse, S. S., J. A. K. Mazet, M. Woolhouse, C. R. Parrish, D. Carroll, W. B. Karesh, C. Zambrana-Torrelio, et al. 2012. "Prediction and Prevention of the Next Pandemic Zoonosis." *The Lancet* 380 (9857): 1956–65.

Nicolo, M., E. Kawaguchi, A. Ghanem-Uzqueda, D. Soto, S. Deva, K. Shanker, R. Lee, et al. 2023. "Characteristics Associated with Attitudes and Behaviors towards Mask Wearing during the COVID-19 Pandemic: The Trojan Pandemic Response Initiative." *BMC Public Health* 23 (1): 1968.

Pannu, J., S. Gebauer, G. McKelvey, A. Cicero, and T. Inglesby. 2024. "AI Could Pose Pandemic-Scale Biosecurity Risks. Here's How to Make It Safer." *Nature* 635 (8040): 808–11.

Patel A. 2020. "Initial Public Health Response and Interim Clinical Guidance for the 2019 Novel Coronavirus Outbreak—United States, December 31, 2019–February 4, 2020." *Morbidity and Mortality Weekly Report* 69 (5): 140–46. https://www.cdc.gov/mmwr/volumes/69/wr/mm6905e1.htm.

Peacock, T. P., L. Moncla, G. Dudas, D. VanInsberghe, K. Sukhova, J. O. Lloyd-Smith, M. Worobey, et al. 2025. "The Global H5N1 Influenza Panzootic in Mammals." *Nature* 637 (8045): 304–13.

Pellejero-Sagastizábal, G., C. Bulescu, N. Gupta, P. Jokelainen, E. Gkrania-Klotsas, A. Barac, A. Goorhuis, et al. Forthcoming. "Delayed Correct Diagnoses in Emerging Disease Outbreaks: Historical Patterns and Lessons for Contemporary Responses." *Clinical Microbiology and Infection*. https://www.clinicalmicrobiologyandinfection.com/article/S1198-743X%2825%2900169-7/fulltext.

Rushton, J., R. Viscarra, E. G. Bleich, and A. McLeod. 2005. "Impact of Avian Influenza Outbreaks in the Poultry Sectors of Five South East Asian Countries (Cambodia, Indonesia, Lao PDR, Thailand, Viet Nam) Outbreak Costs, Responses and Potential Long Term Control." *World's Poultry Science Journal* 61 (3): 491–514.

Sachs, J. D., S. S. A. Karim, L. Aknin, J. Allen, K. Brosbøl, F. Colombo, G. Barron, et al. 2022. "The *Lancet* Commission on Lessons for the Future from the COVID-19 Pandemic." *The Lancet* 400 (10359): 1224–80.

Sanjak, J. S., E. M. McAuley, J. Raybern, R. Pinkham, J. Tarnowski, N. Miko, B. Rasmussen, et al. 2024. "Wastewater Surveillance Pilot at US Military Installations: Cost Model Analysis." *JMIR Public Health and Surveillance* 10. https://www.sciencedirect.com/org/science/article/pii/S2369296024002576.

Simoneau, M., S. Hirshfield, and M. Speer. 2024. "The United States Needs to Step Up Its Response to Bird Flu." Center for Strategic and International Studies, December 19, 2024. https://features.csis.org/US-bird-flu-response.

Smallwood, C. A. H., I. Perehinets, J. S. Meyer, and D. Nitzen. 2021. "WHO's Emergency Response Framework: A Case Study for Health Emergency Governance Architecture." *Eurohealth* 27 (1): 20–25. https://iris.who.int/handle/10665/344935.

Talic, S., S. Shah, H. Wild, D. Gasevic, A. Maharaj, Z. Ademi, X. Li, et al. 2021. "Effectiveness of Public Health Measures in Reducing the Incidence of COVID-19, SARS-CoV-2 Transmission, and COVID-19 Mortality: Systematic Review and Meta-analysis." *BMJ* 375: e068302.

The Independent Panel (The Independent Panel for Pandemic Preparedness and Response). 2021. "COVID-19: Make It the Last Pandemic." The Independent Panel. https://theindependentpanel.org/wp-content/uploads/2021/05/COVID-19-Make-it-the-Last-Pandemic_final.pdf.

Torabi, F., G. Li, C. Mole, G. Nicholson, B. Rowlingson, C. R. Smith, R. Jersakova, et al. 2023. "Wastewater-Based Surveillance Models for COVID-19: A Focused Review on Spatio-temporal Models." *Heliyon* 9 (11): e21734.

Viner, R. M., S. J. Russell, H. Croker, J. Packer, J. Ward, C. Stansfield, O. Mytton, et al. 2020. "School Closure and Management Practices during Coronavirus Outbreaks including COVID-19: A Rapid Systematic Review." *The Lancet Child & Adolescent Health* 4 (5): 397–404.

Vora, N. M., L. Hannah, C. Walzer, M. M. Vale, S. Lieberman, A. Emerson, J. Jennings, et al. 2023. "Interventions to Reduce Risk for Pathogen Spillover and Early Disease Spread to Prevent Outbreaks, Epidemics, and Pandemics." *Emerging Infectious Diseases* 29 (3):e221079.

Wheeler, N. E. 2025. "Responsible AI in Biotechnology: Balancing Discovery, Innovation and Biosecurity Risks." *Frontiers in Bioengineering and Biotechnology* 13 (February). https://www.frontiersin.org/journals/bioengineering-and-biotechnology/articles/10.3389/fbioe.2025.1537471/full.

WHO (World Health Organization). 2021. *Genomic Sequencing of SARS-CoV-2: A Guide to Implementation for Maximum Impact on Public Health.* Geneva: WHO. https://www.who.int/publications-detail-redirect/9789240018440.

Wright, K., N. Aagaard, A. Y. Ali, C. Atuire, M. Campbell, K. Littler, A. Mandil, et al. 2023. "Preparing Ethical Review Systems for Emergencies: Next Steps." *BMC Medical Ethics* 24 (1): 92.

Zweig, S. A., A. J. Zapf, H. Xu, Q. Li, S. Agarwal, A. B. Labrique, D. H. Peters, et al. 2021. "Impact of Public Health and Social Measures on the COVID-19 Pandemic in the United States and Other Countries: Descriptive Analysis." *JMIR Public Health Surveillance* 7 (6): e27917.

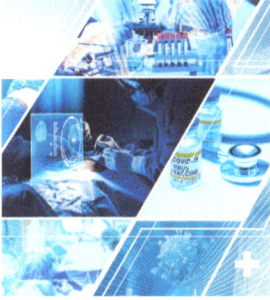

# 2

# Estimated Future Mortality from Pathogens of Epidemic and Pandemic Potential

Nita K. Madhav, Ben Oppenheim, Nicole Stephenson, Rinette Badker, Dean T. Jamison, Cathine Lam, and Amanda Meadows

## ABSTRACT

Epidemics and pandemics pose a sporadic and sometimes severe threat to human health. How should policy makers prioritize preventing and preparing for such events, relative to other needs? To answer that question, this chapter uses computational epidemiology and extreme events modeling simulations to estimate the risk of future mortality from low-frequency, high-severity epidemics and pandemics in two important categories: respiratory diseases (particularly those caused by pandemic influenza viruses and novel coronaviruses) and viral hemorrhagic fevers such as Ebola and Marburg virus diseases. The simulations estimate global annual averages of 2.5 million deaths attributed to respiratory pandemics and 26,000 viral hemorrhagic fever deaths, 72 percent of which are estimated to occur in Africa. Annual averages conceal vast year-by-year variation, and the reported analyses convey that variation, as well as variation across regions and by age. The estimates suggest higher frequency and severity of such events than previously believed and that this chapter likely provides a lower-bound estimate given the chapter's focus on deaths caused by a subset of pathogens. The simulations suggest that an event with the mortality level of COVID-19 (coronavirus) should not be considered a "once in a century" risk, but rather as having an annual probability of 2–3 percent (that is, occurring on average once in 33–50 years). Despite the substantial uncertainty in heavy-tail distributions, policy makers can use these estimates to develop risk-informed financing, prevention, preparedness, and response plans.

## INTRODUCTION

Long before the emergence of COVID-19 (coronavirus), policy analysts described pandemics as a "neglected dimension" of global security because of the persistent underfinancing of fundamental aspects of prevention and preparedness (Jamison et al. 2013; Sands, Mundaca-Shah, and Dzau 2016). Several high-level panels convened in the midst of the COVID-19 pandemic called for large increases in global spending on health system strengthening, surveillance, and preparedness (Sirleaf and Clark 2021). Although vital, these recommendations contend with an entrenched pattern of panic and neglect marked by a strong tendency for sporadic health emergencies to spark short-term attention and investment, which tails off all too rapidly once the crisis has passed.

The slide from panic to neglect happens in part because policy makers operate under uncertainty; they lack estimates of the probability of epidemics—including pandemics—that would enable them to prioritize preparedness for such events relative to other needs (refer to table 2.1 for definitions of epidemic, pandemic, and other terms used in this chapter). Consequently, epidemics and pandemics tend to be treated as random and unpredictable phenomena rather than events for which decision-makers can perform rigorous analysis, estimate costs, and prioritize investments.

**Table 2.1** Key Terms and Abbreviations

| Term | Definition used in this chapter |
| --- | --- |
| Average annual loss | The expected loss (in this chapter, deaths) per year. Refer to annex 2A for further details on its calculation. |
| COVID-19 | A coronavirus disease caused by SARS-CoV-2, beginning in 2019. |
| Direct mortality (or direct deaths) | Deaths caused by primary infection with a pathogen and any immediate secondary effects resulting directly from that infection. This chapter measures direct mortality from the time when an epidemic begins to when transmission ceases. |
| Epidemic | "The occurrence in a community or region of cases of an illness . . . clearly in excess of normal expectancy" (Porta 2014, 93). |
| Event catalog | A collection of historical or modeled events and associated data on event parameters and outcome estimates (Madhav, Stephenson, and Oppenheim 2021). |
| Exceedance probability function, annual | A function, also known as an "EP curve," providing the probability that an event of a given severity or worse will begin within a given year. For the purposes of this chapter, severity is measured in terms of deaths. |
| Excess mortality (or excess deaths) | "The mortality above what would be expected based on the non-crisis mortality rate in the population of interest."[a] |
| Normalized deaths | Deaths per 10,000 population. Also referred to in this chapter as population normalized deaths. |
| Pandemic | "An epidemic occurring over a very wide area, crossing international boundaries, and usually affecting a large number of people" (Porta 2014, 209). References in this chapter to epidemics include pandemics as well. That is, all pandemics are epidemics, but not all epidemics reach the level of becoming pandemics. |
| Respiratory diseases | Diseases that affect the lungs and other parts of the respiratory system.[b] Respiratory diseases of pandemic potential constitute one of the two disease categories modeled in this chapter. The modeled pathogens include pandemic influenza and novel/epidemic coronaviruses. |

*table continues next page*

**Table 2.1** Key Terms and Abbreviations (continued)

| Term | Definition used in this chapter |
|------|--------------------------------|
| Return period | Inverse of annual exceedance probability—that is, the average time between events of a given magnitude or greater (also known as return time or recurrence interval). (Refer also to box 2.2.) |
| Risk | The quantitative combination of the following information: (1) what can occur, (2) the probability that it can occur, and (3) the potential magnitude of consequences that can result (Kaplan and Garrick 1981). |
| Spread risk | Risk that a pathogen spreads from person to person. |
| Tail risk | Risk of low-probability, high-impact events (Cirillo and Taleb 2020). (Refer also to box 2.1.) |
| Viral hemorrhagic fevers (VHFs) | Diseases caused by viruses that damage organ systems, leading to hemorrhaging.[c] VHF epidemics constitute one of the two disease categories of events modeled in this chapter. The modeled pathogens include Ebola, Marburg, and Nipah viruses. |
| Zoonotic pathogen | "An infectious pathogen or parasite that originates in (or is maintained in the wild by) one or more non-human hosts, but can be transmitted to and cause disease in humans" (Han, Kramer, and Drake 2016, 567). The process by which a zoonotic pathogen is transmitted to a human being is called "zoonotic spillover." |
| Zoonotic spillover (or "spark") risk | Risk of transmission of an animal pathogen to a human. (Refer also to the definition of "zoonotic pathogen" in this table.) |

*Source:* Original table created for this publication.

a. World Health Organization, "Global excess deaths associated with COVID-19 (modelled estimates)," https://www.who.int/data/sets/global-excess-deaths-associated-with-covid-19-modelled-estimates.

b. National Cancer Institute, *NCI Dictionary of Cancer Terms*, "Respiratory disease," https://www.cancer.gov/publications/dictionaries/cancer-terms/def/respiratory-disease.

c. US Centers for Disease Control, "About Viral Hemorrhagic Fevers," https://www.cdc.gov/viral-hemorrhagic-fevers/about/?CDC_AAref_Val=https://www.cdc.gov/vhf/about.html.

Moreover, because the benefits of preparing for infrequent events are often invisible, policy makers often choose to prioritize preparedness for high-probability events rather than for rare ones (Lempert and Light 2009). To grapple with the threat posed by infrequent, severe epidemics, analysts should adopt a risk-based approach to decision-making, more akin to methods used for other natural catastrophes. Emergency planners and policy makers are already accustomed to thinking about natural catastrophes, such as floods and earthquakes, in terms of their frequency and severity (FEMA 2016); however, this discipline has not generally translated into public health planning.

A key objective of this chapter is to reduce some dimensions of uncertainty in the analysis of epidemics and pandemics by applying principles of risk management. To do so, it presents a framework through which probabilities can be estimated sufficiently to guide decision-making.

Although not typically used to plan for epidemics, this framework could be used to change the dominant paradigm for risk assessment and preparedness planning.

Adopting the most cost-effective strategies to prevent, prepare for, and respond to epidemics requires an understanding of their anticipated frequency and severity—that is, the level of risk that they pose. Interventions such as strengthening disease surveillance systems, investing in lab and diagnostic capacity, and developing new vaccine platforms, production systems, and supply chains might have a modest benefit-cost ratio if severe pandemics are merely a "once in a century" risk. If the risk is substantially greater, however, such interventions might be very cost-effective strategies to protect global health and reduce mortality. The risk estimates in this chapter allow decision-makers to approximate the necessary level of epidemic preparedness measures, and to identify which measures would be most cost-effective, both during and between epidemic periods.

This chapter presents estimates of the mortality risk of potential future epidemics caused by key respiratory pathogens and viral hemorrhagic fevers (VHFs). It offers new estimates and analyses of simulations, underscoring the substantial risk posed by epidemics. In the third edition of *Disease Control Priorities* (*DCP3*), Madhav et al. (2017) presented risk estimates focusing on pandemic influenza—only one, albeit critical, pathogenic risk with pandemic potential. This chapter expands on that foundation and updates the risk estimates provided in *DCP3* to include estimates for a broader set of epidemic risks. It incorporates new data and scientific advances into model enhancements, developed in part to support multilateral agencies, governments, philanthropic organizations, and the private sector. These enhancements also account for underreporting in epidemiological data and adjust for demographic changes since Madhav et. al (2017) was originally published.

Although many pathogens are capable of sparking large infectious disease events (for example, pandemic influenza viruses, Zika virus, coronaviruses, HIV, cholera, dengue virus, and more [Madhav et al. 2017]), the focus of the analysis in this chapter is based in part on the framework of Fraser et al. (2004) for assessing the controllability of epidemics caused by different pathogenic threats. In that framework, risk of an uncontrollable epidemic increases with human-to-human transmission efficiency and decreases with detection probability. This chapter therefore focuses on a subset of pathogens that meet these criteria and account for the majority of risk: respiratory diseases, notably those caused by pandemic influenza viruses and epidemic or novel coronaviruses. It also presents estimates for VHFs, encompassing filoviruses (such as Ebola and Marburg viruses) and Nipah virus. These pathogens are of global concern and meet some aspects of the criteria in Fraser et al. (2004) because of their potential for causing asymptomatic infection (Diallo et al. 2019) and evading detection (Glennon et al. 2019).

Several other categories of infectious disease threats, although recognized as important, were considered to be outside the scope of this chapter and were thus not included in the analysis:

- *Endemic diseases*, even if they can enter epidemic phases (for example, seasonal influenza, HIV/AIDS, and malaria), because these diseases have well-understood, frequently occurring patterns of losses
- *Vector-borne diseases* (for example, Zika and dengue), because their geographic ranges are constrained by climatic and ecological factors
- *Bacterial diseases*, including those arising from antimicrobial resistance, because treatment methods exist (although this chapter's estimates of direct deaths for viral respiratory diseases include bacterial co-infections)

- *Other nonviral diseases* (for example, prions and fungi), because they have limited geographies, modes of transmission, and transmission efficiency
- *"Unknown unknowns,"* or diseases caused by pathogens not thought to have the potential to infect humans, or those wholly unknown to science. It is important to bear fully in mind the significance of unknown unknowns: not so very long ago, HIV/AIDS would have fallen into this category.

The chapter also does not model risk from bioterror (deliberate release of infectious agents) or bio-error (accidental release of infectious agents, for example from laboratory accidents), because doing so would require additional modeling efforts incorporating, for example, the characteristics, capabilities, and strategies of terrorist organizations, and biosafety protocols and practices within specific laboratories. These factors can be explicitly modeled and linked with the broader risk modeling framework presented here but are beyond the scope of the present analysis (refer to chapter 4 in this volume for a discussion of biosafety and biosecurity).

Although epidemics can lead to many adverse outcomes—including infections, hospitalizations, deaths, societal disruption, educational delays, and economic shocks—this chapter focuses on deaths. It includes neither morbidity estimates nor estimates of the impacts of long-term sequelae, although they are important topics. The considerable welfare losses caused by epidemics and pandemics—including economic damages (refer to Fan, Jamison, and Summers 2017) as well as losses to education and to livelihoods, and trauma and psychological damages—require distinct modeling techniques and are beyond the scope of this chapter. This chapter focuses on deaths because they are the most readily measurable, observable, and reported metric, and therefore provide a less biased indicator of epidemic severity than other metrics such as infections or hospitalizations.

Given all of these considerations, the estimates presented in this chapter are not intended to capture the totality of epidemic risk. Rather, they should be interpreted as a lower-bound estimate of the potential loss from such events.

### Drivers of Epidemic Risk

Risk modeling is not simply an exercise in mathematics; it must appropriately represent real-world processes, and modelers should have familiarity with the complex web of underlying factors shaping the risk. The modeling framework for this chapter therefore explicitly incorporates several critical drivers of epidemic risk, including zoonotic spillover, global travel patterns, and governance challenges. The following paragraphs provide background information about these processes; annex 2A provides specific details of how they are incorporated into the models for this chapter.

Nearly all modern pandemics have sparked when zoonotic pathogens have jumped from animals to humans, often through activities such as hunting, habitat encroachment, and intensive livestock farming (Jones et al. 2013; Olival et al. 2017).

Multiple studies show that epidemics, especially those caused by zoonotic spillover events, are increasing in both frequency and severity (Jones et al. 2008; Smith et al. 2014). For a subset of high priority viruses, this trend is exponential, meaning not only that epidemics are becoming more frequent and more severe but also that spillover-driven epidemics are occurring at an accelerating rate (Meadows et al. 2023). Climate change and other forms of anthropogenic environmental change, such as deforestation and habitat fragmentation, are predicted to increase the frequency of zoonotic spillover events because they increase the frequency of contact between humans and animal reservoir species (Carlson et al. 2022).

Increasing human population density and connectivity through global travel and trade facilitate the spread of the outbreaks (Baker et al. 2021). The accessibility of global air travel makes effective containment of emerging outbreaks increasingly difficult because infected individuals can disperse over large geographic distances before cases are detected and reported to public health officials (Meslé et al. 2022). For example, rapid geographical spread was well-documented in the severe acute respiratory syndrome (SARS, caused by SARS-CoV-1) outbreak of 2003. In a hotel in Hong Kong SAR, China, 1 individual infected 10 others, 6 of whom took international flights to Australia, Canada, the Philippines, Singapore, and Viet Nam. These traveling secondary cases subsequently led to SARS outbreaks in Hanoi, Singapore, and Toronto within a few days of the first reported case in Hong Kong SAR, China (Cherry 2004). Similarly, during the COVID-19 pandemic, early detection of SARS-CoV-2 variants occurred in airline passengers (Wegrzyn et al. 2022). Spread by air travel also occurred during the 2014 West Africa Ebola epidemic (Gomes et al. 2014).

Evidence from serial infectious disease epidemics occurring in fragile and conflict-affected areas, perhaps most notably the 2018 North Kivu Ebola virus disease epidemic in the Democratic Republic of Congo, provides a clear reminder that conflict and instability can facilitate infectious disease transmission. Armed conflict can degrade disease surveillance systems, creating blind spots and lengthening the period during which disease transmission can occur before it is detected and mitigation measures are put in place (Wise and Barry 2017). Insecurity and violence can also increase the risk of disease transmission by facilitating population displacement (Price-Smith 2001) and by impeding public health response activities through operational disruptions, destruction of public health facilities and equipment, and direct attacks on public health personnel (Jombart et al. 2020). Public distrust of government institutions can also reduce compliance with disease control measures such as immunization campaigns and contact tracing, potentially leading to increased morbidity and mortality (Bargain and Aminjonov 2020; Farzanegan and Hofmann 2022; Vinck et al. 2019).

### Techniques for Estimating Risk

Apart from research published in *DCP3*, scant scientific literature exists dedicated to estimating the frequency and severity of infrequent, high-consequence epidemics

(Fan, Jamison, and Summers 2017; Madhav et al. 2017). In contrast to the well-described methods for estimating risk and burden of endemic and frequently occurring diseases, major public health or infectious disease epidemiology textbooks do not explore the quantification of risk—especially tail risk (refer to box 2.1)—from more sporadically-occurring epidemics (Bennett, Dolin, and Blaser 2019; Nelson and Williams 2014). Contributions on this topic have instead come from interdisciplinary research teams or the private sector (Cirillo and Taleb 2020; Marani et al. 2021; Wilkinson 2021). The relatively limited public health literature on the prospective analysis of risk and burden posed by epidemics is perhaps attributable to the multidisciplinary nature of the problem, and the development of estimation techniques within fields that have had limited interaction with public health researchers.

Following the conventions from *DCP3*, this chapter provides risk estimates in the form of exceedance probability functions (EPFs) (Madhav et al. 2017). An EPF can be analyzed to estimate the probability that an event of a given severity or worse will start in a given year, and other metrics of interest, such as the average annual loss (AAL). Modelers can estimate EPFs using empirical data from historical events, or use simulated data from modeled events. Empirical EPFs derived from historical data are most appropriate for pathogens that cause frequent outbreaks or that have a recurrent or seasonal pattern (for example, seasonal influenza or meningococcal meningitis). A historically derived empirical EPF may be misleading when historical data are sparse, marked by underreporting, or include unincorporated trends that could influence future expected losses (Madhav, Stephenson, and Oppenheim 2021). For those reasons, the EPFs for this chapter were generated using a probabilistic modeling approach that generates an event catalog containing simulated events.

## Historical Data Analysis

Historical data are often the first point of reference for evaluating future risk. Although historical data can offer valuable insights, constructing a view of future risk based on empirical data can be misleading, especially for infrequent events. This section highlights the factors that can make historical data an unreliable indicator of future risk, demonstrating the rationale for taking an extreme events modeling approach to quantify the risk.

Figure 2.1 shows a hypothetical time series of historical data. In the graph, it is possible to see the differences between endemic disease patterns as compared to pandemic disease patterns. In this hypothetical 360 weeks—roughly seven years—of data, the endemic disease occurs regularly throughout the time period in a relatively well-characterized pattern. By contrast, a pandemic event occurs in a single spike spanning approximately one year. Interestingly, in this graph, both the endemic disease and the pandemic disease actually have similar AALs, but have very different characteristics of frequency and severity that lead to those annual average values.

Figure 2.1 Example Comparison of Timing and Magnitude of Endemic versus Pandemic Deaths

Deaths (thousand)

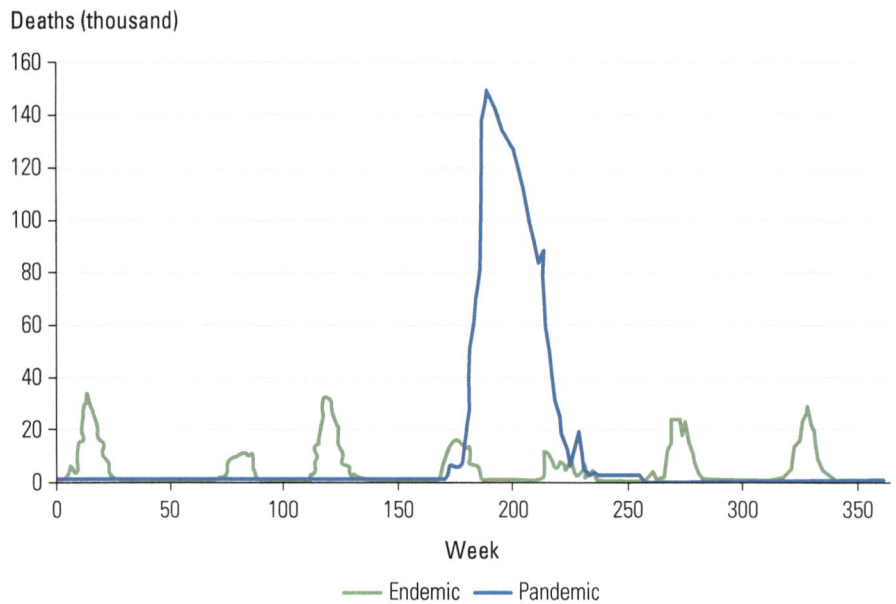

*Source:* Original figure created for this publication.

For frequently occurring infectious diseases with well-characterized historical patterns, historical data can yield acceptable estimates of future risk. For instance, the historical record on pandemic influenza, despite having important limitations, does provide evidence of several major events per century (Morens et al. 2010). Historical data analysis can reveal changes over time, such as increasing frequency and severity of events, rate of increase, and factors that drive this dynamic (Meadows et al. 2023). Techniques for estimating risk solely on the basis of historical data include, for example, statistical and actuarial modeling and parametric curve fitting (Embrechts, Resnick, and Samorodnitsky 1999).

The historical record, however, represents only a small subset of the possible events that can occur, especially for low-probability, high-severity events. It therefore represents a limited sample size, which can lead to erroneous conclusions about what could occur in the future (box 2.1). The absence of empirical data in the form of observed events can be mitigated somewhat by considering counterfactual events (Resolve to Save Lives 2021), but such events do not necessarily provide information about how severe an event would have been had it occurred. Pandemics are relatively rare, and they show large variations in severity. For example, consider the vast difference in mortality between the 1918 and 2009 influenza pandemics.

## The Importance of Tail Risk

The severity distribution of epidemics is highly skewed, exhibiting a very long "tail," consisting of very rare, severe events. When a highly skewed distribution provides only a small sample of data points (in this case, historical events), the "heaviness" of the tail is often underestimated. This underestimation is problematic because appropriately planning for future events requires an accurate understanding of expected losses—especially those caused by less frequent, highly damaging events.

Figure B2.1.1 shows the distributions of cases from historical high-consequence, zoonotic spillover events (Meadows et al. 2023), and how the fitted distribution changes over time with the addition of more events. As more events occur over time, the tail of the distribution (defined as the upper 1 percent) gets longer and heavier, which shifts the expected value (mean) of the distribution as well as the range and expected value of the tail, to the right. There are two explanations for this finding: (1) as the sample size increases over time, the sample distribution and mean get closer to the true distribution, or (2) the true distribution becomes more skewed over time, meaning that events get more severe. The true cause is likely a combination of these two factors. This shift could be further influenced by changes in diagnostic capacity, which may increase detection of less severe outbreaks and would push the mean of the distribution toward a lower value, but could also increase the number of identified cases in larger outbreaks, pushing the mean higher.

The estimation of tail risk affects decision-makers' preparedness planning. When decision-makers have limited resources and need to directly weigh epidemic impact against other health risks, properly accounted-for tail risk is critical to understanding the expected value of future losses. In addition, carefully quantifying tail risk can help decision-makers assess and properly plan for low-frequency, high-severity events. Using epidemiological data and computational modeling makes it possible to supplement historical data with simulated events. These simulations can then provide additional data points on which to base the loss distribution, and allow for a more robust estimation of the tail.

**Figure B2.1.1** Distributions of Historical High-Consequence, Zoonotic Spillover Cases per Outbreak over Time, 1970–2020

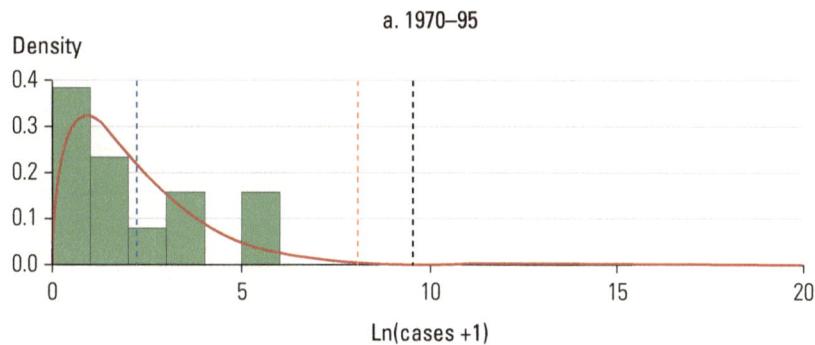

*box and figure continue next page*

**Box 2.1  The Importance of Tail Risk** (continued)

**Figure B2.1.1** Distributions of Historical High-Consequence, Zoonotic Spillover Cases per Outbreak over Time, 1970–2020 (continued)

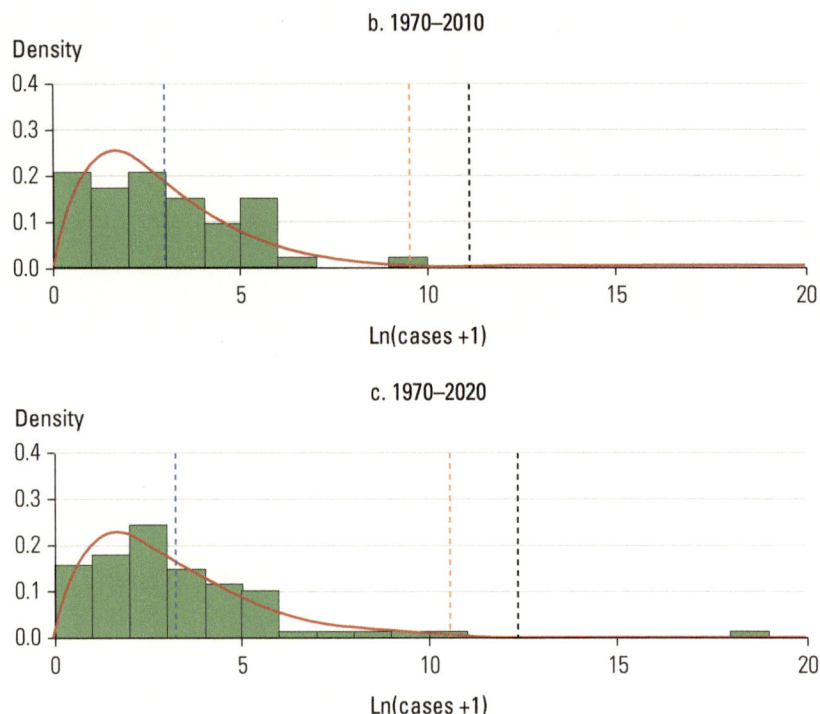

*Source:* Original figure created for this publication.

*Note:* The x-axis shows a natural log transformation of the number of cases +1. The "tail" is defined as the upper 1 percent of the probability density function. The red line shows the fitted probability density function, the blue line shows the expected value, the orange line shows the 99th quantile, and the black line shows the expected value of the tail. Ln = natural log.

The many challenges and biases found in reported epidemiological statistics further complicate the construction of a historical view of epidemic risk (Badker et al. 2021). These factors can lead to data inconsistencies and lack of comparability across different information sources, which further compounds the uncertainty in these estimates. These challenges occur for all types of epidemic data, including for respiratory and VHF events.

In addition to data challenges, the underreporting of many diseases leads to biased estimates of severity and is particularly problematic in resource-limited settings (Glennon et al. 2019). Underreporting is driven by many factors including disease symptomology and severity; contextual conditions (such as local clinical capacity), which can influence mortality rates; public health and disease surveillance infrastructure; sociocultural factors (such as stigma attaching to particular symptoms or diseases); and government censorship (Meadows et al. 2022).

**Extreme Events Modeling**

Extreme events (or "catastrophe") modeling can overcome the challenges of using historical data to develop risk estimates for infrequent, high-severity events, known as "tail risk" (Cirillo and Taleb 2020). For example, the (re)insurance industry routinely consults with modeling experts in natural hazard fields such as meteorology, seismology, hydrology, and volcanology for this purpose (Kozlowski and Mathewson 1995). However, these extreme event modeling techniques tend to be taught within, and used by, intellectual communities that have limited cross-pollination with public health actors.

Extreme event modeling techniques build on historical data as a starting point and use extensive mechanistic modeling and simulation to fill in the gaps beyond the available historical data. The extreme events modeling framework also enables analysts to assess the influence of inputs that may not exist in the historical record but are biologically and epidemiologically plausible. For example, even if a vaccine or treatment option has not yet been widely used but could potentially be deployed in reaction to an outbreak, simulation models can include this intervention when appropriate.

When extreme event modeling techniques are applicable, effective use of this modeling approach still involves substantial technical and analytical requirements. Extreme event models typically require significant computational infrastructure and resources, have many parameters to estimate, and for epidemics, unlike for natural hazards, must account for the effects of human behavior in shaping the course of events.

## METHODS USED IN THIS CHAPTER

This section provides details about the multidisciplinary modeling approach used to generate risk estimates and associated metrics including AALs and EPFs. It also discusses important considerations for modeling total deaths rather than excess deaths or reported deaths, and provides information on potential limitations and uncertainty in the modeled estimates.

**Risk Estimation Process**

The risk modeling approach used to develop the estimates in this chapter draws from principles in computational epidemiology, social science, extreme events modeling, actuarial science, and other fields to produce millions of simulated epidemics and pandemics. The process requires developing probability distributions for each model parameter, statistically sampling values from these parameter distributions, seeding each simulation with these parameter values as initial conditions, and then simulating the spatio-temporal spread of the events through a global, stochastic, metapopulation disease spread model that incorporates information about population vulnerability, mobility patterns, medical technology, preparedness levels, and intervention measures. Annex 2A provides comprehensive details of the methods used for this chapter.

In these simulations, an event is considered to be active until transmission ceases, whether through stochastic die-off, herd immunity, public health and social measures (formerly called nonpharmaceutical interventions), or other phenomena. The simulations include only the acute portion of the events and do not include any transition to an endemic state. This assumption reflects the lack of consistent epidemiological standards to select cutoff points indicating the transition from epidemic to endemic state. Consequently, the loss estimates represent a lower bound; they do not capture ongoing mortality from endemic transitions, in which a pathogen enters a seasonal or cyclic pattern with an ongoing and persistent mortality burden, as occurred during the 1918 influenza (Taubenberger and Morens 2006) and COVID-19 pandemics (Contreras, Iftekhar, and Priesemann 2023).

The simulation process results in model event catalogs, each containing 100,000 simulated years and encompassing millions of infectious disease scenarios, which are used to estimate the risk from epidemics. Note that the event catalogs for this chapter do not project 100,000 years into the future but, rather, represent 100,000 versions of "next year." These catalogs are generated separately for both respiratory diseases and VHFs, and the results are also divided in this way. This division is maintained for ease of interpretation, because deaths from respiratory diseases account for the vast majority of expected deaths from the epidemics modeled. There are orders of magnitude of difference between the levels of potential losses caused by these disease categories, and combining them would obscure this asymmetry. Additionally, different types of response measures may be more relevant and cost-effective for combatting each disease category—for example, mass vaccination efforts and medical oxygen for respiratory diseases versus ring vaccination and safe burials for VHFs—and are easier to tease apart when loss estimates are separated.

These event catalogs are used to produce several estimates, including AAL (measured in deaths), population normalized deaths, exceedance probabilities (EPs), and age- and region-specific mortality estimates (region definitions are shown in map 2.1 and annex 2B). The AAL estimates—that is, the expected value of annual losses—are shown as normalized deaths per 10,000 population and deaths in thousands. Population numbers come from the United Nations' World Population Prospects 2022 release, using a reference year of 2020, for a total estimated global population of 7.8 billion (UN DESA 2022).

In addition to annual estimates, cumulative exceedance probabilities (CEPs) are also estimated over periods of $y$ years using the formula

$$CEP = 1 - (1 - EP)^y \qquad \text{(Equation 2.1)}$$

where $y$ is the time horizon of interest. In this chapter, the time periods of interest are 5, 10, and 25 years; however, the CEP can be computed over any potential time period (for example, over the lifetime of a person born next year and expected to live to the current global life expectancy of approximately 73 years). The CEP is thus another, potentially more useful, way of conveying the same information as the annual EP estimates. It demonstrates the potentially large cumulative risk posed by rare events and estimates risk for time durations of greater interest to policy makers.

The CEP estimates for this chapter contain significant assumptions but likely represent a reasonable lower bound for medium-term pandemic risk. The CEP formula assumes that the risk remains constant at current levels and that each year of the time period is independent. The CEP estimates therefore assume that there are no changes to underlying drivers of risk that could affect the frequency and severity of future epidemics. Current trends, however, suggest that infectious disease risk is increasing (Meadows et al. 2023), driven by increasing human-wildlife contact, deforestation, urbanization, intensifying demand for animal protein, and intensifying international travel (Baker et al. 2021; Carlson et al. 2022). The estimates here likewise do not incorporate assumptions about the potential beneficial impact of new vaccine platforms, improvements to global infectious disease surveillance, early warning, and preparedness. On balance, though, the risk is probably higher over the medium-term future than the assumption of constant risk implies. Annex 2C contains a sensitivity analysis that shows how differing assumptions of future risk would change the estimated CEP.

## Direct Deaths versus Excess Mortality

The modeled deaths presented in this chapter are total direct deaths, rather than reported deaths or excess deaths. For the purposes of this chapter, direct epidemic deaths are considered to be those caused directly by primary infection with the pathogen and any immediate secondary effects resulting directly from that infection (for example, pneumonia resulting from infection with pandemic influenza).

It is important to be explicit about what counts as a direct death in this chapter. The chapter adopts nomenclature from the assessment of the World Health Organization (WHO) of the number of deaths associated with COVID-19 (Msemburi et al. 2023). WHO begins with the concept of "excess deaths," which it defines as the difference between an estimate of actual deaths in the period under consideration and an estimate of what the number of deaths would have been had past trends continued. WHO's COVID-19 excess mortality estimates were calculated by taking the difference between observed all-cause mortality and expected mortality in 2020–21. Expected mortality was modeled by projecting monthly all-cause mortality data from 2015–19 to 2021. Msemburi and colleagues estimate global excess deaths in the COVID-19 years of 2020 and 2021 to have been 14.8 million—2.7 times the 5.42 million reported global deaths from COVID-19 during that same time period (table 2.2). They partition these excess deaths into four categories, A–D:

A. Strictly non-COVID-19 deaths (for example, from other external events such as wars or natural disasters)
B. Indirect COVID-19 deaths (for example, deaths occurring from health system overload)
C. Direct COVID-19 deaths that were not reported
D. Direct COVID-19 deaths that were reported (5.42 million).

**Table 2.2** Excess Death and Reported COVID-19 Death Totals, by Region, January 2020–December 2021

| Region | Excess deaths per 10,000 population (WHO modeled) | Reported deaths per 10,000 population | Excess-to-reported death multiplier |
|---|---|---|---|
| Global | 19 | 7.0 | 2.7 |
| India | 34 | 3.4 | 10 |
| Sub-Saharan Africa | 11 | 1.3 | 8.5 |
| Central Asia | 14 | 2 | 7 |
| Western Pacific and Southeast Asia | 12 | 3.4 | 3.5 |
| Middle East and North Africa | 19 | 6.6 | 2.9 |
| Central and Eastern Europe | 59 | 24 | 2.6 |
| Latin America and the Caribbean | 35 | 24 | 1.5 |
| North Atlantic | 18 | 17 | 1.1 |
| United States | 28 | 25 | 1.1 |
| China[a] | −0.37 | 0.04 | −9.2 |

*Source:* Original calculations based on Msemburi et al. 2023 (excess deaths per 10,000 population) and WHO 2022 (reported deaths per 10,000 population).

*Note:* Numbers in the table are rounded to two significant digits. For details on regional groupings, refer to map 2.1 and annex 2B. WHO = World Health Organization.

a. Excess mortality in China greatly increased in December 2022 (after the time frame of the analysis) following decisions to end a national policy that incorporated extensive testing and public health and social measures to reduce transmission, and excess deaths for the entirety of the pandemic would be substantially higher than these estimates.

The excess mortality estimates also account for any deaths that were averted thanks to pandemic-related changes in social conditions and personal behaviors (for example, fewer traffic deaths because of reduction in travel and working from home, or fewer influenza deaths because of COVID-19 mitigation strategies such as masking and stay-at-home orders). In some countries (such as Australia, China, Japan, and New Zealand), it was estimated that a higher number of deaths were averted because of pandemic-related behavioral changes than were directly or indirectly attributable to COVID-19, resulting in a net negative excess mortality during the 2020–21 study time period. However, substantial changes in disease control policies and disease transmission from 2022 onward led to substantial increases in mortality; incorporating data from this time period could substantially alter the understanding of the regional distribution of excess mortality from COVID-19.

The WHO analysis attempts no estimate of the division of the 9.4 million excess deaths not reported as COVID-19 deaths (14.8 million – 5.4 million) among the categories (A), (B) and (C). Msemburi et al. (2023, 136) do observe that "the greater proportion of excess deaths can be attributed to COVID-19 directly." The risk modeling results provided in this chapter include both reported and unreported direct deaths; that is, they represent the sum of categories (C) and (D). Although WHO does not report that sum directly, a number consistent with Msemburi et al. (2023) would be 11 million to 12 million direct COVID-19 deaths in 2020–21.

**Map 2.1** Regional Grouping of Countries

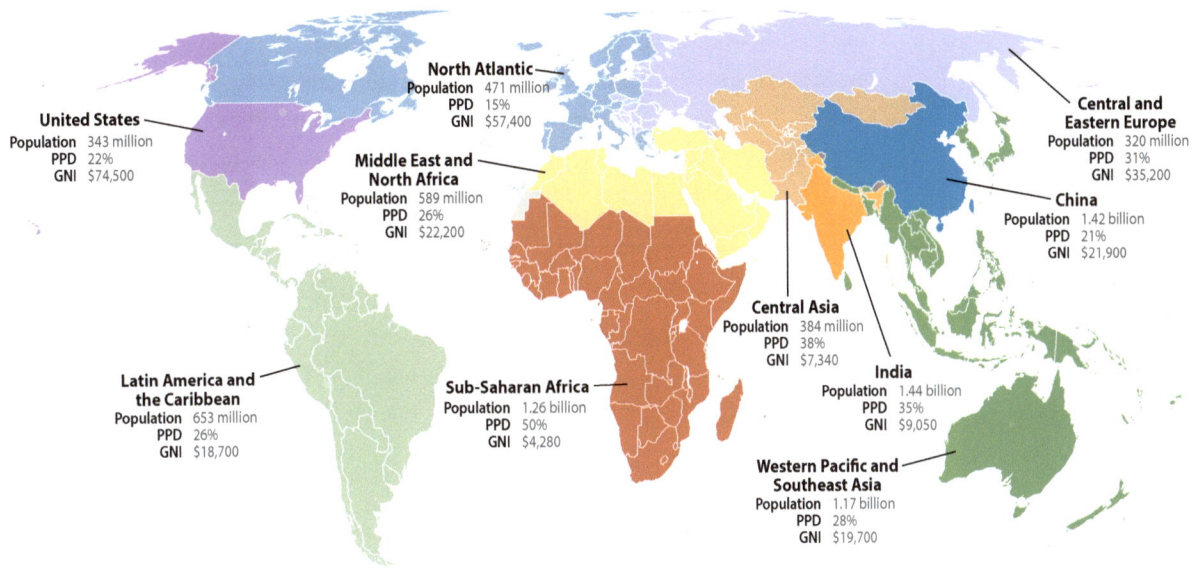

**North Atlantic**
Population 471 million
PPD 15%
GNI $57,400

**United States**
Population 343 million
PPD 22%
GNI $74,500

**Middle East and North Africa**
Population 589 million
PPD 26%
GNI $22,200

**Central and Eastern Europe**
Population 320 million
PPD 31%
GNI $35,200

**China**
Population 1.42 billion
PPD 21%
GNI $21,900

**Central Asia**
Population 384 million
PPD 38%
GNI $7,340

**India**
Population 1.44 billion
PPD 35%
GNI $9,050

**Latin America and the Caribbean**
Population 653 million
PPD 26%
GNI $18,700

**Sub-Saharan Africa**
Population 1.26 billion
PPD 50%
GNI $4,280

**Western Pacific and Southeast Asia**
Population 1.17 billion
PPD 28%
GNI $19,700

IBRD 48894 | MAY 2025

*Source:* Image based on Jamison et al. 2024.

*Note:* Annex 2B lists the countries in each region. GNI = gross national income per person, 2021 international dollars; PPD = probability of premature death, dying before age 70 (2023); PPP = purchasing power parity.

## Limitations and Uncertainty in Model Estimates

Models are abstractions of the real world. Therefore, the approach taken for this chapter has, by necessity, some limitations. First, historic data are limited; and, despite the great care taken to mitigate this challenge with the modeling approach, it is not possible to fully account for gaps and biases in historical data. Second, there are many parameters to estimate, all of which have substantial uncertainty. Third, the outcomes of pandemics are affected by human behavior and movement patterns, which can vary substantially in specific socioeconomic contexts and subpopulations, or could change over time in surprising ways that may not be fully accounted for or characterized in the model. Fourth, models do not fully account for secular trends such as the apparent increase in zoonotic spillover events that can spark pandemics, or amplification patterns that could arise from the intersection of trends in spillover with the intensification of climate change.

It is worth emphasizing that, despite extensive model diagnostics and validation—including sensitivity analyses, benchmarking of historical events, and cross-referencing against other data sources—substantial uncertainty attaches to the estimates in this chapter. This uncertainty results in part from the historically informed probability distributions from which key parameters for the simulations are drawn. Additionally, substantial uncertainties exist in the underlying structure of the models and factors used here, which might influence the future evolution of parameters in ways poorly reflected in history.

In this chapter, 95 percent confidence intervals (CIs) for deaths are estimated by sampling one thousand subsets of 10,000 years each from the broader 100,000-year model event catalogs and estimating the 2.5th and 97.5th percentiles from the samples. As such, the CIs convey the uncertainty in catalog sampling, rather than the full universe of uncertainty. Because of the relatively small width of the estimated CIs for the AAL estimates, and the larger uncertainties that surround the analysis, the chapter does not report CIs for the AAL, because it has the potential for conveying false precision.

CIs associated with the EP estimates are also calculated; these CIs typically fall in the range of 5–20 percent of estimated values, and expand to 40 percent or more of estimated values as one goes further into the tail of the EPF. An important feature of the EPF is that the CIs widen markedly as one moves further out in the tail of the curve. This widening is expected; estimates for extremely rare, massive pandemics are inherently uncertain, given their sparsity.

Further uncertainty is found in the extreme tail of the EPF because of the model's assumptions regarding socio-behavioral responses during epidemics. These assumptions might not hold true under extreme, high-severity scenarios. For example, in a truly massive event, there could potentially be very intense governmental and societal responses to curtail transmission. Major social change could occur (for example, mass quarantine or compulsory licenses of vaccine intellectual property), leading to better outcomes than estimated here. Conversely, the possibility exists that, during a truly massive pandemic, there could be a total societal collapse, which would lead to vastly worse outcomes than estimated here.

Because of the deep underlying uncertainties, the estimates in this chapter—particularly estimates of risk decades into the future—should not be interpreted as conveying great precision. Rather, the headline numbers reflect broad ranges consistent with historical evidence and state-of-the-art modeling.

## RESULTS: RESPIRATORY DISEASES

The following subsections provide estimates of global mortality from future epidemics and pandemics caused by the modeled respiratory diseases. These estimates are presented in terms of AALs, EPFs, and the distribution of loss estimates, demonstrating the skewed nature of the distribution. The subsections also present regional mortality estimates and mortality distributions by age groups.

### Global Respiratory Mortality

The estimated AAL from future epidemics and pandemics caused by the modeled respiratory diseases is approximately 2.5 million deaths. The AAL provides a summary measure of the scale of potential losses. Rather than representing the number of deaths that occur each year, the AAL arises from a pattern of events that exhibit larger amounts of deaths that occur more sporadically and in a punctuated manner, including years having 0 or very low levels of loss (figure 2.1). Within the respiratory event catalog, pandemic influenza viruses are the predominant contributors to the losses, contributing nearly twice as much to the AAL as epidemic/novel coronaviruses (table 2.3).

An inspection of the EPF shows a heavily skewed (that is, asymmetrically overdispersed) distribution of loss estimates (figure 2.2 and table 2.4). Smaller events are more likely to occur, but larger events—even larger than those historically observed—are also possible and represented further out in the tail of the distribution. As the probability decreases (or return period increases—refer to box 2.2), the number of deaths shows an initial, rapid increase, but then decelerates as one moves further into the tail of the distribution. The steep rise in event severity is apparent in the higher-frequency (that is, lower return period) portion of the curve, perhaps most visibly in the large jump in the number of deaths between the 10- and 20-year return periods. Although the steepness of the rise decreases further out in the tail, the tail events contribute substantially to the skewness of the distribution (box 2.2). The steep rise and heavy tail of the curve are consistent with the potential for wide transmission and global spread of respiratory diseases.

**Table 2.3** Global Average Annual Deaths Based on Respiratory Event Catalog

|  | Average annual deaths | |
|---|---|---|
|  | Count (thousand) | Per 10,000 population |
| Pandemic influenza | 1,600 | 2.0 |
| Epidemic/novel coronaviruses | 890 | 1.1 |
| Total | 2,500 | 3.2 |

*Source:* Ginkgo Biosecurity simulations.

**Figure 2.2** Global Respiratory Exceedance Probability Function Based on Respiratory Event Catalog

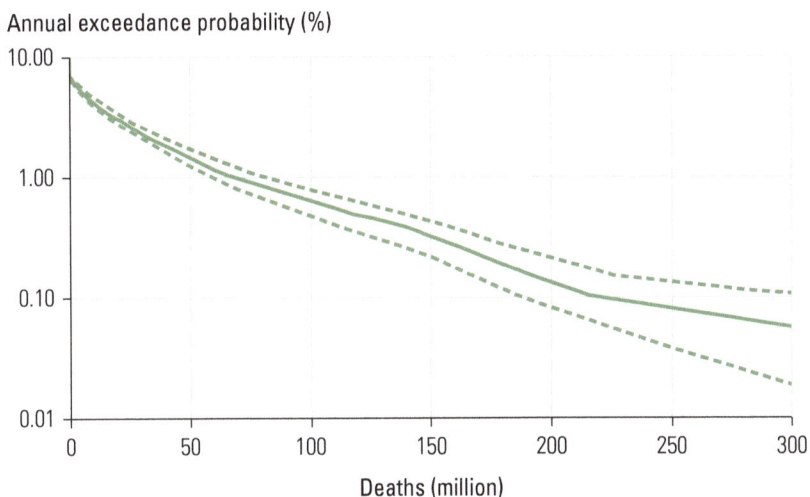

Annual exceedance probability (%)

*Source:* Original figure created for this publication.
*Note:* The solid line depicts the point estimates, and the dashed lines depict the 95 percent confidence interval.

**Table 2.4** Selected Exceedance Probabilities and Associated Global Deaths Based on Respiratory Event Catalog

| Return period (years) | Exceedance probability | Deaths per 10,000 population (95% CI) | Death counts (thousand) (95% CI) |
|---|---|---|---|
| 5 | 0.20000 | 0.001 (0.001, 0.001) | 0.53 (0.50, 0.55) |
| 10 | 0.10000 | 0.002 (0.002, 0.002) | 1.4 (1.2, 1.5) |
| 20 | 0.05000 | 7.2 (5.4, 10) | 5,600 (4,300, 7,700) |
| 35 | 0.02857 | 28 (23, 32) | 22,000 (18,000, 25,000) |
| 50 | 0.02000 | 45 (39, 53) | 35,000 (30,000, 42,000) |
| 100 | 0.01000 | 86 (74, 100) | 68,000 (58,000, 80,000) |
| 200 | 0.00500 | 150 (120, 180) | 110,000 (100,000, 140,000) |
| 333 | 0.00300 | 200 (160, 220) | 150,000 (130,000, 170,000) |
| 500 | 0.00200 | 220 (200, 260) | 170,000 (150,000, 200,000) |
| 667 | 0.00150 | 250 (210, 290) | 190,000 (170,000, 220,000) |
| 1,000 | 0.00100 | 280 (240, 390) | 220,000 (190,000, 300,000) |

*Source:* Ginkgo Biosecurity simulations.

*Note:* CI = confidence interval.

## Box 2.2

### Rolling the Dice

Mathematically, the return period is the inverse of the exceedance probability (the probability that an event of a given severity or worse will begin within a given year). For example, a 1 percent annual exceedance probability—that is, a 1 percent chance of observing an event of a given severity (or worse) in a year—translates to a 100-year return period or, alternatively, a "1-in-100 year event" (FEMA 2016). Although the return period is a convenient way to conceptualize the estimates presented in this chapter, it can also be misinterpreted in ways that encourage decision-makers to underinvest in preparing for low-probability, high-severity events, by assuming (implicitly or explicitly) that the risk is "tomorrow's problem."

It is all too easy for even informed analysts to misinterpret frequency estimates for rare events. A 100-year return period does *not* mean that the level of loss occurs once per 100 years, nor does it mean that the losses are evenly spaced out at 100 year intervals. A "1-in-100 year event" simply means that the event statistically has a 1 percent chance of starting in any given year. That is, a given event is expected to occur, on average, once in repeated samples of 100 year time periods. It is even possible to have multiple "100-year" events occur during a 100-year period. With this explanation in mind, any given year is a roll of the dice.

The EPF is also used to estimate the level of mortality found at different EPs (table 2.5). Box 2.3 presents an in-depth look at the likelihood of an event having mortality of a comparable magnitude to the COVID-19 pandemic.

**Table 2.5** Exceedance Probabilities for Selected Global Death Levels Based on Respiratory Event Catalog

| Global severity | | Likelihood | |
|---|---|---|---|
| Death counts | Deaths per 10,000 population | Return period (years) | Exceedance probability (%) |
| > 800 | > 0.001 | 7 | 14 |
| > 80,000 | > 0.01 | 15 | 6.8 |
| > 8,000,000 | > 10 | 22 | 4.5 |
| > 80,000,000 | > 100 | 120 | 0.8 |

*Source:* Ginkgo Biosecurity simulations.

## Box 2.3

### COVID-19: Not a "Once in a Century" Pandemic

The panic and neglect cycle is driven, at least in part, by the historic fact that severe pandemics occur infrequently. Although the twenty-first century has seen multiple pandemics, including the 2009 pandemic influenza and Zika virus, the last public health crisis seemingly comparable in impact to COVID-19 was the Great Influenza of 1918 (Johnson and Mueller 2002). Because COVID-19 occurred nearly 100 years after the 1918 pandemic, some commentators have described pandemics of this scale as occurring "once in a lifetime" (Guterres 2020) or even "once in a century" (Cruickshank and Shaban 2020; Gates 2020; WHO 2020) .

At the end of December 2022, the end of the third year of the pandemic, there were over 660 million reported cases and 6.5 million reported deaths globally from COVID-19.[a] Based on our simulated event catalog, the annual probability of an event of this mortality level or larger is estimated to be 2–3 percent. In other words, every year there is a 2–3 percent chance that an event equal to or more severe than COVID-19 (in terms of mortality) could occur. Expressed in terms of return periods, it would be a 33- to 50-year event, rather than a 100-year event (box 2.2). Assuming that the level of risk does not change, the chance (cumulative exceedance probability) that an event having a mortality level as severe as or worse than COVID-19 will occur over the next 5 years is estimated at 10–14 percent, over the next decade at 18–26 percent, and over the next 25 years at 40–53 percent.

COVID-19 was more severe than other recent respiratory pandemics, such as the 1957, 1968, and 2009 influenza pandemics. However, comparing COVID-19 to the 1918 influenza pandemic, which many have done, sets up a false equivalency. As a percent of global population mortality, the 1918 pandemic was orders of magnitude more severe than COVID-19. It led to the deaths of up to 5 percent of the global population as compared to the estimated 0.08 percent global mortality from COVID-19 as of December 2022, based on reported deaths (refer to table 2A.13 in annex 2A).

The estimates in this chapter of the frequency and severity of pandemics, rooted in extreme events modeling techniques, demonstrate that COVID-19 is not likely to be a "once in a century" pandemic. On the contrary, over the next 25 years, a pandemic with a mortality level similar to or worse than COVID-19 has a roughly 50 percent probability of occurrence, similar to flipping a coin.

a. Ginkgo Biosecurity, "Spatiotemporal Data for 2019-Novel Coronavirus Covid-19 Cases and deaths," Humanitarian Data Exchange, https://data.humdata.org /dataset/2019-novel-coronavirus-cases.

Because severe respiratory pandemics occur sporadically and have a relatively low (perceived) probability of occurrence in any given year, policy makers tend to underinvest in preparedness (Sands, Mundaca-Shah, and Dzau 2016). Viewed over a longer time horizon—but one still relevant to policy makers and planners—the substantial magnitude of the risk from rare, potentially catastrophic events becomes more apparent (table 2.6). For example, the annual probability of a respiratory pandemic killing at least 10 million people worldwide is estimated at 4.2 percent; however, over a 10-year period, the probability of such an event occurring is 35 percent. Extrapolated further, the results suggest that, over the next 25 years, there is a 66 percent probability of a respiratory pandemic that would kill 10 million people or more, with the caveat that many of the assumptions in the risk modeling approach have greater uncertainty over a longer time period (refer to table 2C.1 in annex 2C).

Although the respiratory model event catalog contains a wide range of event sizes, the vast majority of the risk from respiratory disease pandemics is estimated to fall in the tail of the EPF: low-probability, high-impact events. Approximately 50 percent of the simulated events in the catalog are very small, with an average magnitude of 120 global deaths. Roughly 4 percent of events have 8 million or more global deaths. Only 0.6 percent of events have global death tolls exceeding 100 million. Strikingly, however, the comparatively small number of high-magnitude events heavily drive the estimates of expected mortality. The 1.4 percent of catalog events with death totals exceeding 50 million account for 68 percent of all deaths in the respiratory catalog (figure 2.3 and table 2.7). And, although the higher-frequency events (return periods of 35 years or less) make the lowest contribution to AAL as measured in deaths, they can still cause substantial economic disruption (Madhav et al. 2017).

### Respiratory Mortality by Region

Respiratory diseases have a substantial expected impact on all geographies, but risk is unevenly distributed (refer to map 2.1 and annex 2B for information on the regional country groupings). To reduce the effects of different population age structures by region, in addition to the counts and normalized AALs, the age-standardized AALs per 10,000 population were also calculated, using the WHO 2000–25 Standard Population (Ahmad et al. 2001). The highest age-standardized AAL occurs in Sub-Saharan Africa and the lowest in the North Atlantic region (figure 2.4 and table 2.8).

Table 2.6 Annual, 5-Year, 10-Year, and 25-Year EP Estimates for Selected Global Event Sizes Based on Respiratory Event Catalog

| Deaths | Annual EP (%) | 5-year EP (%) | 10-year EP (%) | 25-year EP (%) |
|---|---|---|---|---|
| 1,000,000 | 6.3 | 28 | 48 | 80 |
| 10,000,000 | 4.2 | 19 | 35 | 66 |
| 25,000,000 | 2.6 | 12 | 23 | 48 |
| 100,000,000 | 0.6 | 3.0 | 5.8 | 14 |

*Source:* Ginkgo Biosecurity simulations.

*Note:* EP = exceedance probability.

**Figure 2.3** Respiratory Event Catalog Composition: Simulated Event Sizes and Their Contribution to Expected Losses

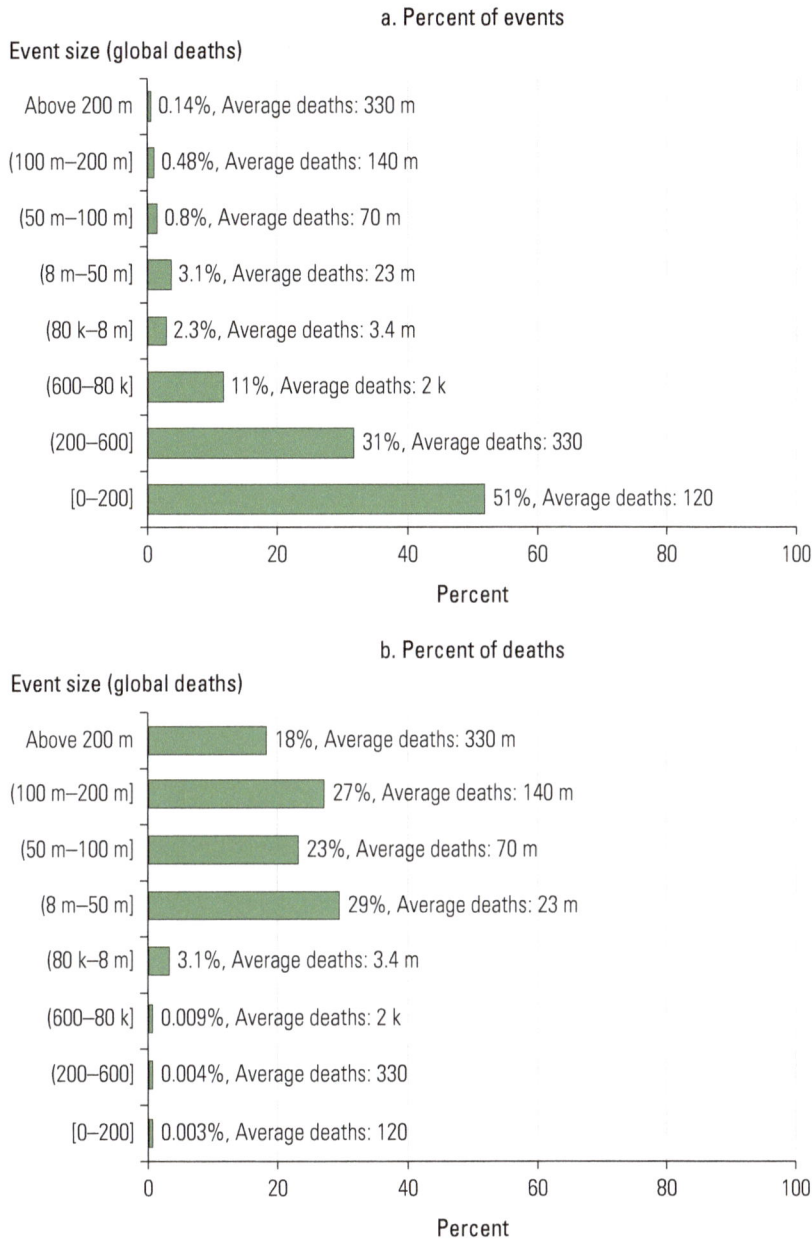

a. Percent of events

Event size (global deaths)

Above 200 m — 0.14%, Average deaths: 330 m
(100 m–200 m] — 0.48%, Average deaths: 140 m
(50 m–100 m] — 0.8%, Average deaths: 70 m
(8 m–50 m] — 3.1%, Average deaths: 23 m
(80 k–8 m] — 2.3%, Average deaths: 3.4 m
(600–80 k] — 11%, Average deaths: 2 k
(200–600] — 31%, Average deaths: 330
[0–200] — 51%, Average deaths: 120

Percent (0, 20, 40, 60, 80, 100)

b. Percent of deaths

Event size (global deaths)

Above 200 m — 18%, Average deaths: 330 m
(100 m–200 m] — 27%, Average deaths: 140 m
(50 m–100 m] — 23%, Average deaths: 70 m
(8 m–50 m] — 29%, Average deaths: 23 m
(80 k–8 m] — 3.1%, Average deaths: 3.4 m
(600–80 k] — 0.009%, Average deaths: 2 k
(200–600] — 0.004%, Average deaths: 330
[0–200] — 0.003%, Average deaths: 120

Percent (0, 20, 40, 60, 80, 100)

*Source:* Original figure created for this publication.

*Note:* The parentheses and brackets notation follows the international standard ISO 80000-2:2019(en) Quantities and units—Part 2, which conveys the following meaning. The "(" indicates the range is exclusive of the number, while "[" and "]" indicate the range is inclusive; k = thousand; m = million.

**Table 2.7** Composition of AAL for Respiratory Event Catalog, by Event Severity and Event Frequency

| AAL, by event severity | | AAL, by event frequency | |
|---|---|---|---|
| **Severity, millions of deaths globally** | **Contribution to AAL, thousand (%)** | **Frequency indicated by return period, years** | **Contribution to AAL, thousand (%)** |
| 200+ | 450 (18) | ≤ 10 | 0.23 (0.01) |
| 100–200 | 670 (27) | 10–35 | 310 (13) |
| 50–100 | 560 (23) | 35–100 | 720 (29) |
| 8–50 | 720 (29) | 100–200 | 440 (18) |
| < 8 | 77 (3.1) | 200+ | 1,000 (40) |
| Total | 2,500 (100) | Total | 2,500 (100) |

*Source:* Ginkgo Biosecurity simulations.

*Note:* AAL = average annual loss.

**Figure 2.4** Age-Standardized Average Annual Respiratory Disease Deaths, by Region, Based on Respiratory Event Catalog

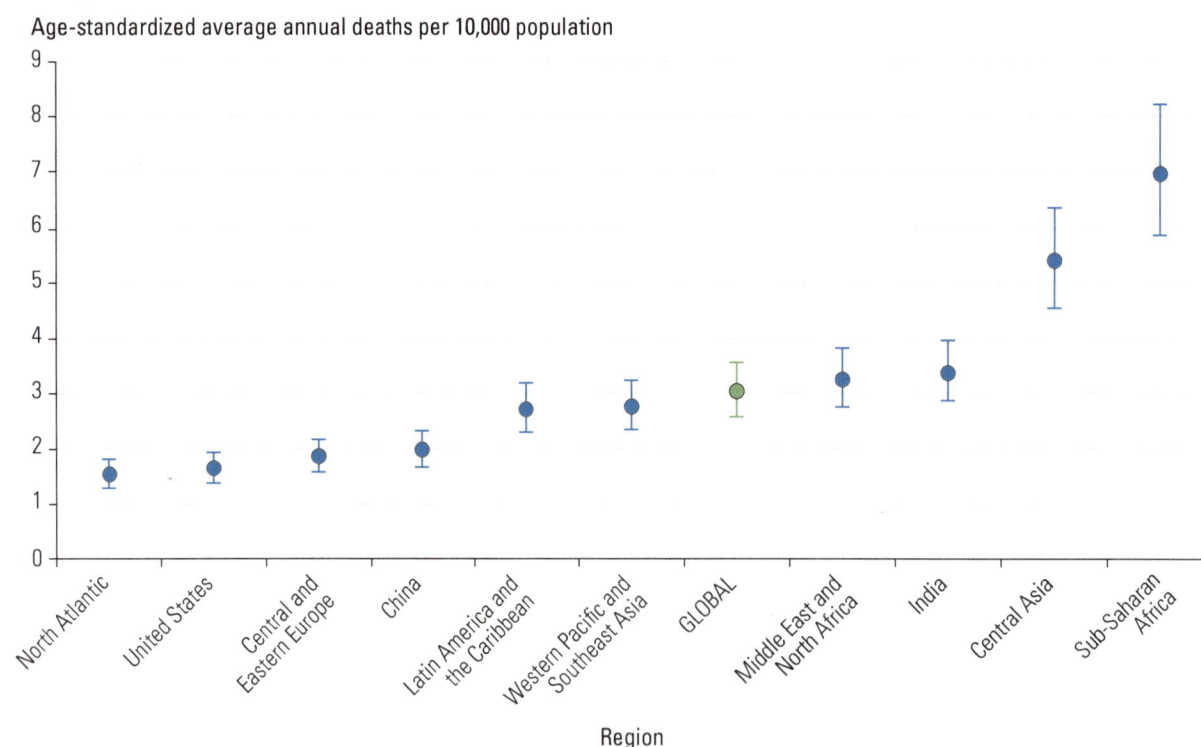

Age-standardized average annual deaths per 10,000 population

*Source:* Original figure created for this publication, based on Ginkgo Biosecurity simulations and World Health Organization 2000–25 Standard Population (Ahmad et al. 2001).

*Note:* For details on regional groupings, refer to map 2.1 and annex 2B. The dots depict the point estimates, and the lines depict the 95 percent confidence intervals.

**Table 2.8** Average Annual Deaths, by Region, Based on Respiratory Event Catalog

| Region | Standardized average annual deaths per 10,000[a] | Average annual deaths per 10,000 population | Average annual deaths (thousand) |
|---|---|---|---|
| Global | 3.0 | 3.2 | 2,500 |
| Central and Eastern Europe | 1.9 | 2.5 | 82 |
| Central Asia | 5.4 | 4.4 | 160 |
| China | 2.0 | 2.4 | 340 |
| India | 3.4 | 3.2 | 450 |
| Latin America and the Caribbean | 2.7 | 2.8 | 180 |
| Middle East and North Africa | 3.3 | 3.0 | 160 |
| North Atlantic | 1.5 | 2.3 | 100 |
| Sub-Saharan Africa | 7.0 | 5.0 | 580 |
| United States | 1.7 | 2.2 | 71 |
| Western Pacific and Southeast Asia | 2.8 | 3.0 | 340 |

*Source:* Ginkgo Biosecurity simulations.

*Note:* For details on regional groupings, refer to map 2.1 and annex 2B.

a. Based on World Health Organization 2000–25 Standard Population (Ahmad et al. 2001).

At first glance, the findings of higher expected mortality in Sub-Saharan Africa may appear inconsistent with the relatively low levels of reported mortality from the COVID-19 pandemic in that region, as compared to others. Notably, the ratio of the age-standardized AAL between Sub-Saharan Africa and the North Atlantic region as derived from table 2.8 is roughly 5:1. This ratio contradicts patterns of estimated excess mortality during the COVID-19 pandemic (table 2.2), which show higher mortality levels in the North Atlantic compared to Sub-Saharan Africa.

Multiple factors likely contribute to this apparent discrepancy. First, evidence suggests significant underreporting in the official statistics—more so in Sub-Saharan Africa than in the North Atlantic region. Estimates that draw on seroprevalence data to estimate mortality while correcting for underreporting find a higher mortality burden for Sub-Saharan Africa (Kogan et al. 2023). Second, the age distribution of deaths is likely to play a role. Comparative mortality ratios show a much higher mortality burden for Sub-Saharan Africa, especially when accounting for the region's younger age distribution (Ledesma et al. 2023). Note that this factor could be somewhat specific to COVID-19; a future respiratory pandemic could have a different pattern, potentially leading to a different spread in future expected losses. Third, mortality displacement may play a role. The following subsection discusses both age effects and mortality displacement.

### Respiratory Mortality by Age Group

AAL results by age group are available in the respiratory model event catalog. Figure 2.5 shows a graph of the global normalized average annual deaths per 10,000 population by age group for respiratory pandemics. Table 2.9 contains the graphed values, including median and 95 percent CIs for each age group. These results show that members of the oldest two population groups are most likely to die during a respiratory pandemic, followed by the youngest in the population. The overall mortality rates exhibit a slight W-shaped pattern (Morens, Taubenberger, and Fauci 2021), but respiratory diseases can exhibit a number of different mortality patterns (for example, U or J). Although not well understood, the determinants of this pattern may be related to immunity patterns in the population (van Wijhe et al. 2018).

Increased mortality, especially in older age groups, can lead to what is known as mortality displacement, or the "harvesting effect." Such a situation involves a compensatory decrease in mortality after a pandemic, because the individuals who died in the pandemic would have been likely to die whether or not the pandemic occurred. This effect has been observed during influenza pandemics (Hoffman and Fox 2019) as well as the COVID-19 pandemic (Astengo et al. 2021).

Beyond the oldest and youngest individuals, who are at greatest mortality risk during a respiratory pandemic, the age groups having the next greatest risk are the 20- to 39-year-old and 40- to 59-year-old categories. The increased mortality for the 20–39 age category is especially concerning from the standpoint of fertility, along with economic losses, because this age category includes prime members of the labor force who would be conducting economically productive activities. Therefore, epidemics having a W-shaped mortality pattern are more likely to cause the greatest economic loss (Ma, Dushoff, and Earn 2011).

Although these results are averaged over the entire set of simulations, the age distribution can take many different forms for any single epidemic. These forms may differ from distributions observed in previous epidemics. For illustrative examples of various age distributions, refer to figure 2.6.

**Figure 2.5** Average Annual Respiratory Disease Deaths, by Age Group, Based on Respiratory Event Catalog

Average annual deaths per 10,000 population

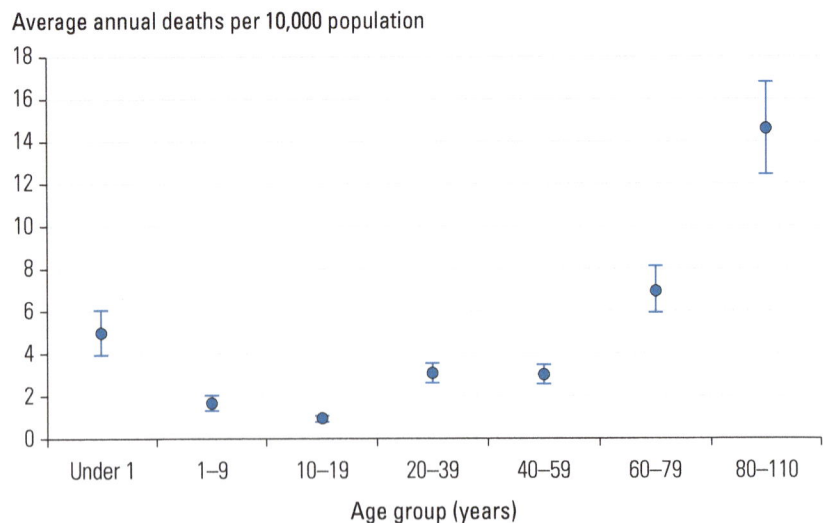

*Source:* Original figure created for this publication, based on Ginkgo Biosecurity simulations.
*Note:* The dots depict the point estimates, and the lines depict the 95 percent confidence intervals.

**Figure 2.6** Age Shapes of Respiratory Disease

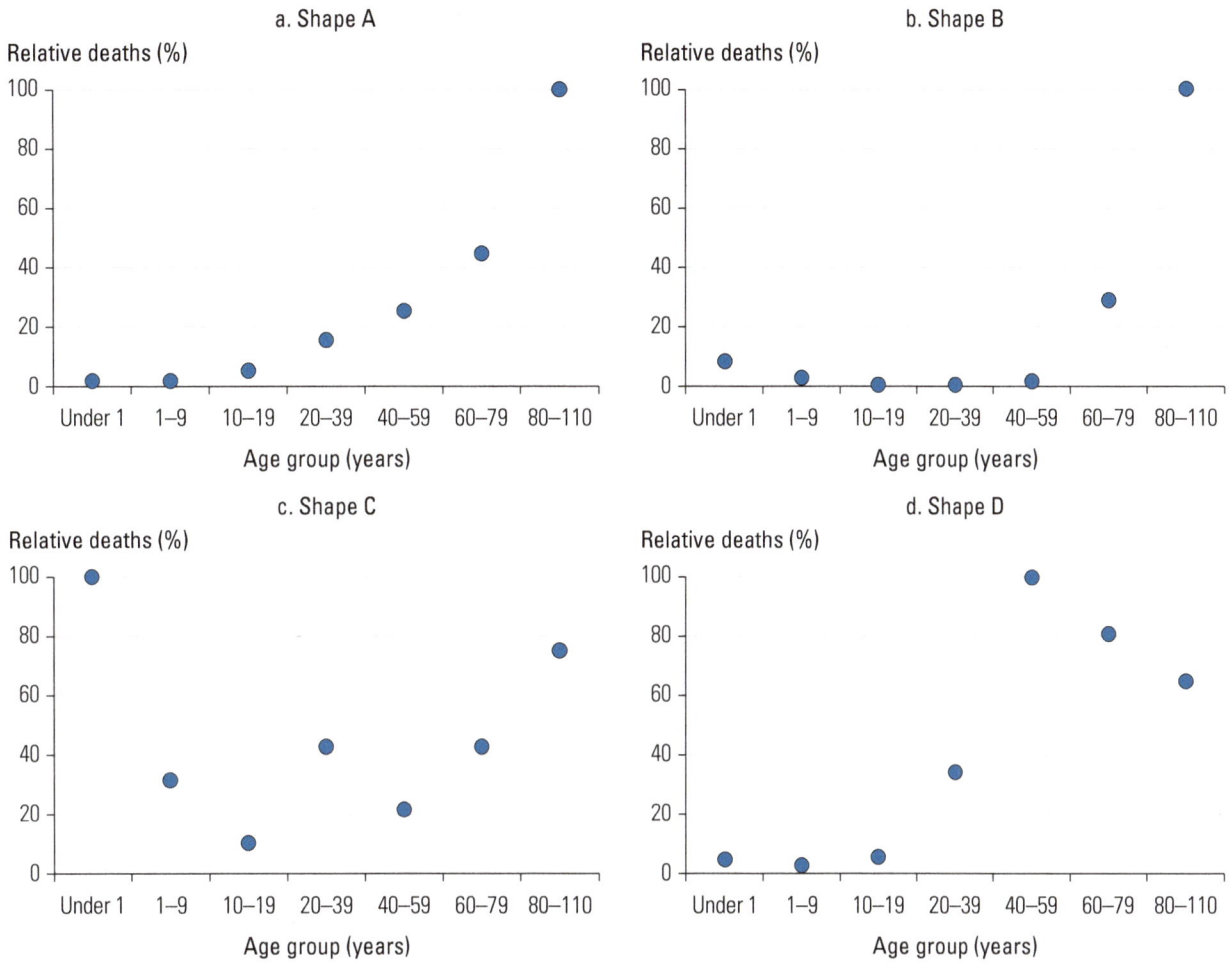

a. Shape A

Relative deaths (%)

Age group (years)

b. Shape B

Relative deaths (%)

Age group (years)

c. Shape C

Relative deaths (%)

Age group (years)

d. Shape D

Relative deaths (%)

Age group (years)

*Source:* Original figure created for this publication.

*Note:* Relative deaths represent the percent of normalized deaths in an age category compared to the age category with the highest number of normalized deaths. These are illustrative examples of how pandemics could have varying levels of severity in different age groups, which could be related, for example, to pathogen characteristics, immunity levels in the affected populations, or differing contact patterns.

**Table 2.9** Global Average Annual Deaths, by Age Group, Based on Respiratory Event Catalog

| Age group (years) | Average annual deaths per 10,000 population in that age group | Average annual deaths in that age group (thousand) |
|---|---|---|
| Under 1 | 5.0 | 66 |
| 1–9 | 1.6 | 200 |
| 10–19 | 0.89 | 110 |
| 20–39 | 3.0 | 710 |
| 40–59 | 3.0 | 530 |
| 60–79 | 6.9 | 620 |
| 80–110 | 15 | 220 |
| **Global total** | **3.2** | **2,500** |

*Source:* Ginkgo Biosecurity simulations.

## RESULTS: VIRAL HEMORRHAGIC FEVERS

VHFs, such as those caused by Ebola, Marburg, and Nipah viruses, can be fatal; and human-to-human transmission can spark large, sustained epidemics. However, the severity of disease, distinctive signs and symptoms after the prodromal phase, and direct contact transmission mechanism all reduce the likelihood of wide international spread. The analysis here focuses on Sub-Saharan Africa because it represents the vast majority of global VHF losses—approximately 72 percent. The next subsections present Sub-Saharan Africa regional estimates for the VHF event catalog, including AALs and EPs, along with estimates of mortality by age group.

### VHF Mortality in Sub-Saharan Africa

The AAL from future VHF epidemics in Sub-Saharan Africa is estimated to be approximately 19,000 deaths (table 2.10); this includes years having 0 or very low levels of loss. This number represents a small fraction of expected losses in comparison to respiratory pandemics. The EPF for VHFs exhibits a skewed distribution, albeit less skewed than the heavy-tailed loss distribution for respiratory diseases (figure 2.7 and table 2.11).

**Table 2.10** Sub-Saharan Africa Average Annual Deaths Based on VHF Event Catalog

|  | Average annual deaths | |
| --- | --- | --- |
|  | **Per 10,000 population** | **Counts (thousand)** |
| VHFs | 0.17 | 19 |

*Source:* Ginkgo Biosecurity simulations.

*Note:* VHF = viral hemorrhagic fever.

**Figure 2.7** Viral Hemorrhagic Fever Exceedance Probability Function, Sub-Saharan Africa, Based on VHF Event Catalog

Annual exceedance probability (%)

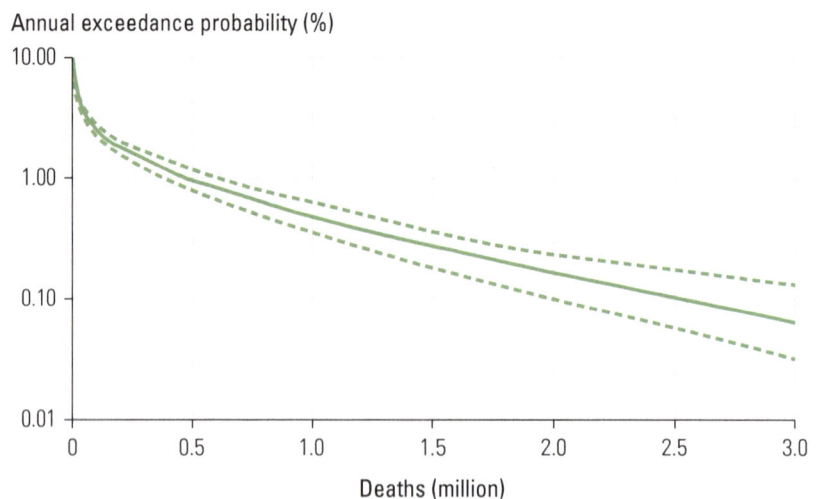

*Source:* Original figure created for this publication.

*Note:* The solid line depicts the point estimates, and the dashed lines depict the 95 percent confidence interval; VHF = viral hemorrhagic fever.

**Table 2.11** Sub-Saharan Africa Deaths at Selected Exceedance Probability Points Based on VHF Event Catalog

| Return period, years | Exceedance probability | Deaths per 10,000 population (95% CI) | Death counts, thousand (95% CI) |
|---|---|---|---|
| 5 | 0.20000 | 0.01 (0.01, 0.01) | 1.3 (1.2, 1.4) |
| 10 | 0.10000 | 0.05 (0.05, 0.06) | 6.3 (5.6, 7.1) |
| 20 | 0.05000 | 0.24 (0.21, 0.28) | 28 (24, 33) |
| 35 | 0.02857 | 0.69 (0.59, 0.85) | 80 (68, 98) |
| 50 | 0.02000 | 1.4 (1.1, 1.8) | 160 (130, 210) |
| 100 | 0.01000 | 4.2 (3.3, 5.3) | 480 (380, 610) |
| 200 | 0.00500 | 8.4 (6.7, 11) | 970 (770, 1,200) |
| 333 | 0.00300 | 12 (9.6, 15) | 1,400 (1,100, 1,700) |
| 500 | 0.00200 | 16 (13, 20) | 1,800 (1,400, 2,300) |
| 667 | 0.00150 | 18 (14, 24) | 2,100 (1,600, 2,800) |
| 1,000 | 0.00100 | 22 (17, 30) | 2,500 (2,000, 3,400) |

*Source:* Ginkgo Biosecurity simulations.

*Note:* CI = confidence interval; VHF = viral hemorrhagic fever.

EPF estimates generated for this chapter suggest that outbreaks such as the Ebola virus disease epidemics in West Africa (2014) and North Kivu (2018 and 2021) are not aberrant events but instead reflect the risk profile of the region. The modeling framework here produces simulated events on the scale and duration of these events, along with events much larger than historically observed. The model results suggest that larger VHF epidemics are more likely to occur than might be assumed if one derives risk estimates based on historical data alone (box 2.2). Furthermore, the frequency and severity of VHF epidemics in Sub-Saharan Africa have increased in recent years (Stephens et al. 2022); if this trend continues, the risk of VHF events in Sub-Saharan Africa will increase even more over time.

As shown in table 2.12, a VHF epidemic causing approximately 10,000 deaths has an estimated 8 percent annual probability of occurrence; viewed over a 10-year period, the risk that such an event will occur is roughly 57 percent. An event five times that magnitude, causing 50,000 deaths within Sub-Saharan Africa, has a roughly 3.7 percent annual probability. Such an event lies outside the range of historical experience and appears improbable given the small annual probability; however, viewed over a 10-year time period, it has a 31 percent probability of occurrence. Over a 25-year period, this probability of occurrence increases to 61 percent. Refer to table 2C.2 in annex 2C for results of sensitivity testing around trend assumptions of future risk.

In the VHF model event catalog for Sub-Saharan Africa, total event sizes in death counts are smaller in magnitude than the respiratory catalog. Even so, about 2.5 percent of the events in the VHF model event catalog have at least 100,000 deaths in Sub-Saharan Africa, whereas nearly 50 percent of all deaths in the catalog are from events having 1 million deaths or more in Sub-Saharan Africa (figure 2.8).

**Table 2.12** Annual, 5-Year, 10-Year, and 25-Year EP Estimates for Selected Sub-Saharan Africa Event Sizes Based on VHF Event Catalog

| Deaths | Annual EP (%) | 5-year EP (%) | 10-year EP (%) | 25-year EP (%) |
|---|---|---|---|---|
| 10,000 | 8.1 | 34 | 57 | 88 |
| 50,000 | 3.7 | 17 | 31 | 61 |
| 100,000 | 2.6 | 12 | 23 | 48 |

*Source:* Ginkgo Biosecurity simulations.

*Note:* EP = exceedance probability; VHF = viral hemorrhagic fever.

**Figure 2.8** VHF Event Catalog Composition: Simulated Event Sizes and Contribution to Expected Losses

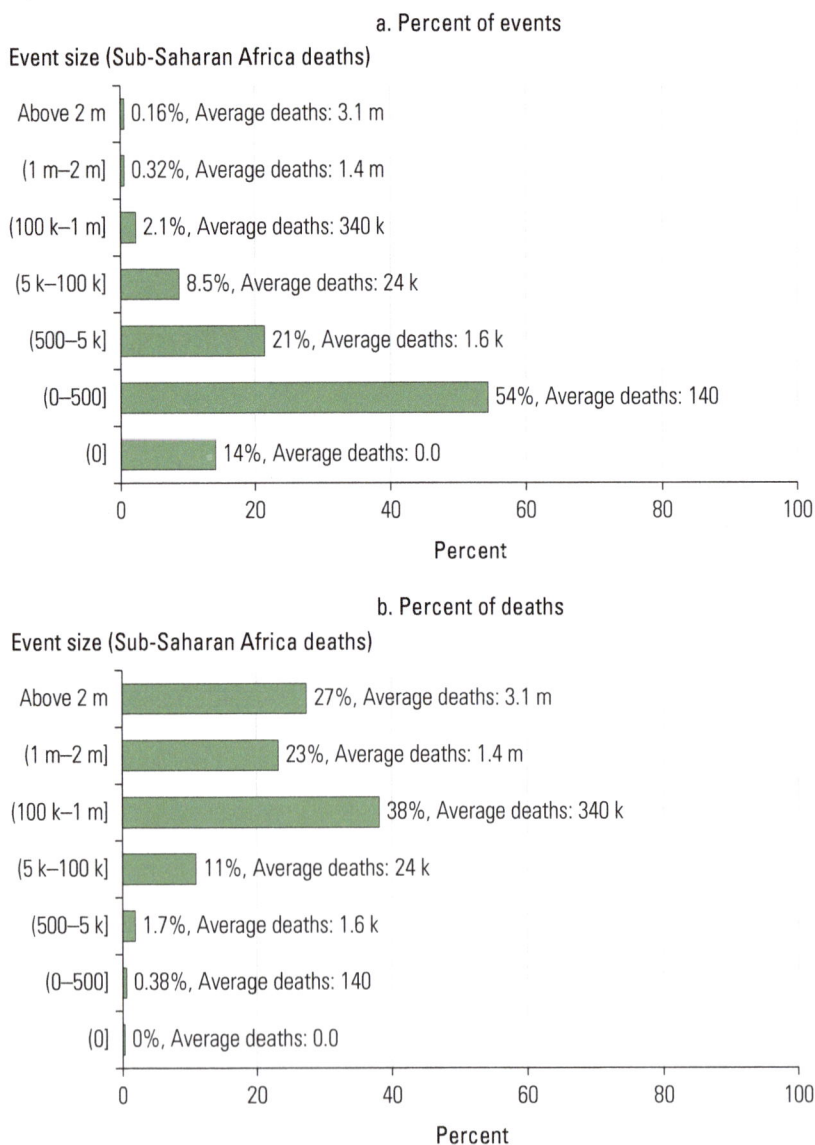

a. Percent of events

Event size (Sub-Saharan Africa deaths)

b. Percent of deaths

Event size (Sub-Saharan Africa deaths)

*Source:* Original figure created for this publication.

*Note:* The parentheses and brackets notation follows the international standard ISO 80000-2:2019(en) Quantities and units—Part 2, which conveys the following meaning. The "(" indicates the range is exclusive of the number, while "[" and "]" indicate the range is inclusive; k = thousand; m = million; VHF = viral hemorrhagic fever.

## VHF Mortality by Age Group

AAL was calculated for each of the modeled age groups. In contrast to the respiratory disease catalog, the normalized average annual deaths per 10,000 population varies considerably less across age groups. Figure 2.9 contains a graph of the normalized average annual deaths per 10,000 population for the VHF modeled event catalog in Sub-Saharan Africa. Table 2.13 presents the graphed values. This analysis suggests that VHFs are more universally fatal, with mortality less differentiated by age than as seen with respiratory diseases (Garske et al. 2017; Rosello et al. 2015).

**Figure 2.9** Average Annual Viral Hemorrhagic Fever Deaths, by Age Group, Based on VHF Event Catalog

Average annual deaths per 10,000 population

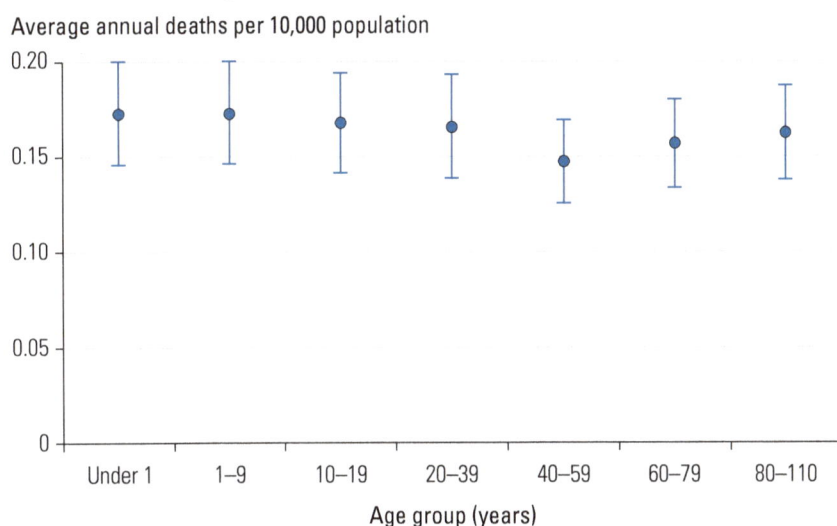

*Source:* Original figure created for this publication.

*Note:* The dots depict the point estimates, and the lines depict the 95 percent confidence intervals; VHF = viral hemorrhagic fever.

**Table 2.13** Sub-Saharan Africa Average Annual Deaths, by Age Group, Based on VHF Event Catalog

| Age group (years) | Average annual deaths per 10,000 population in that age group | Average annual deaths in that age group (thousand) |
|---|---|---|
| Under 1 | 0.17 | 0.66 |
| 1–9 | 0.17 | 5.3 |
| 10–19 | 0.17 | 4.4 |
| 20–39 | 0.17 | 5.5 |
| 40–59 | 0.15 | 2.2 |
| 60–79 | 0.16 | 0.80 |
| 80–110 | 0.16 | 0.07 |
| **Sub-Saharan Africa Total** | **0.17** | **19** |

*Source:* Ginkgo Biosecurity simulations.

*Note:* VHF = viral hemorrhagic fever.

## DISCUSSION

The simulation-based results presented in this chapter demonstrate the scale of the risk posed by pathogens of epidemic potential. The estimated global AAL of 2.5 million deaths represents a larger and more comprehensive accounting of the risk than was presented in *DCP3* (Fan, Jamison, and Summers 2017; Madhav et al. 2017). The view of risk presented here—particularly the focus on losses in terms of deaths—also clearly represents a lower-bound estimate of total potential impact because it does not include other sources of loss to human health and livelihoods (for example, infections, hospitalizations, long-term sequelae, economic shocks, impacts on education, and societal disruption), nor—as noted earlier—does it include all sources of epidemic risk, such as vector-borne pathogens, bacterial infections, and viral threats presently unknown to science.

The results also suggest that, among the diseases modeled, respiratory diseases are the dominant driver of epidemic risk, with VHFs representing a relatively modest global risk in terms of expected deaths. Although deadlier on an individual level, VHFs are less prone to spread than respiratory diseases. Their risk is not negligible, however, especially in Sub-Saharan Africa, and merits attention because of the direct and indirect impacts of these events on lives and livelihoods (Sochas, Channon, and Nam 2017).

### Magnitude of Epidemic and Pandemic Risk

Effective priority setting in global health requires the comparison of disparate burdens and risks, some of which operate on different timescales. As such, it may be helpful to understand how the mortality estimates here compare to other risks. It might seem intuitive to compare epidemic AAL to the annual mortality burden caused by endemic diseases, because both represent average deaths per year. For example, the average annual deaths estimated here for respiratory epidemics is comparable in magnitude to the annual number of deaths caused by routinely occurring endemic lower respiratory infections—approximately 2.4 million deaths (Troeger et al. 2018). When comparing such estimates, however, it is important to keep in mind the very different underlying patterns leading to these averages. Whereas the average annual deaths from endemic diseases are made up of moderate levels of loss that occur regularly, the epidemic AAL represents much larger spikes in losses that occur sporadically, punctuating stretches of nonepidemic years. Mortality spikes caused by low-frequency, high-severity events are potentially more economically disruptive than regularly occurring endemic disease, suggesting that, even when AALs may be similar between both types of diseases, planning efforts for high-impact epidemics should at least be equal to, if not greater than, endemic diseases.

The model results also show that tail risk cannot be ignored. Low-frequency, high-severity events—the tail in the results for this chapter—heavily drive expected deaths. It is all too easy to unconsciously discount the risk that the tail represents. The underrepresentation of extreme events in small sample sizes can lead policy makers to underweight their probability, especially when relying on a limited and biased historical data set (Slovic and Weber 2011). Moreover, because of cognitive biases that draw attention to the frequency component of risk rather than the joint product of frequency *and* severity, the low annual probability of such extreme events tends to cause policy makers to round this probability down toward zero.

To compensate for this discounting bias, this chapter has presented risk estimates for key points on the EPFs in terms of probability of occurrence over the next 5, 10, and 25 years. The results demonstrate how seemingly minute risks are far more substantial when viewed over a somewhat longer time horizon but still relevant in terms of policy making and budgeting. Over a 10-year view, an event on the scale of COVID-19 has a roughly 25 percent probability of occurrence; over the next 25 years, such an event has a likelihood roughly equivalent to a coin toss. These estimates demonstrate that future epidemic risk is more substantial than commonly believed and that severe events are likely to occur much more frequently than once in a century.

## Prevention, Mitigation, and Response Strategies

The estimates presented in this chapter do not, on their face, provide much cause for optimism. The expected losses from epidemic risk are enormous, and the results point to the considerable potential for pandemics that dwarf COVID-19 in terms of human impacts. Expectations can change, however. The risk estimates presented are not immutable. Risk could increase if the global community does not take meaningful steps to address the underlying drivers of risk. Conversely, risk can be reduced through investments in prevention (for example, spillover risk reduction), surveillance, preparedness, and response, which can be achieved through investments from basic necessities to technological innovations.

General investments in health system strengthening can significantly reduce epidemic losses, including those caused by respiratory diseases and VHFs. Because severe events occur sporadically, it is difficult to compare the benefits of improving preparedness between crises: other important determinants, such as technologies to produce medical countermeasures, may also have changed over time. These investments can easily appear to be wasted on threats that do not materialize, but investments to prepare for severe epidemics can also support effective responses to smaller events and other infectious disease risks, even in interpandemic periods. Such general investments having far-reaching benefits include improved laboratory capacity for rapid detection and confirmation of infectious disease threats (Wacharapluesadee et al. 2020), and border monitoring programs to track the importation risk of high-consequence pathogens (Wegrzyn et al. 2022). These improvements can also keep surveillance and response infrastructure "warm"—that is, in continuous operational performance so it may persist in a constant state of readiness. Surveillance and response systems need to operate continuously, both between and during epidemics, so that they can be constantly used and stress-tested, and also so they can detect epidemics in the earliest days of their spark and emergence, because early action has the potential for greatest impact. Ultimately, building these capacities will provide the greatest opportunity to stop an outbreak before it becomes an epidemic or a globally catastrophic pandemic.

Localized outbreaks and smaller epidemics provide additional risk mitigation possibilities. For example, because of the more localized nature of VHFs, the spark location is more influential to the overall mortality for VHFs than for respiratory diseases (Madhav et al. 2020), and potential spark locations are good candidates for spillover reduction efforts. Additionally, for VHFs, interventions often are implemented with a more localized approach than respiratory diseases. For example, health officials have employed ring vaccination, in contrast to mass vaccination, with *Zaire ebolavirus* vaccines and Marburg vaccine candidates (Cross et al. 2022). Furthermore, localized epidemics are more geographically constrained, leading to greater likelihood for international cooperation because neighboring countries and the international community can spare more resources—such as workforce, supplies, and financial assistance—for the affected country, which can greatly improve outcomes.

**Importance of a Risk-Informed Lens**

Although it is impossible to predict the timing and magnitude of the next epidemic, risk modeling can provide informed views of the potential frequency and severity of future epidemics. The key question is what exactly the world should be preparing for. Effectively preparing for an event as severe as the 1918 influenza pandemic could require very different strategies and levels of investment than would be needed, for example, to prepare for a COVID-19-level event. Although it is infeasible and resource-inefficient to plan for every epidemic that could possibly occur, plans should be flexible and adaptable, to handle a wide range of possibilities. Careful consideration of the full range of potential epidemic scenarios—by guiding discussions about the types of surveillance and response systems that must be built, and the level of financing required—can ensure that preparedness and response plans are commensurate with the level of risk. A risk-informed approach can help governments make better decisions around preparedness, ensuring that the world is ready for the next pandemic while making efficient use of limited resources.

Decision-makers traditionally have used a risk-informed analysis framework to prepare for other hazards besides epidemics. For example, in the design of wind loads for bridges, engineers often use a 2 percent annual probability (50-year return period) as a guideline (Garlich et al. 2015). Similarly, engineers may build urban road drainage systems to handle the flood risks from a precipitation event with a 2 percent annual probability (50-year return period) but may build high-risk levees to withstand floods up to a 0.1 percent annual probability (1,000-year return period) because of the catastrophic consequences of failure (Ponce 2008). Discussion of the suitability of these particular risk tolerance thresholds, and whether they should be adopted in planning for epidemic and pandemic risk, is important for risk-informed policy making and effective resource allocation, but is beyond the scope of this chapter. Further discussion may be found elsewhere (for example, refer to Strouth et al. 2019).

Planners and decision-makers can likewise develop risk-informed epidemic preparedness, mitigation, and response plans, relying on EPFs to provide necessary metrics. In practice, depending on country resources and risk tolerance, decision-makers would work to a preparedness target for their country—for example, to be ready for an epidemic with a 5 percent annual probability (20-year return period). Preparedness at this level would imply that a country could effectively respond to an epidemic of that magnitude and bring it under containment. Countries could determine their acceptable risk thresholds for epidemics by using existing frameworks such as the precautionary principle or as low as reasonably practicable (Pike, Khan, and Amyotte 2020).

To meet these risk thresholds, risk models can provide further details to help design and calibrate specific investments. Risk modeling shows that transmissibility and case fatality ratio greatly influence overall epidemic severity for both respiratory pathogens and VHFs. Thus, the intervention measures with the most impact for reducing mortality should target investments that reduce these factors. Toward this aim, risk modeling can be used to estimate stockpile sizes and resource needs for personal protective equipment, diagnostic tests, vaccine doses, antiviral drugs, and other therapeutics, as well as the effects of intervention timing and the costs associated with implementing these measures. Risk models can also help countries develop financing strategies, including risk transfer mechanisms, to offload portions of risk and response that are beyond their immediate budgetary capacity (Asian Development Bank 2022; Madhav et al. 2020).

Larger epidemics require higher-level planning and may need to include provisions for regional cooperation to have the greatest chance at success. For example, developing regional vaccine manufacturing facilities may be a cost-effective and politically viable approach to building surge production capacity (Jha et al. 2021).

International standards for preparedness could also take a risk-informed approach, such as by setting benchmarks for risk tolerance and minimum preparedness levels to counter the potential for a "weakest link" effect. Such a model could, for example, require that all countries be prepared to respond effectively to a respiratory event at least at the 5 percent annual probability level. This type of requirement could augment assessments such as the Joint External Evaluation, which sets standards for the prevention, preparedness, and response capacities that countries must have in place, but does not specify what level of risk mitigation or reduction those capacities can achieve. Countries should strive to take a data-driven and modeling-informed approach to assess their level of risk and risk tolerance, along with their country context, to set the appropriate thresholds for their own country following a common standard.

Requiring that countries meet a common standard for risk tolerance and preparedness would also require sustained financing to meet and maintain the necessary capacities. Many low- and middle-income countries face challenges in financing preparedness and response capacities because of budgeting constraints and competing health system priorities, such as high-burden endemic diseases. However, early detection and mitigation of pathogens with epidemic and pandemic potential represent a global public good that protects the health, national security, and economic prosperity of all countries. Given the scale of the risk, the G20 High Level Independent Panel on Financing the Global Commons for Pandemic Preparedness and Response proposed a dramatic scale-up of financing, including substantial aid for low- and middle-income countries (Shanmugaratnam et al. 2021), which would allow these countries to meet minimum preparedness and response thresholds. One of the primary barriers to effective, and effectively scaled, collective action is uncertainty regarding the magnitude and timing of future pandemics. This type of uncertainty has the well-characterized problem of leading to market failure (Arrow 1963)—in this case, underinvestment in global public goods such as surveillance and response capacities.

A risk-informed view can also prevent policy makers from falling victim to recency bias and overcalibrating to historical experience. For years, historical influenza pandemics were the planning benchmark for pandemic preparedness (US Department of Health and Human Services 2005). The experience of the relatively mild 2009 influenza pandemic led some analysts to conclude that the global community had overplanned and overinvested (Low and McGeer 2010). That conclusion may have even fueled the complacency and neglect that led to shortcomings in the global COVID-19 response. As the most recent severe pandemic, COVID-19 will likely become a de facto planning benchmark. The modeling results presented here suggest that doing so would be short-sighted. Multiple pandemics have occurred over the past century, with varying characteristics and magnitudes. Extreme events modeling shows that a wider range of scenarios is possible and should be taken into consideration to limit the risk of strategic surprise (Fukuyama 2008). Furthermore, the model results in this chapter suggest, and historical experience corroborates, that events more severe than previous historical observations can and do occur. The 2014 West Africa Ebola epidemic, which exceeded deaths during prior Ebola outbreaks by two orders of magnitude, vividly illustrates this point.

The results presented in this chapter strongly suggest that epidemic risk is far more persistent and substantial than is commonly believed. The probability exists that an epidemic—or even a large pandemic—could start in any year. The results demonstrate the urgency and priority of action to mitigate the risk. Armed with this knowledge, the world can be ready for the next major pandemic, which, in all likelihood, will not wait 100 years to find us.

## ACKNOWLEDGMENTS

This content was prepared for publication as this chapter in *Disease Control Priorities, Fourth Edition*, Volume 2, and as a background paper for the *Lancet* Commission on Investing in Health (Jamison et al., 2024).

The authors thank Ben Ash, Stefano Bertozzi, Matteo Chinazzi, Jason Euren, Mike Gahan, Mark Gallivan, Daniel Katz, Seri Lee, Melissa Lesh, Matthew McKnight, Kierste Miller, Ole F. Norheim, Chris Pardee, Ana Pastore y Piontti, Patrick Savage, Volodymyr Serhiyenko, Siddhanth Sharma, Vikram Sridharan, Cristina Stefan, Lawrence Summers, Swati Sureka, Alessandro Vespignani, and Qian Zhang for their valuable programmatic, technical, and editorial contributions. They also thank the participants of prior DCP4 meetings and convenings who provided valuable feedback on various iterations of the manuscript.

The authors gratefully acknowledge the University of Bergen Centre for Ethics and Priority Setting in Health and the Norwegian Agency for Development Cooperation (NORAD) (RAF-18/0009) for providing funding support. Certain supporting data and code are publicly available in the following repositories:

- Zoonotic disease data: https://github.com/concentricbyginkgo/zoonotic_spillover _trend
- Underreporting: https://github.com/metabiota-ameadows/underreporting
- COVID-19 data set: https://data.humdata.org/dataset/2019-novel-coronavirus -cases.

Other data and model code are considered commercial/proprietary and cannot be publicly released. Nita K. Madhav, Ben Oppenheim, Nicole Stephenson, Rinette Badker, Cathine Lam, and Amanda Meadows are or have been employed by Ginkgo Bioworks.

## REFERENCES

Ahmad, O. B., C. Boschi-Pinto, A. D. Lopez, C. J. Murray, R. Lozano, and M. Inoue. 2001. "Age Standardization of Rates: A New WHO Standard." GPE Discussion Paper No. 31, World Health Organization, Geneva.

Arrow, K. J. 1963. "Uncertainty and the Welfare Economics of Medical Care." *The American Economic Review* 53 (5): 941–73.

Asian Development Bank. 2022. *Building Resilience to Future Outbreaks: Infectious Disease Risk Financing Solutions for the Central Asia Regional Economic Cooperation Region.* Manila, Asian Development Bank. http://dx.doi.org/10.22617/TCS220010-2.

Astengo, M., F. Tassinari, C. Paganino, S. Simonetti, D. Gallo, D. Amicizia, M. F. Piazza, et al. 2021. "Weight of Risk Factors for Mortality and Short-Term Mortality Displacement during the COVID-19 Pandemic." *Journal of Preventive Medicine and Hygiene* 62 (4): E864.

Badker, R., K. Miller, C. Pardee, B. Oppenheim, N. Stephenson, B. Ash, T. Philippsen, et al. 2021. "Challenges in Reported COVID-19 Data: Best Practices and Recommendations for Future Epidemics." *BMJ Global Health* 6 (5): e005542.

Baker, R. E., A. S. Mahmud, I. F. Miller, M. Rajeev, F. Rasambainarivo, B. L. Rice, S. Takahashi, et al. 2021. "Infectious Disease in an Era of Global Change." *Nature Reviews Microbiology* 20: 193–205.

Bargain, O., and U. Aminjonov. 2020. "Trust and Compliance to Public Health Policies in Times of COVID-19." *Journal of Public Economics* 192 (December): 104316.

Bennett, J. E., R. Dolin, and M. J. Blaser. 2019. *Mandell, Douglas, and Bennett's Principles and Practice of Infectious Diseases E-book*. Elsevier Health Sciences. https://www.us .elsevierhealth.com/mandell-douglas-and-bennetts-principles-and-practice-of-infectious -diseases-9780323482554.html.

Carlson, C. J., G. F. Albery, C. Merow, C. H. Trisos, C. M. Zipfel, E. A. Eskew, K. J. Olival, et al. 2022. "Climate Change Increases Cross-Species Viral Transmission Risk." *Nature* 607 (7919): 555–62.

Cherry, J. D. 2004. "The Chronology of the 2002–2003 SARS Mini Pandemic." *Paediatric Respiratory Reviews* 5 (4): 262–69.

Cirillo, P., and N. N. Taleb. 2020. "Tail Risk of Contagious Diseases." *Nature Physics* 16 (6): 606–13.

Contreras, S., E. N. Iftekhar, and V. Priesemann. 2023. "From Emergency Response to Long-Term Management: The Many Faces of the Endemic State of COVID-19." *The Lancet Regional Health–Europe* 30: 100664.

Cross, R. W., I. M. Longini, S. Becker, K. Bok, D. Boucher, M. W. Carroll, J. V. Díaz, et al. 2022. "An Introduction to the Marburg Virus Vaccine Consortium, MARVAC." *PLOS Pathogens* 18 (10): e1010805.

Cruickshank, M., and R. Z. Shaban. 2020. "COVID-19: Lessons to be Learnt from a Once-in-a-Century Global Pandemic." *Journal of Clinical Nursing* 29 (21–22): 3901.

Diallo, M. S. K., M. Rabilloud, A. Ayouba, A. Touré, G. Thaurignac, C. Butel, C. Kpamou, et al. 2019. "Prevalence of Infection among Asymptomatic and Paucisymptomatic Contact Persons Exposed to Ebola Virus in Guinea: A Retrospective, Cross-Sectional Observational Study." *The Lancet Infectious Diseases* 19 (3): 308–16.

Embrechts, P., S. I. Resnick, and G. Samorodnitsky. 1999. "Extreme Value Theory as a Risk Management Tool." *North American Actuarial Journal* 3 (2): 30–41.

Fan, V. Y., D. Jamison, and L. H. Summers. 2017. "The Loss from Pandemic Influenza Risk." In *Disease Control Priorities: Improving Health and Reducing Poverty*, Vol. 9, edited by D. Jamison. Washington, DC: World Bank.

Farzanegan, M. R., and H. P. Hofmann. 2022. "A Matter of Trust? Political Trust and the COVID-19 Pandemic." *International Journal of Sociology* 52 (6): 476–99.

FEMA (US Federal Emergency Management Agency). 2016. "The 100 Year Flood Myth." FEMA, https://biotech.law.lsu.edu/blog/AGENCY-The-100-Year-Flood-Myth.pdf.

Fraser, C., S. Riley, R. M. Anderson, and N. M. Ferguson. 2004. "Factors That Make an Infectious Disease Outbreak Controllable." *Proceedings of the National Academy of Sciences of the United States of America* 101 (16): 6146–51.

Fukuyama, F. 2008. *Blindside: How to Anticipate Forcing Events and Wild Cards in Global Politics*. Rowman & Littlefield.

Garlich, M. J., T. H. Pechillo, J. M. Schneider, T. Helwig, M. A. O'Toole, S.-L. C. Kaderbek, M. A. Grubb, and J. Ashton. 2015. *Engineering for Structural Stability in Bridge Construction*. United States. Federal Highway Administration. Office of Bridge Technology.

Garske, T., A. Cori, A. Ariyarajah, I. M. Blake, I. Dorigatti, T. Eckmanns, C. Fraser, et al. 2017. "Heterogeneities in the Case Fatality Ratio in the West African Ebola Outbreak 2013–2016." *Phil. Trans. R. Soc. B* 372 (1721): 20160308.

Gates, B. 2020. "Responding to Covid-19—A Once-in-a-Century Pandemic?" *New England Journal of Medicine* 382 (18): 1677–79.

Glennon, E. E., F. L. Jephcott, O. Restif, and J. L. N. Wood. 2019. "Estimating Undetected Ebola Spillovers." *PLOS Neglected Tropical Diseases* 13 (6): e0007428.

Gomes, M. F. C., A. Pastore y Piontti, L. Rossi, D. Chao, I. Longini, M. E. Halloran, and A. Vespignani. 2014. "Assessing the International Spreading Risk Associated with the 2014 West African Ebola Outbreak." *PLOS Currents*. https://pmc.ncbi.nlm.nih.gov/articles /PMC4169359/.

Guterres, A. 2020. "All Hands on Deck to Fight a Once-in-a-Lifetime Pandemic." *The United Nations COVID-19 Response,* April 2, 2020. https://www.un.org/en/un-coronavirus -communications-team/all-hands-deck-fight-once-lifetime-pandemic.

Han, B. A., A. M. Kramer, and J. M. Drake. 2016. "Global Patterns of Zoonotic Disease in Mammals." *Trends in Parasitology* 32 (7): 565–77.

Hoffman, B. L., and D. P. Fox. 2019. "The 1918–1920 H1N1 Influenza A Pandemic in Kansas and Missouri: Mortality Patterns and Evidence of Harvesting." *Transactions of the Kansas Academy of Science* 122 (3–4): 173–92.

Jamison, D. T., L. H. Summers, G. Alleyne, K. J. Arrow, S. Berkley, A. Binagwaho, F. Bustreo. 2013. "Global Health 2035: A World Converging within a Generation." *The Lancet* 382 (9908): 1898–955.

Jamison, D. T., L. H. Summers, A. Y. Chang, O. Karlsson, W. Mao, O. F. Norheim, O. Ogbuoji, et al. 2024. "Global Health 2050: The Path to Halving Premature Death by Mid-Century. *The Lancet* 404 (10462): 1561–1614. https://www.thelancet.com/journals/lancet/article /PIIS0140-6736(24)01439-9/fulltext.

Jha, P., D. T. Jamison, D. A. Watkins, and J. Bell. 2021. "A Global Compact to Counter Vaccine Nationalism." *The Lancet* 397 (10289): 2046–47.

Johnson, N. P. A. S., and J. Mueller. 2002. "Updating the Accounts: Global Mortality of the 1918–1920 'Spanish' Influenza Pandemic." *Bulletin of the History of Medicine* 76 (1): 105–15.

Jombart, T., C. I. Jarvis, S. Mesfin, N. Tabal, M. Mossoko, L. M. Mpia, A. A. Abedi, et al. 2020. "The Cost of Insecurity: From Flare-Up to Control of a Major Ebola Virus Disease Hotspot during the Outbreak in the Democratic Republic of the Congo, 2019." *Eurosurveillance* 25 (2): 1900735.

Jones, B. A., D. Grace, R. Kock, S. Alonso, J. Rushton, M. Y. Said, D. McKeever, et al. 2013. "Zoonosis Emergence Linked to Agricultural Intensification and Environmental Change." *Proceedings of the National Academy of Sciences* 110 (21): 8399–404.

Jones, K. E., N. G. Patel, M. A. Levy, A. Storeygard, D. Balk, J. L. Gittleman, and P. Daszak. 2008. "Global Trends in Emerging Infectious Diseases." *Nature* 451 (7181): 990–93.

Kaplan, S., and B. J. Garrick. 1981. "On the Quantitative Definition of Risk." *Risk Analysis* 1 (1): 11–27.

Kogan, N. E., S. Gantt, D. Swerdlow, C. Viboud, M. Semakula, M. Lipsitch, and M. Santillana. 2023. "Leveraging Serosurveillance and Postmortem Surveillance to Quantify the Impact of Coronavirus Disease 2019 in Africa." *Clinical Infectious Diseases* 76 (3): 424–32.

Kozlowski, R. T., and S. B. Mathewson. 1995. "Measuring and Managing Catastrophe Risk." *Journal of Actuarial Practice* 3: 211–32. https://digitalcommons.unl.edu/joap/132/.

Ledesma, J. R., C. R. Isaac, S. F. Dowell, D. L. Blazes, G. V. Essix, K. Budeski, J. Bell, and J. B. Nuzzo. 2023. "Evaluation of the Global Health Security Index as a Predictor of COVID-19 Excess Mortality Standardised for Under-Reporting and Age Structure." *BMJ Global Health* 8 (7): e012203.

Lempert, R. J., and P. C. Light. 2009. "Evaluating and Implementing Long-Term Decisions." *The RAND Frederick S. Pardee Center*, 11.

Low, D. E., and A. McGeer. 2010. "Pandemic (H1N1) 2009: Assessing the Response." *CMAJ* 182 (17): 1874–78.

Ma, J., J. Dushoff, and D. J. Earn. 2011. "Age-Specific Mortality Risk from Pandemic Influenza." *Journal of Theoretical Biology* 288: 29–34.

Madhav, N., H. K. Bosa, R. D. Agyarko, N. Stephenson, K. Miller, M. Gallivan, C. Lam, et al. 2020. "Development of a Risk Modeling Approach to Enhance the Effectiveness of Epidemic Preparedness, Response, and Financing Strategies in African Countries." *International Journal of Infectious Diseases* 101: 212–13.

Madhav, N., B. Oppenheim, M. Gallivan, P. Mulembakani, E. Rubin, and N. Wolfe. 2017. "Pandemics: Risks, Impacts, and Mitigation." In *Disease Control Priorities* (third edition), Volume 9, *Improving Health and Reducing Poverty*, edited by D. T. Jamison, H. Gelband,

S. Horton, P. Jha, R. Laxminarayan, C. N. Mock, and R. Nugent. Washington, DC: World Bank. http://www.ncbi.nlm.nih.gov/books/NBK525302/.

Madhav, N., N. Stephenson, and B. Oppenheim. 2021. "Multipathogen Event Catalogs Technical Note." World Bank, Washington, DC. https://documents1.worldbank.org/curated /en/181791625232959415/pdf/Multi-Pathogen-Event-Catalogs-Technical-Note.pdf.

Marani, M., G. G. Katul, W. K. Pan, and A. J. Parolari. 2021. "Intensity and Frequency of Extreme Novel Epidemics." *Proceedings of the National Academy of Sciences* 118 (35): e2105482118. https://doi.org/10.1073/pnas.2105482118.

Meadows, A. J., B. Oppenheim, J. Guerrero, B. Ash, R. Badker, C. K. Lam, C. Pardee, et al. 2022. "Infectious Disease Underreporting Is Predicted by Country-Level Preparedness, Politics, and Pathogen Severity." *Health Security* 20 (4): 331–38.

Meadows, A. J., N. Stephenson, N. K. Madhav, and B. Oppenheim. 2023. "Historical Trends Demonstrate a Pattern of Increasingly Frequent and Severe Epidemics of High-Consequence Zoonotic Viruses." *BMJ Global Health* 8 (11): e012026.

Meslé, M. M., R. Vivancos, I. M. Hall, R. M. Christley, S. Leach, and J. M. Read. 2022. "Estimating the Potential for Global Dissemination of Pandemic Pathogens Using the Global Airline Network and Healthcare Development Indices." *Scientific Reports* 12 (1): 3070a.

Morens, D. M., J. K. Taubenberger, and A. S. Fauci. 2021. "A Centenary Tale of Two Pandemics: The 1918 Influenza Pandemic and COVID-19, Part I." *American Journal of Public Health* 111 (6): 1086–94.

Morens, D. M., J. K. Taubenberger, G. K., Folkers, and A. S. Fauci. 2010. "Pandemic Influenza's 500th Anniversary." *Clinical Infectious Diseases* 51 (12): 1442–44.

Msemburi, W., A. Karlinsky, V. Knutson, S. Aleshin-Guendel, S. Chatterji, and J. Wakefield. 2023. "The WHO Estimates of Excess Mortality Associated with the COVID-19 Pandemic." *Nature* 613 (7942): 130–37.

Nelson, K. E., and C. M. Williams. 2014. *Infectious Disease Epidemiology: Theory and Practice.* Jones & Bartlett Publishers.

Olival, K. J., P. R. Hosseini, C. Zambrana-Torrelio, N. Ross, T. L. Bogich, and P. Daszak. 2017. "Host and Viral Traits Predict Zoonotic Spillover from Mammals." *Nature* 546 (7660): 646–50.

Pike, H., F. Khan, and P. Amyotte. 2020. "Precautionary Principle (PP) versus As Low As Reasonably Practicable (ALARP): Which One to Use and When." *Process Safety and Environmental Protection* 137: 158–68.

Ponce, V. M. 2008. "Q & A on the Return Period to Be Used for Design." San Diego State University, CA. https://ponce.sdsu.edu/return_period.html.

Porta, M. 2014. *A Dictionary of Epidemiology.* Oxford University Press.

Price-Smith, A. T. 2001. *The Health of Nations: Infectious Disease, Environmental Change, and Their Effects on National Security and Development.* MIT Press.

Resolve to Save Lives. 2021. *Epidemics That Didn't Happen.* New York: Resolve to Save Lives. https://preventepidemics.org/epidemics-that-didnt-happen-2021/.

Rosello, A., M. Mossoko, S. Flasche, A. J. V. Hoek, P. Mbala, A. Camacho, S. Funk, et al. 2015. "Ebola Virus Disease in the Democratic Republic of the Congo, 1976–2014." *ELife* 4: e09015.

Sands, P., C. Mundaca-Shah, and V. J. Dzau. 2016. "The Neglected Dimension of Global Security—A Framework for Countering Infectious-Disease Crises." *New England Journal of Medicine* 374 (13)" 1281–87.

Shanmugaratnam, T., L. Summers, N. Okonjo-Iweala, A. Botin, M. El-Erian, J. Frenkel, R. Grynspan, et al. 2021. *A Global Deal for Our Pandemic Age.* Report of the G20 High Level Independent Panel on Financing the Global Commons for Pandemic Preparedness and Response. Pandemic Financing. https://pandemic-financing.org/wp-content/uploads /2021/07/G20-HLIP-Report.pdf.

Sirleaf, E. J., and H. Clark. 2021. "Report of the Independent Panel for Pandemic Preparedness and Response: Making COVID-19 the Last Pandemic." *The Lancet* 398 (10295): 101–3.

Slovic, P., and E. U. Weber. 2011. "Perception of Risk Posed by Extreme Events." In *Regulation of Toxic Substances and Hazardous Waste, 2nd Edition,* edited by J. S. Applegate, J. G. Laitos, J. M. Gaba, and N. M. Sachs. Foundation Press.

Smith, K. F., M. Goldberg, S. Rosenthal, L. Carlson, J. Chen, C. Chen, and S. Ramachandran. 2014. "Global Rise in Human Infectious Disease Outbreaks." *Journal of the Royal Society Interface* 11 (101): 20140950.

Sochas, L., A. A. Channon, and S. Nam. 2017. "Counting Indirect Crisis-Related Deaths in the Context of a Low-Resilience Health System: The Case of Maternal and Neonatal Cealth during the Ebola Epidemic in Sierra Leone." *Health Policy and Planning* 32 (suppl_3): iii32–iii39.

Stephens, P. R., M. Sundaram, S. Ferreira, N. Gottdenker, K. F. Nipa, A. M. Schatz, J. P. Schmidt, and J. M. Drake. 2022. "Drivers of African Filovirus (Ebola and Marburg) Outbreaks." *Vector-Borne and Zoonotic Diseases* 22 (9): 478–90.

Strouth, A., S. McDougall, M. Jakob, K. Holm, and E. Moase. 2019. "Quantitative Risk Management Process for Debris Flows and Debris Floods: Lessons Learned in Western Canada." 7th International Conference on Debris-Flow Hazards Mitigation. https://repository.mines.edu/server/api/core/bitstreams/f82115dc-54af-4296-86dd-6d869961987d/content.

Taubenberger, J. K., and D. M. Morens. 2006. "1918 Influenza: The Mother of All Pandemics." *Emerging Infectious Diseases* 12 (1): 15–22.

Troeger, C., B. Blacker, I. A. Khalil, P. C. Rao, J. Cao, S. R. Zimsen, S. B. Albertson, et al. 2018. "Estimates of the Global, Regional, and National Morbidity, Mortality, and Aetiologies of Lower Respiratory Infections in 195 Countries, 1990–2016: A Systematic Analysis for the Global Burden of Disease Study 2016." *The Lancet Infectious Diseases* 18 (11): 1191–210.

UN DESA (United Nations Department of Economic and Social Affairs). 2022. "World Population Prospects 2022: Data Sources." UN DESA/POP/2022/DC/NO. 9, United Nations, New York. https://www.un.org/development/desa/pd/sites/www.un.org.development.desa.pd/files/undesa_pd_2022_wpp-data_sources.pdf.

US Department of Health and Human Services. 2005. "HHS Pandemic Influenza Plan." US Department of Health and Human Services, Washington, DC. https://www.cdc.gov/pandemic-flu/media/hhspandemicinfluenzaplan.pdf.

van Wijhe, M., M. M. Ingholt, V. Andreasen, and L. Simonsen. 2018. "Loose Ends in the Epidemiology of the 1918 Pandemic: Explaining the Extreme Mortality Risk in Young Adults." *American Journal of Epidemiology* 187 (12): 2503–10.

Vinck, P., P. N. Pham, K. K. Bindu, J. Bedford, and E. J. Nilles. 2019. "Institutional Trust and Misinformation in the Response to the 2018–19 Ebola Outbreak in North Kivu, DR Congo: A Population-Based Survey." *The Lancet Infectious Diseases* 19 (5): 529–36.

Wacharapluesadee, S., S. Iamsirithawon, W. Chaifoo, T. Ponpinit, C. Ruchisrisarod, C. Sonpee, P. Katasrila, et al. 2020. "Identification of a Novel Pathogen Using Family-Wide PCR: Initial Confirmation of COVID-19 in Thailand." *Frontiers in Public Health* 8: 598.

Wegrzyn, R. D., G. D. Appiah, R. Morfino, S. R. Milford, A. T. Walker, E. T. Ernst, W. W. Darrow, et al. 2022. "Early Detection of SARS-CoV-2 Variants Using Traveler-Based Genomic Surveillance at Four US Airports, September 2021–January 2022." *MedRxiv* 2022.03.21.22272490.

WHO (World Health Organization). 2020. "COVID-19 Emergency Committee Highlights Need for Response Efforts over Long Term." News release, August 1, 2020. https://www.who.int/news/item/01-08-2020-covid-19-emergency-committee-highlights-need-for-response-efforts-over-long-term.

WHO (World Health Organization). 2022. WHO Coronavirus (COVID-19) Dashboard. https://covid19.who.int.

Wilkinson, C. 2021. "Pandemic Data Drives Risk Modeling." *Business Insurance*, February 2, 2021. https://www.businessinsurance.com/pandemic-data-drives-risk-modeling-covid-19-coronavirus/.

Wise, P. H., and M. Barry. 2017. "Civil War & the Global Threat of Pandemics." *Daedalus* 146 (4): 71–84.

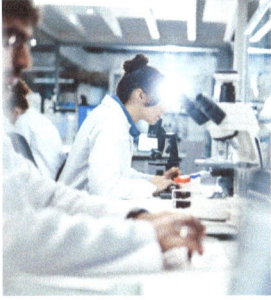

# 3

# One Health: A Comprehensive Approach to Improving Global Health in a Changing World

Jonna Mazet, Franck Berthe, Jane Fieldhouse, Tracey Goldstein, Karli Tyance Hassell, Sean Hillier, Catherine Machalaba, Alexandra Penn, Nistara Randhawa, Jonathan Rushton, Eri Togami, Supaporn Wacharapluesadee, Jakob Zinsstag, and Elizabeth Mumford

## ABSTRACT

The world is facing interconnected crises: pandemics, inequities, climate change, and biodiversity loss. The One Health approach, recognizing links between human, animal, plant, and environmental health, offers solutions. Benefits include reducing zoonotic risks and improving surveillance through collaboration, equity, and stakeholder engagement. Endorsed internationally, the approach has recognized economic benefits through prevention. Consistent integration, capacity building, interdisciplinary teamwork, and Indigenous knowledge inclusion are crucial, and expanding the application to address antimicrobial resistance and food systems is necessary. Recognizing interdependencies and multisectoral cooperation through a One Health lens can lead to efficient and equitable solutions and contribute to sustainable development.

## THE ONE HEALTH APPROACH

Our world is facing critical and converging crises that can no longer be ignored. Attempts to control deadly viruses—such as Middle East respiratory syndrome (MERS) coronavirus, severe acute respiratory syndrome (SARS)-related coronaviruses, and pandemic influenza viruses—have been, out of necessity, almost entirely reactionary. Because of recent devastating events, the world is poised to move beyond that costly approach, which measures impact in death tolls and money spent on diagnosis, treatment, and containment. The time is right for a more proactive paradigm that allows for use of knowledge on what diseases might be emerging and the development of interventions to prevent or at least control the pathogens at their source.

Before the COVID-19 (coronavirus) pandemic, the World Bank (2012) documented that, from 1997 to 2009, at least US$80 billion was spent responding to just six outbreaks of deadly zoonotic diseases, caused by viruses shared between people and animals. It also estimated that a pandemic would reach costs above a trillion US dollars. As evidenced by the COVID-19 crisis, forecasts not only were correctly cautionary but also far underestimated actual costs; they did not begin to anticipate the long-term costs to economies and societies of a severe pandemic.

For decades, scientists and policy makers have advocated for the One Health approach and proactive surveillance to identify all viruses of pandemic risk. They foresaw a relatively modest global cost of US$4 billion, should that work have been conducted and the data used to prepare for a SARS-related coronavirus outbreak in advance (Carroll et al. 2018). Application of One Health approaches could drastically reduce economic and human losses as the public health community drives surveillance and interventions upstream and predicts the risk from these diseases before they emerge.

In addition to recurring epidemics and pandemic threats, we face many interrelated and escalating societal challenges, such as equity and justice, clearly illustrated by disparities in access to health services among and within countries, as well as unjust food systems that fail to equitably deliver nutrition and thus health resilience. The planet itself faces a climate change crisis and an unprecedented loss of ecosystems and biodiversity that humans are—or should be—racing to slow. Current proposed actions to address these challenges are most often siloed, addressing only the clear and specific causes of a single crisis, or the symptom(s) of one, without holistic examination of the inextricably linked drivers of these challenges and thus without the identification of implementable solutions that address the complexity of the current global situation. In addition, single-problem approaches often fail to acknowledge human behavior as the root of all of these problems and human behavior change as the only real solution. If we cannot stop these accelerating processes before we reach identifiable tipping points, life on earth could fundamentally change for us all (Rockström et al. 2009). At the highest levels of international policy making, organizations and confederations such as the World Bank and World Health Organization (WHO), and now the Group of Seven and Group of Twenty, have all begun to advocate for a more integrated approach to health and climate policy—One Health.

Multisectoral collaboration has long been recognized as important for health outcomes (Watkins et al. 2017). The concept of One Health, however, directly acknowledges the connections among the health of humans, animals, plants, and the environment and prioritizes relevant outcomes for each. In 2021, a harmonized definition developed by the One Health High-Level Expert Panel was endorsed by the four organizations that now form the "Quadripartite" (the Food and Agriculture

Organization of the United Nations [FAO], the United Nations Environment Programme [UNEP], WHO, and the World Organisation for Animal Health [WOAH], founded as the Office International des Epizooties [OIE]):

> **One Health** is an integrated, unifying approach that aims to sustainably balance and optimize the health of people, animals and ecosystems. It recognizes the health of humans, domestic and wild animals, plants, and the wider environment (including ecosystems) are closely linked and inter-dependent. The approach mobilizes multiple sectors, disciplines and communities at varying levels of society to work together to foster well-being and tackle threats to health and ecosystems, while addressing the collective need for clean water, energy and air, safe and nutritious food, taking action on climate change, and contributing to sustainable development (OHHLEP et al. 2022). [Emphasis in original.]

The definition is accompanied by underlying principles that reinforce the importance of reducing trade-offs and increasing co-benefits, including through equity, sociopolitical parity, the notion of a socioecological equilibrium, stewardship, and transdisciplinarity and inclusion of stakeholder voices including traditional knowledge forms (OHHLEP et al. 2022).

Similar to equity concerns in other domains, guidance for ethical use and governance is often established without inclusion of all appropriate marginalized communities and does not always include consideration of sovereign rights. Like all nation states, Indigenous Tribal/Nation governing entities require reliable, relevant, and current data to make sensible health policy decisions (Barrett et al. 2022). International frameworks (for example, the Convention on Biological Diversity, Cartagena Protocol on Biosafety, and Nagoya Protocol) and a series of legal instruments have been developed to inform, operationalize, and protect Indigenous Peoples' rights to free, prior, and informed consent—a specific right that pertains to Indigenous Peoples. The United Nations Declaration on the Rights of Indigenous Peoples reaffirms and asserts Indigenous Peoples' rights to self-governance and self-determination over their collection, use, and ownership of data (FAO 2016; United Nations 2007). These rights, coupled with the universal right to self-determination, are the foundation to give and withhold consent to participate in research projects, promote equitable participation, and protect Indigenous knowledge in light of the open science/open data movement. Despite the identification of Indigenous data stewardship practices (refer to Carroll et al. 2021), digital platforms, big data, and open science databases present new international challenges and further inequities (Ross-Hellauer 2022). For instance, the use of digital tools requires technical capacity and resources to ensure protection of confidential information and health identifiers, especially during health crises (Hiraldo, James, and Carroll 2021; Johnson et al. 2021). Indigenous and other marginalized communities often face health data invisibility because of a lack of data collection and because of bias or misrepresentation resulting from data collection using a "deficit" lens, which reinforces dysfunction and marginalization (Barrett et al. 2022).

Although the One Health concept dates back to the time of Hippocrates, historians have described the modern history of One Health (Woods et al. 2017), tracing the term "One World-One Health" to the Wildlife Conservation Society's Manahattan principles of 2003. "One Health" as a term appeared for the first time in the biomedical literature in 2005 (Zinsstag et al. 2005). The approach gained traction as a unifying international paradigm during a pre-COVID-19 time of global crisis, when the international public health community had concerns that the avian influenza A (H5N1) virus, identified in Asia and spreading across continents, would spark a pandemic of severe disease in people and the food supply. Further, this influenza A (H5N1) virus emerged at a time of already-high global health concerns about other zoonotic disease, caused by pathogens shared by people and animals. For myriad reasons, including disruption of previously stable ecosystems and better surveillance and disease detection capacity in countries, there had been increasing reports of outbreaks of new zoonotic disease pathogens, such as bovine spongiform encephalopathy, SARS-related coronaviruses, influenza A (H5N1) virus, influenza A (H1N1) virus, and henipaviruses; reemerging zoonotic pathogens, such as Rift Valley Fever Virus, ebolaviruses, Zika Virus, and West Nile Virus; foodborne diseases; and antimicrobial resistance (AMR) (map 3.1).

**Map 3.1** Notable Disease Outbreaks and Pathogen Emergence and Key Animals Involved in Disease Transmission, by Year

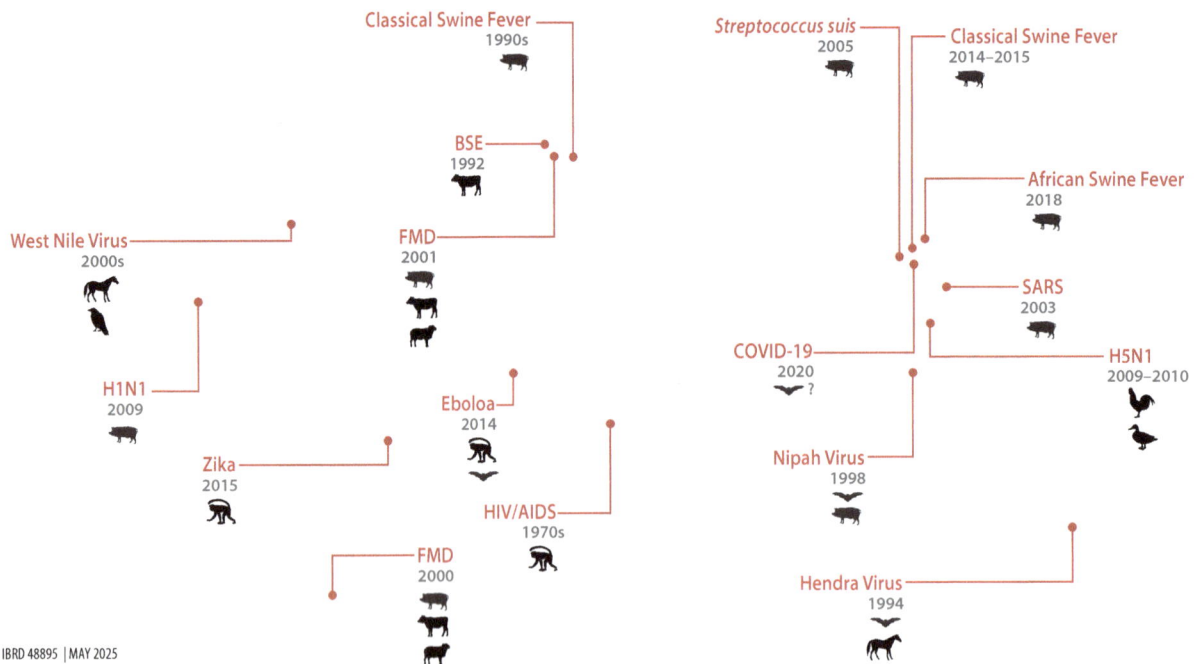

IBRD 48895 | MAY 2025

*Source:* Adapted from Patterson et al. 2020.

*Note:* BSE = bovine spongiform encephalitis; COVID-19 = coronavirus disease 2019; FMD = foot and mouth disease; HIV/AIDS = human immunodeficiency virus and acquired immune deficiency syndrome; SARS = severe acute respiratory syndrome.

In this context, the Tripartite (the One Health platform initially explored by WHO, WOAH, and FAO in 2008 and formalized in 2010) and global health partners, including the World Bank and the newly established United Nations System Influenza Coordination office, convened a series of meetings beginning in 2005. These International Ministerial Conferences on Avian and Pandemic Influenza brought together ministers primarily from the animal health and public health sectors to discuss and agree on the need for intersectoral action to reduce national and global risks from this and other zoonotic influenza viruses (UNSIC and World Bank 2010). In 2008, at the meeting in Sharm el Sheikh, the group broadened the scope to include other emerging and endemic zoonotic diseases in line with the new framework "Contributing to One World, One Health: A Strategic Framework for Reducing Risks of Infectious Diseases at the Animal–Human–Ecosystems Interface" (World Bank et al. 2008). International convenings continued as part of the Global Health Security Agenda and as instigated by large-scale projects, such as those supported by the US Agency for International Development. The term "One Health" began to be widely used to describe the new international policy recommendation of working across sectors and disciplines to address influenza and other zoonotic diseases and AMR. A clear definition of One Health as added value of a closer cooperation between human and animal health was proposed in 2015 (Zinsstag et al. 2015), showing incremental benefits of joint human and animal vaccinations in pastoralist settings in Chad (Schelling et al. 2005) and incremental benefits of zoonoses control (refer to table 3.1).

The new policies and funding established by the World Bank and other development partners sparked an exponential increase in activities using this newly recognized collaborative, multisectoral approach. Many countries have established national mechanisms for coordination using the One Health approach, and ministries now routinely work together on operational activities. They have a variety of tools and processes to support implementation and assessment of One Health capacity, infrastructure, and activities available to them (Pelican et al. 2019; WHO, FAO, and OIE 2019).[1] In 2022, UNEP formally joined the Tripartite, creating the Quadripartite (FAO et al. 2022).

Despite mainstreaming of One Health policy and gains in multisectoral collaboration at the international level and in some countries, especially between the public health and animal health sectors, functional capacity to identify new emerging diseases, especially those evolving in animals, is still limited. We may never truly know the timeline, geography, and species involved in the emergence of the SARS-CoV-2 virus. We do know, however, that global capacity to address the emergence and spillover of novel viruses into humans or into new animal hosts that could act as reservoirs for human exposure, as well as those that could be vulnerable to losses that could severely affect the human food supply, is weak. Since the emergence of SARS-CoV-2, other pathogens have similarly emerged or reemerged, including mpox virus and influenza A (H5N1) virus, with devastating consequences in human and animal populations. These viruses illustrate the ongoing threats from zoonotic pathogens and reinforce the need to change the way we approach their management (FAO 2023; WHO 2022). A handful of large-scale projects have provided the proof of concept that viruses of concern can be identified and ranked for risk mitigating action. Before the COVID-19 pandemic, however, the lack of a global agreement to pursue preparedness left global society's fate in the hands of disconnected public health systems not designed to handle a pandemic caused by a novel disease, now designated as Disease X (Carroll et al. 2018; Grange et al. 2021; PREDICT Consortium 2020).

Working across sectors on surveillance is critical, including sharing information that may increase vigilance and that could provide early alerts of a pending threat; however, simply working together using mainstream scientific approaches to public and animal health is insufficient. We must begin to understand and more holistically address the complexity of the broader social, cultural, and ecological systems involved in disease emergence and control and consider the potential for spillover events in the contexts in which they occur (Daszak, Cunningham, and Hyatt 2000; Kelly et al. 2017; Mumford 2023). Specific efforts to better empower rural and suburban municipalities and include community-based organizations and social scientists, who can help with effective communication and combat misinformation, are essential, as evidenced by the dramatic losses, measured in lives and financial damages, resulting from societal choices and human behavior in response to the COVID-19 pandemic.

## WHY USE A ONE HEALTH FRAMEWORK?

One Health offers not only a theoretical construct but also a practical, solution-oriented approach providing added value over those that do not recognize the interconnected nature of health. Although providing a general structure for collaboration, application of the One Health approach is context specific. Accordingly, the objectives, stakeholders, information needs, and strategies will differ with the particular issues under consideration and local context (Berger-Gonzalez et al. 2020). At the beginning of a process to address a complex problem, the One Health approach can help determine who needs to be at the table and the most efficient and effective ways to address an issue or to pursue a desired outcome (Berthe et al. 2018).

The application of One Health in numerous contexts has resulted in an existing and growing body of knowledge. For example, the development and use of a "Living Safely with Bats" visual booklet supported a One Health approach to risk communication and community education in villages and primary schools in over 20 countries. It increased knowledge about practical strategies for reducing zoonotic disease risks in daily living, while protecting bats and the important ecosystem services they provide in African and Asian countries (Martinez et al. 2022). Monitoring and detection of disease in animals have also helped inform alerts or other action to reduce public health risk. For example, investigation of reports of howler monkey deaths in Bolivia led to detection of Yellow Fever virus circulation and a preventive vaccination campaign in humans (Kelly et al. 2020). Similarly, One Health surveillance has been enhanced within and across countries through regional networking approaches; for example, the MATRIX project on foodborne pathogens and emerging health threats in 12 European countries, funded by the One Health European Joint Programme and the PREDICT project, supported systems strengthening for emerging infectious diseases in 30 countries across Africa and Southeast Asia. Although these case studies show the potential value addition from such an approach, the systems to routinely collect and use this information more systematically across disciplines, sectors, and stakeholders are not widely in place.

Countries are increasingly developing national One Health coordination mechanisms or platforms that provide a multisectoral coordination for ministries and a wider group of stakeholders. In Liberia, for example, a platform was launched in 2016 with a governance manual and five Technical Working Groups; chairing of the platform by the Vice President provided high-level political support. In addition to a goal of more frequent and routine sharing of information and collaboration, these platforms have been mobilized during disease events and in the planning and implementation of strategies. For example, in Tanzania, One Health Rapid Response Teams have been established at the district and regional levels to promote multisectoral disease investigation and outbreak control (Mtui-Malamsha et al. 2020). With national platforms in place, many countries are now working to enable subnational coordination. The establishment of similar coordination mechanisms at the country and regional levels is part of the indicators of projects, such as the World Bank–supported Regional Disease Surveillance Systems Enhancement for West and Central Africa.

The One Health approach also appears to be gaining traction from key commitments by other sectors. For example, the Global Biodiversity Framework adopted by parties to the Convention of Biological Diversity in 2022 states the value of One Health and other integrated approaches to help meet its 23 targets, which span aspects of ecosystem protection, conservation of biodiversity, and prevention of spillover. As power imbalances across ministries remain and must be further addressed, financing mechanisms must be designed to support implementation and to broaden the source of investments and the recipients contributing to One Health. This One Health implementation, in turn, will help support a whole of government and ideally a whole of society approach.

## THE ECONOMIC CASE FOR ONE HEALTH

The economic case for One Health is based on the assumption that closer cooperation between human and animal health and other sectors leads to incremental net benefits that cannot be achieved if the sectors work in isolation (Zinsstag et al. 2015). All the same, such collaborations across the different sectors and disciplines come with costs that need to be understood, described, and estimated, as well as a stream of benefits from improved overall health management and better efficiencies in resource management (Rushton et al. 2012). To prove incremental benefits of a closer cooperation, novel methods must establish the effect of the interventions at the environmental-animal-human interface through statistical or mathematical models that are combined with cross-sectoral economic analyses (refer to example in figure 3.1). A difficulty with such work is the need to estimate crises that do not happen because a One Health approach embodies preventive rather than curative health management.

Given that One Health is an approach, the ways it can be applied and situations in which it could be useful are numerous. Therefore, generating evidence of benefit will always require some interpretation in the specific context. Despite the desperate need for much better systematic understanding of the role of individual ministries and subnational stakeholders in the policy process and analyses of political economy and associated power (Garritzmann and Siderius 2024), good practices are increasingly becoming visible. Such good practices include stakeholder analysis and consultation to ensure sufficient engagement of those who need to be at the table and part of co-design or implementation (table 3.1).

**Table 3.1** Studies Examining the Benefits of Disease Prevention through a One Health Approach

| Study topic | Key finding | Source |
|---|---|---|
| Strengthening human and animal systems | US$1.9 billion to US$3.4 billion per year invested in building up human and animal health system yields. | World Bank 2012 |
| | >US$30 billion annually in avoided costs of epidemics, based on costs of major zoonotic diseases incurred between 1997 and 2009. | |
| Joint vaccination services for animals and humans | Joint vaccination of animals and humans in pastoralist areas of Chad saves 15 percent of the operation cost, compared to separate services. | Schelling et al. 2005 |
| Brucellosis vaccination in livestock | Societal benefits from mass vaccination of livestock to control brucellosis in Mongolia are three times higher than the intervention cost (figure 3.2). | Roth et al. 2003; Zinsstag et al. 2005 |
| Rabies vaccination in dogs | The cumulative cost of mass vaccination of dogs at 70 percent coverage and postexposure prophylaxis is lower than human postexposure prophyslaxis alone in 10-year period. | Mindekem et al. 2017 |
| Benefit-cost analysis of eliminating rabies in Africa | Coordinated mass dog vaccination between countries and PEP would lead to the elimination of canine rabies in Africa, with a total welfare gain of US$9.5 billion (95 percent CI: 8.1 billion to 11.4 billion). Uncoordinated mass vaccination of dogs between countries and incomplete PEP in humans result in lower welfare gains and do not lead to the elimination of canine rabies. | Bucher et al. 2023 |
| Assessing socioeconomic impacts of infectious diseases using a multisector approach | Case studies of Ebola virus disease, Zika virus infection, and others identify wider socioeconomic consequences than traditional public health costs and identify private sector organizations as important and underrecognized stakeholders. | Smith et al. 2019 |

*Source:* Original table compiled for this publication using the indicated sources.

*Note:* CI = confidence interval; PEP = post-exposure prophylaxis.

**Figure 3.1** Schematic Relationship of Time to Detection of an Emerging Pathogen and Its Cumulative Cost of Control

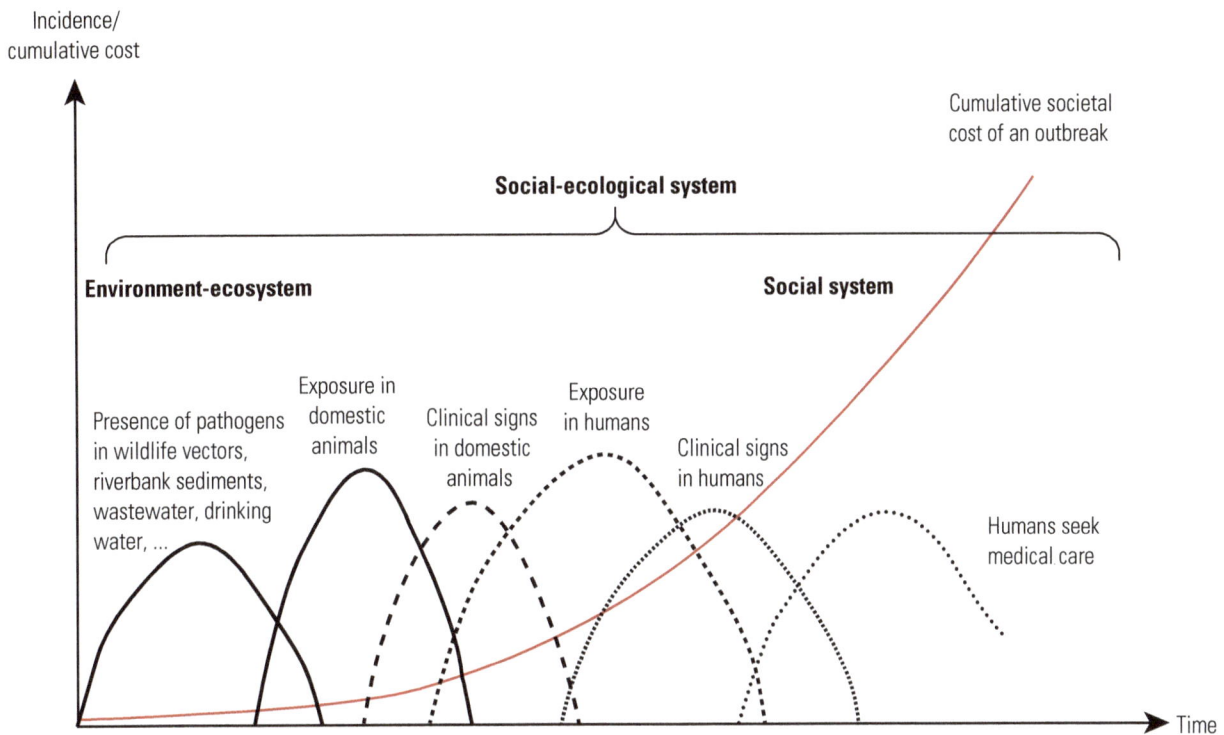

*Source:* Adapted and expanded by Zinsstag, Utzinger et al. 2020 from World Bank 2012.

## IDENTIFYING NONFINANCIAL METRICS

Elinor Ostrom (2015, 15) notes in *Governing the Commons*, "We can consider freedom of disease in its non-rivalrous and non-excludable quality as a common or public good." By analogy, unhindered spread of disease, leading to outbreaks, or endemic stable transmission of disease can be considered a "tragedy of the commons," as described by Garrett Hardin (Zinsstag, Schelling, et al. 2020, chapter 31).

### Local and Global Public Goods

Reducing pandemic risk—although a global public good—requires local actions to curb spillover risk and prevent local outbreaks from spreading. Demonstrating impact at national and local levels may resonate in national and subnational budgets. Investments in One Health–based prevention, detection, response, and recovery can generate local and global public goods relevant for domestic financing. As with other avoided illness or avoided events, however, intervening on pandemic risk, in terms of likelihood or impact, may be considered to have an invisible value of prevention that makes it unattractive for financing and measurement at a national level when considered in isolation. Thus, existing co-benefits may offer more amenable options as a starting point for measurement; in some cases, they can be considered a good proxy for overall systems strengthening that also have broader effects of reduced disease risk. Such metrics must be identified and agreed upon in order to help track outcomes, refine approaches as needed, and demonstrate value for society as well as return on money invested.

Timeliness metrics provide an example of a practical evaluation tool designed to strengthen public and animal health systems by assessing outbreak performance. Strengthening capacities ahead of outbreaks and tracking and measuring the time between key outbreak detection and response milestones provide countries and regions with a systematic and quantifiable method to identify gaps that can be targeted for improvement. Several timeliness metrics frameworks have been proposed, including the One Health timeliness metrics (Salzburg Global Seminar 2020), the 7-1-7 targets piloted by Resolve to Save Lives (Frieden et al. 2021), and the Joint External Evaluations (refer to chapter 5) under the International Health Regulations Monitoring and Evaluation Framework (WHO 2016). The WHO Regional Office for Africa recently adopted the 7-1-7 indicators as a target for timeliness in its 2022–2030 Regional Strategy for Health Security and Emergencies (WHO Regional Committee for Africa 2022).

Anticipating and containing complex outbreaks of priority and novel diseases require tracking and measuring metrics through equitable collaborations between the human, animal, environmental, and plant sectors at the local, national, and regional levels. Recognizing that a multisectoral approach is optimal for detecting and mounting a coordinated response, both the 7-1-7 approach and the One Health timeliness metrics framework support joint after-action reviews as an opportunity to review performance and share data among relevant stakeholders. The One Health timeliness metrics framework additionally proposes that, when possible, dates be tracked for predictive alerts of potential outbreaks and preventive responses to early signals.

Combining sustainable use of natural resources and human and animal health expands One Health methods toward strategy analysis using game theory (Bucher et al. 2023). For global public goods with overwhelming benefits outside of isolated countries, financing often requires international cooperation and solidarity, especially for issues that have global externalities, such as climate change or pandemic risk. At the other end of the spectrum, some of the co-benefits generated by a One Health approach are private goods, such as improved on-farm biosecurity that might improve profitability and resilience of livestock operations (refer to the example in figure 3.2).

**Figure 3.2** Synoptic View of the Costs and Benefits of Mass Animal Vaccination against Brucellosis in Mongolia

US dollars (million)

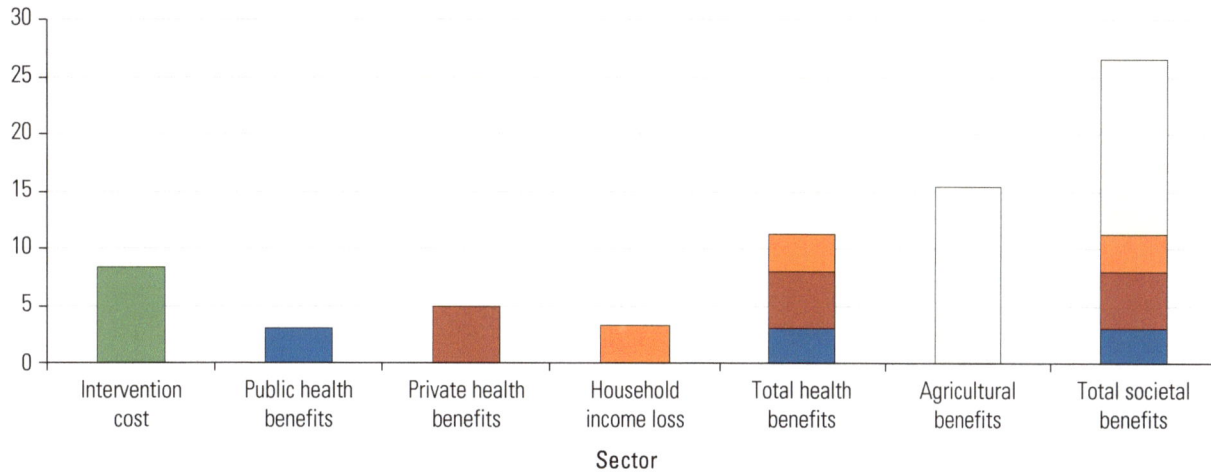

*Source:* Roth et al. 2003.

*Note:* Cost sharing between public health and animal health makes the intervention extremely cost-effective and efficient.

## Investing in Prevention

Part of the attention to One Health involves growing interest in the prevention element of the prevention, detection, response, and recovery spectrum. Calls to action have highlighted possible pathways aimed at reducing risk, such as the elimination of live animal markets. At the same time, these broad-stroke prevention measures create concerns about equity, unintended consequences, and disempowering local stakeholders who need to be part of the design and buy-in for successful uptake. Social inclusion is particularly relevant to these dialogues. For example, Indigenous Peoples make up approximately 5 percent of the population and steward land encompassing 80 percent of the world's biodiversity but are not adequately included and prioritized in decision-making processes (Masaquiza Jerez 2021).

In addition, although not routinely tracked, spending on prevention is widely recognized to result in magnitudes lower costs relative to the response required when diseases are not prevented. Prevention can be highly cost-saving, but the current level of investment is inadequate to produce intended effects. Analysis published in 2022 found that a One Health–based approach to pandemic prevention would cost an estimated US$10.3 billion to US$11.5 billion each year for three core areas of focus: strengthening animal health and veterinary services, improving on-farm biosecurity, and reducing deforestation or forest degradation and improving conservation (World Bank 2022). This cost represents 30 percent of the cost of pandemic preparedness (US$30.1 billion per year) and less than 1 percent of the cost of COVID-19 in 2020, estimated by the Group of Twenty Joint Finance and Health Taskforce. In addition, such investments in prevention have clear potential co-benefits, among them reducing emissions, addressing AMR, improving animal welfare, and limiting risky contact between animals and people. Improved preparedness ensures that systems are in place to both anticipate and reduce risks, as well as to effectively respond when disease events occur. Investing in enhanced preparedness is recognized as key to resilience.

## CHALLENGES TO ONE HEALTH IMPLEMENTATION

In addition to the difficulties of enumerating benefits from prevention, implementation of the One Health approach also has challenges and limitations. The timing of the emergence of One Health internationally meant that it evolved in an emergency and development context, and so has maintained the ethos of development paradigms, including challenges to equitable collaborative governance and power imbalances, as well as restrictions to the scope of stakeholders and actors and methodologies included (Mumford 2023). Engagements have subsequently left out many essential sectors, simply because their representatives weren't at the table when the approach was first developed for emergency response. For example, a long-standing issue involves properly recognizing the role of plants and the environment, and integrating the relevant ministries and departments into planning and activities. This problem is often compounded by underrepresented agencies and ministries being simultaneously underfunded and unable to adjust priorities to health collaborations, especially when budgets are compared to human health and animal agriculture sectors.

The COVID-19 pandemic has highlighted how changes in the environment affect human health. Despite this improved recognition and heightened interest from all sectors, there has been little change in the relative distribution of funds in most countries to allow for equitable multisectoral implementation of the One Health approach. Some signals indicate promise for needed improvements, including specific mention of using the One Health approach in important guidance documents, such as the Pandemic Fund, WHO's Pandemic Treaty, revisions to the International Health Regulations (2005), the US Biden-Harris Administration's bold 100 Days Mission, and numerous statements and convening documents from the Group of Seven and Group of Twenty. Thus, we are in a critical moment for One Health, with a window of opportunity for broad application but with a need to measure and clearly articulate the tangible benefits to improve the health of animals, people, plants, and ecosystems.

### Funding for Global Health Security

Before the COVID-19 pandemic, the US government invested in global health primarily through a lens of specific diseases. Examples include the President's Emergency Plan for AIDs Relief, with over US$100 billion invested since 2003 in the global HIV/AIDS response; the President's Malaria Initiative, with over

US$16.4 billion invested since 2005 to combat malaria in the hardest hit nations in Africa; international tuberculosis activities, with over US$45 million invested since 2013 for global tuberculosis control; and the Global Fund to Fight AIDS, Tuberculosis and Malaria, with over US$53 billion contributed since 2013. US federal appropriations have been earmarked to these specific funds to ensure support for the intended efforts. These efforts, of course, contribute to the strengthening of public health systems in general and to improved capacities to combat these diseases, but they do not go far enough to encourage holistic strategies to plan for, prevent, and respond to Disease X. Flexibility in the use of funds under these programs could go a long way in building and supporting health systems that desperately need to be strengthened across diseases. After suffering impediments to implementation and losses in service delivery during the COVID-19 pandemic, many of these programs are ready to get back to previous activities. Their focus, however, should be shifted to strengthening public health systems in general to try to regain both the services lost and improve public health resilience in general.

Although the COVID-19 pandemic heightened awareness of zoonotic disease transmission, by the time investments in response were made, the disease had already become a human-to-human concern. Thus, emergency investments, rightly so, were made to strengthen public health systems for humans only. The fact that the disease-causing virus initially spilled over from animals is often forgotten or ignored when considering how to best prepare for the next emerging health threat of significance, similar to what has happened for HIV. A major concern remains that future funding will continue to focus on human-oriented public health systems only and overlook the strengthening of animal health and food systems, including through the distribution of Global Health Security funds. We cannot continue to repeat this mistake if we are going to be ready to prevent and respond to future spillover events that will cause large-scale epidemics and pandemics without intervention. The evidence for global health security shows that

> One Health approaches appear to be most effective and sustainable in the prevention, preparedness, and early detection and investigation of evolving risks and hazards; the evidence base for their application is strongest in the control of endemic and neglected tropical diseases. For benefits to be maximized and extended, improved One Health operationalization is needed by strengthening multisectoral coordination mechanisms at national, regional, and global levels (Zinsstag et al. 2023).

## Ongoing Needs

For most countries that are actively advancing and integrating their public and animal health systems, opportunities to develop in the following areas remain:

- *Capability strengthening.* Knowledge and skill development in study design, study implementation, transdisciplinary collaboration, field sampling, pathogen detection, and data management and analysis, as well as workforce development in all sectors using a One Health approach.

- *Capacity improvements.* Public and veterinary laboratory advancements and establishment of laboratory networks, biobank maintenance, surveillance system innovation, biosafety and biosecurity controls, and multisectoral engagement competencies.
- *Gap assessments* using lessons learned from health projects outside of emergency responses to identify areas for improvement on an ongoing basis. Identified gaps can be used to plan for improvements if an easy mechanism exists to feed data and suggestions into public health planning.
- *Relationship strengthening and partnerships with Indigenous Peoples and community partners* to learn from and incorporate previously underappreciated research, longstanding knowledge, and lived experiences.
- *Networking with global experts* to maintain trusting relationships across geopolitical boundaries and to allow for collaboration during the next emergency.
- *Regional response systems*, composed of neighboring countries with similar environments and risks, for early alert action, regional knowledge-sharing, and support.
- *Strengthening coordination and information sharing within one country* among local, subnational, and national human health and animal health reporting systems.
- *Community engagement* to engender trust with science and health systems, combat misinformation, deliver practical training, and co-develop effective intervention plans.
- *Effective use of One Health platforms* to coordinate and improve systems and to leverage synergistic funding.

**Workforce Essentials**

Despite the increased recognition and endorsement of the importance of One Health by international organizations and governments in the wake of the COVID-19 pandemic, the One Health workforce remains difficult to characterize because One Health is an approach to complex health problem-solving rather than an occupation. Efforts to characterize the workforce have most often focused on a single sector or discipline, such as human medicine. No accreditation exists for One Health training, such as that for public health, and no centralized registries exist for One Health workers, as are common in dentistry or veterinary medicine.

To begin to fill this gap, a multinational cross-sectional online survey of students, graduates, workers, and employers in One Health identified essential training areas especially valued in the One Health workforce: interpersonal communication, communication with nonscientific audiences, and the ability to work in transdisciplinary teams (Togami et al. 2023). Survey participants deemed the ability to clarify the expectations, roles, and responsibilities in a transdisciplinary team early on in project development; avoid the use of jargon or technical terms when communicating in a multisectoral team; and seeking opportunities to work across disciplines and organizations for collaborative team building important for a One

Health worker. They also noted the importance for trainees of seeking out positions even if not explicitly advertised as One Health, because the One Health approach is essential to most jobs within the relevant sectors. For employers, hiring candidates with an interdisciplinary and collaborative approach was deemed essential, and it was suggested to use the term "One Health" and associated competencies in job descriptions for recruitment.

Training and workforce programs are beginning to fill gaps. The One Health Workforce project—funded by the United States Agency for International Development and implemented by partners in Africa, Asia, and North America—has strengthened the One Health workforce across 17 countries since 2009. In the most recent One Health Workforce–Next Generation project, One Health university networks in Africa and Southeast Asia have strengthened core competencies and workforce capacities through programs at more than 110 universities. In addition, One Health training is no longer limited to formal degree-granting programs at universities. As massive open online courses continue to gain popularity, open-access online modules on employing and operationalizing the One Health approach have become available. For example, OpenWHO, universities in North America and Europe through platforms, such as Coursera and FutureLearn, and One Health Workforce Academies, among others, offer foundational knowledge and evidence-based case studies of One Health through structured online modules.[2]

## CONSIDERATIONS FOR OPERATIONALIZED AND EFFECTIVE ONE HEALTH

The world's land and water uses are now completely dominated by people and our preferences for certain plants, terrestrial animals, and aquatic species. Humans have modified the global ecology for our benefit; at the same time, however, we have introduced risks to our own health, as well as to that of the plants, animals, and environment on which we all depend. This major change has resulted in the greater frequency of pandemics and epidemics of people and animals, principally associated with livestock food systems (refer to map 3.1).

One Health is continuing to evolve to address complex challenges, including and beyond infectious diseases, such as the climate crisis and how to feed our growing global population. Many of these complex problems are driven by major modifications of land use, especially through encouragement of cropping and grassland systems that support grain, vegetable, and fruit production for human food, as well as grass and crops to support animals needed for food consumption and for companionship and sport. Consequently, plant health, a previously underrepresented discipline in One Health, is now increasingly recognized as critical in employing the approach. Improving plant health is closely linked to safer foods and greater food availability associated with increased crop yield (Rizzo et al. 2021). In addition, the needs for the One Health approach are becoming more apparent in addressing the complexity of food systems and the problems generated from their antiquated designs. For example, our systems are generating an obesogenic environment in societies that have reduced need for manual labor and exercise. This powerful combination has led to a rapid rise in obesity and associated major health issues, with crippling impacts on health systems.

Similarly, the inappropriate use of antimicrobials, driven by the presence of infectious diseases in populations, is leading to shifts in resistance of pathogens to known pharmaceuticals and major problems and costs in health care, life expectancy, and potentially food systems. Although One Health has been employed to study AMR, more holistic interventions are needed to prevent the exacerbation of and to mitigate the impact of antimicrobial resistant pathogens, including good antimicrobial stewardship across human, animal, and environmental health (WHO 2019, 2023). Examples of good stewardship include responsible prescribing practices in human medicine, limiting use of antimicrobials in animals for growth promotion, and improving the management of human and animal waste and byproducts from manufacturing to avoid the contamination of water, soil, and other environments with resistant microbes and those that easily incorporate resistance factors (Larsson and Flach 2021; WHO 2023).

In contrast to overdeveloped, extraction-based food systems, Indigenous communities in remote and rural regions often rely in part or whole on subsistence living in which they acquire, prepare, preserve, and consume food via hunting, fishing, and gathering from the lands and waters (Burnette, Clark, and Rodning 2018). Efforts to improve global food systems should employ the Tribal knowledge and Indigenous research that has led to better sustainability in these systems; however, Tribal and Indigenous systems continue to face their own significant challenges. Ending hunger and disease, and improving health, wellness, and resilience based on subsistence in these regions requires the following approaches:

- Affirming and upholding subsistence rights and activities, often limited by historical and contemporary oppression and persecution, or federal and state legislation, policy, and management of land (Burnette and Figley 2017; McKinley 2022)
- Expanding traditional knowledge applications for food safety and surveillance that reduce and eliminate zoonotic illness and disease (Hueffer et al. 2013)
- Offsetting economic marginalization, enabling improved and sustained access and practice of subsistence lifeways not only to survive but also to thrive and promote healthy communities (Burnette, Clark, and Rodning 2018; Reo and Whyte 2011)
- Coordinated efforts with representation from Indigenous traditional knowledge and rights-holders, policy makers, appropriate agencies or organizations (such as health departments, centers for disease control, and research and education institutions), and infrastructure to support ongoing, culturally responsive training, monitoring, diagnostics, and preventive measures (Hueffer et al. 2013).

As noted earlier, negative externalities of public health are being increasingly recognized, and the associated impacts of the land and water use changes of food production are also now well documented (Rushton et al. 2021). Only relatively recently, however, have methods to capture these impacts been developed and applied in a system called the True Cost Accounting for Food (Gemmill-Herren, Baker, and Daniels 2021). This approach begins to address what needs to be measured in order to understand more carefully the impact of human activity on the ecological system in which we live and work and on which we are completely dependent. Thus, limiting the negatives of emerging threats, endemic diseases, and environmental change—at the same time that we optimize food systems to provide affordable, acceptable, and high-quality foods—requires advancing the One Health approach to improve metrics in all applications, as well as to optimize evaluation and decision-making processes.

One promising development is the push for greater focus on the health of the planet, rather than simply measuring outcomes with regard to human health and associated costs or savings. The holistic and interdisciplinary approach promoted by One Health links nicely with this more recent planetary health movement: "solutions-oriented, transdisciplinary field and social movement focused on analyzing and addressing the impacts of human disruptions to Earth's natural systems on human health and all life on Earth."[3] One Health and planetary health have both gained popularity and been recognized by health practitioners as essential in recent years. These concepts can help highlight the complexity of systems involved in the world's problems and, therefore, can be used to more thoughtfully address the adverse outcomes associated with the drivers of global health challenges, such as the changing climate, population growth, health disparities, fossil fuel consumption, and changes in land use.

### The Importance of Addressing Complexity When Using the One Health Approach

Both biological systems—those for which One Health approaches have been applied—and the larger socioecological systems in which they sit are considered complex adaptive systems. In Systems Science, which is its own scientific field, the interconnections and relationships between the elements or variables, not the variables themselves, are of the most interest. The terms "systems" and "complexity" are used inconsistently in One Health policy and technical discourse. When used to refer to One Health assessment or analysis, "systems" analysis tends to refer to mechanistic modeling methods used to understand causal relationships among variables in the system, such as for prediction.

In contrast to mechanistic systems, "complex" systems—for example animal bodies and the global internet—are by definition nonlinear (although some of the relationships inside them may be linear) and are unpredictable because of certain characteristics, such as adaptation, emergence, self-organization, and tipping points. Using both qualitative and quantitative Systems Science methodologies can be useful for understanding potentially unexpected components and relationships in the broad system and exploring the sometimes-distant impacts of manipulating them.

Given the complex and converging global challenges which One Health is now poised to help solve, there is a pressing need to expand the approach in three dimensions, namely scope, methodologies (or approach), and worldview (Mumford et al. 2023). An evolution in *scope* refers to the plurality of stakeholders and the expertise, experience, knowledge, and perspectives they bring, and, in particular, the need to expand effective and engaged partnerships to include affected communities, including Indigenous Peoples and voices from marginalized populations. An evolution in *methodologies* means inclusion of new or existing but underutilized methodologies and approaches to address some of the challenges in collaborative governance, inclusion of knowledge, and management of complexity inherent in One Health activities, and for which current, mainstream Western scientific methodologies are insufficient. An evolution in *worldview* means authentic consideration and respect for diverse and potentially conflicting worldviews in the planning and implementation of activities (Mumford 2023).

## The Role of Culturally Responsive Education in One Health

A paradigm shift to the inclusion of Indigenous knowledge and methodologies in predominantly Western education systems is well under way, but addressing power relations that view Indigenous knowledge as a tool in existing Western scientific and bureaucratic processes will require work (Barnhardt and Kawagley 1999; Nadasdy 1999). The 2030 Agenda for Sustainable Development calls for the empowerment of Indigenous Peoples, inclusive and equitable education for all, and engagement of Indigenous Peoples in implementing the Agenda, including "equal access to all levels of education and vocational training."[4] Comparatively, however, very few mainstream or Western education frameworks and programs include Indigenous Peoples and cultural competency in core curricula, required courses, or classroom settings (Barnhardt and Kawagley 1999).[5] In light of the ongoing and disproportionate effects of climate change on Indigenous and other marginalized communities, local education and capacity strengthening based on community needs and priorities is crucial to strengthening the next generation of human-animal-plant-environment health practitioners and stewards. Increasing the diversity of perspectives within One Health curriculum and associated degree programs is an area that needs to be improved to combat systemic racism, barriers, and health inequities among underrepresented and underserved groups.

Many Indigenous Peoples consider the land a resource that behaves as a living being and provides the life support system for animals and humans to thrive (Montesanti and Thurston 2016). This connection to the land emphasizes how the health of the land is central to Indigenous communities' health and wellness (Montesanti and Thurston 2016). Indigenous views of health take a holistic approach based on interconnected social and ecological systems (Hueffer et al. 2019). Integrating Indigenous knowledge means moving away from the current westernized model of health to include knowledge that is fundamentally relational—linked to the land, language, and the intergenerational transmission of songs, ceremonies, protocols, and ways of life (Greenwood and Lindsay 2019).

As a term, "One Health" can be seen as yet another colonial term that does not fully reflect Indigenous Peoples' worldviews. Indigenous worldviews and knowledge about holistic health and well-being preceded the evolving concept of One Health in veterinary and human medicine. Within the One Health framing, human health is usually listed first, and this order provides the passive presumption that the preservation of human health is the primary driver of actions (OHHLEP et al. 2022).[6] This prioritization runs counter to the worldview of humans as stewards of the natural world, protecting the health of our ecosystems and waterways, ensuring the continued care of animals and plants, and living in balance rather than over harvesting. Only through reordering our priorities may we start to bring One Health into alignment with traditional understandings of balance.

Indigenous early learning frameworks (for example, Canada's Indigenous Early Learning and Child Care Framework, established in 2018) founded on Indigenous climate action and land-based education, coupled with mainstream One Health principles, can improve science literacy, dissemination, and communication and ultimately enhance resiliency, wellness, and health outcomes. One Health programs grounded in cultural identity and local languages can support community mechanisms for experiential and intergenerational learning. Culture-based and co-learning among elders and K–12 youth can initiate knowledge exchanges across various spatiotemporal dimensions, including scalability in individual and community well-being.

## Co-production of Knowledge

"Through scientists entering into dialogue and mutual learning with societal stakeholders, science becomes part of societal processes, contributing explicit and negotiable values and norms in society and science, and attributing meaning to knowledge for societal problem-solving," a process known as transdisciplinarity (Hirsch Hadorn et al. 2008, 3). It is a pillar of One Health approaches, with scientists and nonacademic actors from several disciplines, including authorities and communities, collaborating in the co-production of academic and practical knowledge for the solving of societal problems (Schelling et al. 2008).

## Tapping the Power of Data Science

Similarly, effective and judicious use of artificial intelligence (AI) and its subset, machine learning (ML) can greatly improve One Health research and interventions. Both AI and ML are being used with increasing frequency in domains across science. Accessing all the necessary data and ensuring the capacity to integrate them to address global challenges will require that One Health approaches include computational scientists along with relevant subject matter experts. The recent advances in generative AI, such as ChatGPT, have transformed discourse on the future of AI-driven applications in modern human life, but they come with ethical, legal, environmental, and social concerns (Harrer 2023).

Contributions of AI/ML models to human, animal, and environmental health span a variety of applications:

- *Disease surveillance and control.* ML techniques have been used with different data types (for example, geospatial, remote sensing textual, genomic, and network data) to predict transmission patterns and outbreaks of pathogens and diseases, such as Zika virus (Jiang et al. 2018), dengue (Scavuzzo et al. 2018), and malaria (Haddawy et al. 2018); to forecast transmission of SARS-CoV-2 (Ward et al. 2022); to determine relevant disease outbreak information (Freifeld et al. 2008); and to predict host-virus interactions to identify potentially zoonotic viruses (Brownstein et al. 2023; Pandit et al. 2022; Poisot et al. 2023).
- *Human health policy and planning.* Algorithms such as XGBoost have been used to identify patients who potentially have long COVID-19 and warrant care at specialty clinics (Pfaff et al. 2022). ML models have also been used to predict length of stay among health care workers in underserved communities in South Africa, providing a means for planning and optimizing public health care recruitment (Moyo et al. 2018).
- *Food safety.* AI-assisted detection of potential bacterial contamination in food products opens up the possibilities of a framework for automated bacterial detection for earlier detection and prevention of foodborne illnesses and outbreaks (Ma et al. 2022).
- *Food security and agriculture.* Deep learning models have been used for image-based plant disease detection, opening up the potential for crop disease diagnosis on a global scale (Mohanty, Hughes, and Salathé 2016). Similarly, many other applications of ML in agriculture include use for weed detection and soil management (Coopersmith et al. 2014; Liakos et al. 2018; Pantazi et al. 2017).
- *Wildlife health and conservation.* Automation of animal identification in data sets of upward of 3 million images has been demonstrated with deep learning algorithms, with an accuracy similar to crowdsourced teams of human volunteers. This method has the potential to reduce cost and to free up human labor to solve more complex questions on animal behavior, ecosystem dynamics, and wildlife conservation (Norouzzadeh et al. 2018).
- *Climate.* Cowls et al. (2021) discuss the many roles of AI in combatting climate change, including for forecasting events associated with climate change, such as prediction of wildlife probabilities (Jaafari et al. 2019). In addition, ML and natural language processing methods have been used to systematically map global research on climate and health (Berrang-Ford et al. 2021).

Big data and AI will drastically alter how worldwide monitoring systems operate to detect pathogens and disease transmission (Osterhaus et al. 2020). Along with the increased reliance and proliferation of AI models come associated challenges that range from ethics underpinning AI models and the data they use to transparency, fairness, and the "possible exacerbation of social and ethical challenges already associated with AI" (Cowls et al. 2021; refer also to Harrer 2023).

Digitization of data raises important concerns over the protection of Indigenous knowledge and intellectual property rights, a longstanding issue across Indigenous communities. Presently, however, no international accountability and transparency measures or processes exist to assess whether global One Health research meets Indigenous standards and principles of protection (Carroll et al. 2021). Consequently, open data processes must follow Indigenous sovereignty and assertions outlined by both Tribal communities and individual rights. New applications of One Health could serve as a catalyst to assess multisectoral data challenges, improve intersectoral collaboration, and develop or improve Indigenous data protection metrics for collective and individual rights.

One Health programs, initiatives, and operations can protect Indigenous knowledge and cultural integrity by establishing a shared Indigenous community-based process for review and authorization of research, including explicit recognition, acknowledgment, and adequate compensation to Indigenous partners, knowledge holders, and culture-bearers. For example, the Alaska Native Knowledge Network provides guidelines for "documentation, representation, and utilization of traditional cultural knowledge as they relate to the role of various participants, including Elders, authors, curriculum developers, classroom teachers, publishers and researchers" (ANKN 2022, 3). One Health guidelines for incorporation of Indigenous knowledge systems in health mandates; diversity, equity, and inclusivity efforts; and teaching within classrooms can prevent misuse and appropriation of knowledge.

In consideration of the ethical concerns regarding the use of AI for health, WHO (2021) has put forth five principles to support the adoption of ethical approaches by governments and interested parties:

1. *Protecting human autonomy.* Use of AI should not undermine human autonomy and should ensure protection of privacy and confidentiality. Valid informed consent should be obtained through appropriate legal frameworks for data protection.
2. *Promoting human well-being and safety and the public interest.* Use of AI technologies should not cause harm, either mental or physical, to people.
3. *Ensuring transparency, explainability, and intelligibility.* AI technologies should be transparent in their design, intelligible or understandable to the concerned parties (including users), and appropriately explainable to those to whom they are explained.
4. *Fostering responsibility and accountability.* AI use should be supervised by humans, and in case of problems associated with AI technology, accountability should be ensured via appropriate mechanisms.
5. *Ensuring inclusiveness and equity.* AI for health should be designed to "encourage the widest possible appropriate, equitable use and access, irrespective of age, sex,

gender, income, race, ethnicity, sexual orientation, ability or other characteristics protected under human rights codes" (WHO 2021, xiii). In addition, AI technologies should not be biased, especially against already marginalized groups.

Keeping the principles for the ethical use of AI in mind, it is imperative that governments, academic institutions, and organizations also fund research to support the development of software tools in parallel with other academic and research outputs (Jombart 2021). As seen during the COVID-19 pandemic, outbreak analytics and disease modeling results inform the response to infectious disease outbreaks (Kucharski, Funk, and Eggo 2020). Ensuring the impact and sustainability of these tools will require prioritizing and supporting the development of high-quality scientific software, including but not limited to that incorporating AI approaches, especially for genomics.

### Financing Mechanisms

Although ministries of health, agriculture and livestock, and the environment are recognized as core to One Health implementation at the country level, ministries of finance play perhaps the most critical function through their allocation and supervision of national budgets. Even when political will for One Health is high, the absence of domestic or donor financing hinders implementation of activities and can lead to unsustainable programs. Lack of equity in financing—including donor-driven projects that target specific issues but may not always address local priorities—has resulted in uneven effort or focus from the concentration of available resources.

From global to local levels, enabling coordination among sectors (ministries, departments, and their stakeholders) in and between emergencies requires simplifying budget and administrative procedures. Maintaining collaborations and long-term commitments presents a critical challenge. Despite the devastating multigenerational socioeconomic impacts of the COVID-19 pandemic, the attention of global leaders is already being diverted to other issues, with a demonstrable reversion of ministry and agency activities to prepandemic siloed approaches. Improved coordination and cross-sectoral investments must continue and should be paired with investments in sector-specific activities and programs that support efficiency and effectiveness, including as part of existing and future plans and priorities. Aside from epidemiological plausibility, a key consideration for interventions must be feasibility, shaped in part by acceptability to stakeholders. Factors including preference, values, and priorities can play a role in willingness to accept (and, in some cases, pay for) interventions or other strategies. Resourcing for subnational implementation is also crucial, including enabling action at local levels. The local workforce, such as community human and animal health workers and eco-guards, should be equipped and incentivized to work together. The role of veterinary services can hardly be overemphasized, yet they are most often underresourced.

Although some financing gaps are likely to require new or additional resources, existing resources can also be leveraged or repurposed under a One Health approach, for example to develop synergies in programs for human, animal, plant, and environmental health systems. The improvements of laboratories, information systems, and immunization schedules offer potential examples.

## CONCLUSIONS

The message is clear: the key to modern health problem-solving is to foster effective partnerships and collaborations across sectors at local, national, regional, and global levels and holistic identification of equitable solutions to complex global problems. Those problems include local land use changes that affect living systems globally, the climate crisis, food system instability, and challenges linked to infectious diseases. Humanity can no longer ignore the suffering of the world's poor and marginalized peoples, the silencing of Indigenous Peoples' voices, nor can we continue our Western mainstream culture of inequities, colonialism, and oppression that contributes to health and social inequities. We cannot continue to burn fossil fuels and forests to support a lifestyle of excess that is rapidly becoming unsustainable. And we cannot continue to address individual and global health using linear, reductionist approaches that fail to consider or address the complexity of the social and ecological systems that influence it (Mumford 2023; Mumford et al. 2023).

Despite the growing evidence base for the benefits of One Health and the recognized need for greater coordination to maximize resources, uptake is still limited (Zinsstag et al. 2023). The typical siloed ways of working result in budgets that are not readily equipped to direct resources where needed, across sectors. Departments and ministries have long histories of scope and operational arrangements that often end up creating vertical programs with limited horizontal, agile capacities, especially when roles and responsibilities are fragmented across multiple agencies, leaving gaps and, in some cases, overlaps. Consequently, the typical starting point is "What can I do?" versus "What needs to be done?" (Berthe et al. 2018). These issues of mandates, capacity, and poor coordination affect ability to deliver on commitments. Equipping key players to act and addressing gaps will require alignment across agencies, reinforced by budget mechanisms (Berthe et al. 2018).

In 2022, the Quadripartite launched a One Health Joint Plan of Action with six action tracks: (1) One Health capacities for health systems; (2) emerging and reemerging zoonotic epidemics; (3) endemic zoonotic, neglected tropical, and vector-borne diseases; (4) food safety risks; (5) antimicrobial resistance; and (6) integrating the environment into One Health (FAO et al. 2022). The plan provides concrete activities and metrics from which to build, with country and regional implementation envisioned, as well as translation of the plan to the local context. To support a coherent approach from agency engagement at the country level, Resident Coordinators that oversee United Nations operations at the country level are being engaged. This engagement and the role of National One Health

Coordination Platforms, working closely with local champions, could potentially increase the impact of One Health approaches across the sustainable development agenda. These plans could be expanded to include activities that incorporate Indigenous Peoples and their knowledge into all engagements, and increasing focus on the inter-related issues of land use change, biodiversity loss, unsustainable food systems (beyond food safety), and the climate crisis.

## NOTES

1. Refer also to the US Centers for Disease Control and Prevention's "One Health" web page, https://www.cdc.gov/one-health/?CDC_AAref_Val=https://www.cdc.gov/onehealth/global-activities/prioritization.html.
2. For more on One Health Workforce Academies, refer to the organization's home page, https://onehealthworkforceacademies.org; refer also to World Health Organization, "Your New OpenWHO.org," https://openwho.org/.
3. Planetary Health Alliance, "Planetary Health," https://www.planetaryhealthalliance.org/planetary-health (accessed April 7, 2023).
4. United Nations, Department of Economic and Social Affairs, Social Inclusion, "2030 Agenda and Indigenous Peoples," https://www.un.org/development/desa/indigenouspeoples/focus-areas/post-2015-agenda/the-sustainable-development-goals-sdgs-and-indigenous.html.
5. For examples of One Health degree pathways across institutions or institutes, refer to Frankson et al. (2016), Hillier et al. (2021), Riley et al. (2021), and Togami et al. (2018).
6. Refer also to the US Centers for Disease Control and Prevention's "One Health Zoonotic Disease Prioritization (OHZDP)" web page, https://www.cdc.gov/one-health/php/prioritization/index.html.

## REFERENCES

ANKN (Alaska Native Knowledge Network). 2022. "Guidelines for Respecting Cultural Knowledge." ANKN, University of Alaska Fairbanks. http://ankn.uaf.edu/publications/knowledge.html.

Barnhardt, Ray, and Oscar Kawagley. 1999. "Education Indigenous to Place: Western Science Meets Indigenous Reality." In *Ecological Education in Action*, edited by G. Smith and D. Williams. New York: SUNY Press.

Barrett, Andy, Amber Budden, S. Jeanette Clark, Natasha Haycock-Chavez, Noor Johnson, Matthew B. Jones, Peter Pulsifer, et al. 2022. "Open Science: Best Practices, Data Sovereignty and Co-production." Arctic Data Center, Navigating the New Arctic Community Office, and ELOKA. https://learning.nceas.ucsb.edu/2022-03-assw/index.html.

Berger-Gonzalez, Monica, Katey Pelikan, Jakob Zinsstag, Seid Mohamed Ali, and Esther Schelling. 2020. "Transdisciplinary Research and One Health." In *One Health: the Theory and Practice of Integrated Health Approaches* (second edition), edited by J. Zinsstag, E. Schelling, L. Crump, M. Whittaker, M. Tanner, and C. Stephen, 57–70. CAB International.

Berrang-Ford, Lea, Anne J. Sietsma, Max Callaghan, Jan C. Minx, Pauline F. D. Scheelbeek, Neal R. Haddaway, Andy Haines, and Alan D. Dangour. 2021. "Systematic Mapping of Global Research on Climate and Health: A Machine Learning Review." *The Lancet Planetary Health* 5 (8): e514–25. https://doi.org/10.1016/S2542-5196(21)00179-0.

Berthe, Franck, Timothy Bouley, William B. Karesh, Francois G. Le Gall, Catherine Christina Machalaba, Caroline Aurelie Plante, and Richard M. Seifman. 2018. "Operational Framework for Strengthening Human, Animal and Environmental Public Health Systems

at their Interface." World Bank, Washington, DC. http://documents.worldbank.org
/curated/en/703711517234402168/Operational-framework-for-strengthening-human
-animal-and-environmental-public-health-systems-at-their-interface.

Brownstein, John S., Benjamin Rader, Christina M Astley, and Huaiyu Tian. 2023. "Advances
in Artificial Intelligence for Infectious-Disease Surveillance." *The New England Journal of
Medicine* 388 (17): 1597–607. https://doi.org/10.1056/nejmra2119215.

Bucher, A., A. Dimov, G. Fink, N. Chitnis, B. Bonfoh, and J. Zinsstag. 2023. "Benefit-
Cost Analysis of Coordinated Strategies for Control of Rabies in Africa." *Nature
Communications* 14: 5370. https://doi.org/10.1038/s41467-023-41110-2.

Burnette, Catherine E., and Charles R. Figley. 2017. "Historical Oppression, Resilience,
and Transcendence: Can a Holistic Framework Help Explain Violence Experienced by
Indigenous People?" *Social Work* 62 (1): 37–44. https://doi.org/10.1093/sw/sww065.

Burnette, Catherine E., Caro B. Clark, and Christopher B. Rodning. 2018. "'Living off the
Land': How Subsistence Promotes Well-Being and Resilience among Indigenous Peoples
of the Southeastern United States." *Social Service Review* 92 (3): 369–400. https://doi.org
/10.1086/699287.

Carroll, Stephanie Russo, Edit Herczog, Maui Hudson, Keith Russell, and Shelley Stall. 2021.
"Operationalizing the CARE and FAIR Principles for Indigenous Data Futures."
*Scientific Data* 8 (1). https://doi.org/10.1038/s41597-021-00892-0.

Carroll, Dennis, Peter Daszak, Nathan Wolfe, George F. Gao, Carlos Medicis Morel,
Subhash Morzaria, Ariel Pablos-Mendez, Oyewale Tomori, and Jonna A. K. Mazet. 2018.
"The Global Virome Project." *Science* 359 (6378): 872–74. https://doi.org/10.1126/science
.aap7463.

Coopersmith, Evan J., Barbara S. Minsker, Craig E. Wenzel, and Brian J. Gilmore.
2014. "Machine Learning Assessments of Soil Drying for Agricultural Planning."
*Computers and Electronics in Agriculture* 104 (June): 93–104. https://doi.org/10.1016/j
.compag.2014.04.004.

Cowls, Josh, Andreas Tsamados, Mariarosaria Taddeo, and Luciano Floridi. 2021. "The AI
Gambit: Leveraging Artificial Intelligence to Combat Climate Change—Opportunities,
Challenges, and Recommendations." *AI & Society* 38 (1): 283–307. https://doi.org/10.1007
/s00146-021-01294-x.

Daszak, Peter, Andrew A. Cunningham, and Alex D. Hyatt. 2000. "Emerging Infectious
Diseases of Wildlife—Threats to Biodiversity and Human Health." *Science* 287 (5452):
443–49. https://doi.org/10.1126/science.287.5452.443.

FAO (Food and Agriculture Organization of the United Nations). 2016. "Free Prior
and Informed Consent, An Indigenous Peoples' Right and a Good Practice for
Local Communities: Manual for Project Partners." FAO, Rome. https://www.un.org
/development/desa/indigenouspeoples/publications/2016/10/free-prior-and-informed
-consent-an-indigenous-peoples-right-and-a-good-practice-for-local-communities-fao/.

FAO (Food and Agriculture Organization of the United Nations). 2023. "Ongoing Avian
Influenza Outbreaks in Animals Pose Risk to Humans." News, July 12, 2023. https://www
.fao.org/animal-health/news-events/news/detail/ongoing-avian-influenza-outbreaks-in
-animals-pose-risk-to-humans/en.

FAO (Food and Agriculture Organization of the United Nations), UNEP (United Nations
Environment Programme), WHO (World Health Organization), and WOAH (World
Organisation for Animal Health). 2022. *One Health Joint Plan of Action (2022-2026):
Working Together for the Health of Humans, Animals, Plants and the Environment.* Rome:
FAO, UNEP, WHO, and WOAH. https://doi.org/10.4060/cc2289en.

Frankson, Rebekah, William D. Hueston, Kira A Christian, Debra K Olson, Mary Lee, Linda
Valeri, Raymond R. Hyatt, Joseph Annelli, and Carol Rubin. 2016. "One Health Core
Competency Domains." *Frontiers in Public Health* 4 (September). https://doi.org/10.3389
/fpubh.2016.00192.

Freifeld, Clark C., Kenneth D. Mandl, Ben Y. Reis, and John S. Brownstein. 2008. "HealthMap: Global Infectious Disease Monitoring through Automated Classification and Visualization of Internet Media Reports." *Journal of the American Medical Informatics Association* 15 (2): 150–57. https://doi.org/10.1197/jamia.m2544.

Frieden, Thomas R., Christopher T. Lee, Aaron F. Bochner, Marine Buissonnière, and Amanda McClelland. 2021. "7-1-7: An Organising Principle, Target, and Accountability Metric to Make the World Safer from Pandemics." *The Lancet* 398 (10300): 638–40. https://doi.org/10.1016/s0140-6736(21)01250-2.

Garritzmann, Julian, and Katrijn Siderius. 2024. "Introducing 'Ministerial Politics': Analyzing the Role and Crucial Redistributive Impact of Individual Ministries in Policy-Making." *Governance* 31 (1): e12859. https://doi.org/10.1111/gove.12859.

Gemmill-Herren, B., L. E. Baker, and P. A. Daniels, eds. 2021. *True Cost Accounting for Food. Balancing the Scale*. Oxford: Routledge.

Grange, Zoe, Tracey Goldstein, Christine K. Johnson, Simon J. Anthony, Kirsten Gilardi, Peter Daszak, Tammie O'Rourke, et al. 2021. "Ranking the Risk of Animal-to-Human Spillover for Newly Discovered Viruses." *PNAS* 118 (15). https://doi.org/10.1073/pnas.2002324118.

Greenwood, Margo, and Nicole Lindsay. 2019. "A Commentary on Land, Health, and Indigenous Knowledge(s)." *Global Health Promotion* 26 (3_suppl): 82–86. https://doi.org/10.1177/1757975919831262.

Haddawy, Peter, Ali Hussein Hasan, Rangwan Kasantikul, Saranath Lawpoolsri, Patiwat Sa-Angchai, Jaranit Kaewkungwal, and Pratap Singhasivanon. 2018. "Spatiotemporal Bayesian Networks for Malaria Prediction." *Artificial Intelligence in Medicine* 84 (January): 127–38. https://doi.org/10.1016/j.artmed.2017.12.002.

Harrer, Stefan. 2023. "Attention Is Not All You Need: The Complicated Case of Ethically Using Large Language Models in Healthcare and Medicine." *EBioMedicine* 90 (April): 104512. https://doi.org/10.1016/j.ebiom.2023.104512.

Hillier, Sean, Abdul Taleb, Elias Chaccour, and Cécile Aenishaenslin. 2021. "Examining the Concept of One Health for Indigenous Communities: A Systematic Review." *One Health* 12 (June): 100248. https://doi.org/10.1016/j.onehlt.2021.100248.

Hiraldo, Danielle, Kyra James, and Stephanie Russo Carroll. 2021. "Case Report: Indigenous Sovereignty in a Pandemic: Tribal Codes in the United States as Preparedness." *Frontiers in Sociology* 6 (March). https://doi.org/10.3389/fsoc.2021.617995.

Hirsch Hadorn, Gertrude, Holger Hoffmann-Reim, Susette Biber-Klemm, Walter Grossenbacher, Dominique Joye, Christian Pohl, Urs Wiesmann, and Elisabeth Zemp, eds. 2008. *Handbook of Transdisciplinary Research*. Springer.

Hueffer, Karsten, Mary F. Ehrlander, Kathy Etz, and Arleigh J. Reynolds. 2019. "One Health in the Circumpolar North." *International Journal of Circumpolar Health* 78 (1): 1607502. https://doi.org/10.1080/22423982.2019.1607502.

Hueffer, Karsten, Alan J. Parkinson, Robert F. Gerlach, and James Berner. 2013. "Zoonotic Infections in Alaska: Disease Prevalence, Potential Impact of Climate Change and Recommended Actions for Earlier Disease Detection, Research, Prevention and Control." *International Journal of Circumpolar Health* 72 (1): 19562. https://doi.org/10.3402/ijch.v72i0.19562.

Jaafari, Abolfazl, Eric K. Zenner, Mahdi Panahi, and Himan Shahabi. 2019. "Hybrid Artificial Intelligence Models Based on a Neuro-Fuzzy System and Metaheuristic Optimization Algorithms for Spatial Prediction of Wildfire Probability." *Agricultural and Forest Meteorology* 266–267 (March): 198–207. https://doi.org/10.1016/j.agrformet.2018.12.015.

Jiang, Dong, Mengmeng Hao, Fang Ding, Jingying Fu, and Meng Li. 2018. "Mapping the Transmission Risk of Zika Virus Using Machine Learning Models." *Acta Tropica* 185 (September): 391–99. https://doi.org/10.1016/j.actatropica.2018.06.021.

Johnson, Noor, Matthew L. Druckenmiller, Finn Danielsen, and Peter Pulsifer. 2021. "The Use of Digital Platforms for Community-Based Monitoring." *BioScience* 71 (5): 452–66. https://doi.org/10.1093/biosci/biaa162.

Jombart, Thibaut. 2021. "Why Development of Outbreak Analytics Tools Should Be Valued, Supported, and Funded." *The Lancet Infectious Diseases* 21 (4): 458–59. https://doi.org/10.1016/s1473-3099(20)30996-8.

Kelly, Terra, William Karesh, Christine Kreuder Johnson, Kirsten Gilardi, Simon Anthony, Tracey Goldstein, Sarah Olson, et al. 2017. "One Health Proof of Concept: Bringing a Transdisciplinary Approach to Surveillance for Zoonotic Viruses at the Human-Wild Animal Interface." *Journal of Preventive Veterinary Medicine* 137(Pt B): 112–18. https://doi.org/10.1016/j.prevetmed.2016.11.023.

Kelly, Terra, Catherine Machalaba, William Karesh, Paulina Zielinska Crook, Kirsten Gilardi, Julius Nziza, Marcela Uhart, et al. 2020. "Implementing One Health Approaches to Confront Emerging and Re-Emerging Zoonotic Disease Threats: Lessons from PREDICT." *One Health Outlook* 2 (1). https://doi.org/10.1186/s42522-019-0007-9.

Kucharski, Adam J., Sebastian Funk, and Rosalind M Eggo. 2020. "The COVID-19 Response Illustrates That Traditional Academic Reward Structures and Metrics Do Not Reflect Crucial Contributions to Modern Science." *PLOS Biology* 18 (10): e3000913. https://doi.org/10.1371/journal.pbio.3000913.

Larsson, D. G. Joakim, and Carl-Fredrik Flach. 2021. "Antibiotic Resistance in the Environment." *Nature Reviews Microbiology* 20 (5): 257–69. https://doi.org/10.1038/s41579-021-00649-x.

Liakos, Konstantinos, Patrizia Busato, Dimitrios Moshou, Simon Pearson, and Dionysis Bochtis. 2018. "Machine Learning in Agriculture: A Review." *Sensors* 18 (8): 2674. https://doi.org/10.3390/s18082674.

Ma, Luyao, Jiyoon Yi, Nicharee Wisuthiphaet, Mason Earles, and Nitin Nitin. 2022. "Accelerating the Detection of Bacteria in Food Using Artificial Intelligence and Optical Imaging." *Applied and Environmental Microbiology* 89 (1). https://doi.org/10.1128/aem.01828-22.

Martinez, Stephanie, Ava Sullivan, Emily Hagan, Jonathan Goley, Jonathan H. Epstein, Kevin J. Olival, Karen Saylors, et al. 2022. "Living Safely with Bats: Lessons in Developing and Sharing a Global One Health Educational Resource." *Global Health, Science and Practice* 10 (6): e2200106. https://doi.org/10.9745/ghsp-d-22-00106.

Masaquiza Jerez, Mirian. 2021. "Challenges and Opportunities for Indigenous Peoples' Sustainability." United Nations Department of Economic and Social Affairs. https://www.un.org/development/desa/dspd/wp-content/uploads/sites/22/2021/04/PB_101.pdf.

McKinley, Catherine E. 2022. "'We Were Always Doing Something Outside. … I Had a Wonderful, Wonderful Life': U.S. Indigenous Peoples' Subsistence, Physical Activity, and the Natural World." *SSM – Qualitative Research in Health* 2 (December): 100170. https://doi.org/10.1016/j.ssmqr.2022.100170.

Mindekem, Rolande, Monique Léchenne, Kemdongarti Service Naissengar, Assandi Oussiguéré, Bidjeh Kebkiba, Doumagoum Moto Daugla, Idriss Oumar Alfaroukh, et al. 2017. "Cost Description and Comparative Cost Efficiency of Post-Exposure Prophylaxis and Canine Mass Vaccination against Rabies in N'Djamena, Chad." *Frontiers in Veterinary Science* 4 (April).

Mohanty, Sharada P., David Hughes, and Marcel Salathé. 2016. "Using Deep Learning for Image-Based Plant Disease Detection." *Frontiers in Plant Science* 7 (September). https://doi.org/10.3389/fpls.2016.01419.

Montesanti, S., and W. E. Thurston. 2016. "Engagement of Indigenous Peoples in One-Health Education and Research." In *One Health Case Studies: Addressing Complex Problems in a Changing World*, 346–55. 5M Publishing.

Moyo, Sangiwe, Tuan Nguyen Doan, Jessica Yun, and Ndumiso Tshuma. 2018. "Application of Machine Learning Models in Predicting Length of Stay among Healthcare Workers in Underserved Communities in South Africa." *Human Resources for Health* 16 (1). https://doi.org/10.1186/s12960-018-0329-1.

Mtui-Malamsha, Niwael, Justine A. Assenga, Emmanuel S. Swai, Faraja Msemwa, Selemani Makungu, Harrison Chinyuka, Jubilate Bernard, et al. 2020. "Subnational Operationalization of One Health: Lessons from the Establishment of One Health Rapid Response Teams in Tanzania." *Transactions of the Royal Society of Tropical Medicine and Hygiene* 114 (7): 538–40. https://doi.org/10.1093/trstmh/trz138.

Mumford, Elizabeth. 2023. "One Health Policy and Practice: Evolution towards More Sustainable Impact." PhD Thesis, University of Surrey, U.K.

Mumford, Elizabeth, Deniss J. Martinez, Karli Tyance-Hassell, Alasdair Cook, Gail R. Hansen, Ronald Labonté, Jonna A. K. Mazet, et al. 2023. "Evolution and Expansion of the One Health Approach to Promote Sustainable and Resilient Health and Well-Being: A Call to Action." *Frontiers in Public Health* 10 (January). https://doi.org/10.3389/fpubh .2022.1056459.

Nadasdy, Paul. 1999. "The Politics of Tek: Power and the 'Integration' of Knowledge." *Arctic Anthropology* 36 (1/2): 1–18. http://www.jstor.org/stable/40316502.

Norouzzadeh, Mohammad Sadegh, Anh Nguyen, Margaret Kosmala, Alexandra Swanson, Meredith S. Palmer, Craig Packer, and Jeff Clune. 2018. "Automatically Identifying, Counting, and Describing Wild Animals in Camera-Trap Images with Deep Learning." *PNAS* 115 (25). https://doi.org/10.1073/pnas.1719367115.

OHHLEP (One Health High-Level Expert Panel), Wiku Adisasmito, Salama Almuhairi, Casey Barton Behravesh, Pépé Bilivogui, Salome A. Bukachi, Natalia Casas, et al. 2022. "One Health: A New Definition for a Sustainable and Healthy Future." *PLOS Pathogens* 18 (6): e1010537. https://doi.org/10.1371/journal.ppat.1010537.

Osterhaus, Albert D. M. E., Chris Vanlangendonck, Maurizio Barbeschi, Christianne J. M. Bruschke, Renee Christensen, Peter Daszak, Frouke De Groot, et al. 2020. "Make Science Evolve into a One Health Approach to Improve Health and Security: A White Paper." *One Health Outlook* 2 (1). https://doi.org/10.1186/s42522-019-0009-7.

Ostrom, Elinor. 2015. *Governing the Commons: The Evolution of Institutions for Collective Action.* Cambridge University Press. http://www.loc.gov/catdir/enhancements/fy1606 /2015487909-d.html.

Pandit, Pranav, Simon J. Anthony, Tracey Goldstein, Kevin J. Olival, Megan Doyle, Nicole R. Gardner, Brian H. Bird, et al. 2022. "Predicting the Potential for Zoonotic Transmission and Host Associations for Novel Viruses." *Communications Biology* 5 (1). https://doi .org/10.1038/s42003-022-03797-9.

Pantazi, Xanthoula Eirini, Alexandra A. Tamouridou, Thomas Alexandridis, Anastasia L. Lagopodi, Javid Kashefi, and Dimitrios Moshou. 2017. "Evaluation of Hierarchical Self-Organising Maps for Weed Mapping Using UAS Multispectral Imagery." *Computers and Electronics in Agriculture* 139 (June): 224–30. https://doi.org/10.1016/j .compag.2017.05.026.

Patterson, Grace T., Lian F. Thomas, Lucy Coyne, and Jonathan Rushton. 2020. "Moving Health to the Heart of Agri-Food Policies; Mitigating Risk from Our Food Systems." *Global Food Security* 26 (September): 100424. https://doi.org/10.1016/j.gfs.2020.100424.

Pelican, Katharine M., Stephanie J. Salyer, Casey Barton Behravesh, Guillaume Belot, Maud Carron, F. Caya, Stéphane De La Rocque, et al. 2019. "Synergising Tools for Capacity Assessment and One Health Operationalisation." *Revue Scientifique et Technique de l'Office International des Epizooties* 38 (1): 71–89. https://doi.org/10.20506/rst.38.1.2942.

Pfaff, Emily, Andrew T. Girvin, Tellen D. Bennett, Abhishek Bhatia, Ian M. Brooks, Rachel Deer, Jonathan Dekermanjian, et al. 2022. "Identifying Who Has Long COVID in the USA: A Machine Learning Approach Using N3C Data." *The Lancet Digital Health* 4 (7): e532–41. https://doi.org/10.1016/s2589-7500(22)00048-6.

Poisot, Timothée, Marie-Andrée Ouellet, Nardus Mollentze, Maxwell J. Farrell, Daniel Becker, Liam Brierley, Gregory F. Albery, et al. 2023. "Network Embedding Unveils the Hidden

Interactions in the Mammalian Virome." *Patterns* 4 (6): 100738. https://doi.org/10.1016/j
.patter.2023.100738.

PREDICT Consortium. 2020. *Advancing Global Health Security at the Frontiers of Disease
Emergence*. One Health Institute, University of California, Davis.

Reo, Nicholas J., and Kyle Powys Whyte. 2011. "Hunting and Morality as Elements of
Traditional Ecological Knowledge." *Human Ecology* 40 (1): 15–27. https://doi.org/10.1007
/s10745-011-9448-1.

Riley, Tamara, Neil Anderson, Raymond Lovett, Anna Meredith, Bonny Cumming, and
Joanne Thandrayen. 2021. "One Health in Indigenous Communities: A Critical Review of
the Evidence." *International Journal of Environmental Research and Public Health* 18 (21):
11303. https://doi.org/10.3390/ijerph182111303.

Rizzo, David M., Maureen Y. Lichtveld, Jonna A. K. Mazet, Eri Togami, and Sally A.
Miller. 2021. "Plant Health and Its Effects on Food Safety and Security in a One Health
Framework: Four Case Studies." *One Health Outlook* 3 (1). https://doi.org/10.1186/s42522
-021-00038-7.

Rockström, Johan, Will Steffen, Kevin J. Noone, Åsa Persson, F. Stuart Chapin, Eric F.
Lambin, Timothy M. Lenton, et al. 2009. "A Safe Operating Space for Humanity." *Nature*
461 (7263): 472–75. https://doi.org/10.1038/461472a.

Ross-Hellauer, Tony. 2022. "Open Science, Done Wrong, Will Compound Inequities." *Nature*
603 (7901): 363. https://doi.org/10.1038/d41586-022-00724-0.

Roth, Felix, Jakob Zinsstag, Dontor Orkhon, G. Chimed-Ochir, Guy Hutton, Ottorino Cosivo,
Guy Carrin, and Joachim Otte. 2003. "Human Health Benefits from Livestock Vaccination
for Brucellosis: Case Study." *Bulletin of the World Health Organization*. 81 (12): 867–76.

Rushton, Jonathan, Barbara Häsler, Nicoline De Haan, and Ruth Rushton. 2012. "Economic
Benefits or Drivers of a "One Health" Approach: Why Should Anyone Invest?"
*Onderstepoort Journal of Veterinary Research* 79 (2): a461. https://doi.org/10.4102/ojvr
.v79i2.461.

Rushton, Jonathan, Barry J. McMahon, Mary E. Wilson, Jonna A. K. Mazet, and Bhavani
Shankar. 2021. "A Food System Paradigm Shift: From Cheap Food at Any Cost to
Food within a One Health Framework." *NAM Perspectives* 11 (November). https://doi
.org/10.31478/202111b.

Salzburg Global Seminar. 2020. "New Timeliness Metrics Seek to Improve Pandemic
Preparedness." Salzburg Global Seminar, May 04, 2020. https://www.salzburgglobal
.org/news/latest-news/article/new-timeliness-metrics-seek-to-improve-pandemic
-preparedness.

Scavuzzo, Juan M., Francisco Trucco, Manuel Espinosa, Carolina B. Tauro, Marcelo Abril,
Carlos M. Scavuzzo, and Alejandro C. Frery. 2018. "Modeling Dengue Vector Population
Using Remotely Sensed Data and Machine Learning." *Acta Tropica* 185 (September):
167–75. https://doi.org/10.1016/j.actatropica.2018.05.003.

Schelling, Esther, Kaspar Wyss, Mahamat Bechir, Doumagoum Moto Daugla., and Jakob
Zinsstag. 2005. "Synergy between Public Health and Veterinary Services to Deliver
Human and Animal Health Interventions in Rural Low Income Settings." *BMJ* 331 (7527):
1264–67. https://doi.org/10.1136/bmj.331.7527.1264.

Schelling, Esther, Kaspar Wyss, Colette Diguimbaye, Mahamat Bechir, Moustapha Ould
Taleb, Bassirou Bonfoh, Marcel Tanner, and Jakob Zinnstag. 2008. "Towards Integrated
and Adapted Health Services for Nomadic Pastoralists." In *Handbook of Transdisciplinary
Research*, edited by G. Hirsch Hadorn, H. Hoffmann-Reim, S. Biber-Klemm,
W. Grossenbacher, D. Joye, C. Pohl, U. Wiesmann, and E. Zemp, 277–91. Springer.

Smith, Kristine, Catherine C. Machalaba, Richard Seifman, Yasha Feferholtz, William B.
Karesh. 2019. "Infectious Disease and Economics: The Case for Considering Multi-sectoral
Impacts." *One Health* 7 (June): 100080. https://doi.org/10.1016/j.onehlt.2018.100080.

Togami, Eri, Casey Barton Behravesh, Tracey Dutcher, Gail R. Hansen, Lonnie King, Katharine
M. Pelican, and Jonna A. K. Mazet. 2023. "Characterizing the One Health Workforce to

Promote Interdisciplinary, Multisectoral Approaches in Global Health Problem-Solving." *PLOS One* 18 (5): e0285705. https://doi.org/10.1371/journal.pone.0285705.

Togami, Eri, Jennifer L. Gardy, Gail R. Hansen, George Poste, David M. Rizzo, Mary E. Wilson, and Jonna A. K. Mazet. 2018. "Core Competencies in One Health Education: What Are We Missing?" *NAM Perspectives* 8 (6). https://doi.org/10.31478/201806a.

United Nations. 2007. "Resolution Adopted by the General Assembly, 13 September 2007: United Nations Declaration on the Rights of Indigenous Peoples." A/RES/61/295, United Nations, New York. https://social.desa.un.org/sites/default/files/migrated/19/2018/11/UNDRIP_E_web.pdf.

UNSIC (United Nations System Influenza Coordination) and World Bank. 2010. "Animal and Pandemic Influenza: A Framework for Sustaining Momentum. Fifth Global Progress Report." United Nations and World Bank. https://openknowledge.worldbank.org/handle/10986/18202.

Ward, Thomas, Alexander Johnsen, Stanley Ng, and François Chollet. 2022. "Forecasting SARS-CoV-2 Transmission and Clinical Risk at Small Spatial Scales by the Application of Machine Learning Architectures to Syndromic Surveillance Data." *Nature Machine Intelligence* 4 (10): 814–27. https://doi.org/10.1038/s42256-022-00538-9.

Watkins, David A., Rachel Nugent, Helen Saxenian, Gavin Yamey, Kristen Danforth, Eduardo González-Pier, Charles N. Mock, et. al. 2017. "Intersectoral Policy Priorities for Health." Chapter 2 in *Disease Control Priorities* (third edition), Volume 9, edited by D. T. Jamison, H. Gelband, S. Horton, P. Jha, R. Laxminarayan, C. N. Mock, and R. Nugent. Washington, DC: World Bank.

WHO (World Health Organization). 2019. "Antimicrobial Stewardship Programmes in Health-Care Facilities in Low- and Middle-Income Countries: A WHO Practical Toolkit." World Health Organization, Geneva. https://apps.who.int/iris/handle/10665/329404.

WHO (World Health Organization). 2016. "International Health Regulations (2005), 3rd ed." World Health Organization, Geneva. https://apps.who.int/iris/handle/10665/246107.

WHO (World Health Organization). 2021. *Ethics and Governance of Artificial Intelligence for Health: WHO Guidance.* Geneva: World Health Organization. https://www.who.int/publications-detail-redirect/9789240029200.

WHO (World Health Organization). 2022. "Mpox (Monkeypox) Outbreak 2022." World Health Organization, Geneva. https://www.who.int/emergencies/situations/monkeypox-oubreak-2022.

WHO (World Health Organization). 2023. "Global Research Agenda for Antimicrobial Resistance in Human Health." World Health Organization, Geneva. https://www.who.int/publications/m/item/global-research-agenda-for-antimicrobial-resistance-in-human-health.

WHO (World Health Organization), FAO (Food and Agriculture Organization of the United Nations), and OIE (World Organisation for Animal Health). 2019. *Taking a Multisectoral, One Health Approach: A Tripartite Guide to Addressing Zoonotic Diseases in Countries.* Geneva: WHO. https://apps.who.int/iris/handle/10665/325620.

WHO (World Health Organization) Regional Committee for Africa, 72. 2022. "Regional Strategy for Health Security and Emergencies 2022-2030: Report of the Secretariat." WHO, Lomé, Republic of Togo. https://apps.who.int/iris/handle/10665/361858.

Woods, A., M. Bresalier, A. Cassidy, and R. Mason Dentinger. 2017. *Animals and the Shaping of Modern Medicine: One Health and Its Histories.* Springer.

World Bank. 2012. "People, Pathogens and Our Planet: The Economics of One Health." World Bank, Washington, DC. http://documents.worldbank.org/curated/en/612341468147856529/People-pathogens-and-our-planet-the-economics-of-one-health.

World Bank. 2022. "Putting Pandemics behind Us: Investing in One Health to Reduce Risks of Emerging Infectious Diseases." World Bank, Washington, DC.

World Bank, World Health Organization, Food and Agriculture Organization of the United Nations, United Nations Children's Fund, United Nations System Influenza Coordination, and World Organisation for Animal Health. 2008. "Contributing to One World, One Health: A Strategic Framework for Reducing Risks of Infectious Diseases at the Animal–Human–Ecosystems Interface." Consultation Document. https://www.preventionweb .net/publication/contributing-one-world-one-health-strategic-framework-reducing-risks -infectious.

Zinsstag, Jakob, Andrea Kaiser-Grolimund, Kathrin Heitz-Tokpa, Rajesh Sreedharan, Juan Lubroth, Francois Caya, Matthew Stone, et al. 2023. "Advancing One Human-Environmental-Animal Health for Global Health Security: What Does the Evidence Say?" *The Lancet*. https://doi.org/10.1016/S0140-6736(22)01595-1.

Zinsstag, Jakob, Esther Schelling, Lisa Crump, Maxine Whittaker, Marcel Tanner, and Craig Stephen, eds. 2020. *One Health: The Theory and Practice of Integrated Health Approaches* (second edition). CAB International.

Zinsstag, Jakob, Esther Schelling, David Waltner-Toews, Maxine Whittaker, and Marcel Tanner, eds. 2015. *One Health: The Theory and Practice of Integrated Health Approaches*. CAB International.

Zinsstag, Jakob, Esther Schelling, Kaspar Wyss, and Mahamat Béchir Mahamat. 2005. "Potential of Cooperation between Human and Animal Health to Strengthen Health Systems." *The Lancet* 366 (9503): 2142–45. https://doi.org/10.1016/s0140-6736(05)67731-8.

Zinsstag, Jakob, Jurg Utzinger, Nicole Probst-Hensch, L. V. Shan, and Xiao-Nong Zhou. 2020. "Towards Integrated Surveillance-Response Systems for the Prevention of Future Pandemics." *Infectious Diseases of Poverty* 9 (1): 140. https://doi.org/10.1186/s40249-020 -00757-5.

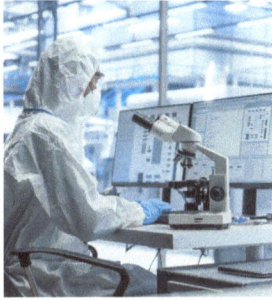

# 4

# Biosafety and Biosecurity

Bridget Williams, Gregory Lewis, Sophie Rose, Rassin Lababidi, and Geoffrey Otim

## ABSTRACT

The amount and scope of biological research being conducted are increasing.
These increases, and the greater diversity in who is conducting research, bring many
opportunities to improve health. Research carries risks, however, making it vital
to establish measures to mitigate those risks. Laboratory accidents and intentional
misuse of research have occurred in the past, but few data exist to quantify the
frequency and impact of such events. Improving monitoring and expanding the
evidence base are key priorities for addressing biosafety and biosecurity risks.
Current expert opinion suggests the importance of implementing laboratory
standards and investing in workforce development and research governance.

## INTRODUCTION

With increasing research funding, laboratory space, research institutions, and higher
education access, biosciences research is being conducted at an unprecedented scale,
leading to great advances in fields such as medicine, agriculture, and veterinary
sciences. The increasing volume of biomedical research, and greater diversity in who
is conducting it, will likely create many opportunities to improve health. Research
also carries risks, particularly of sparking outbreaks of disease, including of diseases
with pandemic potential, which makes it vital to establish measures to mitigate those
risks. Because the risks are not limited to the biomedical laboratory setting, biosafety
and biosecurity measures must also encompass life sciences research conducted in
the field, and in agricultural or animal health laboratories.

This chapter examines the role of biosafety and biosecurity in pandemic prevention, preparedness, and response. It uses the term "biosafety" to refer to efforts to reduce the risk of accidental exposure to biological organisms and "biosecurity" to refer to efforts to reduce the misuse of biological organisms. The chapter reviews the risks from inadequate biosafety and biosecurity measures, relevant global and regional governance initiatives, and options for improving biosafety and biosecurity.

## HEALTH RISKS FROM INADEQUATE BIOSAFETY AND BIOSECURITY

Quantifying the risk of biosafety and biosecurity failures is difficult, partly because the true historical rate of relevant incidents is unknown and partly because it is unclear how the rate and type of incidents may change in the future. The historical record suggests that these risks were relatively minor compared to other threats to health security during the twentieth century, but advancing technology could make them major ones in the twenty-first century.

### History of Biosafety and Biosecurity Incidents

The global incidence of biosafety and biosecurity failures remains opaque, with the evidence base amounting to an incomplete and sometimes disputed case series. The outcomes of a failure of laboratory containment can range from zero (or subclinical) infections to a major outbreak. The former may go unnoticed, but attributing the latter is difficult: it is easy to make false accusations, and responsible parties have strong incentives to conceal their involvement. Surviving evidence is therefore biased to cases of intermediate severity, to countries with relatively stronger norms of openness and transparency, and to pathogens for which there would not be a credible competing hypothesis of natural infection.

Laboratory-acquired infections (LAIs) are sporadically reported in academic and gray literature as well as the media. Few attempts have been made to compile these events, and those attempts have had varying inclusion criteria (Manheim and Lewis 2022; Wurtz et al. 2016). Certainly, the observed record dramatically undercounts the true event rate.

The greatest public health threat arises from the potential for LAIs to seed an outbreak. That danger increases with the location of most high-containment laboratories in major cities with airports, the use of pathogens to which the local population is immunologically naive, and some research aiming to modify "wild-type" behavior. Despite some clearly established cases of lab origin outbreaks, in other cases origins are fiercely contested. The most prominent and controversial outbreak with contested origins, the COVID-19 (coronavirus) pandemic, highlights the importance of timely and unimpeded investigation to determine an outbreak's source (Gostin and Gronvall 2023). A 2024 study found that most experts believe that COVID-19 likely had a natural zoonotic origin, but roughly 20 percent put a greater than 50 percent probability on some other origin (Ackerman et al. 2024). Another outbreak with

**Table 4.1** Examples of Biosafety Events

| Year | Event | Description |
|---|---|---|
| 1967 | Marburg virus outbreak | Marburg virus was discovered after synchronous outbreaks in Freiberg and Marburg, Germany, and Belgrade, Serbia, with 32 confirmed cases and 7 deaths. The outbreaks arose from a contaminated monkey shipment that resulted in the infection of laboratory workers (Brauburger et al. 2012). |
| 1978 | UK smallpox outbreak | Janet Parker, the last recorded smallpox death, was infected by smallpox virus at Birmingham Medical School, where she worked. How she became infected is uncertain (Shooter et al. 1980). |
| 1979 | Sverdlovsk anthrax leak | At least 68 deaths resulted from anthrax released from a Soviet military research facility. The cause of the accident was a fault in air handling of a spray-dryer exhaust (Meselson et al. 1994). |
| 2004 | SARS outbreak | The last 9 cases of SARS occurred because of an outbreak originating from research on the virus conducted by a researcher and postgraduate student (Walgate 2004). |
| 2007 | UK foot and mouth outbreak | A faulty effluent pipe at a BSL4 facility led to environmental contamination and a subsequent epidemic of foot and mouth virus. The economic cost of the outbreak was estimated at £47 million (HSE, n.d.). |
| 2022 | Netherlands poliovirus outbreak | Wastewater surveillance detected shedding of WPV3. The source was later found to be an asymptomatic laboratory worker (Duizer et al. 2023). |

*Source:* Original table based on the sources cited.

*Note:* BSL4 = biosafety level 4; SARS = severe acute respiratory syndrome; WPV3 = wild poliovirus type 3.

contested origins, the 1977 influenza pandemic, involved a strain that circulated in the 1950s. Leading hypotheses are that the outbreak resulted from a laboratory accident or a vaccine trial escape (Rozo and Gronvall, 2015). Table 4.1 presents some events that are generally agreed to have been caused by biosafety breaches.

In terms of biological attacks rather than accidents, the data are scarcer still. Although many states pursued biological weapons over the twentieth century, they seldom used those weapons in conflict. The most notorious case was Japanese biological weapon attacks in China during World War II, which killed (at least) tens of thousands (Frischknecht 2003). The other cases involved small-scale use—often with limited effect—predominantly in the context of irregular warfare (Carus 2017).

Pursuit of biological weapons by nonstate actors is rare, and attacks still rarer. Aum Shinrikyo attempted biological attacks with anthrax and botulinum toxin, but the attacks were ineffective (Monterey Institute of International Studies 2001). The 2001 US anthrax attacks, which killed five, were likely caused by an individual employed at a biodefense laboratory misappropriating anthrax samples from it (US Department of Justice 2010). The Rajneeshee cult caused 751 cases of salmonellosis in an attempt to sway a local election (Török et al. 1997). Outside of those events, biological weapon activity by nonstate actors primarily comprises abortive attempts at development—most notably by Al Qaeda before the invasion of Afghanistan (Salama and Hansell 2005)—and smaller-scale attempts to use biological toxins (Carus 2001). Table 4A.1 in the annex provides more detail on biowarfare and bioterrorism incidents.

### Evolving Biosafety and Biosecurity Risks

Advances in science and biotechnology, a potential lack of adequate biosafety, and the growing number of labs handling dangerous pathogens all contribute to increased frequencies of high-risk events.

#### *Increasing Prevalence of Biomedical Research*

As of 2022, the world has about 69 maximum-containment laboratories (also referred to as biosafety level 4, or BSL4, labs) either in operation or under construction (King's College London and Schar School of Policy and Government 2023)—refer to map 4.1. This number reflects an increase from only a few known maximum-containment labs in the 1980s. BSL4 labs are designed to house work with pathogens that cause life-threatening disease and for which limited or no treatment or vaccines exist.

The number of these high-containment laboratories designed for lower-risk work (such as BSL3 and BSL3+ labs) has also increased in recent years, with at least 460 current laboratories (Schuerger, Abdulla, and Puglisi 2022). Some of this growth has occurred in low- and middle-income countries, which housed 12 maximum-biocontainment laboratories as of 2022. Most biomedical research labs, however, are either BSL1 or BSL2 labs that may conduct research on pathogens deemed low-risk, such as E. coli bacteria. Those labs have lower biosafety standards and relatively high accessibility, which may also give nefarious actors greater access to dangerous or modified pathogens.

**Map 4.1** Countries with BSL4 Laboratories

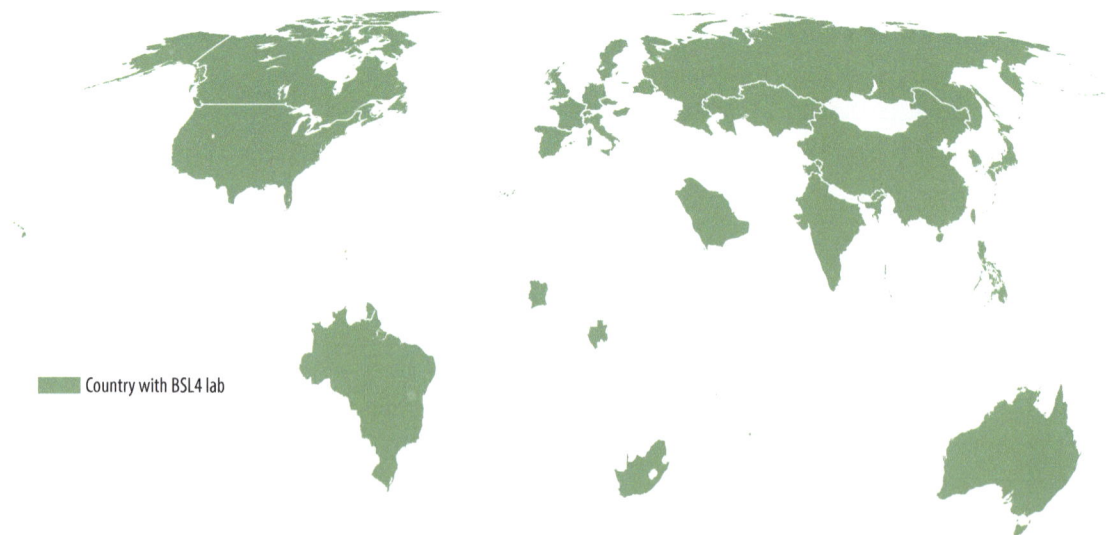

Country with BSL4 lab

IBRD 48896 | MAY 2025

*Source:* King's College London and Schar School of Policy and Government 2023.
*Note:* BSL4 = biosafety level 4.

## Increasing Capabilities in Biological Research

Biotechnologies such as the use of CRISPR-Cas9 for genetic modification and de novo DNA synthesis have already brought health benefits. They have contributed to the development of novel diagnostics and treatments (Frangoul et al. 2021; Myhrvold et al. 2018), and greatly sped up vaccine research, contributing to the relatively rapid development of the COVID-19 vaccine (Dolgin 2020). They can also, however, be used to synthesize dangerous pathogens (Cello, Paul, and Wimmer 2002; Noyce, Lederman, and Evans 2018; Tumpey et al. 2005), make pathogens more deadly or transmissible, and synthesize modified pathogens from nucleotide building blocks (Xie et al. 2021).

Increasing capabilities in artificial intelligence in the biosciences may also present risks to biosecurity (Sandbrink 2023). The ability to predict the folding of different proteins, for example, may enable novel drug discovery but can also facilitate the design of modified biological agents that can avoid detection and be more toxic or virulent (Boiko, MacKnight, and Gomes 2023; Ekins et al. 2023; Urbina et al. 2022). The makers of large language models such as ChatGPT have also voiced concern that more powerful language models could provide dangerous help to those wishing to use biology research techniques to cause harm (Amodei 2023; OpenAI 2023).

As synthetic biology continues to evolve, it is also becoming significantly cheaper and more accessible, allowing countries with lower research and development funding to elevate their capabilities for positive gains in research and development. De novo DNA synthesis, for example, can now potentially cost less than US$100 for the synthesis of most RNA viral genomes or fragments, and costs will probably continue to decline (Kosuri and Church 2014; Song et al. 2021). In addition, standardized protocols or methods to use technologies for pathogen assembly are increasingly accessible to technically proficient actors (Lee 2014; Maroun et al. 2017; Thi Nhu Thao et al. 2020). Although the need for fundamental tacit knowledge from performing biological research may still represent an important barrier to such experimentation (Ben Ouagrham-Gormley 2014), increasing capabilities and access have made deliberate or accidental misuse of these technologies likelier.

## Attempts at Risk Assessment

Assessing the likelihood and impact of future breaches of biosafety or biosecurity is difficult. The available evidence is typically uncertain, data are almost surely missing, and it is unclear how future developments will influence risk. The assessments surveyed in this section vary markedly. All should be considered extremely tentative.

One approach to quantifying risk is developing a crude event rate by tracking known events over a given time interval. Different researchers using this approach have suggested a historical rate of 0.68, or one bioterrorist event per year, 0.21 event of state biowarfare use, and 1.73 events of accidental or deliberate exposure to a pathogenic agent (Gryphon Scientific 2015; Manheim and Lewis 2022; Millet and

Snyder-Beattie 2017).[1] Challenges to that approach range from underreporting to difficulties defining ambiguous events as cases of misuse: Should a letter containing razor blades contaminated with (supposedly) infected blood be considered an attack or a threat? Results also depend on how events are individuated—for example, whether a single source's multiple releases on the same day counts as one event or many. Finally, the typical LAI does not result in a large epidemic, and the typical bioterrorist attack kills no one. The overwhelming public health concern attaches to atypical events that threaten mass casualties, making assessment sensitive to the hard-to-determine question of how atypical such events are.

An alternative approach is judgmental forecasting—that is, asking people to provide their best guess, all things considered, of the likelihood of events of a given magnitude. This approach substitutes concerns about the interpretation of scarce data with concerns about the reliability and representativeness of the forecasts. The accuracy of long-run forecasts of the rate of rare (or unprecedented) events is largely unproven, and forecaster selection may involve biases.

The most comprehensive effort thus far is the Existential Risk Persuasion Tournament, which elicited forecasts from domain experts for a variety of risks. The experts included both biosecurity experts and "superforecasters," individuals selected for their strong performance in making geopolitical forecasts (Karger et al. 2023). The superforecasters predicted a 1 percent chance of a catastrophe[2] due to engineered pathogens before 2100, whereas the biosecurity experts predicted a 3 percent chance (Karger et al. 2023). Forecasters primarily arrived at their estimates by identifying the rate of comparable events in the past and adjusting up or down on the basis of factors such as the representativeness and accuracy of data, and expected societal and technological changes.

## CURRENT STATE OF GLOBAL BIOSAFETY AND BIOSECURITY

In recognition of the serious threat that inadequate biosafety and biosecurity pose to countries' health, well-being, and economic stability, several global policy instruments aim to improve global capacity for strengthening biosafety and biosecurity. Notable examples include the 2005 International Health Regulations (IHR)—an international agreement administered by the World Health Organization (WHO) to monitor, report on, and respond to any events that could pose a threat to international public health (WHO 2016)—and the Biological and Toxin Weapons Convention, which prohibits the development, production, acquisition, transfer, stockpiling, and use of biological and toxin weapons.[3] In addition, various multilateral initiatives and global bodies are working to further the management of global biosafety and biosecurity risks. They include the Global Health Security Agenda, the Global Preparedness Monitoring Board, and the International Federation of Biosafety Associations, to name just a few. Refer to boxes 4A.1 and 4A.2 in the annex for more detail on these and other initiatives.

## Global Biosafety and Biosecurity Performance

The IHR require all WHO State Parties to develop core public health capacities to detect and respond to health threats. The Joint External Evaluation (JEE) tool, developed in 2016 as a mechanism for assessing the IHR capacities, has since been updated twice, most recently in 2022. A voluntary, collaborative process between countries and external experts, the JEE assesses 19 technical capacities, including biosafety and biosecurity. It uses two indicators to assess biosafety and biosecurity: (1) assessing whether the country has in place a whole-of-government[4] biosafety and biosecurity system for human, animal, and agriculture health; and (2) assessing biosafety and biosecurity training and practices.

As of August 2023, JEE reports from 108 countries were publicly available, 14 countries were listed as having completed a JEE but no data were available, and a further 8 countries were listed as having a JEE in process. The global average score for the biosafety and biosecurity capacity was 43.6 (out of 100), and the global average for each of the two indicators was 2.2 (out of 5). Table 4.2 shows scores by income group and region, and map 4.2 shows country scores.

Table 4.2 JEE Global Biosecurity and Biosafety Capacities for Countries, by Income Classification and Region, 2023

| | Capacity score (max. score = 100) | Indicator score (max. score = 5) | |
| --- | --- | --- | --- |
| | Biosafety and Biosecurity | Whole-of-government biosafety and biosecurity system | Biosafety and biosecurity training and practices |
| **Global average** | 43.6 | 2.2 | 2.2 |
| **Income group** | | | |
| Low | 31.7 | 1.6 | 1.6 |
| Lower-middle | 35.6 | 1.7 | 1.9 |
| Upper-middle | 44.5 | 2.2 | 2.2 |
| High | 70.0 | 3.5 | 3.5 |
| **Region** | | | |
| East Asia and Pacific | 58.4 | 3.0 | 2.8 |
| Europe and Central Asia | 53.7 | 2.5 | 2.8 |
| Latin America and the Caribbean | — | — | — |
| Middle East and North Africa | 50.0 | 2.4 | 2.6 |
| North America | 85.0 | 4.5 | 4.0 |
| South Asia | 33.3 | 1.7 | 1.7 |
| Sub-Saharan Africa | 31.0 | 1.6 | 1.6 |

*Source:* Based on IHR score per capacity from the World Health Organization's "Electronic IHR State Parties Self-Assessment Annual Reporting Tool" (accessed January 30, 2024), https://extranet.who.int/e-spar#capacityscore.

*Note:* IHR = International Health Regulations; JEE = Joint External Evaluation; — = not available.

**Map 4.2** JEE Biosafety and Biosecurity Capacity Score, by Country, 2023

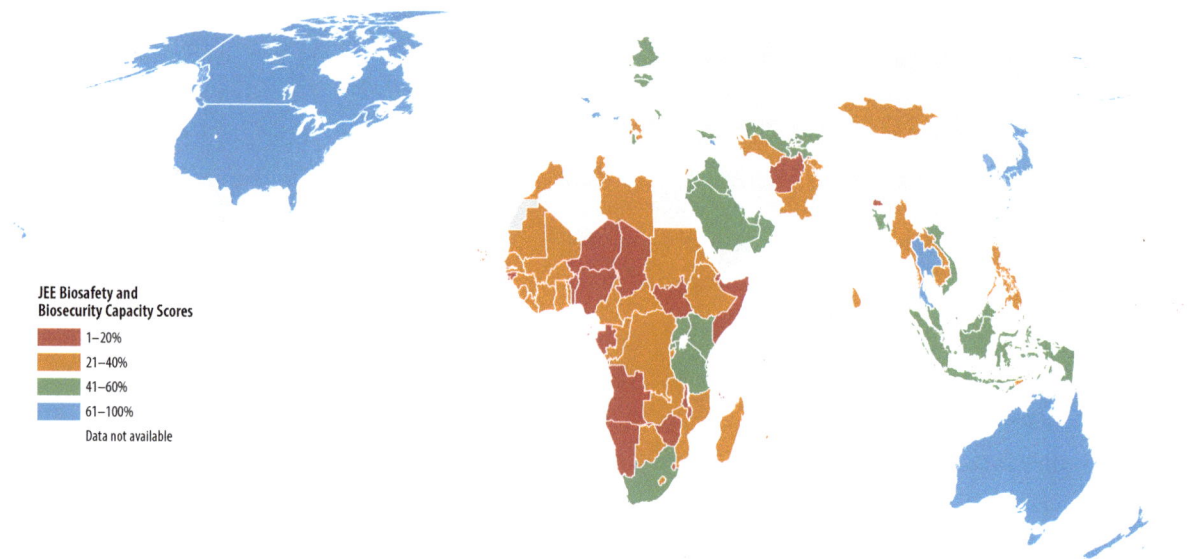

IBRD 48897 | MAY 2025

*Source:* Based on IHR score per capacity from the World Health Organization's "Electronic IHR State Parties Self-Assessment Annual Reporting Tool" (accessed January 30, 2024), https://extranet.who.int/e-spar#capacityscore.

*Note:* IHR = International Health Regulations; JEE = Joint External Evaluation.

A supplement to the JEE is the Global Health Security Index (GHSI), which also evaluates countries' capacities to prevent and respond to biological threats, but relies on publicly available data to do so. Compared to the JEE, the GHSI has scores for a greater number of countries: 195. Like the JEE, the GHSI assesses biosafety and biosecurity capacities, but it uses slightly different indicators. The GHSI also assesses a country's oversight of dual-use research. Table 4.3 shows the GHSI scores for these capacities.

These evaluations show that most countries lack at least some important biosafety and biosecurity capacities. Although lower-income countries, in particular, lack these capacities, higher-income countries do as well, especially when it comes to oversight of dual-use research. The lower scores among lower-income countries may not reflect inadequate priorities, given that relatively less research currently occurs in these settings. As the biological research base of low- and middle-income countries expands, however, improving oversight of laboratories and research will become increasingly important.

**Table 4.3** GHSI Global Biosecurity and Biosafety Capacities for Countries, by Income Classification and Region, 2021

| | Capacity score (max. score = 100) | | |
|---|---|---|---|
| | **Biosecurity capacity** | **Biosafety capacity** | **Dual-use research and culture of responsible science** |
| **Global average** | 18.7 | 20.9 | 2.6 |
| **Income classification** | | | |
| Low | 3.6 | 0 | 0 |
| Lower-middle | 8.6 | 5.6 | 0 |
| Upper-middle | 19.2 | 26.4 | 3.3 |
| High | 34.2 | 39.4 | 5.6 |
| **Region** | | | |
| East Asia and Pacific | 14.0 | 14.1 | 2.6 |
| Europe and Central Asia | 41.7 | 48.6 | 5.1 |
| Latin America and the Caribbean | 12.1 | 19.7 | 1.0 |
| Middle East and North Africa | 8.8 | 7.5 | 1.7 |
| North America | 88.0 | 100 | 50.0 |
| South Asia | 11.5 | 0 | 0 |
| Sub-Saharan Africa | 3.8 | 2.1 | 0 |

*Source:* Global Health Security Index, 2021, https://ghsindex.org/#l-section--exploreindexsect.

*Note:* GHSI = Global Health Security Index.

Over half of the 26 countries that host a BSL4 laboratory did not have JEE data publicly available from WHO. Of those for which data were available, roughly 40 percent received a score of 60 or below on the JEE assessment of biosafety and biosecurity capacities. On the GHSI, roughly half of the countries with BSL4 labs had a score below 40 for biosafety and biosecurity capacities. The GHSI assessed only 6 of the 26 countries as having regulations in place for oversight of research with especially dangerous pathogens or of other dual-use research.

## IMPROVING LABORATORY BIOSAFETY AND BIOSECURITY

Given that few events are recognized and promptly investigated, there is scant evidence to inform where existing biosafety and biosecurity practice falls short and how it could be improved. The cases that are thoroughly investigated are presumably prone to considerable selection bias, so their findings may not fully represent the true pattern of risk. Thus, guidance and recommendations tend to rely on expert opinion or analogy to other safety-critical fields, such as aviation and nuclear power (Dettmann et al. 2022; King's College London and Schar School of Policy and Government 2023; Palmer, Fukuyama, and Relman 2015).

This section discusses suggestions for ways to improve laboratory biosafety and biosecurity, acknowledging, however, the absence of data on the relative effectiveness and cost-effectiveness of these methods. Filling this evidence gap would help countries prioritize actions to reduce risk, although the details of local settings also matter to an intervention's effectiveness. Importantly, these suggestions apply to laboratories at all biosafety levels, not just BSL3 and BSL4 laboratories. They also apply to animal health and agricultural laboratories, in addition to laboratories focused on human health and basic biology research.

### Improving Monitoring and Expanding the Biorisk Management Evidence Base

The highest priority is gaining better evidence on the quantity and quality of risks, and on the effectiveness of strategies to reduce them. We currently know too little about how frequently laboratory biosafety and biosecurity breaches occur, their impacts, and contributing causal factors. Without this information, it is difficult to make recommendations for how to invest resources to reduce biosafety and biosecurity risks, and how to weigh these investments against others aiming to protect health (Dettmann et al. 2022; Health Security Threats Subcommittee on Laboratory Biosafety and Biosecurity 2022; Kimman, Smit, and Klein 2008; King's College London and Schar School of Policy and Government 2023; Palmer, Fukuyama, and Relman 2015).

The best opportunity lies in more rigorous monitoring to detect incidents and near misses, with greater transparency in reporting. Ideally, national governments would require mandatory reporting of significant biosafety and biosecurity breaches, and investigate to identify causal factors in the incident. Data on incidents and near misses, and the results of any investigations, would ideally be made publicly available to improve public trust and facilitate research. Public availability of this information may also help the spread of good practice between labs, and a richer data set may reveal rarer faults or milder shortcomings that an individual lab could not detect alone. In the absence of national systems for reporting, high-containment laboratories should provide public records of all incidents experienced, but currently only some do (Manheim 2021). Standardized reporting would allow comparison and would facilitate research. Potential disincentives to reporting should be addressed (Manheim 2021). In particular, it is important to ensure that concern about losing employment or funding doesn't prevent incident reporting, and that reporting systems are simple and easy to use.

Emerging technologies could aid laboratory biosafety and biosecurity, and pioneering them in this context may aid their development for other public health applications. The wild poliovirus type 3 case in the Netherlands offers a success story for environmental biosurveillance focused on laboratory facilities: wastewater detection discovered an asymptomatic member of staff shedding infectious poliovirus (Duizer et al. 2023). Other opportunities on this frontier include staff serosurveillance, metagenomic environmental biodetection, and telemetry. Besides their potential in detecting breaches that could otherwise go unnoticed, such approaches can shape incentives to encourage individuals or labs to promptly report accidents they are aware of, because the accident will likely be detected regardless.

### Developing and Implementing Standards and Building Laboratory Oversight

A key intervention for improving biosafety and biosecurity is to ensure that laboratories handling harmful pathogens operate according to existing safety standards. Although no international body has standardized principles for biosafety or biosecurity, or monitors compliance with these standards, several documents offer useful guidance.

The International Organization for Standardization (ISO) has developed the ISO 35001 standard, a voluntary standard-setting biorisk management system for laboratories and other related organizations, which provides recommendations for laboratory leadership, planning, support, operation, performance evaluation, and improvement (ISO 2020).

Although they do not provide standards, WHO's *Laboratory Biosafety Manual* and *Laboratory Biosecurity Guidance* both provide broad guidance on best practices in biosafety and biosecurity for use in all settings (WHO 2020, 2024). They offer guidance for conducting biosafety and biosecurity risk assessments, and implementing core features and higher-risk measures for laboratory biosafety, biosafety program management, and laboratory biosecurity measures. WHO has also produced several subject-specific monographs that provide more detail on implementation of biosafety measures (WHO 2020). This guidance should be used to develop laboratory-specific standard operating procedures and best practices.

A national laboratory oversight system that involves registration of high-containment labs would allow for the communication and enforcement of standards, and for monitoring LAIs and other laboratory incidents. Several groups have suggested national laboratory governance measures as an important step in reducing biorisk (Dettmann et al. 2022; King's College London and Schar School of Policy and Government 2023; Palmer, Fukuyama, and Relman 2015).

### Building the Biorisk Workforce and Developing a Culture of Safety

Biosafety incident reports are consonant with the hard-won lessons in other safety-critical fields. Major incidents emerge from a chain of milder faults, which in turn arise from the erosion of good practice and the normalization of deviation from standards (Wurtz et al. 2016). This pattern suggests the likely value of ensuring that laboratory workers are adequately trained or retrained in good practice.

A 2008 study found that only 3 out of 57 universities (across 29 countries) offered a module focused specifically on biosecurity for students of life sciences (Mancini and Revill 2008). Surveys have found gaps in the knowledge of students working in laboratories (Abu-Siniyeh and Al-Shehri 2021; Liu et al. 2021). Providing biosafety and biosecurity education as part of life sciences studies would be a useful step in reducing risk. Standardized continuing professional development training can refresh knowledge and convey updated understanding of best practice (Dettmann et al. 2022). Because of the risk-management approach of many laboratory safety guidelines (including the WHO laboratory safety manual and ISO standard), biorisk management has been identified as a key training area. Training should ideally be a component of standards and accreditation processes, and should incorporate guidelines for conduct of the life sciences, including WHO's *Global Guidance Framework for Responsible Use of the Life Sciences* (WHO 2022) and the "Tianjin Biosecurity Guidelines for Codes of Conduct for Scientists" (Wang, Song, and Zhang 2021).

## IMPROVING GOVERNANCE OF RESEARCH AND TECHNOLOGY

Another important aspect of biosafety and biosecurity is the choice of what research to conduct and what technology to develop. The term "dual-use" describes research and technology that can bring benefit or cause harm. A subset of dual-use research, described as "dual-use research of concern" or DURC, poses serious risks of harm. WHO describes DURC as "research that is conducted for peaceful and beneficial purposes, but could easily be misapplied to do harm with no, or only minor, modification." (WHO 2022, p. xx).

In an example of DURC, research aimed to generate a version of the H5N1 influenza virus that would transmit between mammals (Resnik 2013). This flu virus causes severe disease with significant mortality in humans, but there has not been a known case of human-to-human transmission. The scientists conducting this work aimed to inform the development of countermeasures and public health strategies (Kawaoka 2012), but concerns arose that this research, if successful, could cause harm either through accidental or deliberate misuse (Lipsitch and Inglesby 2014).

It may not always be the case that DURC should not occur. Having a system to govern such research, however, is important. This section describes some approaches to dual-use research governance and outlines some challenges for governance of biotechnologies with dual-use potential.

### Research Governance

WHO's *Global Guidance Framework for Responsible Conduct of the Life Sciences* outlines principles for the governance of biological research (WHO 2022). It gives examples of policies and tools that different stakeholders—including national governments, scientists, research funders, and editors of scientific journals—can use. These governance measures span the life cycle of research, from idea generation to funding, conduct, and results reporting.

Although many countries have policies that influence the conduct of some dual-use research (such as export control and biosafety regulations), few countries have regulations specifically for governing DURC (Lev 2019). The United States is an exception: its May 2024 United States Government Policy for Oversight of Dual Use Research of Concern and Pathogens with Enhanced Pandemic Potential requires investigators at any federally funded institution to prepare a risk-benefit assessment and mitigation plan for (1) listed experiment types involving specified high-risk agents or (2) work reasonably anticipated to create or use a pathogen with enhanced pandemic potential (OSTP 2024). When countries are determining how to manage dual-use research, it would be important to consider all research, including agriculture and animal health research, privately funded research, and research conducted outside of the laboratory.

Training aimed at improving scientists' understanding of, and their approach to minimizing risk from, DURC has been suggested as a way to reduce research risks. Unfortunately, little evidence exists on the effectiveness of training programs to guide the choice of format. However, case studies of DURC education in several countries suggest that training should be tailored to fit local environments (Arfin Qasmi, Sarwar, and Azheruddin 2021; Minehata et al. 2013; Revill et al. 2012).

Scientific journals also have a role to play in reducing dual-use risks. Journals could require that methodology sections of published studies include details of biorisk management steps taken (Dettmann et al. 2022). Journal editors could play an important part in governing the publication of information that might pose security risks, including through choosing not to publish research that has a high risk of misuse, or publishing it only in part.

An important challenge for governance of scientific research is balancing the reduction of risks with the minimization of barriers to conducting useful scientific research (Wurtz, Grobusch, and Raoult 2014). As such, risk assessments should carefully consider benefits and risks.

## Governance of Biotechnologies

New technologies are expanding the scope of what can be done with biology, and are lowering the barriers to conducting biological research by simplifying or conducting parts of the research process. For instance, synthetic DNA can be purchased online and used to construct viruses, although doing so still requires significant technical skill (Noyce, Lederman, and Evans 2018). Automated laboratories are becoming more common and promise to automate much of the biological research process (Arnold 2022). Artificial intelligence can already assist with many parts of the research process, including the design of novel chemicals that pose safety and security risks (Boiko, MacKnight and Gomes 2023; Urbina et al. 2022). These technologies are largely developed in private industry, so they fall outside the scope of research governance, focused as it is on government-funded research.

The synthetic DNA industry has been proactive in considering the potential harms from its product. In 2009 the International Gene Synthesis Consortium was established with the goal of encouraging synthetic DNA companies to voluntarily screen the orders they receive, including screening of customer identities and the specific sequences requested.[5] Although this industry-led governance is promising, not all companies conduct screening. According to 2021 GHSI data, only two countries have regulations in place to require synthetic DNA companies to screen orders (NTI and Johns Hopkins Center for Health Security 2021). This absence of regulation may result partly from industry concern about global competitiveness but may also reflect the complexity of establishing processes to determine when screening is adequate. Similarly, there is no governance for automated laboratories and artificial intelligence with biosecurity implications. These biotechnology industries will expand in the coming years, and many countries will need to consider how to regulate them.

## BIOSAFETY AND BIOSECURITY IN PANDEMIC PLANNING

The increasing volume of biological research suggests that we should not ignore the possibility of epidemics or pandemics that result from it. The optimal response to an epidemic from a laboratory source may differ from the optimal response to a naturally emerging epidemic. Protocols and tabletop exercises designed to improve outbreak response should include pathogen escape scenarios.

### Planning for Outbreaks Due to Laboratory-Escaped Pathogens

Reporting laboratory accidents promptly will make it much more likely that a health agency can take appropriate measures to prevent an outbreak from spreading. As well as standard outbreak response plans, it would be valuable for health departments to have access to information on what pathogens are being studied in laboratories in their jurisdiction. With that information, they can be alert to the possibility of an outbreak due to a LAI that a laboratory might not have noticed or recorded.

### Planning for Outbreaks Due to Intentionally Released Pathogens

Deliberate misuse of pathogens, such as the intentional release of an engineered pathogen, could have catastrophic consequences. Several tabletop exercises simulating bioterrorist attacks have explored such scenarios (MacIntyre et al. 2019; Yassif, O'Prey, and Isaac 2021).[6] Compared to a naturally emerging pathogen, an intentionally released pathogen is more likely to be associated with multiple locations, altering the approach to controlling the outbreak.

Effective communication with security agencies is important. Researchers and laboratory staff should be trained to recognize potential security threats and report any suspicious activity to the appropriate authorities.[7] Doing so can help prevent intentional release of dangerous pathogens, as well as identify potential vulnerabilities in laboratory security protocols. In addition, security agencies can provide guidance on how to safely handle and transport dangerous pathogens.

## CONCLUSION

The risks of laboratory containment or security breaches are low and uncertain, and the risks of high-consequence breaches leading to epidemics or pandemics are still lower and more uncertain. Nevertheless, these risks are not low enough to be negligible, and the merit of research conducted in high-containment facilities, and efforts to improve biosafety and biosecurity, turn on their likelihood and severity.

A key step in improving biosafety and biosecurity would be improving the monitoring of LAIs and using the data to evaluate current approaches to biosafety and biosecurity. This monitoring would ideally form part of a comprehensive biosafety and biosecurity system that incorporates implementation of laboratory standards, biosafety and biosecurity training for laboratory staff, systems for the governance of DURC and emerging technologies, and inclusion of pathogen escape scenarios in pandemic preparedness planning. As the magnitude and scope of biological research increase, an important task for national governments and the international research community will be to gain a better understanding of the magnitude of the risk posed by inadequate biosafety and biosecurity, as well as the cost-effectiveness of alternative pathways to reducing that risk.

## ANNEX 4A. SUPPLEMENTARY MATERIALS

**Table 4A.1** Selected Biological Weapon Incidents

| Year | Event | Description |
|---|---|---|
| *State bioweapon attacks* | | |
| 1915–18 | German biological sabotage campaign | Clandestine attacks with anthrax and glanders on livestock in Argentina, Finland, France, and the United States (Wheelis 1999). |
| 1939–45 | Japanese bioweapons attacks | Attacks throughout World War II with plague, anthrax, typhoid, cholera, and others. The deadliest incidents occurred with concerted use during the Zhe-Gan campaign, killing tens of thousands (Harris 1999). |
| Approximately 1975–80 | Rhodesian bioweapons campaign | Rudimentary chemical and biological weapons campaign by Rhodesian authorities against African nationalists. Alleged use of cholera and anthrax were coincident with major outbreaks, but attribution is uncertain (Cross 2017). |
| 1981–95 | Project Coast | Clandestine chemical and biological weapon program conducted by apartheid South Africa from 1981 to 1995. Most uses were chemical agents for assassination purposes, but use of salmonella and cholera has been alleged (Gould and Folb 2002). |
| *Nonstate actor bioweapon attacks* | | |
| 1984 | Rajneeshee Salmonella attack | 751 cases of salmonellosis through restaurant salad bar contamination by members of the Rajneeshee religious community, with the goal to incapacitate them from voting in a local election (Török et al. 1997). |
| 1990–95 | Aum Shinrikyo attacks | Numerous attacks with what Aum Shinrikyo believed to be botulinum toxin and anthrax. Failure to acquire the pathogenic strains rendered these attacks ineffectual (Monterey Institute of International Studies 2001). |
| 2001 | American anthrax attacks | 5 deaths and 17 injuries due to letters contaminated with anthrax spores (US Department of Justice 2010). |

*Sources:* Original table based on the sources cited.

**Table 4A.2** Selected Biosafety and Biosecurity Risk Estimates

| Source | Estimate | Notes |
|---|---|---|
| *Crude rate calculations* | | |
| Manheim and Lewis (2022) | 1.73 events/year of accidental or purposeful exposure to a pathogenic agent | 71 events between 1975 and 2016. List developed through a search of news stories, books, gray literature, and academic journal articles. |
| Global Terrorism Database[a] | 0.68 event/year of bioterrorism | 34 events between 1970 and 2020. Notably, most of the events classed as bioterror events in this database did not result in any fatalities or injuries. |
| Gryphon Scientific (2015) | 0.96 event/year of biocrimes | 24 events between 1990 and 2015. Both this list and the list of bioterrorist events was collated from secondary sources. |
| | 1 event/year of bioterrorism | 42 events between 1972 and 2014. |
| Millet and Snyder-Beattie (2017) | 0.21 event/year of state biowarfare use | 18 events of "use or possible use" between 1915 and 2000. |
| *Judgmental forecasting* | | |
| Global Challenges Foundation (Pamlin and Armstrong 2015) | 1 in 1 million risk of existential catastrophe from synthetic biology | Literature review and workshop assessment. |
| Existential Risk Persuasion Tournament (Karger et al. 2023) | 1 percent risk of catastrophe and 1 in 10,000 risk of extinction from engineered pathogens by 2100 | Only superforecaster estimates reported.<br><br>The researchers defined a catastrophe as >10 percent of the population dying within a five-year period.<br><br>The term "expected event" is to account for uncertainty in the origin of a pathogen (for example, if a panel of experts estimated a 30 percent chance a pathogen would escape from a laboratory, it would be considered 0.3 expected event). |
| | 0.68 expected event of a laboratory escape killing more than 1,000 people by 2050 | |
| | 1 expected event of a nonstate actor killing >1,000 people, and 0.038 event of killing >100,000 by 2050 with a biological weapon | |
| | 1 expected event of a state actor killing >1,000, and 0.15 event of killing >100,000 by 2050 with a biological weapon | |

*Sources:* Original table based on the sources cited.

a. National Consortium for the Study of Terrorism and Responses to Terrorism, *Global Terrorism Database (GTD)*, University of Maryland (accessed September 1, 2023), https://www.start.umd.edu/gtd/.

**Box 4A.1**

## Examples of Global Biosecurity and Biosafety Governance Instruments

**International Health Regulations.** A 2005 international agreement overseen by the World Health Organization, which took effect in 2007, between 194 State Parties and the World Health Organization to monitor, report on, and respond to any events that could pose a threat to international public health (WHO 2016). Countries had until 2012 to fully implement the regulations, but many gaps in compliance remain as of 2022.

**Biological and Toxin Weapons Convention.** The first multilateral disarmament treaty to prohibit an entire class of weapons of mass destruction upon its signing in 1972. It prohibits the development, production, acquisition, transfer, stockpiling, and use of biological and toxin weapons. The 185 State Parties to the convention meet approximately every five years to review the treaty and attempt to strengthen its relevance and effectiveness.[a]

*box continues next page*

**Box 4A.1  Examples of Global Biosecurity and Biosafety Governance Instruments** (continued)

**Australia Group.** An informal group of countries that aim to coordinate national export control laws around chemical precursors and biological agents, in order to mitigate the risk of further chemical and biological weapons proliferation.[b]

**Cartagena Protocol on Biosafety.** A protocol adopted in 2000 with the aim of limiting the adverse effects of modified organisms on biodiversity by governing their safe handling, transport and use.[c]

a.  United Nations Office of Disarmament Affairs, "Biological Weapons," https://disarmament.unoda.org/biological-weapons/.
b.  The Australia Group, "Fighting the Spread of Chemical and Biological Weapons: Strengthening Global Security," https://www.dfat.gov.au/publications/minisite/theaustraliagroupnet/site/en/index.html.
c.  Convention on Biological Diversity, "The Cartagena Protocol on Biosafety" (accessed April 27, 2023), https://bch.cbd.int/protocol/.

**Box 4A.2**

## Multilateral Initiatives and Global Bodies Working on the Management of Biosafety and Biosecurity Risks

**Global Health Security Agenda.** A partnership of more than 70 countries that matches donors with recipients to accelerate capacity-building efforts to improve countries' resilience to emerging infectious disease threats. It has a specific focus on whole-of-government national biosafety and biosecurity capacity building.[a]

**Global Partnership Against the Spread of Weapons of Mass Destruction.** An international forum that coordinates projects to prevent chemical, biological, radiological, and nuclear terrorism and proliferation. The partnership's Biosecurity Working Group focuses on implementing projects to combat biological weapons proliferation, including the Signature Initiative to Mitigate Deliberate Biological Threats in Africa.[b]

**Global Preparedness Monitoring Board.** An independent monitoring and accountability body to ensure robust preparedness for global health crises, including emerging infectious disease threats.[c]

**International Experts Group of Biosafety and Biosecurity Regulators.** A group composed of biosafety and biosecurity regulatory authorities from 11 member countries. It provides a forum for the sharing of best practices for overseeing biosecurity issues involving human and zoonotic pathogens.[d]

**Biosafety Level 4 Zoonotic Laboratory Network.** A network of public health and animal organizations across five countries—Australia. Canada, Germany, the United Kingdom, and the United States—established to respond to emerging high-consequence biological threats and facilitate international partnerships.[e]

**ABSA International.** An association of biosecurity and biosafety professionals that runs events and credentialing courses and publishes the journal *Applied Biosafety*.[f]

**International Federation of Biosafety Associations.** A nongovernmental organization of regional and national biosafety associations that runs certification courses, a mentoring program, and a conference.[g]

a.  US Centers for Disease Control and Prevention, "What Is the Global Health Security Agenda?" https://www.cdc.gov/global-health/topics-programs/global-health-security.html.
b.  Global Partnership Against the Spread of Weapons and Materials of Mass Destruction, "About Us," https://www.gpwmd.com.
c.  Global Preparedness Monitoring Board, https://www.gpmb.org.
d.  International Experts Groups of Biosafety and Biosecurity Regulators, https://iegbbr.org/.
e.  Government of Canada, "Biosafety Level 4 Zoonotic Laboratory Network," https://inspection.canada.ca/science-and-research/science-collaborations/biosafety-level-4-zoonotic-laboratory-network/eng/1597148065020/1597148065380.
f.  ABSA International, "Who We Are," https://absa.org/about/.
g.  International Federation of Biosafety Associations, https://internationalbiosafety.org/.

## NOTES

1. Refer also to National Consortium for the Study of Terrorism and Responses to Terrorism, *Global Terrorism Database (GTD)*, University of Maryland (accessed September 1, 2023), https://www.start.umd.edu/gtd/.
2. The study defined "catastrophe" as more than 10 percent of the population dying as a result of the event.
3. United Nations Office of Disarmament Affairs, "Biological Weapons," https://disarmament.unoda.org/biological-weapons/.
4. A "whole-of-government" approach is defined as "one in which public service agencies work across portfolio boundaries, formally and informally, to achieve a shared goal and an integrated government response to particular issues" (WHO 2015).
5. International Gene Synthesis Consortium, https://genesynthesisconsortium.org/.
6. Refer also to Johns Hopkins Center for Health Security, "Our Work: Tabletop Exercises," https://centerforhealthsecurity.org/our-work/tabletop-exercises.
7. World Health Organization, Global Outbreak Alert and Response Network, https://goarn.who.int/.

## REFERENCES

Abu-Siniyeh, A., and S. S. Al-Shehri. 2021. "Safety in Medical Laboratories: Perception and Practice of University Students and Laboratory Workers." *Applied Biosafety* 26 (S1): S-34. https://doi.org/10.1089/apb.20.0050.

Ackerman, G., B. Behlendorf, S. Baum, H. Peterson, A. Wetzel, and J. Halstead. 2024. "The Origin and Implications of the COVID-19 Pandemic: An Expert Survey." Global Catastrophic Risk Institute Technical Report 24-1, Global Catastrophic Risk Institute. https://gcrinstitute.org/papers/069_covid-origin.pdf.

Amodei, D. 2023. "Written Testimony of Dario Amodei, Ph.D., Co-Founder and CEO, Anthropic, for a Hearing on 'Oversight of A.I.: Principles for Regulation.'" Before the Judiciary Committee, Subcommittee on Privacy, Technology, and the Law, United States Senate, July 25. https://www.judiciary.senate.gov/imo/media/doc/2023-07-26_-_testimony_-_amodei.pdf.

Arfin Qasmi, S., S. Sarwar, and M. Azheruddin. 2021. "Capacity Building for the Identification, Mitigation, and Communication of DURC in Pakistan: A Cross-Sectional Study." *Journal of Biosafety and Biosecurity* 3 (2): 141–46. https://doi.org/10.1016/j.jobb.2021.10.004.

Arnold, C. 2022. "Cloud Labs: Where Robots Do the Research." *Nature* 606 (7914): 612–13. https://doi.org/10.1038/d41586-022-01618-x.

Ben Ouagrham-Gormley, S. 2014. *Barriers to Bioweapons: The Challenges of Expertise and Organization for Weapons Development.* Ithaca, NY: Cornell University Press.

Boiko, D. A., R. MacKnight, and G. Gomes. 2023. "Emergent Autonomous Scientific Research Capabilities of Large Language Models." arXiv:2304.05332. https://doi.org/10.48550/arXiv.2304.05332.

Brauburger, K., A. J. Hume, E. Mühlberger, and J. Olejnik. 2012. "Forty-Five Years of Marburg Virus Research." *Viruses* 4 (10): 1878–927. https://doi.org/10.3390/v4101878.

Carus, W. S. 2017. "A Short History of Biological Warfare: From Pre-History to the 21st Century." CSWMD Occasional Paper 12, Center for the Study of Weapons of Mass Destruction, National Defense University, Washington, DC. https://ndupress.ndu.edu/Portals/68/Documents/occasional/cswmd/CSWMD_OccasionalPaper-12.pdf.

Carus, W. S. 2001. "Bioterrorism and Biocrimes: The Illicit Use of Biological Agents Since 1900." Working Paper, Center for Counterproliferation Research, National Defense University, Washington, DC. https://doi.org/10.21236/ADA402108.

Cello, J., A. V. Paul, and E. Wimmer. 2002. "Chemical Synthesis of Poliovirus cDNA: Generation of Infectious Virus in the Absence of Natural Template." *Science* 297 (5583): 1016–18. https://pubmed.ncbi.nlm.nih.gov/12114528/.

Cross, G. 2017. *Dirty War: Rhodesia and Chemical Biological Warfare 1975–1980*. West Midlands: Helion and Company.

Dettmann, R. A., R. Ritterson, E. Lauer, and R. Casagrande. 2022. "Concepts to Bolster Biorisk Management." *Health Security* 20 (5): 376–86. https://doi.org/10.1089/hs.2022.0074.

Dolgin, E. 2020. "Synthetic Biology Speeds Vaccine Development." *Nature Portfolio Milestones*, September 28, 2020. https://www.nature.com/articles/d42859-020-00025-4.

Duizer, E. W. L. M. Ruijs, A. D. P. Hintaran, M. C. Hafkamp, M. van der Veer, and M. J. M. te Wierik. 2023. "Wild Poliovirus Type 3 (WPV3)-Shedding Event Following Detection in Environmental Surveillance of Poliovirus Essential Facilities, the Netherlands, November 2022 to January 2023." *Eurosurveillance* 28 (5): 2300049. https://doi.org/10.2807/1560-7917.ES.2023.28.5.2300049.

Ekins, S., F. Lentzos, M. Brackman, and C. Invernizzi. 2023. "There's a "ChatGPT" for Biology. What Could Go Wrong?" *Bulletin of the Atomic Scientists*, March 24, 2023. https://thebulletin.org/2023/03/chat-gpt-for-biology/.

Frangoul, H., D. Altshuler, M. D. Cappellini, Y.-S. Chen, J. Domm, B. K. Eustace, J. Foell, and S. Corbacioglu. 2021. "CRISPR-Cas9 Gene Editing for Sickle Cell Disease and β-Thalassemia." *New England Journal of Medicine* 384 (3): 252–60. https://doi.org/10.1056/NEJMoa2031054.

Frischknecht F. 2003. "The History of Biological Warfare. Human Experimentation, Modern Nightmares and Lone Madmen in the Twentieth Century." *EMBO Reports* 4: S47–S52. https://doi.org/10.1038/sj.embor.embor849.

Gostin, L. O., and G. K. Gronvall. 2023. "The Origins of Covid-19—Why It Matters (and Why It Doesn't)." *New England Journal of Medicine* 388 (25): 2305–08. https://www.nejm.org/doi/full/10.1056/NEJMp2305081.

Gould, C., and P. Folb. 2002. *Project Coast: Apartheid's Chemical and Biological Warfare Programme*. Geneva: United Nations Institute for Disarmament Research; Cape Town: Centre for Conflict Resolution.

Gryphon Scientific. 2015. "Risk and Benefit Analysis of Gain of Function Research." Work conducted under NIH Contract HHSN263201500002C. http://gryphonsci.wpengine.com/wp-content/uploads/2018/12/Final-Gain-of-Function-Risk-Benefit-Analysis-Report-12.14.2015.pdf.

Harris, S. 1999. "The Japanese Biological Warfare Programme: An Overview." In *Biological and Toxin Weapons: Research, Development and Use from the Middle Ages to 1945*, edited by E. Geissler and J. E. van Courtland Moon, 127–52. Oxford: Oxford University Press.

Health Security Threats Subcommittee on Laboratory Biosafety and Biosecurity. 2022. "Evidence-Based Laboratory Biorisk Management Science & Technology Roadmap." National Science and Technology Council. https://bidenwhitehouse.archives.gov/wp-content/uploads/2022/04/04-2022-NSTC-ST-Biorisk-Research-Roadmap_FINAL.pdf.

HSE (Health and Safety Executive). No date. "Initial Report on Potential Breaches of Biosecurity at the Pirbright Site 2007." Government of United Kingdom. https://web.archive.org/web/20090211174536/http://www.hse.gov.uk/news/archive/07aug/pirbright.pdf.

ISO (International Organization for Standardization). 2020. *ISO 35001:2019: Biorisk Management for Laboratories and Other Related Organisations*. Geneva: ISO. https://www.iso.org/standard/71293.html.

Karger, E., J. Rosenberg, Z. Jacobs, M. Hickman, R. Hadshar, K. Gamin, T. Smith, et al. 2023. "Forecasting Existential Risks: Evidence from a Long-Run Forecasting Tournament." FRI Working Paper 1, Forecasting Research Institute. https://forecastingresearch.org/s/XPT.pdf.

Kawaoka Y. 2012. "H5N1: Flu Transmission Work Is Urgent." *Nature* 482 (7384): 155. https://doi.org/10.1038/nature10884.

Kimman, T. G., E. Smit, and M. R. Klein. 2008. "Evidence-Based Biosafety: A Review of the Principles and Effectiveness of Microbiological Containment Measures." *Clinical Microbiology Reviews* 21 (3): 403–25. https://doi.org/10.1128/CMR.00014-08.

King's College London and Schar School of Policy and Government, George Mason University. 2023. *Global BioLabs Report 2023*. King's College London and George Mason University. https://www.kcl.ac.uk/warstudies/assets/global-biolabs-report-2023.pdf.

Kosuri, S., and G. Church. 2014. "Large-Scale de Novo DNA Synthesis: Technologies and Applications | Nature Methods." *Nature Methods* 11: 499–507. https://www.nature.com/articles/nmeth.2918.

Lee, C.-W. 2014. "Reverse Genetics of Influenza Virus." In *Animal Influenza Virus*, edited by E. Spackman, 37–50. Methods in Molecular Biology Series. Humana. https://doi.org/10.1007/978-1-4939-0758-8_4.

Lev, O. 2019. "Regulating Dual-Use Research: Lessons from Israel and the United States." *Journal of Biosafety and Biosecurity* 1 (2): 80–85. https://doi.org/10.1016/j.jobb.2019.06.001.

Lipsitch, M., and T. V. Inglesby. 2014. "Moratorium on Research Intended to Create Novel Potential Pandemic Pathogens." *mBio* 5 (6): e02366-14. https://doi.org/10.1128/mBio.02366-14.

Liu, Y., Y. Guo, S. Li, B. Liu, J. Wen, and C. Zhao. 2021. "Investigation and Analysis of the Biosafety Awareness of Laboratory Staff Involved in the Detection of Pathogens in Seven Provincial Centers for Disease Control and Prevention in China." *Biosafety and Health* 3 (4): 224–29. https://doi.org/10.1016/j.bsheal.2021.07.001.

MacIntyre, C. R., D. J. Heslop, D. Nand, C. Schramm, M. Butel, W. Rawlinson, M. Baker, et al. 2019. "Exercise Mataika: White Paper on Response to a Smallpox Bioterrorism Release in the Pacific." *Global Biosecurity* 1 (1). https://doi.org/10.31646/gbio.10.

Mancini, G., and J. Revill. 2008. "Fostering the Biosecurity Norm: Biosecurity Education for the Next Generation of Life Scientists." Landau Network-Centro Volta. Como, Italy; Bradford Disarmament Research Centre, Department of Peace Studies, University of Bradford, UK.

Manheim, D., and G. Lewis. 2022. "High-Risk Human-Caused Pathogen Exposure Events from 1975–2016." *F1000Research* 10: 752. https://doi.org/10.12688/f1000research.55114.2.

Manheim, D. B. 2021. "Results of a 2020 Survey on Reporting Requirements and Practices for Biocontainment Laboratory Accidents." *Health Security* 19 (6): 642–51. https://doi.org/10.1089/hs.2021.0083.

Maroun, J., M. Muñoz-Alía, A. Ammayappan, A. Schulze, K.-W. Peng, and S. Russell. 2017. "Designing and Building Oncolytic Viruses." *Future Virology* 12 (4): 193–213. https://doi.org/10.2217/fvl-2016-0129.

Meselson, M., J. Guillemin, M. Hugh-Jones, A. Langmuir, I. Popova, A. Shelokov, and O. Yampolskaya. 1994. "The Sverdlovsk Anthrax Outbreak of 1979." *Science* 266 (5188): 1202–08. https://doi.org/10.1126/science.7973702.

Millett, P., and A. Snyder-Beattie. 2017. "Existential Risk and Cost-Effective Biosecurity." *Health Security* 15 (4): 373–83. https://doi.org/10.1089/hs.2017.0028.

Minehata, M., J. Sture, N. Shinomiya, and S. Whitby. 2013. "Implementing Biosecurity Education: Approaches, Resources and Programmes." *Science and Engineering Ethics* 19 (4): 1473–86. https://doi.org/10.1007/s11948-011-9321-z.

Monterey Institute of International Studies. 2001. "Chronology of Aum Shinrikyo's CBW Activities." James Martin Center for Nonproliferation Studies. https://www.nonproliferation.org/wp-content/uploads/2016/06/aum_chrn.pdf.

Myhrvold, C., C. A. Freije, J. S. Gootenberg, O. O. Abudayyeh, H. C. Metsky, A. F. Durbin, M. J. Kellner, et al. 2018. "Field-Deployable Viral Diagnostics Using CRISPR-Cas13." *Science* 360 (6387): 444–48. https://doi.org/10.1126/science.aas8836.

Noyce, R. S., S. Lederman, and D. H. Evans. 2018. "Construction of an Infectious Horsepox Virus Vaccine from Chemically Synthesized DNA Fragments." *PLOS One* 13 (1): e0188453. https://doi.org/10.1371/journal.pone.0188453.

NTI (Nuclear Threat Initiative) and Johns Hopkins Center for Health Security, Bloomberg School of Public Health. 2021. "Global Health Security Index: Advancing Collective Action and Accountability amid Crisis." NTI, Washington, DC. https://ghsindex.org/wp-content /uploads/2021/12/2021_GHSindexFullReport_Final.pdf.

OpenAI. 2023. "OpenAI's Approach to Frontier Risk: An Update for the UK AI Safety Summit." *OpenAI*, October 26, 2023. https://openai.com/global-affairs/our-approach-to -frontier-risk.

OSTP (Office of Science and Technology Policy). 2024. "United States Government Policy for Oversight of Dual Use Research of Concern and Pathogens with Enhanced Pandemic Potential." United States Government. https://aspr.hhs.gov/S3/Documents/USG-Policy-for -Oversight-of-DURC-and-PEPP-May2024-508.pdf.

Palmer, M. J., F. Fukuyama, and D. A. Relman. 2015. "A More Systematic Approach to Biological Risk." *Science* 350 (6267): 1471–73. https://doi.org/10.1126/science.aad8849.

Pamlin, D., and S. Armstrong. 2015. *Global Challenges: 12 Risks That Threaten Human Civlization—The Case for a New Risk Category.* Global Challenges Foundation. https:// static1.squarespace.com/static/59dc930532601e9d148e3c25/t/59f11eebfe54ef5bd76cb3 8d/1508974382403/12-Risks-that-threaten-human-civilisation-GCF-Oxford-2015.pdf.

Resnik, D. B. 2013. "H5N1 Avian Flu Research and the Ethics of Knowledge." *Hastings Center Report* 43 (2): 22–33. https://doi.org/10.1002/hast.143.

Revill, J., M. D. C. Carnevali, Å. Forsberg, A. Holmström, J. Rath, Z. K. Shinwari, and G. M. Mancini. 2012. "Lessons Learned from Implementing Education on Dual-Use in Austria, Italy, Pakistan and Sweden." *Medicine, Conflict, and Survival* 28 (1): 31–44. https://doi.org/10.1080/13623699.2012.658624.

Rozo, M., and G. K. Gronvall. 2015. "The Reemergent 1977 H1N1 Strain and the Gain-of-Function Debate." *mBio* 6(4): e01013-15. https://doi.org/10.1128/mBio.01013-15.

Salama, S., and L. Hansell. 2005. "Does Intent Equal Capability? Al-Qaeda and Weapons of Mass Destruction." *Nonproliferation Review* 12 (3): 615–53. https://doi .org/10.1080/10736700600601236.

Sandbrink, J. B. 2023. "Artificial Intelligence and Biological Misuse: Differentiating Risks of Language Models and Biological Design Tools." arXiv 2306.13952. https://doi .org/10.48550/arXiv.2306.13952.

Schuerger, C., S. Abdulla, and A. Puglisi. 2022. "Mapping Biosafety Level-3 Laboratories by Publications." CSET Data Brief, Center for Security and Emerging Technology, Georgetown University. https://cset.georgetown.edu/publication/mapping-biosafety-level -3-laboratories-by-publications/.

Shooter, R. A., C. C. Booth, Sir D. Evans, J. R. McDonald, A. J. Tyrrell, and Sir R. Williams. 1980. "Report of the Investigation into the Cause of the 1978 Birmingham Smallpox Occurrence." The House of Commons, Her Majesty's Stationery Office, London. https:// assets.publishing.service.gov.uk/government/uploads/system/uploads/attachment_data /file/228654/0668.pdf.pdf.

Song, L.-F., Z.-H. Deng, Z.-Y. Gong, L.-L. Li, and B.-Z. Li. 2021. "Large-Scale de Novo Oligonucleotide Synthesis for Whole-Genome Synthesis and Data Storage: Challenges and Opportunities." *Frontiers in Bioengineering and Biotechnology* 9. https://www.frontiersin .org/articles/10.3389/fbioe.2021.689797.

Thi Nhu Thao, T., F. Labroussaa, N. Ebert, P. V'kovski, H. Stalder, J. Portmann, J. Kelly, et al. 2020. "Rapid Reconstruction of SARS-CoV-2 Using a Synthetic Genomics Platform." *Nature* 582 (7813): 561–65. https://doi.org/10.1038/s41586-020-2294-9.

Török, T. J., R. V. Tauxe, R. P. Wise, J. R. Livengood, R. Sokolow, S. Mauvais, K. A. Birkness, et al. 1997. "A Large Community Outbreak of Salmonellosis Caused by Intentional Contamination of Restaurant Salad Bars." *JAMA* 278 (5): 389–95. https://doi .org/10.1001/jama.1997.03550050051033.

Tumpey, T. M., C. P. Basler, P. V. Aguilar, H. Zeng, A. Solórzano, D. E. Swayne, N. J. Cox, et al. 2005. "Characterization of the Reconstructed 1918 Spanish Influenza Pandemic Virus." *Science* 310 (5745): 77–80. https://doi.org/10.1126/science.1119392.

Urbina, F., F. Lentzos, C. Invernizzi, and S. Ekins. 2022. "Dual Use of Artificial-Intelligence-Powered Drug Discovery." *Nature Machine Intelligence* 4 (3): 189–91. https://doi.org/10.1038/s42256-022-00465-9.

US Department of Justice. 2010. *Amerithrax Investigative Summary*. US Department of Justice. https://www.justice.gov/archive/amerithrax/docs/amx-investigative-summary.pdf.

Walgate, R. 2004. "SARS Escaped Beijing Lab Twice." *Genome Biology* 4: spotlight-20040427-03. https://doi.org/10.1186/gb-spotlight-20040427-03.

Wang, L., J. Song, and W. Zhang. 2021. "Tianjin Biosecurity Guidelines for Codes of Conduct for Scientists: Promoting Responsible Sciences and Strengthening Biosecurity Governance." *Journal of Biosafety and Biosecurity* 3 (2): 82–83. https://doi.org/10.1016/j.jobb.2021.08.001.

Wheelis, M. 1999. "Biological Sabotage in World War I." *Biological and Toxin Weapons: Research, Development and Use from the Middle Ages to 1945*, edited by E. Geissler and J. E. van Courtland Moon, 5–62. SIPRI Chemical & Biological Warfare Studies 18. Oxford: Oxford University Press.

WHO (World Health Organization). 2015. "Contributing to Social and Economic Development: Sustainable Action across Sectors to Improve Health and Health Equity (Follow-Up of the 8th Global Conference on Health Promotion)." Sixty-Eighth World Health Assembly Provisional Agenda Item 14.5, WHO, Geneva. https://apps.who.int/gb/ebwha/pdf_files/WHA68/A68_17-en.pdf.

WHO (World Health Organization). 2016. *International Health Regulations (2005) Third Edition*. Geneva: WHO. https://www.who.int/publications/i/item/9789241580496.

WHO (World Health Organization). 2020. *Laboratory Biosafety Manual, Fourth Edition*. Geneva: WHO. https://www.who.int/publications-detail-redirect/9789240011311.

WHO (World Health Organization). 2022. *Global Guidance Framework for the Responsible Use of the Life Sciences: Mitigating Biorisks and Governing Dual-Use Research*. Geneva: WHO. https://www.who.int/publications/i/item/9789240056107

WHO (World Health Organization). 2024. *Laboratory Biosecurity Guidance*. Geneva: WHO. https://www.who.int/publications/i/item/9789240095113.

Wurtz, N., M. P. Grobusch, and D. Raoult. 2014. "Negative Impact of Laws Regarding Biosecurity and Bioterrorism on Real Diseases." *Clinical Microbiology and Infection* 20 (6): 507–15. https://doi.org/10.1111/1469-0691.12709.

Wurtz, N., A. Papa, M. Hukic, A. Di Caro, I. Leparc-Goffart, E. Leroy, M. P. Landini, et al. 2016. "Survey of Laboratory-Acquired Infections around the World in Biosafety Level 3 and 4 Laboratories." *European Journal of Clinical Microbiology & Infectious Diseases* 35 (8): 1247–58. https://doi.org/10.1007/s10096-016-2657-1.

Xie, X., K. G. Lukogamage, X. Zhang, M. N. Vu, A. E. Muruato, V. D. Menachery, and P.-Y. Shi. 2021. "Engineering SARS-CoV-2 Using a Reverse Genetic System." *Nature Protocols* 16 (3): 1761–84. https://doi.org/10.1038/s41596-021-00491-8.

Yassif, J., K. O'Prey, and C. R. Isaac. 2021. "Strengthening Global Systems to Prevent and Respond to High-Consequence Biological Threats: Results from the 2021 Tabletop Exercise Conducted in Partnership with the Munich Security Conference." NTI Paper, Nuclear Threat Initiative. https://www.nti.org/wp-content/uploads/2021/11/NTI_Paper_BIO-TTX_Final.pdf.

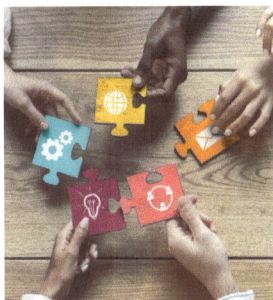

# 5

# Early Outbreak Detection and Control, and Prepandemic Preparedness

Brett N. Archer, Christopher T. Lee, Charles Whittaker, Victoria Y. Fan, Lee M. Hampton, Sabine L. Van Elsland, Olivier le Polain de Waroux, Olaolu M. Aderinola, Kathleen Warren, and Chikwe Ihekweazu

## ABSTRACT

Infectious disease epidemics, disasters, and other public health emergencies are recurring globally with increasing frequency and complexity. Known ecological and anthropogenic drivers of epidemic risks offer opportunities to better predict hot spots and cycles of pathogen (re)emergence, deploy preventive and risk mitigation measures, enhance surveillance for early warning, and target response capacities to more effectively avert and rapidly control outbreaks before they become large and disruptive. Countries must prioritize surveillance strengthening efforts using assessments of risks, capacity, and performance before and during emergencies to build their subnational and national capacities. Moreover, investments are warranted in decision-making—by systematically strengthening surveillance and collaboration among diverse stakeholders to enhance the availability of public health intelligence for action. Such investments may be aided by incentivizing and systematically conducting independent cost analyses of surveillance systems. Ensuring the communication of timely, contextualized, and interpreted data and information to decision-makers can markedly improve the effectiveness and efficiency, and mitigate the unintended negative impacts of prevention and control measures.

## INTRODUCTION

The COVID-19 (coronavirus) pandemic had a devastating impact on all societies. Analyses suggest that excess mortality ranged from two to four times reported confirmed deaths, resulting in over 28 million excess deaths during 2020–23 (Giattino et al. 2020). Estimated impacts on the global economy amount to tens of trillions of dollars (Cutler and Summers 2020; Vardavas et al. 2023;

World Bank 2022), in addition to disruptions to education and climate action as well as exacerbated levels of poverty and humanitarian needs, which disproportionately affected low- and middle-income countries (LMICs) and vulnerable communities globally.

The COVID-19 pandemic, however, also resulted in many public health successes. It galvanized global actors to develop, test, and manufacture vaccines against SARS-CoV-2 in record time, which yielded an estimated US$155 billion in cost savings through infections and deaths averted by September 2021 (Yang et al. 2023). It highlighted the opportunity to leverage ongoing global changes to combat emergencies, such as increasing digital connectivity and declining genomic sequencing costs to track the emergence of SARS-CoV-2 variants, and unprecedented global sharing of sequences and other data for public health benefit (ITU 2022).[1] Moreover, it brought about a renewed programmatic focus on strengthening global public health security to become more resilient to health emergencies (WHO 2023f).

The COVID-19 pandemic should not be viewed as an isolated event. Rather, it occurred in the context of a worrying pattern of concurrent epidemics, disasters, conflicts, resource insecurity, and other major emergencies that are occurring with increasing frequency and complexity (WHO 2023c). Trends suggest a future marked by more extensive insecurity—the number of people forced to flee their homes in 2021 was double that from a decade prior (UNHCR 2023). Recent responses to outbreaks of cholera (Charnley et al. 2022) and Ebola virus disease (Jombart et al. 2020) exemplify the role conflict and insecurity play in the frequency and prolongation of emergencies. Health impacts of climate change are surging, resulting in more frequent and severe extreme weather events, accelerated spread of infectious diseases, and other tolls devastating lives and livelihoods (Romanello et al. 2023). Moreover, emergencies occur amid an increasing burden of chronic diseases that draw upon the same limited health care and public health resources. In the absence of collective and coordinated action to address these challenges, a vicious cycle of compounding impacts of concurrent public health emergencies is likely, and the strain placed on local and global resources will progressively erode the provision of adequate measures required to respond effectively to future crises, in turn intensifying their impacts. For example, disasters due to strong storms cause displacement, resulting in outbreaks among vulnerable populations, many of whom have noncommunicable diseases, leading to worse outcomes. Preparedness must be an integrated approach to address the multipronged needs.

Rapid identification and response to emerging epidemics can potentially avert localized outbreaks or prevent them from becoming global pandemics. Averting outbreaks and pandemics, and minimizing impacts when they inevitably occur, requires establishing robust and flexible collective capacities before the onset of an event. Yet investment in prevention, preparedness, early detection, response and control, and recovery, with good public health decision-making throughout, presents a paradox. That is, when these public health objectives (further explained in figure 5.1) are successfully met, the true and perceived risks associated with the epidemic are diminished, making cost savings difficult to demonstrate. This paradox presents an ongoing challenge to economies when faced with sizable costs of health emergency preparedness and competing demands. One systematic review of studies in the last two decades found that improving health emergency preparedness alone required sustained annual investments ranging from US$1.6 billion among LMICs to US$43 billion worldwide (Clarke et al. 2022). A recent World Health Organization (WHO)–World Bank estimate found that financing effective health emergency preparedness will require approximately US$30 billion per year, with a funding gap of US$10 billion per year (WHO 2023f).

This chapter outlines key considerations for strengthening early detection, control, and preparedness for epidemics, pandemics, and other emergencies. It discusses drivers of risks that may be opportunistically leveraged to inform proactive protection measures, outlines key global frameworks guiding the public health sector, and presents a case for enhanced investment in tools for decision-making to strengthen health emergency preparedness, response, and resilience.

**Figure 5.1** Epidemic Phases and Associated Activity

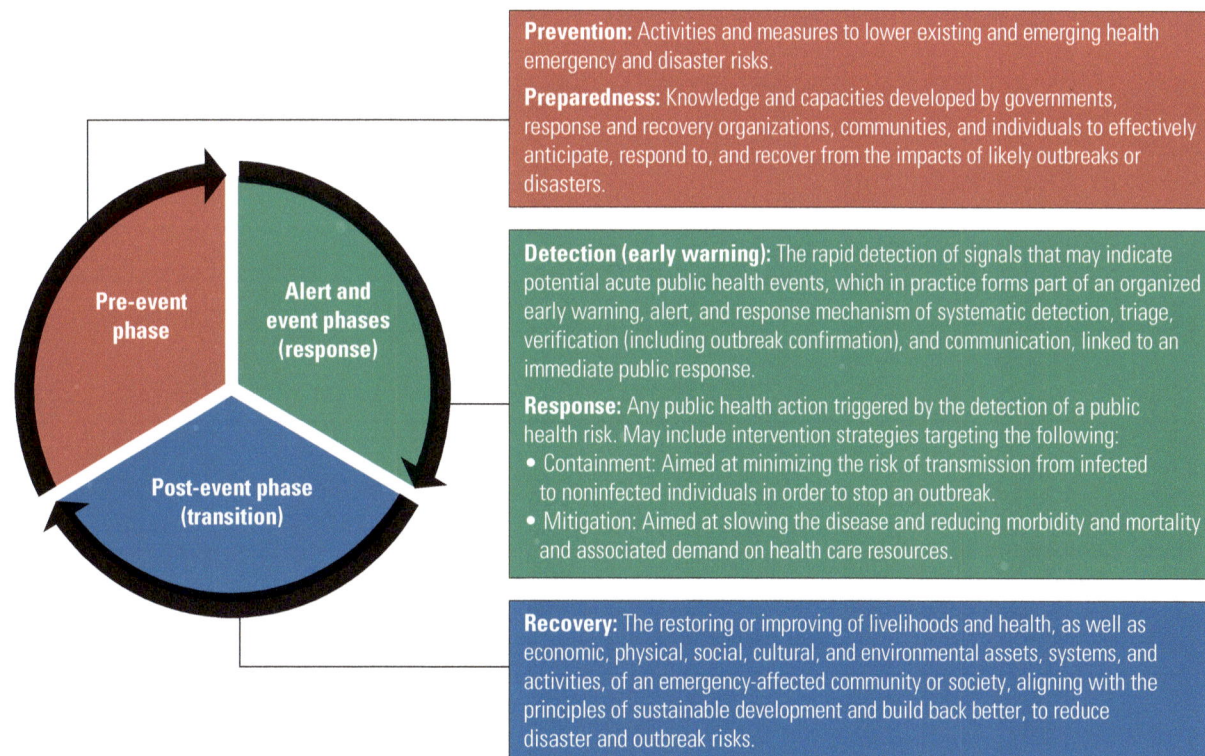

**Prevention:** Activities and measures to lower existing and emerging health emergency and disaster risks.

**Preparedness:** Knowledge and capacities developed by governments, response and recovery organizations, communities, and individuals to effectively anticipate, respond to, and recover from the impacts of likely outbreaks or disasters.

**Detection (early warning):** The rapid detection of signals that may indicate potential acute public health events, which in practice forms part of an organized early warning, alert, and response mechanism of systematic detection, triage, verification (including outbreak confirmation), and communication, linked to an immediate public response.

**Response:** Any public health action triggered by the detection of a public health risk. May include intervention strategies targeting the following:
- Containment: Aimed at minimizing the risk of transmission from infected to noninfected individuals in order to stop an outbreak.
- Mitigation: Aimed at slowing the disease and reducing morbidity and mortality and associated demand on health care resources.

**Recovery:** The restoring or improving of livelihoods and health, as well as economic, physical, social, cultural, and environmental assets, systems, and activities, of an emergency-affected community or society, aligning with the principles of sustainable development and build back better, to reduce disaster and outbreak risks.

Pre-event phase

Alert and event phases (response)

Post-event phase (transition)

*Sources:* Adapted from OECD 2020 and WHO 2020.

Early Outbreak Detection and Control, and Prepandemic Preparedness **129**

## UNDERSTANDING DRIVERS OF EPIDEMIC AND PANDEMIC RISK TO PREDICT RISK AND STRENGTHEN SURVEILLANCE

The public health risk related to infectious disease outbreaks is a function of the characteristics of the pathogen (severity and potential for spread), the probability of exposure, and the context in which they emerge—particularly the vulnerability of the population and the local public health response capacity (Poljanšek et al. 2018). The public health risk from an epidemic often increases with the presence of other hazards because of a combination of overstretched response capacities and increased population vulnerability. This section highlights an exemplary subset of ecological and anthropogenic drivers of pandemic risk, and it demonstrates how our scientific understanding of the impact of these drivers offers opportunities for improvements to public health surveillance and response.

First, among other impacts on health, global climate change intensifies zoonotic risk through changes in the ecology of animal reservoir hosts and vector populations (Thomson and Stanberry 2022), further increasing the frequency of cross-species virus transmission in a growing number of geographic regions (Carlson et al. 2022). Studies have underscored the intricate relationships between climatic dynamics— such as seasonal variations in temperature and precipitation, or larger-scale climatic phenomena like El Niño—in the emergence and spread of Lassa fever, Rift Valley fever, or cholera, for example (Jutla et al. 2013; Redding et al. 2017; Redding et al. 2021). Moreover, land use changes (for example, deforestation and urbanization) may increase the proximity between humans and potential or known environmental reservoirs of infectious diseases, and the risk of spillover (cross-species) transmission events (Gibb et al. 2020; McKee et al. 2021; Redding et al. 2019).

Understanding these risks, and how they drive epidemics, can lead to more targeted and anticipatory approaches to disease surveillance and forecasting, better define risk and potential hot spots based on proxy variables, and better target surveillance and prevention activities in the most vulnerable areas and communities. Examples include adoption of climate models to predict and enhance early warning for zoonotic and vector-borne diseases (Caldwell et al. 2021; Lotto Batista et al. 2023), as well as the use of animal populations as sentinel surveillance systems for diseases like West Nile virus (Gossner et al. 2017).

Second, the increasingly interconnected world facilitates the spread of infectious diseases (Tatem, Rogers, and Hay 2006). Urbanization and population movement amplify epidemic risk of certain pathogens and the potential for rapid global dissemination of pathogens. During the COVID-19 pandemic, population density was a significant driver of transmission intensity (Rader et al. 2020). As such, population mobility data (for example, from air traffic, cell phone usage, and traveler screening) provide opportunities for innovative, data-driven approaches to improve epidemic risk prediction, such as predicting risks posed by a local event on other geographic regions, monitoring the importation of novel SARS-CoV-2 variants, or reconstructing transmission dynamics in settings with otherwise limited surveillance (Chang et al. 2021; Kahn et al. 2019; Kucharski et al. 2023; Oliver et al. 2020; Sharma et al. 2023).

Third, the contexts created by humanitarian crises often amplify epidemic risks. Examples include factors that increase risk of pathogen emergence and transmission (for example, high population density, poor shelters and sanitation, and disruptions to routine vaccinations or vector control), and severity (for example, due to underlying malnutrition or limited access to treatment) (Jones et al. 2008). In the Republic of Yemen, for example, conflict, destruction of infrastructure (such as health, water, or sanitation), chronic malnutrition, displacement, and overcrowding, among other factors, have fueled the largest cholera outbreak in recorded history (Federspiel and Ali 2018). As such, ensuring adequate epidemic surveillance and response in humanitarian settings is paramount to reduce the risk of excess mortality and morbidity in already fragile populations, and beyond. These measures include the development of community-based early warning systems (Kongelf et al. 2016; Ratnayake et al. 2020), supported by agile digital solutions of reporting and monitoring—for instance, WHO's Early Warning Alert and Response System to establish surveillance and response activities in difficult and remote settings without reliable internet and electricity.

Fourth, immunity gaps increase the risk of vaccine-preventable disease outbreaks (Abubakar et al. 2019; Dureab et al. 2019). Monitoring of vaccination coverage and key influences on vaccine uptake (for example, sociocultural factors and a population's ability to access vaccines) is essential not only to improve routine vaccine coverage but also to understand and predict epidemic risks and mobilize strategies and resources for prevention and mitigation. Capturing data at the local level is important because, even in highly vaccinated settings, epidemics of vaccine-preventable diseases are often driven by local clusters of unvaccinated individuals (Masters et al. 2020).

These risks frequently compound. For example, humanitarian crises often exacerbate the risk of measles outbreaks and other vaccine-preventable diseases such as diphtheria by creating immunity gaps (Lam, McCarthy, and Brennan 2015). Disruptions to routine health services during conflict and displacement often result in suboptimal vaccination coverage, and conditions such as overcrowding, poor sanitation, and malnutrition enhance transmission and severity. This susceptibility is further complicated by limited health care infrastructure in crises, with limited surveillance, delayed case detection, and insufficient response capacities potentially leading to higher-than-typical morbidity and mortality (Kouadio, Kamigaki, and Oshitani 2010).

In contexts of past and ongoing outbreaks and limited historical data, serological surveillance or surveys are useful tools to better understand population immunity profiles and associated factors (such as community trust in vaccines), enhance risk prediction, and inform targeted interventions. For example, serological surveillance has been used throughout COVID-19 to predict the size of peaks driven by a novel variant (Buss et al. 2022) as well as to inform relaxation of imposed control measures (Kraay et al. 2021).

## FRAMEWORKS FOR STRENGTHENING GLOBAL HEALTH SECURITY

The International Health Regulations (IHR) have formed a normative basis for global health security implementation since their introduction in 1969. They provide a legally binding agreement among 196 countries to develop, maintain, and monitor implementation of capacities to prevent, detect, and respond to public health threats, as well as to report these events to WHO (WHO 2016). Born out of response to deadly epidemics, the IHR have undergone numerous revisions prompted by increasing risks of disease (re)emergence with international travel and trade, as well as global events such as the SARS (severe acute respiratory syndrome) epidemic in 2003 and, most recently, the COVID-19 pandemic.

The IHR further require State Parties' self-assessment annual reporting, with reports supplemented by tools including Joint External Evaluations, simulation exercises, after-action reviews, and independent measures (for example, the Global Health Security Index), all geared toward assessing country-level preparedness and informing strategies to develop capacity and improve compliance with the IHR. The COVID-19 pandemic, however, highlighted limitations of these accountability mechanisms, which primarily rely on static capacity measures rather than evaluating the functionality of systems under real-world conditions. Research investigating the correlation between preparedness measures and actual population health outcomes has yielded inconsistent results, which may partly be attributed to the sensitivities in model parameters applied and the inherent unpredictability of factors, such as sociopolitical influences, that affect the translation of preparations into a robust response during an emergency (Bollyky et al. 2022; Ledesma et al. 2023; NTI and Johns Hopkins Center for Health Security 2021; Nuzzo and Ledesma 2023). One study found that higher Joint External Evaluations scores were associated with significantly fewer overall communicable disease deaths, but not fewer COVID-19 deaths (Jain et al. 2022).

Despite their importance as a tool to help countries develop capacity-building plans, and despite their revisions during the COVID-19 pandemic, the Joint External Evaluations are not designed to predict future performance in pandemics. Such static measures of capacity provide only one dimension for informing risk assessments. As outlined in the previous section, other highly variable dynamics of risk include the hazard, probability of exposure, and, perhaps most dynamically, vulnerability of individuals, communities, systems, and assets. The triangulation of data across these dynamics provides the means for informing investments to best tackle recurring threats such as pandemics through not only boosting systems' capacities but also reducing population vulnerabilities and exposures to hazards.

Accountability challenges persist for ensuring the timeliness of detection and response. Because of the difficulty in generating counterfactual data on epidemics averted, evaluating the effectiveness of surveillance systems and investigations is challenged by a lack of clear outcome measures. In this context, there has been an increased focus on the promise of timeliness metrics, indicating rapid detection and response to emerging threats as a performance metric of public health surveillance systems, as well as a quality improvement framework (Frieden et al. 2021).

The "7-1-7" target, shown in figure 5.2 and used increasingly to assess country performance in real-world conditions, identifies bottlenecks to rapid detection, notification, and early response (Bochner et al. 2023). Using this approach, countries have begun to use systems analyses for outbreaks that were successfully contained and to identify bottlenecks for larger events to inform systems improvement. As opposed to the aforementioned regulatory performance assessments, the 7-1-7 target can be integrated into functional assessments or "early action reviews" to align stakeholders during the emergence of outbreaks, and to inform targeted measures to prevent and mitigate the impacts of new epidemics and pandemics (Mayigane, Vedrasco, and Chungong 2023). Similarly, after-action reviews have demonstrated potential to assess the what, how, and why of a response to real-world events; identify best practices and challenges encountered; and propose mid- and long-term actions for improvement.

The Independent Panel for Pandemic Preparedness and Response and the IHR Review Committees stressed the importance of new assessments and tools that assess operational capacities in real-world stress situations (IPPPR 2023).[2] Furthermore, numerous independent performance assessments emphasize the need for more predictable and sustainable financing at the international and national levels, as well as stronger frameworks to address international cooperation (WHO 2021b).[3] Notable steps made toward these goals include the launch and ongoing implementation of a framework for strengthening health emergency prevention, preparedness, response, and resilience (HEPR). The HEPR framework addresses governance, systems, and financing issues noted during the COVID-19 pandemic, and offers prioritized solutions (WHO 2023f). Although HEPR addresses all hazards, the solutions proposed are echoed in disease-specific preparedness and surveillance strategies, including current implementation plans for the Pandemic Influenza Preparedness Framework and the associated Global Influenza Surveillance and Response System (WHO 2023e).

Success of these initiatives, however, depends on overcoming numerous challenges. These challenges include delivering and sustaining increased domestic financing to achieve goals set out under national action and investment plans, ensuring stronger alignment of international financing to support national aspirations more synergistically and equitably, and addressing financing mechanisms to improve the scale and speed to access finances for the deployment of large-scale operations and medical countermeasures during emergencies (refer to the policy considerations section later in this chapter).

**Figure 5.2** The 7-1-7 Timeliness Metrics and Targets for Detection, Notification, and Response Related to Public Health Events

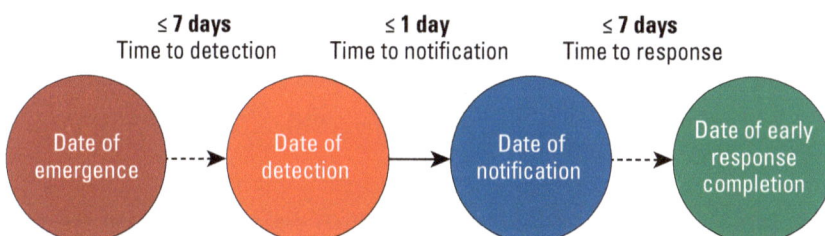

*Source:* WHO 2023d.

## INVESTMENT IN TIMELY PUBLIC HEALTH DECISION-MAKING

Substantial data show the health and economic benefits of public health interventions during emergencies (Juneau et al. 2022). The availability of data and information before and during an epidemic can markedly improve the efficiency of prevention, preparedness, and control efforts by informing the choice, timing, targeting, and impact monitoring of interventions, among other benefits. For example, many diseases can cause acute watery diarrhea clinically indistinguishable from that caused by cholera, but the appropriate application of surveillance and diagnostic tests can enable targeting of cholera-specific vaccinations, leading to sizable cost savings (Hampton, Johnson, and Berkley 2022; Lee et al. 2019; Xu et al. 2024).

It is also well established that timely detection of outbreaks can allow more effective and efficient implementation of measures to contain an outbreak compared to delayed detection and the ensuing costly response. For example, of 12 Ebola virus disease outbreaks detected during 2013–22, the 9 outbreaks confirmed within 33 days were contained to less than 150 cases each. In contrast, the 2013–16 West Africa outbreak, confirmed 110 days after its start, caused 28,610 reported cases and cost international donors alone at least US$1.8 billion. The 2018–20 outbreak predominantly in eastern provinces of the Democratic Republic of Congo was confirmed 93 days after its start, caused 3,470 reported cases, and committed funding from international donors ranging from US$730 million to US$1.18 billion (Hampton et al. 2023; Zeng et al. 2023).

A recurring example is the identification and response to novel influenza subtypes in animals, resulting in an interruption of transmission among the animal population before the first human cases have been detected (Lee et al. 2017). Moreover, outbreaks of Rift Valley fever have demonstrated the value of intersectoral information sharing and response to zooneses, with early detections in animal populations providing an opportunity for preventive interventions, enhanced clinical care, and timely response to mitigate human infections (Archer et al. 2013). Such events exemplify the critical need to apply a One Health approach in identifying and responding to disease threats in people, animals, and plants, with international calls to integrate or interconnect systems and responses, and institutionalize a collaborative effort to disease control (Hayman et al. 2023; WHO 2023b).

A key remaining challenge is the generation and provision of timely and adequate information to appropriate decision-makers to prevent infectious disease outbreaks from becoming catastrophic events (Lipsitch and Santillana 2019; Tan 2006). Adequately answering the diverse array of questions that arise—both in routine monitoring of prioritized public health hazards and risks and throughout the course of an epidemic—requires a range of data. On a routine basis, surveillance supports, for example, monitoring and assessment of endemic disease trends, health care and preventive service provision and resource use, and aberration detection for events of potential clinical or public health importance. Countries typically achieve these aims by deploying a variable array of surveillance methods designed to generate data on the occurrence of a health-related event within human and animal populations, as well as the environment around them, through established systems and chains of communication, coupled with secondary analyses of administrative and other existing data (figure 5.3).

At the onset of an epidemic, when containment is most feasible and cost-effective, the deployment of the most appropriate set of interventions depends on sufficient insights into the causative pathogen and its epidemiological characteristics; the burden and spread within the affected population, and associated health and socioeconomic impacts; an understanding of community enablers of (or barriers to) effective epidemic control; and any major uncertainties across these variables. As the epidemic progresses, there is a need to continuously monitor for major changes in these and other parameters, to assess the impacts of interventions to adjust and better target control strategies, and to continuously right-size these strategies to maximize their impact while minimizing adverse effects on individuals and societies.

**Figure 5.3** Simplified Diagram of Data and Information Flow in Public Health Surveillance Systems

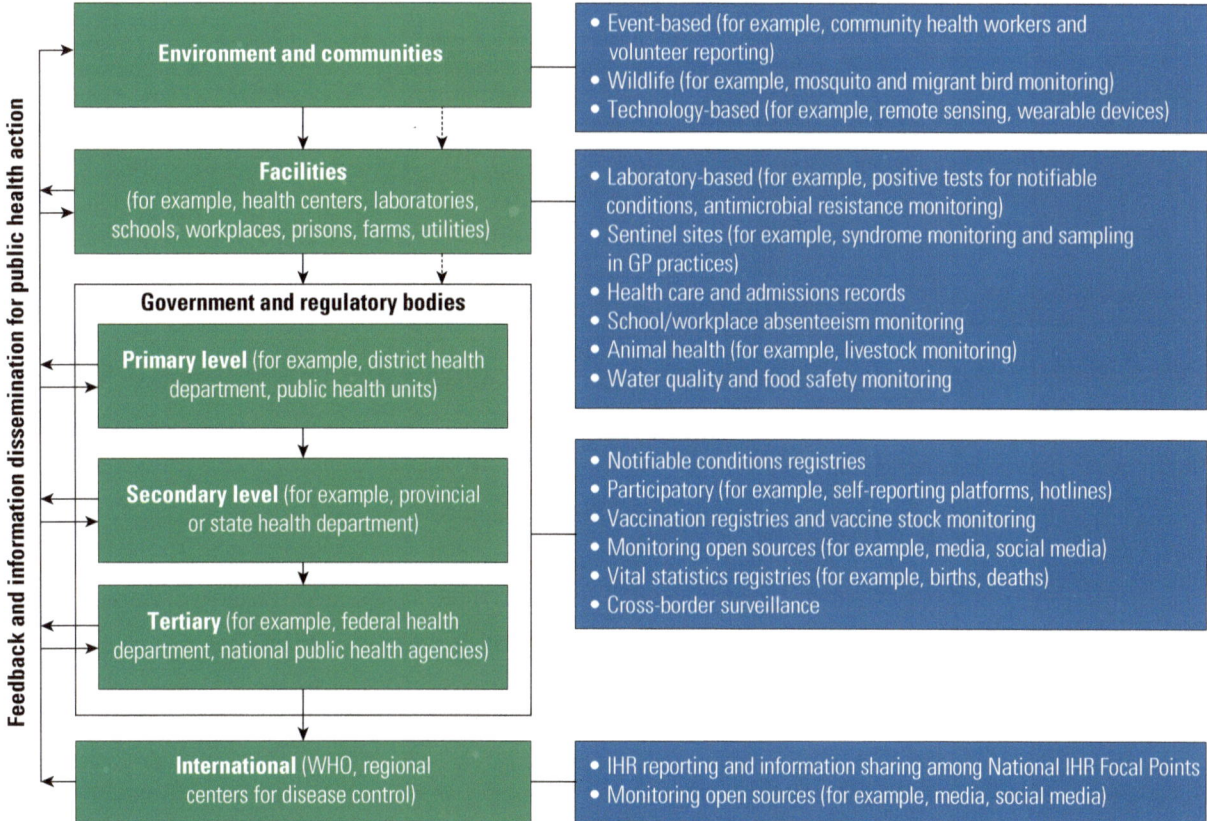

Source: Original figure for this publication.

Note: GP = general practitioner; IHR = International Health Regulations; WHO = World Health Organization.

National and subnational governments are primarily responsible for establishing and managing a suite of surveillance systems to address these diverse information needs while generating or digesting information from other sources (for example, special studies, outbreak investigations, and research) to fill information gaps. In the public health sector, this responsibility typically rests with ministries or departments of health that are variably supported by national public health agencies, other government sectors, academia, nongovernmental and civil society organizations, public and philanthropic funders, foreign governments, and regional and international organizations and agencies. These authorities and partners must collectively operate and flexibly apply a wide range of surveillance systems to address evolving information needs during and outside of public health emergencies (figure 5.4).

**Figure 5.4** Variability and Relative Importance of Different Data and Surveillance Types for Meeting Emergency Preparedness and Response Objectives over the Course of an Epidemic

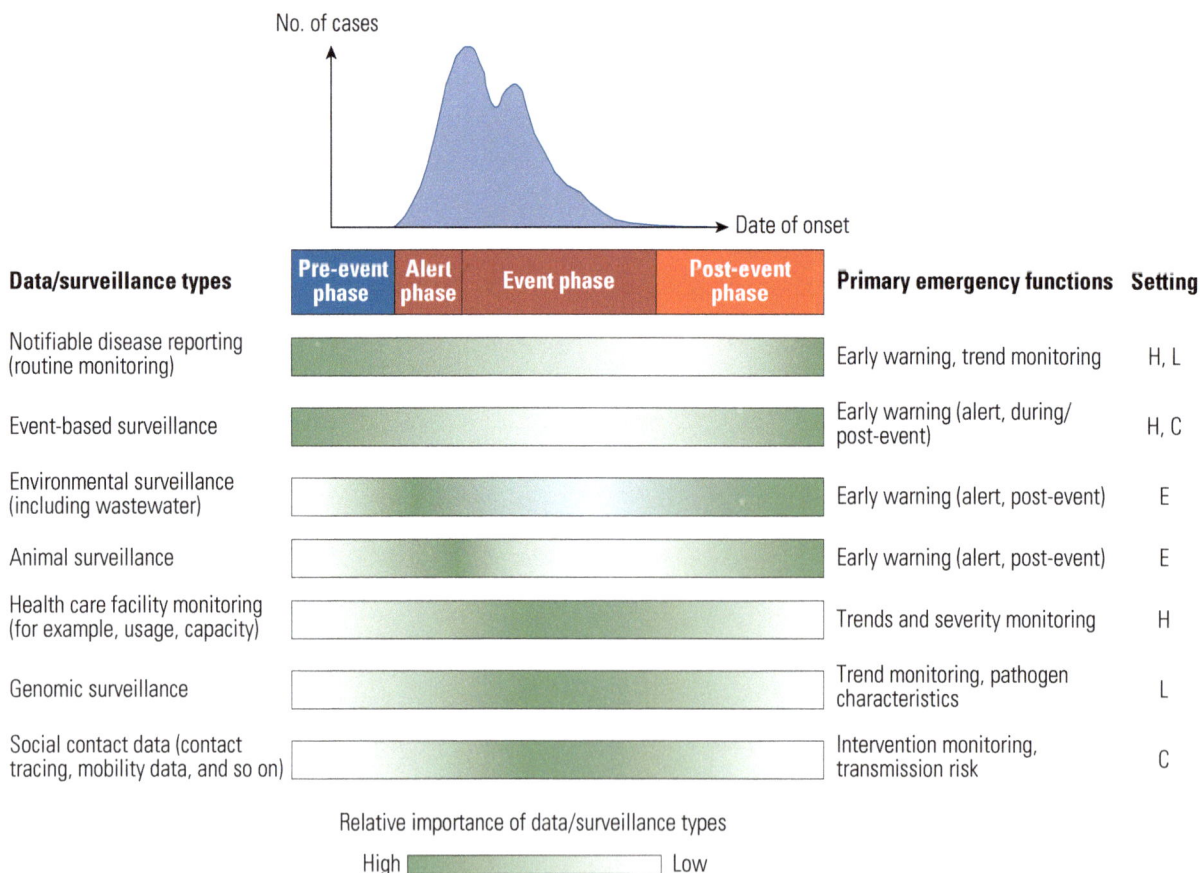

Source: Original figure created for this report.

Note: Data/surveillance types listed are illustrative and nonexhaustive; many other approaches typically exist in countries. The assigned relative importance, primary functions, and settings relate to the outputs and decision themes that each surveillance type may be best placed to inform in or around an epidemic. Surveillance serves many other primary and complementary objectives for both routine monitoring and emergency response, and their relative importance in any given phase is highly variable across different pathogens and contexts. C = community; E = environment; H = health facilities, L = laboratories.

At face value, the task of collecting, analyzing, and interpreting data from multiple sources, and communicating health intelligence, appears simple. In most countries, however, public health surveillance comprises a complex array of systems that have evolved organically over many decades. Health authorities must contend with fragmented and sometimes duplicative and inflexible systems, often characterized by independent silos of unlinked activity across administrative levels, diseases, sectors, and organizations, with most funding earmarked to deliver against a narrow set of surveillance objectives for specific diseases (Choi 2012).

Addressing systems' fragmentation is critical for improving the timeliness and robustness of information available to inform early outbreak detection and control. For over 20 years, strategies for Integrated Disease Surveillance and Response (IDSR) have been prioritized internationally and have demonstrated mixed successes in LMICs (Mremi et al. 2021). The COVID-19 pandemic brought renewed attention to the need to specifically enhance collaboration across the surveillance landscape to address diverse decision-maker needs—termed "collaborative surveillance" (WHO 2023b). The collaborative surveillance approach encompasses prioritizing One Health systems to more cohesively address drivers of disease emergence and surveillance opportunities at the human-animal-environment interface (Hayman et al. 2023). The degree of local application of these global strategies is also context-dependent, and local human, animal, and environmental health authorities must ultimately choose the suite of surveillance approaches and capacities that best address decision-making needs in their local context.

Beyond the specific technical and contextual considerations, domestic financing and international investor interests heavily shape the ultimate design of a country's surveillance systems. Moreover, a tendency exists for individual surveillance systems to overstate their utility and attract investment in limited objectives without considering opportunity costs to other systems, and risking data gaps to address this and other critical surveillance objectives. This practice can result in a lack of (or, worse, misleading) information for making decisions and taking actions at different phases of emergencies. This chapter, therefore, stresses the need for a more holistic outlook on the impacts of investments in surveillance capacities and offers several considerations for strategic improvement (box 5.1).

Surveillance is incomplete without coordinated, multisectoral public health action. Public health emergency operation centers serve as a crucial hub for information exchange and resource coordination (WHO 2015). The establishment of these centers at both national and subnational levels facilitates the timely triangulation and use of data from various sources, interconnected with response mechanisms (Balajee et al. 2017; Oyebanji et al. 2021). However, numerous countries face challenges in fully operationalizing such centers, in part because of a disproportionate focus on physical infrastructure, often at the expense of other vital investments such as the development of robust legal and governance frameworks (Elmahal et al. 2022).

## Box 5.1

### Consideration for Critical Design and Appraisal of Surveillance Investments

- **Define use cases and work backward.** Addressing this full range of informational needs requires an appropriate mosaic of surveillance approaches, with strong coordination and collaboration between systems and their curators. This desired mosaic of many data sources must, however, be balanced against the resource requirements and overheads inherent in maintaining and coordinating across multiple surveillance workflows; accordingly, it requires prioritization and organizational design of surveillance to maximize both impact potential and efficiency. Strategic investments in systems thinking approaches carry the potential to improve overall utility in informing public health decisions and action, for example, by defining data use cases (decision-making objectives) and mapping upstream data best suited to deliver against each use case.

- **Systematically evaluate decision-making and action potential of the system.** The value of public health data lies in their ability to inform impactful decisions and prompt action. The usefulness of collecting specific information depends on the costs and benefits of each option, the relevance of the data to the decision at hand, and how often that decision arises. Decision analysis, widely used to assess the cost-effectiveness in health care, can also be applied to assess surveillance systems, guide outbreak response decisions, and prioritize among different options for investing in improving information available for decision-making.

- **Assess robustness of downstream capacities to effectively use surveillance outputs.** Surveillance must be coupled with the necessary public health intelligence capacities (skilled workforce, established systems and infrastructure, standardized processes, connectivity, and so on) to collate, verify, analyze, contextualize, and interpret information triangulated from multiple health and nonhealth sources; undertake systematic assessments of evolving risks; and effectively communicate findings with relevant response authorities. Efforts to strengthen data collection and technologies for event detection, and to enhance collaboration capacity, will be in vain if not met with an adequately trained workforce and established processes to transform data into actionable intelligence.

- **Prioritize core, routine systems with the flexibility to address multiple hazards and to surge during emergencies.** Attributes inherent in any chosen surveillance approach should inform investments in core or recommended approaches. Other approaches may serve to enhance surveillance when resources allow but should be considered secondary to ensuring the optimization of core surveillance functions. These systems should have flexibility to address multiple, diverse hazards (pathogens and other threats) and surge during emergencies. Such systems and capacities require long-term investments to become a core resource at every level of public health delivery and decrease reliance on contingency surveillance tools introduced midevent.

- **Review the sufficiency of evidence on new surveillance technologies before scaling.** Although investments in emerging technologies offer attractive opportunities to augment surveillance capacities, their introduction must be carefully curated. For example, wastewater and genomic surveillance, coupled with either targeted or pathogen-agnostic laboratory investigations, have the potential for more detection of (re)emerging pathogens. Likewise, digital technologies (such as mobile applications, location tracking, and wearables) have the potential to augment traditional data collection. However, investments must be balanced against core systems while assessing how best to equitably operationalize these technologies in diverse contexts and evaluate the utility and cost-benefit of data generated relative to other approaches.

Given the importance of timely decision-making and action in dealing with outbreak-prone diseases, investments can help ensure that public health decision-making is well structured, and individuals in decision-making positions are competent to make decisions and plans. Notably, because of the fast-evolving nature of outbreaks, decisions and actions must proceed amid a degree of uncertainty. Delays due to indecision—for example, regarding implementation of outbreak responses or requests for outside assistance with responses—can lead to severe negative consequences in outbreak-affected communities (Hassan et al. 2018). Devolving decision-making to the lowest possible level can help address such issues, as can deliberate building and maintaining of relationships and processes among institutions involved with decisions and their implementation, such as scientific advisory groups, government ministries, and international organizations.

## POLICY CONSIDERATIONS FOR UNDERSTANDING THE VALUE OF SURVEILLANCE

Amid a paucity of research and evidence on the cost-effectiveness and value of surveillance, there is a need for global-level investment in understanding both the relative value of individual surveillance approaches and the value of public health surveillance overall. Recent research highlights that very few economic evaluations of infectious disease surveillance systems have been performed (De Vries et al. 2021). When economic evaluations have been undertaken, they have overwhelmingly focused on surveillance systems for individual pathogens (Herida, Dervaux, and Desenclos 2016).

Multiple factors complicate economic evaluations of surveillance systems. First, these evaluations must consider the fact that surveillance systems operate as part of a package of tools. In other words, because disease surveillance's value lies in improving use of medical and nonpharmaceutical interventions at a population level, the potential impact of surveillance must reflect and is limited by the potential impact of those interventions. However, economic evaluations of surveillance are still possible through comparisons of carefully constructed counterfactuals on what would happen with the use of medical and nonpharmaceutical interventions in the presence versus the absence of disease surveillance (WHO 2005). Especially for diseases that can cause socially and economically disruptive outbreaks, such evaluations should incorporate a social perspective.

Second, surveillance systems can potentially collect information on a range of diseases, with synergies across diseases for many of the system components. For example, a given surveillance worker with the right training can potentially identify and report suspected cases of many diseases. Economic evaluations of surveillance systems should ideally reflect the synergies from tracking multiple diseases with a single system despite the increased challenges of assessing the value and costs of surveillance for multiple diseases instead of a single disease. Such joint surveillance can have potentially large economies of scope—that is, for multiple diseases rather than for a single disease.

Third, surveillance systems can address both diseases that occur relatively frequently, such as measles and cholera, and diseases that occur more rarely, such as novel zoonotic diseases like COVID-19. Surveillance systems can potentially have great value in guiding control measures for both relatively frequent and rare diseases, including triggering timely responses to and containment of novel zoonotic outbreaks, which can be devastating if not contained. However, data on the frequency and consequences of rare diseases and the potential impact of surveillance systems in their control can be relatively sparse. Nevertheless, economic evaluations of surveillance systems should ideally capture the value and costs of their addressing both frequent and rare diseases.

Despite these challenges, economic evaluations can be useful for assessing the value of surveillance and delineating what constitutes a menu of "best buys" for surveillance (Fan et al. 2023). One key lesson from efforts to control human immunodeficiency virus and acquired immune deficiency syndrome (HIV/AIDS), tuberculosis, and malaria is the role and importance of expanding the measurement of costs and benefits of disease control efforts, including surveillance of these diseases, and either vertical systems (for a specific disease) or horizontal systems (for multiple diseases). Economic evaluations can provide assessments of previous investments and guide future investment decisions, perhaps most saliently demonstrated in the case of HIV/AIDS and the US President's Emergency Plan for AIDS Relief (Ruiz 2023). In another example, an evaluation conducted in Burkina Faso with a focus on meningitis outcomes found that the implementation of IDSR had a low cost (US$$0.01 per capita) yet was associated with statistically significant reductions in meningitis incidence and mortality and potentially with cost savings (Somda et al. 2010). Given the paucity of economic evaluations of surveillance systems, qualitative assessments of such systems' value, potentially relying on gray literature or the experience of practitioners and public health authorities, can be useful, but rigorous and quantitative independent assessments are preferable whenever possible.

## CONCLUSIONS

The concurrent occurrence of epidemics, natural disasters, humanitarian crises, conflicts, and other emergencies is an everyday reality faced by communities the world over. Further, the continued emergence of pathogens with pandemic potential is a certainty. The cost of indecision and inaction, or delayed and ill-informed actions, is great. Concerted efforts, however, can prevent or greatly mitigate the tremendous impacts of these events on public health and society.

The IHR and WHO's HEPR framework underscore the need to strengthen national and local health systems to achieve global health security. Among the top priorities advocated is the need to strengthen surveillance capacity and collaboration among stakeholders to improve public health decisions. A premise of enhancing local (subnational) insights of evolving risks, applied to inform local decisions and local action, must be at the forefront of capacity development investments and activities. Moreover, the growing global knowledge base of the drivers of epidemic and pandemic risks can be operationalized to better target surveillance and preparedness efforts.

Delivering the diverse and evolving information required for decision-making in both "peace time" and before, during, and after public health emergencies will require a careful selection and organization of a suite of surveillance approaches, interconnected with response capacities. The investment design and appraisal considerations outlined in this chapter can support counteracting some of the inherent fragmentation in surveillance systems.

There remains a pressing need to strengthen the evidence base to support best investments in decision-making capacities. Such strengthening should include systematic and independent evaluations of the effectiveness and cost-effectiveness of surveillance approaches, and the value of surveillance overall. High-quality research is vital for enhancing pandemic and epidemic intelligence, forming the basis for effective collaborative surveillance and informed public health decisions, which should consider internationally prioritized themes, such as the application of technologies (for example, artificial intelligence) and multisectoral approaches (WHO 2024).

The COVID-19 pandemic served as a stark reminder of the profound impact that communicable diseases can have on societies worldwide. It was, however, neither the final pandemic we will face nor an isolated incident—in fact, health emergencies are a daily reality. By strategically investing in the preparation of our health systems and unlocking the potential to generate and act on health intelligence at all levels, we can preempt epidemics and pandemics before they take hold, enable the early detection of emerging risks, and guide targeted response interventions to prevent localized outbreaks from escalating into full-blown catastrophes.

## ANNEX 5A. GLOSSARY

**Global public health security:** The activities required, both proactive and reactive, to minimize the danger and impact of acute public health events that endanger people's health across geographical regions and international boundaries (WHO 2020).

**Hazard:** A process, phenomenon, or human activity that may cause loss of life, injury, or other health impacts; property damage; social and economic disruption; or environmental degradation (WHO 2020). Hazards may be single, sequential, or combined in their origin and effects, and, under the WHO classification of hazards, include natural hazards (biological, extraterrestrial, geophysical, and hydro-meteorological), human-induced hazards (technological and societal), and environmental hazards (environmental degradation).[4]

**One Health:** An integrated, unifying approach that aims to sustainably balance and optimize the health of humans, animals, plants, and ecosystems. It recognizes the close link and interdependence among the health of humans, domestic and wild animals, plants, and the wider environment (including ecosystems). The approach mobilizes multiple sectors, disciplines, and communities at different levels of society to work together to foster well-being and tackle threats to health and ecosystems while addressing the collective need for clean water, energy, and air and safe and nutritious food; taking action on climate change; and contributing to sustainable development (FAO et al. 2022).

**Public health intelligence:** A core public health function responsible for identifying, collecting, connecting, synthesizing, analyzing, assessing, interpreting, and generating a wide range of information for actionable insights and disseminating these insights for informed and effective decision-making to protect and improve the health of populations.[5]

**Risk:** The potential loss of life, injury, or destroyed or damaged assets that could occur to a system, society, or a community in a specific period of time, determined probabilistically as a function of hazard, exposure, vulnerability, and capacity (UN 2016; WHO 2020).

**Surveillance (public health surveillance):** The systematic, ongoing collection, collation, and analysis of data for public health purposes and the timely dissemination of public health information for assessment and public health response, as necessary (WHO 2016, 2020).

**Threat:** A person, place, thing, or development, or a combination of these elements, that can harm health security, either as a real or perceived danger (WHO 2014). Examples include antimicrobial resistance or environmental threats such as climate change. Threats can also refer to deliberate events such as an intent to release a hazardous substance to cause harm. Refer also to the definition of hazard.

**Vulnerability:** The characteristics and circumstances (physical, social, economic, and environmental factors or processes) of an individual, community, system, or asset that make it susceptible to the effects of a hazard (UN 2016; WHO 2021a).

## NOTES

**Disclaimer:** The findings and conclusions in this chapter are those of the authors and do not necessarily represent the official position of the organizations for which they work.

1. Refer also to National Human Genome Research Institute, "DNA Sequencing Costs: Data," https://www.genome.gov/about-genomics/fact-sheets/DNA-Sequencing-Costs-Data.
2. Refer also to WHO, "IHR Review Committees," https://www.who.int/teams/ihr/ihr-review-committees.
3. Refer also to WHO, "WHO Dashboard of COVID-19 Related Recommendations," http://bit.ly/3MGMq3o.
4. United Nations Office for Disaster Risk Reduction, "Definition: Hazard" (accessed April 14, 2023), https://www.undrr.org/terminology/hazard.
5. United Nations Department for General Assembly and Conference Management, "UNTERM: The United Nations Terminology Database," (accessed April 14, 2023), https://unterm.un.org/unterm2/en/.

## REFERENCES

Abubakar, Ahmed, Mahmud Dalhat, Abdulaziz Mohammed, Olayinka Stephen Ilesanmi, Uchenna Anebonam, Nyampa Barau, Sarafadeen Salami, et al. 2019. "Outbreak of Suspected Pertussis in Kaltungo, Gombe State, Northern Nigeria, 2015: The Role of Sub-Optimum Routine Immunization Coverage." *Pan African Medical Journal* 32 (Suppl 1): 9. https://doi.org/10.11604/pamj.supp.2019.32.1.13352.

Archer, Brett N., Juno Thomas, Jacqueline Weyer, Ayanda Cengimbo, Dadja E. Landoh, Charlene Jacobs, Sindile Ntuli, et al. 2013. "Epidemiologic Investigations into Outbreaks of Rift Valley Fever in Humans, South Africa, 2008–2011." *Emerging Infectious Diseases* 19 (12). https://doi.org/10.3201/eid1912.121527.

Balajee, S. Arunmozhi, Omer G. Pasi, Alain Georges M. Etoundi, Peter Rzeszotarski, Trang T. Do, Ian Hennessee, Sharifa Merali, et al. 2017. "Sustainable Model for Public Health Emergency Operations Centers for Global Settings." *Emerging Infectious Diseases* 23 (13). https://doi.org/10.3201/eid2313.170435.

Bochner, Aaron F., Issa Makumbi, Olaolu Aderinola, Aschalew Abayneh, Ralph Jetoh, Rahel L. Yemanaberhan, Jenom S. Danjuma, et al. 2023. "Implementation of the 7-1-7 Target for Detection, Notification, and Response to Public Health Threats in Five Countries: A Retrospective, Observational Study." *The Lancet Global Health* 11 (6): E871–79. https://doi.org/10.1016/S2214-109X(23)00133-X.

Bohl, Jennifer A., Sreyngim Lay, Sophana Chea, Vida Ahyong, Daniel M. Parker, Shannon Gallagher, Jonathan Fintzi, et al. 2022. "Discovering Disease-Causing Pathogens in Resource-Scarce Southeast Asia Using a Global Metagenomic Pathogen Monitoring System." *Proceedings of the National Academy of Sciences* 119 (11): e2115285119. https://doi.org/10.1073/pnas.2115285119.

Bollyky, Thomas J., Erin N. Hulland, Ryan M. Barber, James K. Collins, Samantha Kiernan, Mark Moses, David M. Pigott, et al. 2022. "Pandemic Preparedness and COVID-19: An Exploratory Analysis of Infection and Fatality Rates, and Contextual Factors Associated with Preparedness in 177 Countries, from Jan 1, 2020, to Sept 30, 2021." *The Lancet* 399 (10334): 1489–512. https://doi.org/10.1016/S0140-6736(22)00172-6.

Buss, Lewis, Carlos A. Prete, Charles Whittaker, Tassila Salomon, Marcio K. Oikawa, Rafael H. M. Pereira, Isabel C. G. Moura, et al. 2022. "Predicting SARS-CoV-2 Variant Spread in a Completely Seropositive Population Using Semi-Quantitative Antibody Measurements in Blood Donors." *Vaccines* 10 (9): 1437. https://doi.org/10.3390/vaccines10091437.

Caldwell, Jamie M., A. Desiree LaBeaud, Eric F. Lambin, Anna M. Stewart-Ibarra, Bryson A. Ndenga, Francis M. Mutuku, Amy R. Krystosik, et al. 2021. "Climate Predicts Geographic and Temporal Variation in Mosquito-Borne Disease Dynamics on Two Continents." *Nature Communications* 12 (1): 1233. https://doi.org/10.1038/s41467-021-21496-7.

Carlson, Colin J., Gregory F. Albery, Cory Merow, Christopher H. Trisos, Casey M. Zipfel, Evan A. Eskew, Kevin J. Olival, et al. 2022. "Climate Change Increases Cross-Species Viral Transmission Risk." *Nature* 607 (7919): 555–62. https://doi.org/10.1038/s41586-022-04788-w.

Chang, Serina, Emma Pierson, Pang Wei Koh, Jaline Gerardin, Beth Redbird, David Grusky, and Jure Leskovec. 2021. "Mobility Network Models of COVID-19 Explain Inequities and Inform Reopening." *Nature* 589 (7840): 82–87. https://doi.org/10.1038/s41586-020-2923-3.

Charnley, Gina E. C., Kévin Jean, Ilan Kelman, Katy A. M. Gaythorpe, and Kris A. Murray. 2022. "Association between Conflict and Cholera in Nigeria and the Democratic Republic of the Congo." *Emerging Infectious Diseases* 28 (12): 2472–81. https://doi.org/10.3201/eid2812.212398.

Choi, Bernard C. K. 2012. "The Past, Present, and Future of Public Health Surveillance." *Scientifica* 2012: 1–26.

Clarke, Lorcan, Edith Patouillard, Andrew J. Mirelman, Zheng Jie Marc Ho, Tessa Tan-Torres Edejer, and Nirmal Kandel. 2022. "The Costs of Improving Health Emergency Preparedness: A Systematic Review and Analysis of Multi-Country Studies." *eClinicalMedicine* 44 (February): 101269. https://doi.org/10.1016/j.eclinm.2021.101269.

Cutler, David M., and Lawrence H. Summers. 2020. "The COVID-19 Pandemic and the $16 Trillion Virus." *JAMA* 324 (15): 1495. https://doi.org/10.1001/jama.2020.19759.

De Vries, Linda, Marion Koopmans, Alec Morton, and Pieter Van Baal. 2021. "The Economics of Improving Global Infectious Disease Surveillance." *BMJ Global Health* 6 (9): e006597. https://doi.org/10.1136/bmjgh-2021-006597.

Donelle, Lorie, Leigha Comer, Brad Hiebert, Jodi Hall, Jacob J. Shelley, Maxwell J. Smith, Anita Kothari, et al. 2023. "Use of Digital Technologies for Public Health Surveillance during the COVID-19 Pandemic: A Scoping Review." *DIGITAL HEALTH* 9 (January): 205520762311732. https://doi.org/10.1177/20552076231173220.

Dureab, Fekri, Maysoon Al-Sakkaf, Osan Ismail, Naasegnibe Kuunibe, Johannes Krisam, Olaf Müller, and Albrecht Jahn. 2019. "Diphtheria Outbreak in Yemen: The Impact of Conflict on a Fragile Health System." *Conflict and Health* 13 (1): 19. https://doi.org/10.1186/s13031-019-0204-2.

Elmahal, Osman M., Ali Abdullah, Manal K. Elzalabany, Huda Haidar Anan, Dalia Samhouri, and Richard John Brennan. 2022. "Public Health Emergency Operation Centres: Status, Gaps and Areas for Improvement in the Eastern Mediterranean Region." *BMJ Global Health* 7 (Suppl 4): e008573. https://doi.org/10.1136/bmjgh-2022-008573.

Fan, Victoria Y., Eleni Smitham, Lydia Regan, Pratibha Gautam, Ole Norheim, Javier Guzman, and Amanda Glassman. 2023. "Strategic Investment in Surveillance for Pandemic Preparedness: Rapid Review and Roundtable Discussion." CGD Policy Paper 298, Center for Global Development, Washington, DC. https://doi.org/10.13140/RG.2.2.24442.67520.

FAO (Food and Agriculture Organization of the United Nations), UNEP (United Nations Environment Programme), WHO (World Health Organization), and WOAH

(World Organisation for Animal Health). 2022. *One Health Joint Plan of Action (2022–2026): Working Together for the Health of Humans, Animals, Plants and the Environment.* Rome: FAO, UNEP, WHO, and WOAH. https://doi.org/10.4060/cc2289en.

Federspiel, Frederik, and Mohammad Ali. 2018. "The Cholera Outbreak in Yemen: Lessons Learned and Way Forward." *BMC Public Health* 18 (1): 1338. https://doi.org/10.1186/s12889-018-6227-6.

Frieden, Thomas R., Christopher T. Lee, Aaron F. Bochner, Marine Buissonnière, and Amanda McClelland. 2021. "7-1-7: An Organising Principle, Target, and Accountability Metric to Make the World Safer from Pandemics." *The Lancet* 398 (10300): 638–40. https://doi.org/10.1016/S0140-6736(21)01250-2.

Giattino, Charlie, Hannah Ritchie, Esteban Ortiz-Ospina, Lucas Rodés-Guirao, Joe Hasell, and Max Roser. 2020. "Excess Mortality during the Coronavirus Pandemic (COVID-19)." *Our World in Data*, March 5, 2020. https://ourworldindata.org/excess-mortality-covid.

Gibb, Rory, David W. Redding, Kai Qing Chin, Christl A. Donnelly, Tim M. Blackburn, Tim Newbold, and Kate E. Jones. 2020. "Zoonotic Host Diversity Increases in Human-Dominated Ecosystems." *Nature* 584 (7821): 398–402. https://doi.org/10.1038/s41586-020-2562-8.

Gossner, Céline M., Laurence Marrama, Marianne Carson, Franz Allerberger, Paolo Calistri, Dimitrios Dilaveris, Sylvie Lecollinet, et al. 2017. "West Nile Virus Surveillance in Europe: Moving towards an Integrated Animal-Human-Vector Approach." *Eurosurveillance* 22 (18). https://doi.org/10.2807/1560-7917.ES.2017.22.18.30526.

Hampton, Lee M., Hope L. Johnson, and Seth F. Berkley. 2022. "Diagnostics to Make Immunisation Programmes More Efficient, Equitable, and Effective." *The Lancet Microbe* 3 (4): e242–43. https://doi.org/10.1016/S2666-5247(22)00038-6.

Hampton, Lee M., Francisco Luquero, Alejandro Costa, Anais Legand, and Pierre Formenty. 2023. "Ebola Outbreak Detection and Response since 2013." *The Lancet Microbe* 4 (9): e661–62. https://doi.org/10.1016/S2666-5247(23)00136-2.

Hassan, Assad, G. U. Mustapha, Bola B. Lawal, Aliyu M. Na'uzo, Raji Ismail, Eteng Womi-Eteng Oboma, Oyeronke Oyebanji, et al. 2018. "Time Delays in the Response to the Neisseria Meningitidis Serogroup C Outbreak in Nigeria – 2017." *PLOS One* 13 (6): e0199257. https://doi.org/10.1371/journal.pone.0199257.

Hayman, David T. S., Wiku B. Adisasmito, Salama Almuhairi, Casey Barton Behravesh, Pépé Bilivogui, Salome A. Bukachi, Natalia Casas, et al. 2023. "Developing One Health Surveillance Systems." *One Health* 17 (December): 100617. https://doi.org/10.1016/j.onehlt.2023.100617.

Herida, Magid, Benoit Dervaux, and Jean-Claude Desenclos. 2016. "Economic Evaluations of Public Health Surveillance Systems: A Systematic Review." *European Journal of Public Health* 26 (4): 674–80. https://doi.org/10.1093/eurpub/ckv250.

IPPPR (Independent Panel for Pandemic Preparedness and Response). 2023. "COVID-19: Make It the Last Pandemic." IPPPR. https://theindependentpanel.org/wp-content/uploads/2021/05/COVID-19-Make-it-the-Last-Pandemic_final.pdf.

ITU (International Telecommunication Union). 2022. *Global Connectivity Report 2022.* Geneva: ITU.

Jain, Vageesh, Ashley Sharp, Matthew Neilson, Daniel G. Bausch, and Thomas Beaney. 2022. "Joint External Evaluation Scores and Communicable Disease Deaths: An Ecological Study on the Difference between Epidemics and Pandemics." *PLOS Global Public Health* 2 (8): e0000246. https://doi.org/10.1371/journal.pgph.0000246.

Jombart, Thibaut, Christopher I. Jarvis, Samuel Mesfin, Nabil Tabal, Mathias Mossoko, Luigino Minikulu Mpia, Aaron Aruna Abedi, et al. 2020. "The Cost of Insecurity: From Flare-Up to Control of a Major Ebola Virus Disease Hotspot during the Outbreak in the Democratic Republic of the Congo, 2019." *Eurosurveillance* 25 (2). https://doi.org/10.2807/1560-7917.ES.2020.25.2.1900735.

Jones, Kate E., Nikkita G. Patel, Marc A. Levy, Adam Storeygard, Deborah Balk, John L. Gittleman, and Peter Daszak. 2008. "Global Trends in Emerging Infectious Diseases." *Nature* 451 (7181): 990–93. https://doi.org/10.1038/nature06536.

Juneau, Carl-Etienne, Tomas Pueyo, Matt Bell, Genevieve Gee, Pablo Collazzo, and Louise Potvin. 2022. "Lessons from Past Pandemics: A Systematic Review of Evidence-Based, Cost-Effective Interventions to Suppress COVID-19." *Systematic Reviews* 11 (1): 90. https://doi.org/10.1186/s13643-022-01958-9.

Jutla, Antarpreet, Elizabeth Whitcombe, Nur Hasan, Bradd Haley, Ali Akanda, Anwar Huq, Munir Alam, et al. 2013. "Environmental Factors Influencing Epidemic Cholera." *American Journal of Tropical Medicine and Hygiene* 89 (3): 597–607. https://doi.org/10.4269/ajtmh.12-0721.

Kahn, Rebecca, Ayesha S. Mahmud, Andrew Schroeder, Luis Hernando Aguilar Ramirez, John Crowley, Jennifer Chan, and Caroline O. Buckee. 2019. "Rapid Forecasting of Cholera Risk in Mozambique: Translational Challenges and Opportunities." *Prehospital and Disaster Medicine* 34 (05): 557–62. https://doi.org/10.1017/S1049023X19004783.

Kilaru, Pruthvi, Dustin Hill, Kathryn Anderson, Mary B. Collins, Hyatt Green, Brittany L. Kmush, and David A. Larsen. 2023. "Wastewater Surveillance for Infectious Disease: A Systematic Review." *American Journal of Epidemiology* 192 (2): 305–22. https://doi.org/10.1093/aje/kwac175.

Kongelf, A., T. Tingberg, A. L. McClelland, M. C. Jean, and B. D. Dalziel. 2016. "Community-Based Cholera Surveillance by Volunteers with Mobile Phones: A Case Study from Western Area, Haiti." *International Journal of Infectious Diseases* 53 (December):115–16. https://doi.org/10.1016/j.ijid.2016.11.289.

Kouadio, Isidore K., Taro Kamigaki, and Hitoshi Oshitani. 2010. "Measles Outbreaks in Displaced Populations: A Review of Transmission, Morbidity and Mortality Associated Factors." *BMC International Health and Human Rights* 10 (1): 5. https://doi.org/10.1186/1472-698X-10-5.

Kraay, Alicia N. M., Kristin N. Nelson, Conan Y. Zhao, David Demory, Joshua S. Weitz, and Benjamin A. Lopman. 2021. "Modeling Serological Testing to Inform Relaxation of Social Distancing for COVID-19 Control." *Nature Communications* 12 (1): 7063. https://doi.org/10.1038/s41467-021-26774-y.

Kucharski, Adam J., Kiyojiken Chung, Maite Aubry, Iotefa Teiti, Anita Teissier, Vaea Richard, Timothy W. Russell, et al. 2023. "Real-Time Surveillance of International SARS-CoV-2 Prevalence Using Systematic Traveller Arrival Screening: An Observational Study." *PLOS Medicine* 20 (9): e1004283. https://doi.org/10.1371/journal.pmed.1004283.

Lam, Eugene, Amanda McCarthy, and Muireann Brennan. 2015. "Vaccine-Preventable Diseases in Humanitarian Emergencies among Refugee and Internally-Displaced Populations." *Human Vaccines & Immunotherapeutics* 11 (11): 2627–36. https://doi.org/10.1080/21645515.2015.1096457.

Ledesma, Jorge Ricardo, Christopher R. Isaac, Scott F. Dowell, David L. Blazes, Gabrielle V. Essix, Katherine Budeski, Jessica Bell, and Jennifer B. Nuzzo. 2023. "Evaluation of the Global Health Security Index as a Predictor of COVID-19 Excess Mortality Standardised for Under-Reporting and Age Structure." *BMJ Global Health* 8 (7): e012203. https://doi.org/10.1136/bmjgh-2023-012203.

Lee, Christopher, Sally Slavinski, Corinne Schiff, Mario Merlino, Demetre Daskalakis, Dakai Liu, Jennifer L. Rakeman, et al. 2017. "Outbreak of Influenza A(H7N2) among Cats in an Animal Shelter with Cat-to-Human Transmission—New York City, 2016." *Clinical Infectious Diseases* 65 (11): 1927–29. https://doi.org/10.1093/cid/cix668.

Lee, Elizabeth C., Andrew S. Azman, Joshua Kaminsky, Sean M. Moore, Heather S. McKay, and Justin Lessler. 2019. "The Projected Impact of Geographic Targeting of Oral Cholera Vaccination in Sub-Saharan Africa: A Modeling Study." *PLOS Medicine* 16 (12): e1003003. https://doi.org/10.1371/journal.pmed.1003003.

Lipsitch, Marc, and Mauricio Santillana. 2019. "Enhancing Situational Awareness to Prevent Infectious Disease Outbreaks from Becoming Catastrophic." In *Global Catastrophic*

*Biological Risks*, edited by Thomas V. Inglesby and Amesh A. Adalja, 59–74. Current Topics in Microbiology and Immunology. Cham: Springer International Publishing. https://doi.org/10.1007/82_2019_172.

Lotto Batista, Martín, Eleanor M. Rees, Andrea Gómez, Soledad López, Stefanie Castell, Adam J. Kucharski, Stéphane Ghozzi, et al. 2023. "Towards a Leptospirosis Early Warning System in Northeastern Argentina." *Journal of The Royal Society Interface* 20 (202): 20230069. https://doi.org/10.1098/rsif.2023.0069.

Marais, Gert, Diana Hardie, and Adrian Brink. 2023. "A Case for Investment in Clinical Metagenomics in Low-Income and Middle-Income Countries." *The Lancet Microbe* 4 (3): e192–99. https://doi.org/10.1016/S2666-5247(22)00328-7.

Masters, Nina B., Marisa C. Eisenberg, Paul L. Delamater, Matthew Kay, Matthew L. Boulton, and Jon Zelner. 2020. "Fine-Scale Spatial Clustering of Measles Nonvaccination That Increases Outbreak Potential Is Obscured by Aggregated Reporting Data." *Proceedings of the National Academy of Sciences* 117 (45): 28506–14. https://doi.org/10.1073/pnas.2011529117.

Mayigane, Landry Ndriko, Liviu Vedrasco, and Stella Chungong. 2023. "7-1-7: The Promise of Tangible Results through Agility and Accountability." *The Lancet Global Health* 11 (6): e805–6. https://doi.org/10.1016/S2214-109X(23)00167-5.

McKee, Clifton D., Ausraful Islam, Stephen P. Luby, Henrik Salje, Peter J. Hudson, Raina K. Plowright, and Emily S. Gurley. 2021. "The Ecology of Nipah Virus in Bangladesh: A Nexus of Land-Use Change and Opportunistic Feeding Behavior in Bats." *Viruses* 13 (2): 169. https://doi.org/10.3390/v13020169.

Mremi, Irene R., Janeth George, Susan F. Rumisha, Calvin Sindato, Sharadhuli I. Kimera, and Leonard E. G. Mboera. 2021. "Twenty Years of Integrated Disease Surveillance and Response in Sub-Saharan Africa: Challenges and Opportunities for Effective Management of Infectious Disease Epidemics." *One Health Outlook* 3 (1): 22. https://doi.org/10.1186/s42522-021-00052-9.

NTI (Nuclear Threat Initiative) and Johns Hopkins Center for Health Security, Bloomberg School of Public Health. 2021. "Global Health Security Index: Advancing Collective Action and Accountability amid Crisis." NTI, Washington, DC. https://ghsindex.org/wp-content/uploads/2021/12/2021_GHSindexFullReport_Final.pdf.

Nuzzo, Jennifer B., and Jorge R. Ledesma. 2023. "Why Did the Best Prepared Country in the World Fare So Poorly during COVID?" *Journal of Economic Perspectives* 37 (4): 3–22. https://doi.org/10.1257/jep.37.4.3.

OECD (Organisation for Economic Co-operation and Development). 2020. "Flattening the COVID-19 Peak: Containment and Mitigation Policies." OECD Policy Paper, OECD, Paris. https://www.oecd.org/en/publications/flattening-the-covid-19-peak-containment-and-mitigation-policies_e96a4226-en/full-report.html.

Oliver, Nuria, Bruno Lepri, Harald Sterly, Renaud Lambiotte, Sébastien Deletaille, Marco De Nadai, Emmanuel Letouzé, et al. 2020. "Mobile Phone Data for Informing Public Health Actions across the COVID-19 Pandemic Life Cycle." *Science Advances* 6 (23): eabc0764. https://doi.org/10.1126/sciadv.abc0764.

Oyebanji, Oyeronke, Fatima Ibrahim Abba, Oluwatosin Wuraola Akande, Everistus Chijioke Aniaku, Anwar Abubakar, John Oladejo, Olaolu Aderinola, et al. 2021. "Building Local Capacity for Emergency Coordination: Establishment of Subnational Public Health Emergency Operations Centres in Nigeria." *BMJ Global Health* 6 (10): e007203. https://doi.org/10.1136/bmjgh-2021-007203.

Poljanšek, K., M. Marin-Ferrer, L. Vernaccini, and L. Messina. 2018. *Incorporating Epidemics Risk in the INFORM Global Risk Index*. EUR 29603 EU. Luxembourg: Publications Office of the European Union. https://data.europa.eu/doi/10.2760/990429.

Rader, Benjamin, Samuel V. Scarpino, Anjalika Nande, Alison L. Hill, Ben Adlam, Robert C. Reiner, David M. Pigott, et al. 2020. "Crowding and the Shape of COVID-19 Epidemics." *Nature Medicine* 26 (12): 1829–34. https://doi.org/10.1038/s41591-020-1104-0.

Ratnayake, Ruwan, Meghan Tammaro, Amanda Tiffany, Anine Kongelf, Jonathan A Polonsky, and Amanda McClelland. 2020. "People-Centred Surveillance: A Narrative Review of

Community-Based Surveillance among Crisis-Affected Populations." *The Lancet Planetary Health* 4 (10): e483–95. https://doi.org/10.1016/S2542-5196(20)30221-7.

Redding, David W., Peter M. Atkinson, Andrew A. Cunningham, Gianni Lo Iacono, Lina M. Moses, James L. N. Wood, and Kate E. Jones. 2019. "Impacts of Environmental and Socio-economic Factors on Emergence and Epidemic Potential of Ebola in Africa." *Nature Communications* 10 (1): 4531. https://doi.org/10.1038/s41467-019-12499-6.

Redding, David W., Rory Gibb, Chioma C. Dan-Nwafor, Elsie A. Ilori, Rimamdeyati Usman Yashe, Saliu H. Oladele, Michael O. Amedu, et al. 2021. "Geographical Drivers and Climate-Linked Dynamics of Lassa Fever in Nigeria." *Nature Communications* 12 (1): 5759. https://doi.org/10.1038/s41467-021-25910-y.

Redding, David W., Sonia Tiedt, Gianni Lo Iacono, Bernard Bett, and Kate E. Jones. 2017. "Spatial, Seasonal and Climatic Predictive Models of Rift Valley Fever Disease across Africa." *Philosophical Transactions of the Royal Society B: Biological Sciences* 372 (1725). https://doi.org/10.1098/rstb.2016.0165.

Romanello, Marina, Claudia Di Napoli, Carole Green, Harry Kennard, Pete Lampard, Daniel Scamman, Maria Walawender, et al. 2023. "The 2023 Report of the *Lancet* Countdown on Health and Climate Change: The Imperative for a Health-Centred Response in a World Facing Irreversible Harms." *The Lancet* 402 (10419): 2346–94. https://doi.org/10.1016/S0140-6736(23)01859-7.

Ruiz, Santi. 2023. "How to Save Twenty Million Lives, with Dr. Mark Dybul." *Statecraft*, August 29, 2023. https://www.statecraft.pub/p/saving-twenty-million-lives.

Sharma, Siddhanth, Jaspreet Pannu, Sam Chorlton, Jacob L. Swett, and David J. Ecker. 2023. "Threat Net: A Metagenomic Surveillance Network for Biothreat Detection and Early Warning." *Health Security* 21 (5). https://doi.org/10.1089/hs.2022.0160.

Somda, Zana C., Helen N. Perry, Nancy R. Messonnier, Mamadou H. Djingarey, Salimata Ouedraogo Ki, and Martin I. Meltzer. 2010. "Modeling the Cost-Effectiveness of the Integrated Disease Surveillance and Response (IDSR) System: Meningitis in Burkina Faso." *PLOS One* 5 (9): e13044. https://doi.org/10.1371/journal.pone.0013044.

Tan, Chorh-Chuan. 2006. "SARS in Singapore—Key Lessons from an Epidemic." *Annals of the Academy of Medicine, Singapore* 35 (5): 345–49.

Tatem, A. J., D. J. Rogers, and S. I. Hay. 2006. "Global Transport Networks and Infectious Disease Spread." *Advances in Parasitology* 62: 293–343. https://doi.org/10.1016/S0065-308X(05)62009-X.

Thomson, Madeleine C., and Lawrence R. Stanberry. 2022. "Climate Change and Vectorborne Diseases." *New England Journal of Medicine* 387 (21): 1969–78. https://doi.org/10.1056/NEJMra2200092.

UN (United Nations). 2016. *Report of the Open-Ended Intergovernmental Expert Working Group on Indicators and Terminology Relating to Disaster Risk Reduction. Note by the Secretary-General.* New York: UN.

UNHCR (United Nations High Commissioner for Refugees). 2023. "Global Trends: Forced Displacement in 2022." UNHCR, Geneva. https://www.unhcr.org/global-trends-report-2022.

Vardavas, Constantine, Konstantinos Zisis, Katerina Nikitara, Ioanna Lagou, Valia Marou, Katerina Aslanoglou, Konstantinos Athanasakis, et al. 2023. "Cost of the COVID-19 Pandemic versus the Cost-Effectiveness of Mitigation Strategies in EU/UK/OECD: A Systematic Review." *BMJ Open* 13 (10): e077602. https://doi.org/10.1136/bmjopen-2023-077602.

WHO (World Health Organization). 2005. *Evaluating the Costs and Benefits of National Surveillance and Response Systems: Methodologies and Options.* Geneva: WHO.

WHO (World Health Organization). 2014. *Early Detection, Assessment and Response to Acute Public Health Events: Implementation of Early Warning and Response with a Focus on Event-Based Surveillance: Interim Version.* Geneva: WHO.

WHO (World Health Organization). 2015. *Framework for a Public Health Emergency Operations Centre: November 2015.* Geneva: WHO.

WHO (World Health Organization). 2016. *International Health Regulations (2005)* (third edition). Geneva: WHO.

WHO (World Health Organization). 2020. *Glossary of Health Emergency and Disaster Risk Management Terminology*. Geneva: WHO.

WHO (World Health Organization). 2021a. *Strategic Toolkit for Assessing Risks: A Comprehensive Toolkit for All-Hazards Health Emergency Risk Assessment*. Geneva: WHO.

WHO (World Health Organization). 2021b. *WHA74/9 - WHO's Work in Health Emergencies: Strengthening Preparedness for Health Emergencies*. Geneva: WHO. https://cdn.who.int /media/docs/default-source/documents/emergencies/a74_9add1-en.pdf.

WHO (World Health Organization). 2023a. *"Crafting the Mosaic": A Framework for Resilient Surveillance for Respiratory Viruses of Epidemic and Pandemic Potential*. Geneva: WHO. https://www.who.int/publications/i/item/9789240070288.

WHO (World Health Organization). 2023b. *Defining Collaborative Surveillance: A Core Concept for Strengthening the Global Architecture for Health Emergency Preparedness, Response, and Resilience (HEPR)*. Geneva: WHO. https://apps.who.int/iris/handle/10665 /367927.

WHO (World Health Organization). 2023c. *Global Public Health Intelligence Report 2022*. Geneva: WHO.

WHO (World Health Organization). 2023d. *Guidance for Conducting a Country Early Action Review (EAR): Rapid Performance Improvement for Outbreak Detection and Response, 31 August 2023*. Geneva: WHO.

WHO (World Health Organization). 2023e. *Pandemic Influenza Preparedness Framework: Partnership Contribution High-Level Implementation Plan III 2024-2030*. Geneva: WHO.

WHO (World Health Organization). 2023f. *Strengthening the Global Architecture for Health Emergency Prevention, Preparedness, Response and Resilience*. Geneva: WHO.

WHO (World Health Organization). 2024. *Research Prioritization for Pandemic and Epidemic Intelligence: Technical Brief*. Geneva: WHO.

World Bank. 2022. "The Economic Impacts of the COVID-19 Crisis." Chapter 1 in *World Development Report 2022: Finance for an Equitable Recovery*. Washington, DC: World Bank. https://doi.org/10.1596/978-1-4648-1730-4.

Xu, Hanmeng, Kaiyue Zou, Juan Dent, Kirsten E. Wiens, Espoir Bwenge Malembaka, Godfrey Bwire, Placide Welo Okitayemba, et al. 2024. "Enhanced Cholera Surveillance to Improve Vaccination Campaign Efficiency." *Nature Medicine* 30: 1104–10. https://doi.org/10.1038 /s41591-024-02852-8.

Yang, Jingyan, Shailja Vaghela, Benjamin Yarnoff, Solene De Boisvilliers, Manuela Di Fusco, Timothy Lee Wiemken, Moe H. Kyaw, et al. 2023. "Estimated Global Public Health and Economic Impact of COVID-19 Vaccines in the Pre-Omicron Era Using Real-World Empirical Data." *Expert Review of Vaccines* 22 (1): 54–65. https://doi.org/10.1080/1476058 4.2023.2157817.

Zeng, Wu, Hadia Samaha, Michel Yao, Steve Ahuka-Mundeke, Thomas Wilkinson, Thibaut Jombart, Dominique Baabo, et al. 2023. "The Cost of Public Health Interventions to Respond to the 10th Ebola Outbreak in the Democratic Republic of the Congo." *BMJ Global Health* 8 (10): e012660. https://doi.org/10.1136/bmjgh-2023-012660.

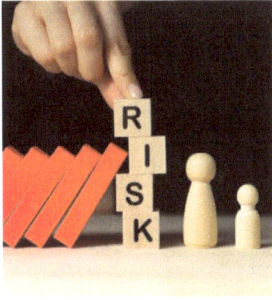

# 6

# Public Health and Social Measures for Respiratory Infections

Hitoshi Oshitani, Victoria Y. Fan, and Ole F. Norheim

## ABSTRACT

Public health and social measures (PHSM) play a crucial role in reducing the transmission of epidemics or pandemics, particularly when pharmaceutical interventions, such as vaccines and therapeutics, are unavailable. For coronavirus disease (COVID-19), PHSM were implemented at an unprecedented level. Scientific evidence on the impact and effectiveness of PHSM remains limited, however, and their effectiveness depends on several factors, including the epidemiological characteristics of the target pathogen, the timing of implementation, and adherence to policies. Implementing stringent PHSM has negative social and economic consequences. Policy makers and other stakeholders should understand potential benefits, limitations, and negative consequences when they implement PHSM.

## INTRODUCTION

Public health and social measures (PHSM), previously referred to as "nonpharmaceutical interventions," are vital strategies for reducing the transmission of pathogens during an epidemic or pandemic. They can be implemented for various infectious diseases, including sexually transmitted infections, vector-borne infections, and waterborne infections. The choice of measures depends on the modes of transmission of target pathogens.

PHSM play a critical role in mitigating the impact of respiratory infections, especially during pandemics. A wide range of PHSM has been implemented for past pandemics, including influenza pandemics and the COVID-19 (coronavirus) pandemic. PHSM for respiratory infections can be categorized according to their targets (refer to table 6.1), including (1) active case finding and contact identification measures, such as isolating symptomatic individuals and quarantining close contacts of infected persons; (2) personal protection measures such as hand hygiene and face masks; (3) environmental measures such as surface cleaning and improved ventilation; (4) social measures such as school and business closures and restrictions on social gatherings; and (5) international travel and trade measures such as entry and exit screenings and travel restrictions (WHO 2024a). This chapter explores general issues and challenges in developing policies for PHSM, specifically for respiratory infections such as COVID-19 and pandemic influenza. For more on active case finding and contact identification measures, also known as "targeted interventions," refer to chapter 7 in this volume; for more on school closures and their negative consequences, refer to chapter 8.

Despite the crucial role of pharmaceutical interventions, including vaccines and therapeutics, in mitigating the effects of epidemics and pandemics, these tools are often unavailable during the initial stages of an outbreak caused by a novel pathogen. For instance, even with the unprecedented speed of vaccine development during

**Table 6.1** Classification of Public Health and Social Measures

| First-level PHSM category | Second-level PHSM category |
|---|---|
| Active case finding and contact identification measures | 1) Active case finding |
| | 2) Case-specific measures (isolation) |
| | 3) Contact-specific measures (quarantine) |
| Personal protection measures | 1) Personal protective equipment (masks, gloves, and so on) |
| | 2) Personal hygiene measures (hand hygiene, respiratory hygiene, cough etiquette, and so on) |
| Environmental measures | 1) Physical infrastructure |
| | 2) Surface cleaning |
| | 3) Indoor air quality |
| Social measures | 1) Social interactions and gathering |
| | 2) Domestic mobility (stay-at-home order, restriction of movement, and so on) |
| | 3) Modifications to activities and services (closures of schools and businesses and so on) |
| International travel and trade measures | 1) Trade measures for imported goods |
| | 2) Trade measures for exported goods |
| | 3) Travel-related screening or testing |
| | 4) International border measures |
| | 5) Quarantine upon arrival |
| | 6) Travel advice or warning |

*Source:* Adapted from WHO 2024a.

*Note:* PHSM = public health and social measures.

**152**    Investing in Pandemic Prevention, Preparedness, and Response | Siddhanth Sharma et al.

the COVID-19 pandemic, saving millions of lives, the vaccine rollout began almost a year after identification of the first COVID-19 cases. A new initiative, known as the 100 Days Mission, aims to develop vaccines and other medical countermeasures within 100 days. Even if this goal is achieved, vaccines will not be available in the earliest stages of a future pandemic, necessitating reliance on PHSM to mitigate impact and gain time for development of medical countermeasures.

Historically, PHSM have played a crucial role in controlling infectious disease outbreaks. For instance, quarantine (separating potentially exposed individuals) was widely implemented during the fourteenth-century plague outbreak known as the "Black Death" (Tognotti 2013). The influenza pandemic of 1918–20 caused devastating impacts, with an estimated 50 million deaths. Various PHSM were used during that pandemic, including bans on public gatherings, school closures, and strict quarantine and isolation measures (Tomes 2010). In the United States, the timing and intensity of PHSM implementation during the influenza pandemic varied between cities. For example, St. Louis, which adopted stringent PHSM, such as closing schools, churches, theaters, and other public places, experienced lower case counts and mortality rates compared to cities like Philadelphia or New York, which were less proactive (Belshe 2012).

Considering the potential effectiveness of PHSM requires evolving and updated knowledge about modes of transmission of respiratory pathogens. During the severe acute respiratory syndrome (SARS) epidemic in 2002–03, vaccines and effective antivirals were unavailable. Nonetheless, SARS was successfully contained using PHSM, primarily active case finding and contact identification measures. Because most individuals infected with SARS exhibited infectiousness only after developing severe clinical symptoms, isolating infected persons after symptom onset proved effective in controlling its spread (Anderson et al. 2004). Affected areas also implemented social measures, such as closing entertainment venues and schools (Pang et al. 2003); however, these measures had limited impact on reducing SARS transmission, because most spread occurred in health care settings, elderly care facilities, and households rather than in the broader community. The swine-origin influenza A (H1N1) 2009 pandemic began with initial cases in Mexico and the United States in April 2009. In Mexico, the government implemented PHSM, including social measures such as suspending most social gatherings and closing schools (Vargas-Parada 2009). Because the clinical severity of the influenza A (H1N1) 2009 pandemic was comparable to that of seasonal influenza (Presanis et al. 2009), most countries did not implement social measures apart from school closures, which were adopted in some regions (Cauchemez et al. 2014).

## PHSM FOR PANDEMIC INFLUENZA IN THE TWENTIETH CENTURY

Three influenza pandemics took place in the twentieth century: the Spanish flu in 1918, the Asian flu in 1957, and the Hong Kong flu in 1968. Because of the devastating impacts of these pandemics, the importance of pandemic preparedness was recognized decades ago. Nonetheless, programs on pandemic preparedness at both global and country levels did not begin until the late 1990s.

The highly pathogenic avian influenza A (H5N1) outbreak, with the first confirmed human cases, including six deaths, occurred in Hong Kong SAR, China, in 1997. Since the end of 2003, highly pathogenic avian influenza A (H5N1) has caused outbreaks worldwide in wild and domestic birds, with sporadic human infections with a high case-fatality ratio (Lai et al. 2016). These epidemics heightened concerns about pandemics with significant mortality impacts.

The World Health Organization (WHO) published its first pandemic preparedness plan in 1999, and revised it in 2005 (WHO 2005). Although the revised plan recommended various PHSM during different phases of a pandemic, evidence related to PHSM was limited. In 2006, the WHO writing group published two review articles summarizing the available evidence on PHSM (Bell et al. 2006a, 2006b). The group concluded that "the knowledge base for use in developing guidance for non-pharmaceutical interventions for influenza is limited" (Bell et al. 2006b, 92).

## STRATEGIC OBJECTIVES FOR PANDEMIC RESPONSE AND ROLES OF PHSM

Before the COVID-19 pandemic, the primary strategic objective for pandemic response in most countries was mitigation. *Mitigation* aims to slow the spread of disease and reduce the peak number of cases, thereby alleviating health care demands on hospitals and infrastructure (figure 6.1). The US government published interim guidance on pandemic influenza mitigation in 2007, which it revised in 2017 (Qualls et al. 2020). This guidance emphasized a pandemic mitigation framework based on "an early, targeted, layered application of multiple partially effective non-pharmaceutical measures" (CDC 2007, 8). It recommended a wide range of PHSM but did not recommend stringent measures such as stay-at-home orders and travel restrictions because of their high economic and social costs.

In general, it is challenging to achieve the two objectives of minimizing the health impact of a pandemic using PHSM and reducing social and economic costs associated with PHSM (Hollingsworth et al. 2011). Mitigation guidelines for pandemics in most countries before COVID-19 focused on avoiding social and economic disruptions. Implementing stringent measures was often considered both unrealistic and unfeasible.

Another possible strategic objective of PHSM for pandemics is *containment*, defined as the interruption of all chains of transmission within a target area. Infectious diseases such as Ebola virus disease and SARS have been successfully contained primarily through active case finding and contact identification measures; however, the feasibility of containment depends on the transmission

**Figure 6.1** Strategic Objectives of Pandemic Response

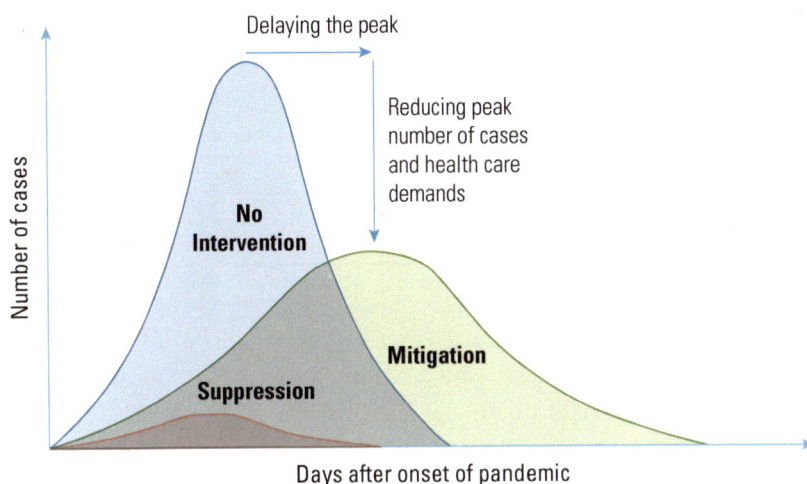

*Source:* Adapted from Qualls et al. 2020 and Wu et al. 2021.

dynamics of the specific disease. If transmissions occur before symptom onset (presymptomatic transmission) or from individuals without symptoms (asymptomatic transmission), and transmissibility is high, containment becomes unfeasible (Fraser et al. 2004). As such, containment has typically been considered only for exceptional situations or during the early stages of an influenza pandemic.

COVID-19 exhibited different epidemiological characteristics from past influenza pandemics. The basic reproduction number ($R_0$), representing the average number of secondary cases generated by a primary case, indicates transmissibility. The estimated $R_0$ of the original strain of COVID-19 exceeds 3.0 (Liu et al. 2020), substantially higher than the estimated $R_0$ of 1.8 for the 1918 Spanish flu pandemic (Biggerstaff et al. 2014). COVID-19 also has a considerable mortality impact, particularly among the elderly. Models predicted significant mortality impacts with adoption of a mitigation approach (Davies et al. 2020; Ferguson et al. 2020). Simultaneously, the high transmissibility of COVID-19 and the presence of presymptomatic and asymptomatic transmissions made containment exceptionally challenging.

Consequently, many countries pursued a third strategic objective, suppression (Wu et al. 2021) (figure 6.1). *Suppression* involves reducing community infections to very low levels by implementing PHSM. Achieving suppression for COVID-19, however, requires stringent measures, such as stay-at-home orders. Even when suppression is attained, a surge in cases is likely once control measures are lifted (Anderson et al. 2020). With rising numbers of severe cases and deaths, most countries eventually adopted this approach, employing strict PHSM, including stay-at-home orders (also called "lockdown"). For example, Italy implemented stringent stay-at-home measures in early March 2020 in response to increasing numbers of severe cases and an overwhelming burden on the health care system (Boccia, Ricciardi, and Ioannidis 2020). The United States had also implemented stay-at-home measures by early April 2020, with significant variations between and within states (Haffajee and Mello 2020). PHSM to suppress the transmission during the COVID-19 pandemic had a critical role in reducing the health care burden when specific treatment and vaccines were not available (Li et al. 2021).

## SCIENTIFIC EVIDENCE FOR PHSM

Significant research has been conducted over the past decades to address the knowledge gaps related to PHSM, especially during the COVID-19 pandemic. WHO established the PHSM Knowledge Hub, which includes the PHSM Bibliographic Library.[1] Despite this effort and others, substantial gaps remain (Majeed et al. 2024). For example, because of ethical and practical constraints, very few randomized controlled trials—considered the gold standard for generating high-quality evidence—were conducted on PHSM for COVID-19 (Enria et al. 2021). Many PHSM, especially social and travel-related measures, are implemented only during severe epidemics and pandemics, resulting in limited real-world data on their impact or effectiveness. Most studies analyzing real-world data are observational and thus prone to various biases and confounding factors. Nonetheless, because they can be conducted rapidly and relatively easily, observational studies provide crucial information during the early stages of epidemics and pandemics. Standardized master protocols developed before epidemics and pandemics can be useful for obtaining more robust evidence (Ricotta et al. 2023).

An additional challenge lies in assessing the effectiveness of individual measures. During severe epidemics or pandemics, the simultaneous implementation of multiple measures makes it difficult or impossible to isolate the impact of each measure. Policy recommendations and decisions must invariably be made under high uncertainty in weighing the benefits and harms of any specific policy. Policy makers are responsible for considering a wide variety of information about the potential impacts of any policy, including considering equity and vulnerable populations when making decisions.

Given the scarcity of real-world data, mathematical modeling has been used extensively to estimate the theoretical impact or effectiveness of PHSM (Ahmed, Zviedrite, and Uzicanin 2018). Applying mathematical models to assess PHSM presents its own set of challenges, however. For instance, these models often rely on parameters that may not be readily available, particularly in the early stages of a pandemic (James et al. 2021). Furthermore, incorporating individual differences as well as population or international differences into mathematical models remains a significant hurdle (Afzal et al. 2022). Integrating both epidemiological and economic information into a model is critical to support evidence-informed policy making (WHO, OECD, and World Bank 2024).

## PHSM IMPLEMENTED FOR COVID-19

The COVID-19 pandemic witnessed an unprecedented level of implementation of PHSM. Among the many studies conducted on PHSM for COVID-19 (Fadlallah et al. 2024), some studies have shown the public health impact of PHSM in reducing transmission and mortality (Haug et al. 2020; Li et al. 2021; Talic et al. 2021). Others have also shown the significant negative social and economic consequences of such measures (Li, Taeihagh, and Tan 2023; Onyeaka et al. 2021). None of the PHSM can entirely eliminate transmission; rather, multiple measures must be combined for effective transmission reduction (Li et al. 2021). Furthermore, the impact of individual PHSM depends on factors such as the timing of implementation, the evolving knowledge and understanding of transmission characteristics of the pathogen in question, and adherence to the policies. Significant knowledge gaps persist in developing effective PHSM policies (Majeed et al. 2024), particularly in the early stages of an outbreak or pandemic when the transmission characteristics are not well understood. Policy makers and other stakeholders must, therefore, carefully consider the benefits, limitations, uncertainties, and potential negative consequences of PHSM when designing strategies for future epidemics or pandemics.

Many countries implemented measures, such as stay-at-home orders and travel restrictions, previously considered unrealistic because of their associated social and economic disruptions. Other extensively implemented PHSM included the widespread use of face masks, surface cleaning, and promotion of hand hygiene. A meta-analysis concluded that, of those measures, hand hygiene, face masks, and physical distancing were effective in reducing transmission and mortality of COVID-19 (Talic et al. 2021); however, changing or inconsistent recommendations from health authorities, particularly regarding the use of face masks, created substantial public confusion (Greenhalgh et al. 2020). Moreover, some measures that had limited effectiveness in reducing transmission, such as surface cleaning, were widely adopted. The following subsections discuss key issues related to the implementation of specific PHSM during COVID-19.

### Lockdowns and Stay-at-Home Measures

During the COVID-19 pandemic, most countries implemented various social measures, such as school and workplace closures, bans on social gatherings, and physical distancing. Many countries also introduced more stringent measures to minimize person-to-person contact, including lockdowns or stay-at-home orders.

*Lockdown* broadly refers to large-scale communitywide measures and movement restrictions imposed during COVID-19; however, no universally accepted definition of lockdown exists (Haider et al. 2020). Historically, lockdowns prohibited the free movement of people within a building or area and were implemented for infectious diseases like the plague and cholera under the concept of "sanitary cordons" (Tognotti 2013). Lockdowns were also implemented for more recent outbreaks, such as SARS in 2003 and Ebola virus disease in 2014; however, the Ebola lockdowns were criticized as violations of human rights and contributors to humanitarian crises (Eba 2014).

On January 23, 2020, a citywide lockdown and other stringent measures—including suspension of outbound transportation, traffic restrictions within the city, and cancellation of social gatherings—were imposed in Wuhan, China, the epicenter of COVID-19. Additional measures, such as stay-at-home orders for all residents, followed on February 2, 2020 (Pan et al. 2020). These actions successfully contained initial outbreaks in Wuhan and other Chinese cities (Tian et al. 2020).

By mid-March 2020, COVID-19 had caused widespread community transmission in Europe and North America. Some Western countries had shifted their strategies from containment to mitigation, deeming containment unfeasible for COVID-19 (Parodi and Liu 2020). For instance, on March 12, 2020, the UK government transitioned from the containment phase to the delay phase, announcing that it would not implement school closures and bans on mass gatherings (Scally, Jacobson, and Abbasi 2020). With a rise in severe cases and deaths, however, the UK government announced a nationwide lockdown on March 23, 2020. Other countries, including the United States, followed suit. As noted earlier, studies show that a combination of PHSM, including stay-at-home measures, effectively reduced COVID-19 transmission (Haug et al. 2020; Li et al. 2021).

## Travel-Related Measures

Another critical but controversial strategy during the COVID-19 pandemic involved travel-related measures, particularly travel restrictions. WHO issued travel advisories for COVID-19, which it revised multiple times. Despite WHO's ongoing recommendation against travel and trade restrictions under the International Health Regulations, most countries imposed some form of travel restriction during the pandemic (Von Tigerstrom and Wilson 2020).

WHO advises that restricting the movement of people and goods is ineffective in most public health emergencies, including infectious disease outbreaks. A systematic review on travel measures for pandemic influenza in 2014 concluded that "extensive travel restrictions may delay the dissemination of influenza but cannot prevent it" (Mateus et al. 2014, 868). However, a mathematical modeling study indicated that Wuhan's lockdown, including restricted movement out of the city, potentially reduced exported cases by approximately 80 percent by mid-February 2020 (Chinazzi et al. 2020). Once considered unfeasible, mandatory quarantine for incoming passengers was also implemented in China and other countries (Tu et al. 2021). A 2021 systematic review concluded that travel measures played a significant role in shaping the early transmission dynamics of COVID-19 (Grépin et al. 2021).

Despite these findings, a modeling study analyzing data from 162 countries indicated that even stringent travel restrictions had limited effects on local transmission in countries with widespread community transmission (Russell et al. 2021). That is, in regions where transmission was suppressed, strict travel measures were beneficial; however, areas with extensive community spread saw minimal benefits. Therefore, reducing the international spread of COVID-19 required a harmonized and coordinated approach (Von Tigerstrom and Wilson 2020).

Travel restrictions during COVID-19 were associated with significant economic and social consequences (Bonaccorsi et al. 2020). The implementation in many countries of restrictions that contradicted WHO guidance based on the International Health Regulations raised concerns about the infringement of fundamental human rights (Sekalala et al. 2020) and violations of international law (Habibi et al. 2020).

## TRANSMISSION DYNAMICS OF COVID-19 AND PHSM POLICIES

Conflicting information and confusion regarding the transmission characteristics and dynamics of COVID-19 affected policies related to PHSM. Early data revealed that presymptomatic transmission was common (Wei et al. 2020), indicating that individuals without symptoms could still act as transmission sources. This finding had significant implications for face mask policies.

Widespread debate and confusion surrounding face masks resulted from conflicting messages and inconsistent recommendations. Initially, WHO and some national authorities recommended the use of face masks only by symptomatic individuals and in health care settings. They did not advise universal masking—that is, wearing face masks by the general public, including those without symptoms (Feng et al. 2020). Their recommendations were based on influenza data, which showed that wearing face masks during illness had some protective effect in reducing onward transmission but provided limited evidence for preventing infection in those who wear masks (Cowling et al. 2010); however, a 2020 systematic review concluded that universal masking in the community could be beneficial (MacIntyre and Chughtai 2020). In June 2020, WHO updated its recommendations, advising governments to encourage the general public to wear masks in specific situations and settings.

Environmental measures, such as surface and object cleaning and disinfection, and personal protective measures, including hand hygiene and cough etiquette, have been widely implemented for seasonal and pandemic influenza as well as for COVID-19. The effectiveness of these measures depends on the mode of transmission of the pathogen. The modes of influenza transmission have long been debated, with three main modes previously considered: droplet, contact, and airborne transmission (Brankston et al. 2007). *Droplet* transmission involves large particles, generated by infected individuals, that travel short distances (less than 1 meter). *Airborne* transmission involves smaller particles suspended in the air and that can travel long distances. *Contact* transmission can occur through direct contact with infected individuals or indirect contact with contaminated surfaces (fomite transmission). Generally, droplet and contact transmission were considered the primary modes for influenza transmission, with airborne transmission playing a limited role (Brankston et al. 2007). A newer concept of *aerosol* transmission emerged, however, suggesting that infected individuals generate particles of varying sizes and that smaller particles can remain suspended in the air, facilitating both short- and long-distance transmission (Tellier 2009).

WHO and some national authorities adopted inconsistent positions regarding the transmission modes of COVID-19 (Jimenez et al. 2022). A scientific brief published by WHO on March 29, 2020, stated that SARS-CoV-2 is primarily transmitted through respiratory droplets and contact transmission, with no reported airborne transmission (WHO 2020). Growing evidence suggested, however, that aerosol transmission could be a significant mode of COVID-19 spread (Morawska and Milton 2020). In December 2021, WHO acknowledged airborne transmission, now referred to as "transmission through the air" (Greenhalgh et al. 2024), as an important mode of spread. This delay in revising WHO's position had significant implications for PHSM policies, particularly in terms of environmental and personal protective measures.

During the early phase of the pandemic, the assumption that fomite transmission was a major route of spread resulted in extensive efforts to implement disinfection, surface cleaning, and hand hygiene—necessary measures in health care facilities and households with confirmed or suspected cases. The risk of fomite transmission in the community was found to be low, however, and surface cleaning had limited effectiveness in reducing transmission (Pitol and Julian 2021). Conversely, increasing ventilation—a highly effective measure to mitigate airborne or aerosol transmission (Tang et al. 2020)— was not widely prioritized during the pandemic's early stages. Understanding the relative importance of different transmission modes is critical for implementing effective environmental and personal protective measures.

## LESSONS FROM COVID-19

The implementation of PHSM during COVID-19 provided several important lessons. Before the COVID-19 pandemic, WHO and most countries focused primarily on influenza pandemics in their preparedness plans. Because the epidemiological characteristics of COVID-19 differed from those of past influenza pandemics, however, strategies for PHSM developed for influenza pandemics proved less effective for COVID-19. Stringent measures, such as lockdowns and travel restrictions, were not considered even for severe influenza pandemics, because mitigation was the primary strategic objective for such scenarios.

COVID-19's much higher transmissibility compared to past pandemics, including the 1918 influenza pandemic, meant that a mitigation approach would not have had a significant impact on mortality. Additionally, China's experience demonstrated the possibility of containment or suppression with highly stringent PHSM. Many countries ultimately implemented stringent measures, such as stay-at-home orders and travel restrictions, although implementation of these measures was delayed in Europe and North America compared to East Asia and the Pacific (Liu et al. 2021).

Europe and North America had significantly higher numbers of reported deaths per population during the first year of the COVID-19 pandemic (Jamison and Wu 2021), suggesting that, generally, early implementation of PHSM is more effective in reducing transmission (Jamison and Wu 2021).

Another unique characteristic of COVID-19 was the emergence of multiple variants and subvariants. Variants or subvariants become dominant when they acquire transmission advantages over previously circulating strains. For SARS-CoV-2, these advantages include increased transmissibility and immune escape capabilities, enabling the virus to evade immunity from previous infections or vaccinations. Immune escape reduces vaccine effectiveness, and increased transmissibility diminishes the effectiveness of PHSM. Higher transmissibility necessitates more stringent PHSM to suppress transmission. After the emergence of the Omicron variant, which was significantly more transmissible than earlier strains, achieving suppression through PHSM alone became unfeasible in many regions, underscoring the importance of understanding transmission characteristics when formulating PHSM policies.

Variations in reporting systems, definitions of COVID-19-associated deaths, and ascertainment practices make comparisons of mortality impacts between countries difficult. Excess death estimates, or deaths attributable to COVID-19, have been used to address this issue. Several such estimates have been published, including by WHO (Callaway 2021). According to the WHO estimates, excess deaths were significantly higher in 2021 (10.36 million) than in 2020 (4.47 million). The highest excess deaths occurred in mid-2021, during the period when the more virulent Delta variant was dominant.

India had particularly high excess deaths in 2021 (3.9 million) compared to 2020 (0.8 million). Despite implementing strict lockdowns in 2020, India was unprepared for the surge in cases caused by the Delta variant, first detected in the country in April 2021. Although India began its vaccine rollout in January 2021, only 6.1 percent of the population had received the second dose by July 2021 (Choudhary, Choudhary, and Singh 2021). Clinical care capacities were also inadequate, with severe shortages of medical oxygen posing significant barriers to saving lives.

When PHSM effectively suppress transmission, most of the population remains susceptible to infection unless vaccinated, because natural exposure to the virus is minimized. In India, this susceptibility allowed the more transmissible and virulent Delta variant to spread rapidly. The experience in India highlights the critical need to accelerate preparedness efforts while transmission is suppressed, including expanding vaccination coverage and enhancing clinical care capacity.

## Adherence to PHSM Policies for COVID-19

Although many countries implemented similar policies of PHSM during the COVID-19 pandemic (Hale et al. 2021), adherence to policies varied between countries and between communities. Studies from various settings conclude that adherence to PHSM depends on multiple interrelated factors. Older adults and women reported higher compliance with measures such as hand hygiene and social distancing (Armitage et al. 2021). Psychological factors also play a prominent role. Higher risk perception and self-efficacy were linked with protective behavior (Murukutla et al. 2022; Savadori and Lauriola 2021). Social determinants further shape behavior. For example, social support and trust in the government facilitate adherence (Han et al. 2023; Smith et al. 2020), whereas economic constraints, cultural norms, and occupation-related demands serve as barriers (Coetzee and Kagee 2020; Nivette et al. 2021). Considering the various factors involved in adherence to PHSM, increasing adherence requires effective risk communication and active community engagement (Gilmore et al. 2020; Heydari et al. 2021).

### Social and Economic Impacts Associated with PHSM for COVID-19

The COVID-19 pandemic and associated PHSM have had significant and uneven socioeconomic impacts across different countries and social groups (Osterrieder et al. 2021; Zhou and Kan 2021), disproportionately affecting vulnerable populations, such as the elderly, children, low-income groups, and minorities (Li, Taeihagh, and Tan 2023). The pandemic has exacerbated existing inequalities and led to increased poverty (Gerszon Mahler, Yonzan, and Lakner 2022) and domestic violence (Kourti et al. 2023). Although effective in controlling virus transmission, social distancing measures have also resulted in negative psychological consequences, including anxiety, depression, and loneliness (Bu, Steptoe, and Fancourt 2020; Fancourt, Steptoe, and Bu 2021).

The COVID-19 pandemic has had a severe and widespread impact on businesses globally, particularly small enterprises (Apedo-Amah et al. 2020). Many businesses experienced significant drops in sales, with some facing temporary closures and layoffs (Bartik et al. 2020). Small businesses, often with limited cash reserves to weather the crisis, were found to be financially fragile (Bartik et al. 2020). In response, many businesses turned to digital solutions and sought government aid, though concerns about accessing such support were common (Apedo-Amah et al. 2020; Bartik et al. 2020).

A systematic review of studies on the cost-effectiveness of control strategies for COVID-19 in Europe and Organisation for Economic Co-operation and Development countries indicated that the cost-effectiveness of physical distancing measures depends on the duration, compliance, and the phase of the epidemic (Vardavas et al. 2023). Implementation of PHSM should involve consideration of the economic costs associated with them.

### Lessons from COVID-19 in Low- and Middle-Income Countries

Most low- and middle-income countries (LMICs) implemented stringent measures, including lockdowns (Haider et al. 2020; Jang et al. 2021). The data indicate that even stringent measures did not successfully contain COVID-19 in LMICs

(Jang et al. 2021). Several reasons could account for that unsuccessful containment. For instance, many LMICs followed measures implemented in high-income countries, and those measures were not always context-specific or evidence-based (Alakija 2023). Sociocultural factors, such as distrust, misinformation, and denial, hindered the implementation of PHSM, and religious and social norms sometimes conflicted with certain measures in LMICs (Mackworth-Young et al. 2021; Zakar et al. 2021). A high proportion of people in LMICs works in the informal sector, making it impossible for them to comply with social distancing measures (Jang et al. 2021). LMICs should invest in research capacity to generate real-time evidence data to inform control policies. Community engagement is critical to implementing effective and context-specific control measures (Shafique et al. 2024).

## PHSM for Future Epidemics and Pandemics

The COVID-19 pandemic offers many lessons because it saw implementation of the most stringent PHSM in history. A comprehensive report from the European Centre for Disease Prevention and Control summarizes the lessons from COVID-19 and recommendations for future pandemics (ECDC 2024). Every epidemic and pandemic is unique, however, and some lessons from COVID-19 may not apply to future events. The public health impact and effectiveness of PHSM depend on the epidemiological characteristics of the target pathogen, including the relative importance of different transmission modes, transmissibility, and population susceptibility.

Most PHSM, particularly social and travel measures, have significant social and economic consequences. Policies regarding PHSM should strike a balance between the benefits of implementation and potential unintended adverse effects. Generally, more stringent measures, such as stay-at-home orders, are more effective in reducing the transmission of the virus; however, such measures often come with high social and economic costs. Another critical factor to consider is the severity of the epidemic or pandemic. For extremely severe events, implementing stringent measures may be justifiable, even if they are associated with significant costs. This was the case during the first year of the COVID-19 pandemic. Conversely, stringent measures may not be implemented for less severe epidemics or pandemics, even if they are effective.

The severity of an epidemic or pandemic is not limited to clinical severity. WHO's Pandemic Influenza Severity Assessment uses four main indicators to evaluate severity: (1) transmissibility, (2) seriousness of the disease, (3) morbidity and mortality, and (4) impact on health care capacity (WHO 2024b). *Transmissibility* refers to the number of individuals who become infected. *Seriousness* is measured by the proportion of severe illnesses among those infected. *Morbidity and mortality* quantify the number of serious diseases and deaths in the population. The *impact on health care capacity* evaluates how an outbreak affects health care systems, including providing care for non-outbreak-related conditions. Because risk can vary between and within countries, risk assessment should be conducted at national and local levels. The International Health Regulations, revised in 2005, request countries to take a risk-based approach in implementing control measures. There is no "one-size-fits-all" approach to PHSM implementation.

The mortality impact of the next pandemic could differ significantly from COVID-19. For example, it could be much lower, as seen in the 2009 A (H1N1) pandemic, or far more devastating, potentially resulting in up to 100 million deaths (Jamison et al. 2024). Age groups vulnerable to severe illness and death may also differ. Whereas COVID-19 predominantly affected the elderly, the 1957 Asian flu caused significant excess deaths in children under five years of age (Viboud et al. 2015). The 1918 Spanish flu had elevated mortality rates among young children, young adults, and the elderly, with nearly half of the deaths occurring in individuals ages 20–40 years (Taubenberger and Morens 2006). If a future pandemic primarily affects younger age groups, it could have substantially greater social impact than COVID-19, and mortality rates could be higher in LMICs, which have younger populations. In such a scenario, preventing devastating mortality impacts may require more stringent PHSM, particularly in LMICs.

## CONCLUSION

PHSM, implemented at an unprecedented level during the COVID-19 pandemic, played critical roles in reducing its impact, particularly before vaccines became available. None of the measures, however, could completely interrupt the transmission. Stringent measures were associated with various unintended negative consequences, with many countries implementing some unnecessary or excessive measures. The effectiveness of each measure depends on several factors, such as transmission characteristics of the target pathogen, the timing of implementation, and people's adherence to policies. High-quality evidence is still lacking for most of the PHSM. There are no "blanket measures" for the next epidemic and pandemic: policies on PHSM should grow from a risk-based approach with comprehensive and real-time risk assessments at global, national, and local levels.

## NOTE

1. For more on the PHSM Knowledge Hub and its resources, refer to its website, https://ephsm.who.int/en.

## REFERENCES

Afzal, A., C. A. Saleel, S. Bhattacharyya, N. Satish, O. D. Samuel, and I. A. Badruddin. 2022. "Merits and Limitations of Mathematical Modeling and Computational Simulations in Mitigation of COVID-19 Pandemic: A Comprehensive Review." *Archives of Computational Methods in Engineering* 29 (2): 1311–37. https://doi.org/10.1007/s11831-021-09634-2.

Ahmed, F., N. Zviedrite, and A. Uzicanin. 2018. "Effectiveness of Workplace Social Distancing Measures in Reducing Influenza Transmission: A Systematic Review." *BMC Public Health* 18 (1). https://doi.org/10.1186/S12889-018-5446-1.

Alakija, A. 2023. "Leveraging Lessons from the COVID-19 Pandemic to Strengthen Low-Income and Middle-Income Country Preparedness for Future Global Health Threats." *The Lancet Infectious Diseases* 23 (8): e310–17. https://doi.org/10.1016/S1473-3099(23)00279-7.

Anderson, R. M., C. Fraser, A. C. Ghani, C. A. Donnelly, S. Riley, N. M. Ferguson, G. M. Leung, et al. 2004. "Epidemiology, Transmission Dynamics and Control of SARS: The 2002–2003 Epidemic." *Philosophical Transactions of the Royal Society B: Biological Sciences* 359 (1447). https://doi.org/10.1098/rstb.2004.1490.

Anderson, R. M., H. Heesterbeek, D. Klinkenberg, and T. D. Hollingsworth. 2020. "How Will Country-Based Mitigation Measures Influence the Course of the COVID-19 Epidemic?" *The Lancet* 395 (10228): 931–34. https://doi.org/10.1016/S0140-6736(20)30567-5.

Apedo-Amah, M. C., B. Avdiu, X. Cirera, M. Cruz, E. Davies, A. Grover, L. Iacovone, et al. 2020. "Unmasking the Impact of COVID-19 on Businesses: Firm Level Evidence from across the World." Policy Research Working Paper 9434, World Bank, Washington, DC. https://documents1.worldbank.org/curated/en/399751602248069405/pdf/Unmasking-the-Impact-of-COVID-19-on-Businesses-Firm-Level-Evidence-from-Across-the-World.pdf.

Armitage, C. J., C. Keyworth, J. Z. Leather, L. Byrne-Davis, and T. Epton. 2021. "Identifying Targets for Interventions to Support Public Adherence to Government Instructions to Reduce Transmission of SARS-CoV-2." *BMC Public Health* 21 (1): 1–6. https://doi.org/10.1186/S12889-021-10574-6/TABLES/2.

Bartik, A. W., M. Bertrand, Z. Cullen, E. L. Glaeser, M. Luca, and C. Stanton. 2020. "The Impact of COVID-19 on Small Business Outcomes and Expectations." *Proceedings of the National Academy of Sciences of the United States of America* 117 (30): 17656–66. https://doi.org/10.1073/PNAS.2006991117/SUPPL_FILE/PNAS.2006991117.SAPP.PDF.

Bell, D., A. Nicoll, K. Fukuda, P. Horby, A. Monto, F. Hayden, C. Wylks, et al. 2006a. "Nonpharmaceutical Interventions for Pandemic Influenza, International Measures." *Emerging Infectious Diseases* 12 (1): 81. https://doi.org/10.3201/EID1201.051370.

Bell, D., A. Nicoll, K. Fukuda, P. Horby, A. Monto, F. Hayden, C. Wylks, et al. 2006b. "Nonpharmaceutical Interventions for Pandemic Influenza, National and Community Measures." *Emerging Infectious Diseases* 12 (1): 88. https://doi.org/10.3201/EID1201.051371.

Belshe, R. B. 2012. "A Century of Influenza Prevention in St. Louis." *Missouri Medicine* 109 (2).

Biggerstaff, M., S. Cauchemez, C. Reed, M. Gambhir, and L. Finelli. 2014. "Estimates of the Reproduction Number for Seasonal, Pandemic, and Zoonotic Influenza: A Systematic Review of the Literature." *BMC Infectious Diseases* 14 (1). https://doi.org/10.1186/1471-2334-14-480.

Boccia, S., W. Ricciardi, and J. P. A. Ioannidis. 2020. "What Other Countries Can Learn from Italy during the COVID-19 Pandemic." *JAMA Internal Medicine* 180 (7): 927–28. https://doi.org/10.1001/jamainternmed.2020.1447.

Bonaccorsi, G., F. Pierri, M. Cinelli, A. Flori, A. Galeazzi, F. Porcelli, A. L. Schmidt, et al. 2020. "Economic and Social Consequences of Human Mobility Restrictions under COVID-19." *Proceedings of the National Academy of Sciences of the United States of America* 117 (27). https://doi.org/10.1073/pnas.2007658117.

Brankston, G., L. Gitterman, Z. Hirji, C. Lemieux, and M. Gardam. 2007. "Transmission of Influenza A in Human Beings." *The Lancet Infectious Diseases* 7 (4): 257–65. https://doi.org/10.1016/S1473-3099(07)70029-4.

Bu, F., A. Steptoe, and D. Fancourt. 2020. "Who Is Lonely in Lockdown? Cross-Cohort Analyses of Predictors of Loneliness before and during the COVID-19 Pandemic." *Public Health* 186 (September): 31–34. https://doi.org/10.1016/J.PUHE.2020.06.036.

Callaway, E. 2021. "Delta Coronavirus Variant: Scientists Brace for Impact." *Nature* 595 (7865): 17–18. https://doi.org/10.1038/d41586-021-01696-3.

Cauchemez, S., M. D. Van Kerkhove, B. N. Archer, M. Cetron, B. J. Cowling, P. Grove, D. Hunt, et al. 2014. "School Closures during the 2009 Influenza Pandemic: National and Local Experiences." *BMC Infectious Diseases* 14 (1). https://doi.org/10.1186/1471-2334-14-207.

CDC (US Centers for Disease Control and Prevention). 2007. "Interim Pre-pandemic Planning Guidance: Community Strategy for Pandemic Influenza Mitigation in the United States—Early, Targeted, Layered Use of Nonpharmaceutical Interventions." CDC, Atlanta. https://stacks.cdc.gov/view/cdc/11425.

Chinazzi, M., J. T. Davis, M. Ajelli, C. Gioannini, M. Litvinova, S. Merler, A. Pastore y Piontti, et al. 2020. "The Effect of Travel Restrictions on the Spread of the 2019 Novel Coronavirus (COVID-19) Outbreak." *Science* 368 (6489): 395–400. https://doi.org/10.1126/science.aba9757.

Choudhary, O. P., P. Choudhary, and I. Singh. 2021. "India's COVID-19 Vaccination Drive: Key Challenges and Resolutions." *The Lancet Infectious Diseases* 21 (11): 1483–84. https://doi.org/10.1016/S1473-3099(21)00567-3.

Coetzee, B. J., and A. Kagee. 2020. "Structural Barriers to Adhering to Health Behaviours in the Context of the COVID-19 Crisis: Considerations for Low- and Middle-Income Countries." *Global Public Health* 15 (8): 1093–102. https://doi.org/10.1080/17441692.2020.1779331.

Cowling, B. J., Y. Zhou, D. K. M. Ip, G. M. Leung, and A. E. Aiello. 2010. "Face Masks to Prevent Transmission of Influenza Virus: A Systematic Review." *Epidemiology and Infection* 138 (4): 449–56. https://doi.org/10.1017/S0950268809991658.

Davies, N. G., A. J. Kucharski, R. M. Eggo, A. Gimma, W. J. Edmunds, T. Jombart, K. O'Reilly, et al. 2020. "Effects of Non-pharmaceutical Interventions on COVID-19 Cases, Deaths, and Demand for Hospital Services in the UK: A Modelling Study." *The Lancet Public Health* 5 (7): e375–85. https://doi.org/10.1016/S2468-2667(20)30133-X.

Eba, P. M. 2014. "Ebola and Human Rights in West Africa." *The Lancet* 384 (9960): 2091–93. https://doi.org/10.1016/S0140-6736(14)61412-4.

ECDC (European Centre for Disease Prevention and Control). 2024. "Public Health and Social Measures for Health Emergencies and Pandemics in the EU/EEA: Recommendations for Strengthening Preparedness Planning." Technical Report, ECDC, Stockholm. https://www.ecdc.europa.eu/en/publications-data/public-health-and-social-measures-health-emergencies-and-pandemics.

Enria, D., Z. Feng, A. Fretheim, C. Ihekweazu, T. Ottersen, A. Schuchat, K. Ungchusak, et al. 2021. "Strengthening the Evidence Base for Decisions on Public Health and Social Measures." *Bulletin of the World Health Organization* 99 (9): 610–10A. https://pmc.ncbi.nlm.nih.gov/articles/PMC8381089/.

Fadlallah, R., F. El-Jardali, L. Bou Karroum, N. Kalach, R. Hoteit, A. Aoun, L. Al-Hakim, et al. 2024. "The Effects of Public Health and Social Measures (PHSM) Implemented during the COVID-19 Pandemic: An Overview of Systematic Reviews." *Cochrane Evidence Synthesis and Methods* 2 (5): e12055. https://doi.org/10.1002/CESM.12055.

Fancourt, D., A. Steptoe, and F. Bu. 2021. "Trajectories of Anxiety and Depressive Symptoms during Enforced Isolation Due to COVID-19 in England: A Longitudinal Observational Study." *The Lancet Psychiatry* 8 (2): 141–49. https://doi.org/10.1016/S2215-0366(20)30482-X.

Feng, S., C. Shen, N. Xia, W. Song, M. Fan, and B. J. Cowling. 2020. "Rational Use of Face Masks in the COVID-19 Pandemic." *The Lancet Respiratory Medicine* 8 (5): 434–36. https://doi.org/10.1016/S2213-2600(20)30134-X.

Ferguson, N. M., D. Laydon, G. Nedjati-Gilani, N. Imai, K. Ainslie, M. Baguelin, S. Bhatia, et al. 2020. "Impact of Non-pharmaceutical Interventions (NPIs) to Reduce COVID-19 Mortality and Healthcare Demand." Report No. 9, Imperial College COVID-19 Response Team, Imperial College London. https://www.imperial.ac.uk/media/imperial-college/medicine/sph/ide/gida-fellowships/Imperial-College-COVID19-NPI-modelling-16-03-2020.pdf.

Fraser, C., S. Riley, R. M. Anderson, and N. M. Ferguson. 2004. "Factors That Make an Infectious Disease Outbreak Controllable." *Proceedings of the National Academy of Sciences of the United States of America* 101 (16): 6146–51.

Gerszon Mahler, D., N. Yonzan, and C. Lakner. 2022. "The Impact of COVID-19 on Global Inequality and Poverty." Policy Research Working Paper 10198, World Bank, Washington, DC. https://openknowledge.worldbank.org/entities/publication/54fae299-8800-585f-9f18 -a42514f8d83b.

Gilmore, B., R. Ndejjo, A. Tchetchia, V. De Claro, E. Mago, A. A. Diallo, C. Lopes, and S. Bhattacharyya. 2020. "Community Engagement for COVID-19 Prevention and Control: A Rapid Evidence Synthesis." *BMJ Global Health* 5 (10): 3188. https://doi.org/10.1136 /BMJGH-2020-003188.

Greenhalgh, T., M. B. Schmid, T. Czypionka, D. Bassler, and L. Gruer. 2020. "Face Masks for the Public during the Covid-19 Crisis." *BMJ* 369 (April). https://doi.org/10.1136/BMJ .M1435.

Greenhalgh, T., C. R. MacIntyre, M. Ungrin, and J. M. Wright. 2024. "Airborne Pathogens: Controlling Words Won't Control Transmission." *The Lancet* 403 (10439): 1850–51. https://doi.org/10.1016/S0140-6736(24)00244-7.

Grépin, K. A., T.-L. Ho, Z. Liu, S. Marion, J. Piper, C. Z. Worsnop, and K. Lee. 2021. "Evidence of the Effectiveness of Travel-Related Measures during the Early Phase of the COVID-19 Pandemic: A Rapid Systematic Review." *BMJ Global Health* 6 (3). https://doi.org/10.1136 /bmjgh-2020-004537.

Habibi, R., G. L. Burci, T. C. de Campos, D. Chirwa, M. Cinà, S. Dagron, M. Eccleston-Turner, et al. 2020. "Do Not Violate the International Health Regulations during the COVID-19 Outbreak." *The Lancet* 395 (10225): 664–66. https://doi.org/10.1016/S0140-6736(20)30373-1.

Haffajee, R. L., and M. M. Mello. 2020. "Thinking Globally, Acting Locally—The U.S. Response to Covid-19." *New England Journal of Medicine* 382 (22). https://doi.org/10.1056 /NEJMP2006740/SUPPL_FILE/NEJMP2006740_DISCLOSURES.PDF.

Haider, N., A. Y. Osman, A. Gadzekpo, G. O. Akipede, D. Asogun, R. Ansumana, R. John Lessells, et al. 2020. "Lockdown Measures in Response to COVID-19 in Nine Sub-Saharan African Countries." *BMJ Global Health* 5 (10): 21. https://doi.org/10.1136/BMJGH-2020 -003319.

Hale, T., N. Angrist, R. Goldszmidt, B. Kira, A. Petherick, T. Phillips, S. Webster, et al. 2021. "A Global Panel Database of Pandemic Policies (Oxford COVID-19 Government Response Tracker)." *Nature Human Behaviour* 5 (4): 529–38. https://doi.org/10.1038/s41562-021 -01079-8.

Han, Q., B. Zheng, M. Cristea, M. Agostini, J. J. Bélanger, B. Gützkow, J. Kreienkamp, et al. 2023. "Trust in Government Regarding COVID-19 and Its Associations with Preventive Health Behaviour and Prosocial Behaviour during the Pandemic: A Cross-Sectional and Longitudinal Study." *Psychological Medicine* 53 (1): 149–59. https://doi.org/10.1017 /S0033291721001306.

Haug, N., L. Geyrhofer, A. Londei, E. Dervic, A. Desvars-Larrive, V. Loreto, B. Pinior, et al. 2020. "Ranking the Effectiveness of Worldwide COVID-19 Government Interventions." *Nature Human Behaviour* 4 (12): 1303–12. https://doi.org/10.1038/s41562-020-01009-0.

Heydari, S. T., L. Zarei, A. K. Sadati, N. Moradi, M. Akbari, G. Mehralian, and K. B. Lankarani. 2021. "The Effect of Risk Communication on Preventive and Protective Behaviours during the COVID-19 Outbreak: Mediating Role of Risk Perception." *BMC Public Health* 21 (1): 1–11. https://doi.org/10.1186/S12889-020 -10125-5/TABLES/5.

Hollingsworth, T. D., D. Klinkenberg, H. Heesterbeek, and R. M. Anderson. 2011. "Mitigation Strategies for Pandemic Influenza A: Balancing Conflicting Policy Objectives." *PLOS Computational Biology* 7 (2). https://doi.org/10.1371/journal.pcbi.1001076.

James, L. P., J. A. Salomon, C. O. Buckee, and N. A. Menzies. 2021. "The Use and Misuse of Mathematical Modeling for Infectious Disease Policymaking: Lessons for the COVID-19 Pandemic." *Medical Decision Making* 41 (4): 379–85. https://doi.org/10.1177/0272989X21990391/ASSET/7476DF9D-B215-405A-B45D-7C2C1C83FAA3/ASSETS/IMAGES/LARGE/10.1177_0272989X21990391-FIG3.JPG.

Jamison, D. T., L. H. Summers, A. Y. Chang, O. Karlsson, W. Mao, O. F. Norheim, O. Ogbuoji, et al. 2024. "Global Health 2050: The Path to Halving Premature Death by Mid-Century." *The Lancet* 404 (10462): 1561–614. https://doi.org/10.1016/S0140-6736(24)01439-9.

Jamison, D. T., and K. B. Wu. 2021. "The East–West Divide in Response to COVID-19." *Engineering* 7 (7). https://doi.org/10.1016/j.eng.2021.05.008.

Jang, S. Y., L. Hussain-Alkhateeb, T. Rivera Ramirez, A. Asa'ad Al-Aghbari, D. J. Chackalackal, R. Cardenas-Sanchez, M. A. Carrillo, et al. 2021. "Factors Shaping the COVID-19 Epidemic Curve: A Multi-country Analysis." *BMC Infectious Diseases* 21 (1): 1–16. https://doi.org/10.1186/S12879-021-06714-3/FIGURES/6.

Jimenez, J. L., L. C. Marr, K. Randall, E. T. Ewing, Z. Tufekci, T. Greenhalgh, R. Tellier, et al. 2022. "What Were the Historical Reasons for the Resistance to Recognizing Airborne Transmission during the COVID-19 Pandemic?" *Indoor Air* 32 (8): e13070. https://doi.org/10.1111/INA.13070.

Kourti, A., A. Stavridou, E. Panagouli, T. Psaltopoulou, C. Spiliopoulou, M. Tsolia, T. N. Sergentanis, and A. Tsitsika. 2023. "Domestic Violence during the COVID-19 Pandemic: A Systematic Review." *Trauma, Violence, and Abuse* 24 (2): 719–45. https://doi.org/10.1177/15248380211038690/SUPPL_FILE/SJ-PDF-2-TVA-10.1177_15248380211038690.PDF.

Lai, S., Y. Qin, B. J. Cowling, X. Ren, N. A. Wardrop, M. Gilbert, T. K. Tsang, et al. 2016. "Global Epidemiology of Avian Influenza A H5N1 Virus Infection in Humans, 1997–2015: A Systematic Review of Individual Case Data." *The Lancet Infectious Diseases* 16 (7): E108–18. https://doi.org/10.1016/S1473-3099(16)00153-5.

Li, L., A. Taeihagh, and S. Y. Tan. 2023. "A Scoping Review of the Impacts of COVID-19 Physical Distancing Measures on Vulnerable Population Groups." *Nature Communications* 14 (1): 1–19. https://doi.org/10.1038/s41467-023-36267-9.

Li, Y., H. Campbell, D. Kulkarni, A. Harpur, M. Nundy, X. Wang, and H. Nair. 2021. "The Temporal Association of Introducing and Lifting Non-pharmaceutical Interventions with the Time-Varying Reproduction Number (R) of SARS-CoV-2: A Modelling Study across 131 Countries." *The Lancet Infectious Diseases* 21 (2): 193–202. https://doi.org/10.1016/S1473-3099(20)30785-4.

Liu, Y., A. A. Gayle, A. Wilder-Smith, and J. Rocklöv. 2020. "The Reproductive Number of COVID-19 Is Higher Compared to SARS Coronavirus." *Journal of Travel Medicine* 27 (2). https://doi.org/10.1093/jtm/taaa021.

Liu, Y., C. Morgenstern, J. Kelly, R. Lowe, J. Munday, C. J. Villabona-Arenas, H. Gibbs, et al. 2021. "The Impact of Non-pharmaceutical Interventions on SARS-CoV-2 Transmission across 130 Countries and Territories." *BMC Medicine* 19 (1): 1–12. https://doi.org/10.1186/S12916-020-01872-8/FIGURES/5.

MacIntyre, C. R., and A. A. Chughtai. 2020. "A Rapid Systematic Review of the Efficacy of Face Masks and Respirators against Coronaviruses and Other Respiratory Transmissible Viruses for the Community, Healthcare Workers and Sick Patients." *International Journal of Nursing Studies* 108: 103629. https://doi.org/10.1016/j.ijnurstu.2020.103629.

Mackworth-Young, C. R. S., R. Chingono, C. Mavodza, G. McHugh, M. Tembo, C. D. Chikwari, H. A. Weiss, et al. 2021. "Community Perspectives on the Covid-19 Response, Zimbabwe." *Bulletin of the World Health Organization* 99 (2): 85–91. https://doi.org/10.2471/BLT.20.260224.

Majeed, A., J. K. Quint, S. Bhatt, F. Davies, and N. Islam. 2024. "Non-pharmaceutical Interventions: Evaluating Challenges and Priorities for Future Health Shocks." *BMJ* 387 (October): e080528. https://doi.org/10.1136/BMJ-2024-080528.

Mateus, A. L. P., H. E. Otete, C. R. Beck, G. P. Dolan, and J. S. Nguyen-Van-Tam. 2014. "Effectiveness of Travel Restrictions in the Rapid Containment of Human Influenza: A Systematic Review." *Bulletin of the World Health Organization* 92 (12): 868. https://doi.org/10.2471/BLT.14.135590.

Morawska, L., and D. K. Milton. 2020. "It Is Time to Address Airborne Transmission of Coronavirus Disease 2019 (COVID-19)." *Clinical Infectious Diseases* 71 (9): 2311–13. https://doi.org/10.1093/cid/ciaa939.

Murukutla, N., A. K. Gupta, M. Maharjan, C. Fabrizio, E. W. Myers, A. Johnson, V. Nkwanzi, et al. 2022. "Psychosocial Determinants of Adherence to Public Health and Social Measures (PHSMs) in 18 African Union Member States during the Early Phase of the COVID-19 Pandemic: Results of a Cross-Sectional Survey." *BMJ Open* 12 (6): e054839. https://doi.org/10.1136/BMJOPEN-2021-054839.

Nivette, A., D. Ribeaud, A. Murray, A. Steinhoff, L. Bechtiger, U. Hepp, L. Shanahan, and M. Eisner. 2021. "Non-compliance with COVID-19-Related Public Health Measures among Young Adults in Switzerland: Insights from a Longitudinal Cohort Study." *Social Science & Medicine* 268 (January): 113370. https://doi.org/10.1016/J.SOCSCIMED.2020.113370.

Onyeaka, H., C. K. Anumudu, Z. T. Al-Sharify, E. Egele-Godswill, and P. Mbaegbu. 2021. "COVID-19 Pandemic: A Review of the Global Lockdown and Its Far-Reaching Effects." *Science Progress* 104 (2). https://doi.org/10.1177/00368504211019854 /ASSET/70E0D950-EFEE-459B-BAF5-64F03CEE3E3F/ASSETS/IMAGES /LARGE/10.1177_00368504211019854-FIG3.JPG.

Osterrieder, A., G. Cuman, W. Pan-Ngum, P. K. Cheah, P. K. Cheah, P. Peerawaranun, M. Silan, et al. 2021. "Economic and Social Impacts of COVID-19 and Public Health Measures: Results from an Anonymous Online Survey in Thailand, Malaysia, the UK, Italy and Slovenia." *BMJ Open* 11 (7). https://doi.org/10.1136/BMJOPEN-2020-046863.

Pan, A., L. Liu, C. Wang, H. Guo, X. Hao, Q. Wang, J. Huang, et al. 2020. "Association of Public Health Interventions with the Epidemiology of the COVID-19 Outbreak in Wuhan, China." *Journal of the American Medical Association* 323 (19): 1915–23. https://doi.org/10.1001/jama.2020.6130.

Pang, X., Z. Zhu, F. Xu, J. Guo, X. Gong, D. Liu, Z. Liu, et al. 2003. "Evaluation of Control Measures Implemented in the Severe Acute Respiratory Syndrome Outbreak in Beijing, 2003." *Journal of the American Medical Association* 290 (24): 3215–21. https://doi.org /10.1001/jama.290.24.3215.

Parodi, S. M., and V. X. Liu. 2020. "From Containment to Mitigation of COVID-19 in the US." *Journal of the American Medical Association* 323 (15): 1441–42. https://doi.org/10.1001 /jama.2020.3882.

Pitol, A. K., and T. R. Julian. 2021. "Community Transmission of SARS-CoV-2 by Surfaces: Risks and Risk Reduction Strategies." *Environmental Science and Technology Letters* 8 (3): 263–69. https://doi.org/10.1021/acs.estlett.0c00966.

Presanis, A. M., D. De Angelis, A. Hagy, C. Reed, S. Riley, B. S. Cooper, L. Finelli, et al. 2009. "The Severity of Pandemic H1N1 Influenza in the United States, from April to July 2009: A Bayesian Analysis." *PLOS Medicine* 6 (12). https://doi.org/10.1371/journal .pmed.1000207.

Qualls, N., A. Levitt, N. Kanade, N. Wright-Jegede, S. Dopson, M. Biggerstaff, C. Reed, and A. Uzicanin. 2020. "Community Mitigation Guidelines to Prevent Pandemic Influenza— United States, 2017." *MMWR Recommendations and Reports* 66 (1): 1–34. https://doi .org/10.15585/MMWR.RR6601A1.

Ricotta, E. E., A. Rid, I. G. Cohen, and N. G. Evans. 2023. "Observational Studies Must Be Reformed before the Next Pandemic." *Nature Medicine* 29 (8): 1903–05. https://doi .org/10.1038/s41591-023-02375-8.

Russell, T. W., J. T. Wu, S. Clifford, W. J. Edmunds, A. J. Kucharski, and M. Jit. 2021. "Effect of Internationally Imported Cases on Internal Spread of COVID-19: A Mathematical Modelling Study." *The Lancet Public Health* 6 (1). https://doi.org/10.1016/S2468-2667(20)30263-2.

Savadori, L., and M. Lauriola. 2021. "Risk Perception and Protective Behaviors during the Rise of the COVID-19 Outbreak in Italy." *Frontiers in Psychology* 11. https://doi.org/10.3389/fpsyg.2020.577331.

Scally, G., B. Jacobson, and K. Abbasi. 2020. "The UK's Public Health Response to Covid-19." *BMJ* 369: n1932. https://doi.org/10.1136/bmj.m1932.

Sekalala, S., L. Forman, R. Habibi, and B. M. Meier. 2020. "Health and Human Rights Are Inextricably Linked in the COVID-19 Response." *BMJ Global Health*, September 15, 2020. https://doi.org/10.1136/bmjgh-2020-003359.

Shafique, S., D. S. Bhattacharyya, I. Nowrin, F. Sultana, M. R. Islam, G. K. Dutta, M. O. Del Barrio, and D. D. Reidpath. 2024. "Effective Community-Based Interventions to Prevent and Control Infectious Diseases in Urban Informal Settlements in Low- and Middle-Income Countries: A Systematic Review." *Systematic Reviews* 13 (1): 253. https://doi.org/10.1186/S13643-024-02651-9/TABLES/3.

Smith, L. E., R. Amlôt, H. Lambert, I. Oliver, C. Robin, L. Yardley, and G. J. Rubin. 2020. "Factors Associated with Adherence to Self-Isolation and Lockdown Measures in the UK: A Cross-Sectional Survey." *Public Health* 187 (October):41–52. https://doi.org/10.1016/J.PUHE.2020.07.024.

Talic, S., S. Shah, H. Wild, D. Gasevic, A. Maharaj, Z. Ademi, X. Li, et al. 2021. "Effectiveness of Public Health Measures in Reducing the Incidence of Covid-19, SARS-CoV-2 Transmission, and Covid-19 Mortality: Systematic Review and Meta-Analysis." *BMJ* 375 (November). https://doi.org/10.1136/BMJ-2021-068302.

Tang, S., Y. Mao, R. M. Jones, Q. Tan, J. S. Ji, N. Li, J. Shen, et al. 2020. "Aerosol Transmission of SARS-CoV-2? Evidence, Prevention and Control." *Environment International* 144. https://doi.org/10.1016/j.envint.2020.106039.

Taubenberger, J. K., and D. M. Morens. 2006. "1918 Influenza: The Mother of All Pandemics." *Emerging Infectious Diseases* 12 (1). https://doi.org/10.3201/eid1201.050979.

Tellier, R. 2009. "Aerosol Transmission of Influenza A Virus: A Review of New Studies." *Journal of the Royal Society Interface* 6 (SUPPL. 6). https://doi.org/10.1098/rsif.2009.0302.focus.

Tian, H., Y. Liu, Y. Li, C. H. Wu, B. Chen, M. U. G. Kraemer, B. Li, et al. 2020. "An Investigation of Transmission Control Measures during the First 50 Days of the COVID-19 Epidemic in China." *Science* 368 (6491). https://doi.org/10.1126/science.abb6105.

Tognotti, E. 2013. "Lessons from the History of Quarantine, from Plague to Influenza A." *Emerging Infectious Diseases* 19 (2).

Tomes, N. 2010. "'Destroyer and Teacher': Managing the Masses During the 1918–1919 Influenza Pandemic." *Public Health Reports* 125 (Suppl 3): 48. https://doi.org/10.1177/00333549101250S308.

Tu, H., K. Hu, M. Zhang, Y. Zhuang, and T. Song. 2021. "Effectiveness of 14 Day Quarantine Strategy: Chinese Experience of Prevention and Control." *BMJ* 375: e066121. https://doi.org/10.1136/BMJ-2021-066121.

Vardavas, C., K. Zisis, K. Nikitara, I. Lagou, V. Marou, K. Aslanoglou, K. Athanasakis, et al. 2023. "Cost of the COVID-19 Pandemic versus the Cost-Effectiveness of Mitigation Strategies in EU/UK/OECD: A Systematic Review." *BMJ Open* 13 (10): e077602. https://doi.org/10.1136/BMJOPEN-2023-077602.

Vargas-Parada, L. 2009. "H1N1: A Mexican Perspective." *Cell* 139 (7): 1203–05. https://doi.org/10.1016/j.cell.2009.12.019.

Viboud, C., L. Simonsen, R. Fuentes, J. Flores, M. A. Miller, and G. Chowell. 2015. "Global Mortality Impact of the 1957–1959 Influenza Pandemic." *Journal of Infectious Diseases* 212 (11). https://doi.org/10.1093/infdis/jiv534.

Von Tigerstrom, B., and K. Wilson. 2020. "COVID-19 Travel Restrictions and the *International Health Regulations (2005)*." *BMJ Global Health* 5 (5). https://doi.org/10.1136/bmjgh-2020-002629.

Wei, W. E., Z. Li, C. J. Chiew, S. E. Yong, M. P. Toh, and V. J. Lee. 2020. "Presymptomatic Transmission of SARS-CoV-2—Singapore, January 23–March 16, 2020." *Morbidity and Mortality Weekly Report* 69 (14): 411–15. https://doi.org/10.15585/MMWR.MM6914E1.

WHO (World Health Organization). 2005. "WHO Global Influenza Preparedness Plan: The Role of WHO and Recommendations for National Measure before and during Pandemics." WHO, Geneva. https://iris.who.int/handle/10665/68998.

WHO (World Health Organization). 2020. "Modes of Transmission of Virus Causing COVID-19: Implications for IPC Precaution Recommendations." Scientific brief, March 29, 2020. https://www.who.int/news-room/commentaries/detail/modes-of-transmission-of-virus-causing-covid-19-implications-for-ipc-precaution-recommendations.

WHO (World Health Organization). 2024a. *Global Guidance on Monitoring Public Health and Social Measures Policies during Health Emergencies.* Geneva: WHO. https://www.who.int/publications/i/item/9789240094444.

WHO (World Health Organization). 2024b. *Pandemic Influenza Severity Assessment (PISA): A WHO Guide to Assess the Severity of Influenza in Seasonal Epidemics and Pandemics, Second Edition.* Geneva: WHO. https://www.who.int/publications/i/item/9789240093881.

WHO (World Health Organization), OECD (Organisation for Economic Co-operation and Development), and World Bank. 2024. *Strengthening Pandemic Preparedness and Response through Integrated Modelling.* WHO, OECD, and World Bank. https://www.who.int/publications/i/item/9789240090880.

Wu, S., R. Neill, C. De Foo, A. Q. Chua, A.-S. Jung, V. Haldane, S. M. Abdalla, et al. 2021. "Aggressive Containment, Suppression, and Mitigation of Covid-19: Lessons Learnt from Eight Countries." *BMJ* 375: e067508. https://doi.org/10.1136/bmj-2021-067508.

Zakar, R., F. Yousaf, M. Z. Zakar, and F. Fischer. 2021. "Sociocultural Challenges in the Implementation of COVID-19 Public Health Measures: Results from a Qualitative Study in Punjab, Pakistan." *Frontiers in Public Health* 9 (July): 703825. https://doi.org/10.3389/FPUBH.2021.703825/FULL.

Zhou, M., and M. Y. Kan. 2021. "The Varying Impacts of COVID-19 and Its Related Measures in the UK: A Year in Review." *PLOS One* 16 (9): e0257286. https://doi.org/10.1371/JOURNAL.PONE.0257286.

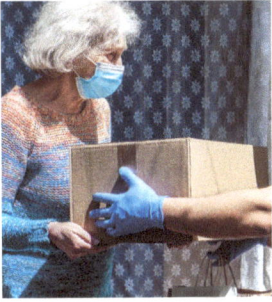

# 7

# Targeted Isolation and Related Measures to Control Epidemic Pathogens

Simiao Chen, Lirui Jiao, Wenjin Chen, Zara Shubber, Victoria Y. Fan, Muhammad Ali Pate, David Canning, Lan Xue, Chen Wang, and Till Bärnighausen

## ABSTRACT

Targeted isolation of infected individuals is an important approach to control epidemics at an early stage. This chapter focuses on strategies for isolating infected individuals to protect the uninfected. It provides an overview of isolation strategies and related measures used in past outbreaks, including the COVID-19 (coronavirus) pandemic. In addition, it presents impact evaluations, including epidemiological and economic evaluations, of different targeted isolation strategies used in past outbreaks based on the existing literature. Finally, it offers recommendations for better control of future epidemics.

## INTRODUCTION

Whereas the previous chapter ("Public Health and Social Measures for Respiratory Infections") focused on population-wide interventions to mitigate outbreaks and epidemics, this chapter focuses on isolation strategies that target infected individuals to protect those who have remained uninfected.[1] Epidemics, such as the recent COVID-19 (coronavirus) pandemic, demonstrate the importance of swift and effective interventions to prevent the spread of infectious diseases. This chapter explores various isolation strategies and related targeted measures that have been used in past epidemics, including those that were used to control the spread of COVID-19. By examining these targeted interventions, we can gain a better understanding of how to prevent and control future epidemics.

The initial stage of an outbreak represents a critical and challenging period with respect to infectious disease control and typically occurs before the development of pathogen-specific pharmaceutical interventions, which take time to develop.

This early epidemic period can be particularly important for low- and middle-income countries (LMICs), which may not gain timely access to pharmaceutical measures even when those measures become available in high-income countries (HICs). Influenza pandemic guidelines have identified the need to implement targeted nonpharmaceutical interventions in the early phases of a potential pandemic to reduce the reproductive number. Doing so can buy time to evaluate the transmissibility and severity of the pandemic pathogen, thereby enabling development of a careful, measured, and customized response strategy (CDC 2007).

Targeted isolation strategies have three key objectives: containment, suppression, and mitigation. According to definitions from the *Lancet* Commission on Investing in Health (Jamison et al. 2024), "containment" aims to halt all transmission pathways, often through rigorous interventions; "suppression" seeks to keep transmission rates very low; and "mitigation" focuses on decelerating the spread of infection to lower the peak number of cases, commonly known as "flattening the curve." When implemented early and comprehensively, targeted isolation can support containment by interrupting all chains of transmission and entirely halting the spread of the pathogen. In settings with ongoing but manageable transmission, targeted isolation can contribute to suppression by reducing the number of active cases to controllable levels. Where widespread transmission cannot be avoided, targeted isolation can play a critical role in mitigation by moderately slowing the rate of spread, thereby protecting vulnerable populations and reducing the strain that pandemic progression puts on already overburdened health care systems (Chen, Rodewald, et al. 2021). Achieving containment is often more feasible in the early stages of an outbreak, whereas mitigation strategies become increasingly important as the epidemic progresses. Achieving any of these three key objectives can yield substantial health and economic benefits.

This chapter mainly evaluates home-based and facility-based targeted isolation strategies. It details six potential isolation strategies and discusses how some of them were used during the recent COVID-19 pandemic. It then reviews isolation strategies and other relevant measures used in epidemics prior to COVID-19. Next, it evaluates the epidemiological and economic impacts of isolation strategies, and discusses ethical and legal considerations. Finally, it concludes with recommendations for potential future epidemics.

## DECISION-MAKING CONSIDERATIONS FOR IMPLEMENTING TARGETED ISOLATION

Public health decision-makers must consider a common set of criteria or questions when determining whether targeted isolation measures should be implemented during an epidemic and, if so, what specific measures are likely to be most effective and contextually appropriate. These criteria reflect the complex and uncertain nature of outbreaks and include the following: First, decision-makers must consider a number of key parameters related to the epidemic pathogen, including the mode of transmission (that is, whether the pathogen spreads via aerosols, droplets, surfaces, person-to-person contact, the fecal-oral route, vectors, or other mechanisms), disease severity (measured, for example, as case fatality or hospitalization rate), transmission speed, and the possibility of asymptomatic spread. In addition, it is important to determine the length of isolation required to be effective, as informed by assessment of the pathogen's infectious period (that is, the time during which an individual can spread a pathogen to others) and incubation period (that is, the time from exposure to onset of symptoms). Second, decision-makers must consider health care system capacity, such as availability of hospital beds and intensive care units, as well as testing and contact tracing capabilities. Third, decision-makers must consider the acceptability and desirability of various targeted isolation strategies, which are often shaped by cultural, economic, legal, and social conditions.

Consideration of these criteria can inform not only whether targeted isolation is warranted but also which specific targeted isolation strategy to choose, what related supportive measures should be implemented, and how targeted isolation should be enforced (each of these additional decision points is discussed in subsequent sections of the chapter). Decision-makers must remain adaptable in implementing targeted isolation strategies, making strategic adjustments guided by real-time epidemiological data—including trends in case counts, test positivity rates, and the secondary attack rate—as well as public sentiment, endorsement, and participation. Moreover, changes in the availability of prevention and treatment options, health care capacity, and economic and social trade-offs can inform either escalation or de-escalation of targeted isolation. Finally, decision-makers must consider their exit strategy from targeted isolation, which may depend on several factors, such as continued epidemic spread, cost, and public participation in the different available prevention and treatment offerings.

## TARGETED ISOLATION STRATEGIES TO CONTROL EPIDEMICS

This section identifies six potential targeted isolation strategies. It examines the use of home-based and facility-based isolation for patients who are asymptomatic or suffer from mild or moderate symptoms and assumes that patients with severe to critical symptoms would receive hospital-based treatment. It also evaluates how the six targeted isolation strategies were used in the COVID-19 context.

### Six Targeted Isolation Strategies

The six targeted isolation strategies discussed in this chapter are voluntary home-based isolation (VHI), voluntary facility-based isolation (VFI), combined voluntary home- and facility-based isolation (C-VHI-VFI), mandatory home-based isolation (MHI), mandatory facility-based isolation (MFI), and combined mandatory home- and facility-based isolation (C-MHI-MFI) (figure 7.1).

**Figure 7.1** Six Targeted Isolation Strategies

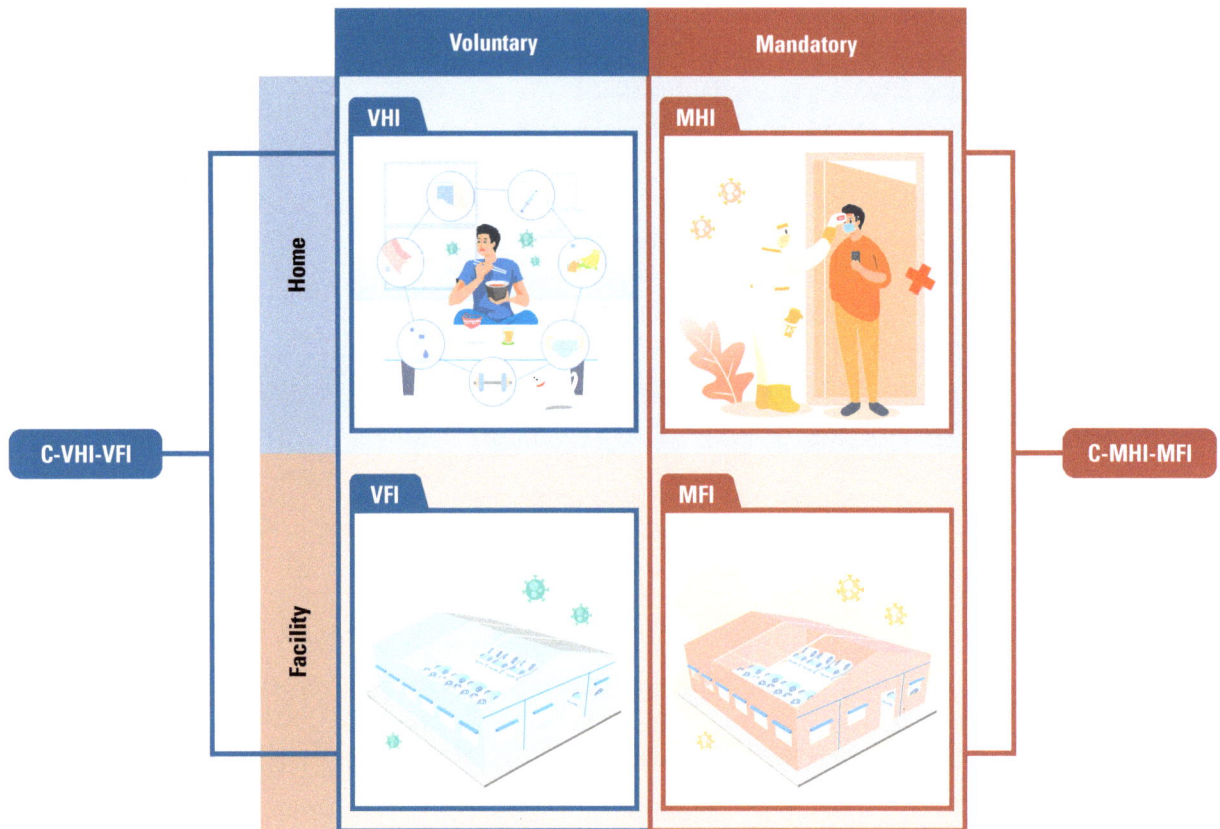

*Source:* Original figure created for this publication.

*Note:* C-MHI-MFI = combined mandatory home- and facility-based isolation; C-VHI-VFI = combined voluntary home- and facility-based isolation; MFI = mandatory facility-based isolation; MHI = mandatory home-based isolation; VFI = voluntary facility-based isolation; VHI = voluntary home-based isolation.

Each of VHI, VFI, and C-VHI-VFI relies exclusively on voluntary measures. Under home-based isolation, infected individuals remain in their homes to avoid contact with other community members. Home-based isolation, particularly VHI, is easy to implement and may contribute positively to the psychological well-being of isolated individuals (Ju et al. 2021). However, adherence to VHI guidelines may be imperfect and is difficult to enforce, threatening its ability to achieve epidemic control (Smith et al. 2020). Facility-based isolation focuses on placing patients with mild or moderate symptoms, as well as asymptomatic patients, in nonhospital care facilities, which provide symptom monitoring and basic health care services (Chen, Chen, et al. 2021; Chia et al. 2021). Facility-based isolation may be more effective than home-based isolation because it relies less on self-imposed adherence to guidelines and does not put uninfected family members at risk (Smith et al. 2020). Although facility-based isolation is likely more expensive for the government than home-based isolation, implementation costs for facility-based isolation can be reduced if isolation facilities are repurposed from existing buildings (for example, stadiums or convention centers), as opposed to being newly constructed. However, facility-based isolation can be challenging to implement in LMICs because of the lack of infrastructure and human resources. Finally, C-VHI-VFI represents a scenario in which governments offer communal isolation centers in addition to encouraging VHI. Offering infected individuals options for how to isolate should make them better-off than if they had only one choice (assuming the number of options is not overwhelming), because they are more likely to find an option that suits their needs and preferences (Lavecchia, Liu, and Oreopoulos 2016).

Mandatory measures include MHI, MFI, and C-MHI-MFI. Mandatory isolation may be enforced when voluntary isolation measures are not effective in controlling the spread of the pathogen to family and community members. MHI involves mandating that infected individuals isolate at home for a specified period. MHI will likely boost the number of people in home-based isolation but may be difficult to comprehensively enforce and carries higher implementation costs than VHI. By contrast, MFI involves mandating facility-based isolation to ensure complete isolation of infected individuals. Finally, under C-MHI-MFI, some form of isolation is mandated, but individuals are allowed to choose whether to isolate at home or in a facility. Mandating isolation may put disproportionate burdens on already disadvantaged populations and may be challenging to implement in resource-poor communities where people depend on uninterrupted incomes for food security and survival.

## Targeted Isolation Strategies during COVID-19

Various targeted isolation strategies were used during the COVID-19 pandemic. This chapter mainly focuses on the strategies implemented during a pandemic's initial stage, though it also references illustrative examples of these strategies from subsequent phases, when relevant. The original strain of SARS-CoV-2, the virus that causes COVID-19, was detected at the end of 2019, and the first officially designated variant of concern (the Alpha variant) was reported in the United Kingdom in December 2020 (Carvalho, Krammer, and Iwasaki 2021). The initial stage of the COVID-19 pandemic in this chapter is therefore defined as the period that spanned approximately from the end of 2019 to the end of 2020 (figure 7.2).

Home-based isolation was a key strategy for reducing the spread of COVID-19 in several countries and regions, as shown in table 7.1. Under home-based isolation, individuals are advised to monitor their symptoms closely, seek medical attention if necessary, and follow strict hygiene practices to prevent transmission of the virus to others in their household (WHO 2022). As outlined in table 7.1, nonadherence diminishes the effectiveness of VHI in controlling disease. Income loss, for example, was a major driver of nonadherence to home-based isolation during the COVID-19 pandemic (Cevik et al. 2021). Income loss is particularly of concern among economically disadvantaged populations in HICs and in general in LMICs, but it may be overcome through supportive measures, discussed in detail later in the chapter. MHI may lead to better disease control than VHI, but fewer countries and regions implemented MHI during the COVID-19 pandemic, likely because of its potentially high enforcement costs, the need for strong administrative capacity, and social acceptability challenges. In addition, intrafamily transmission remains a concern under MHI as well as VHI.

**Figure 7.2** Timeline of COVID-19, 2020–22

Number of new cases per million people                                   Number of new deaths per million people

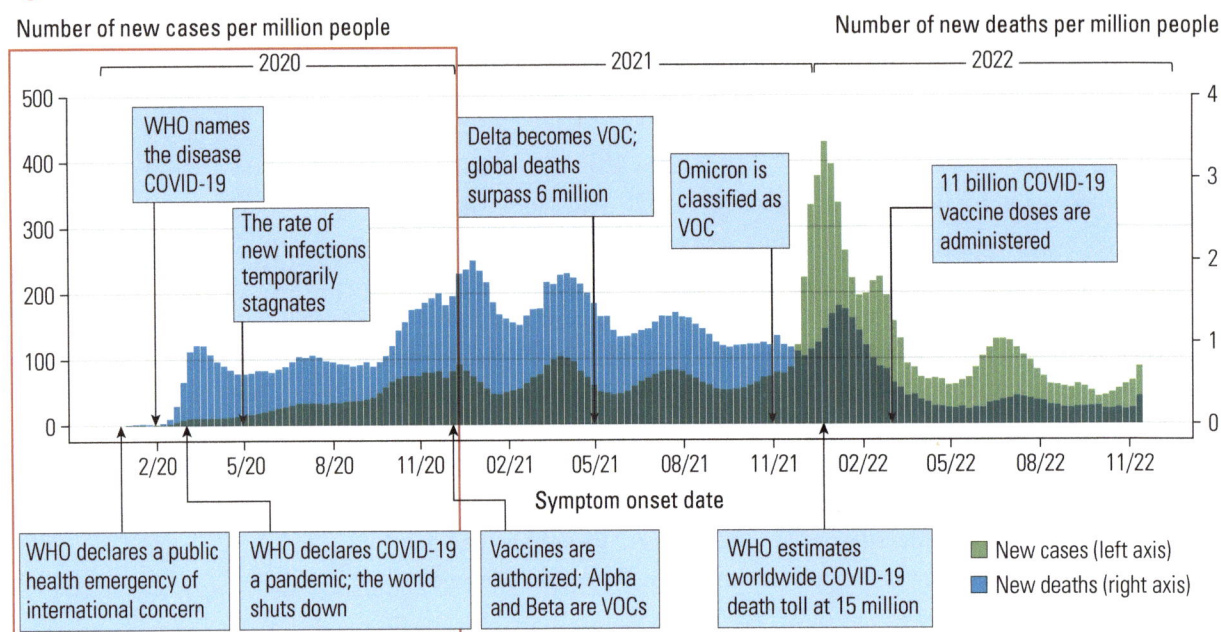

*Source:* Original figure created for this publication based on https://ourworldindata.org/covid-cases.

*Note:* The dark green bars show the overlap between new cases and new deaths. The period marked by the red box shows the early stage of the COVID-19 pandemic, as defined in this chapter. VOC = variant of concern; WHO = World Health Organization.

In addition to home-based isolation, facility-based isolation provided in community care centers was also used during the COVID-19 pandemic. MFI was a common element of packages of rigorous control measures implemented in some Asian countries and regions (table 7.1). In China, Fangcang shelter hospitals for MFI were rapidly established by repurposing public venues (Chen et al. 2020). Later in the pandemic, C-MHI-MFI was also implemented in some locations. In Hong Kong SAR, China, for example, individuals who tested positive for COVID-19 were mandated to isolate either at a designated community isolation facility or at home (The Government of the Hong Kong Special Administrative Region 2022). Furthermore, some countries and regions offered C-VHI-VFI to provide safe alternatives for vulnerable individuals (such as the unhoused or those living in crowded homes) to voluntarily isolate. For example, the Safe Voluntary Isolation Sites Program in Canada helped place infected or exposed individuals (including homeless individuals) in accessible self-isolation sites to prevent household transmission (Public Health Agency of Canada 2021; Tasker and Burke 2020) (table 7.1). In another related example, the Javits Center in New York City was originally set up as an alternative care site to take in non-COVID-19 patients from overburdened hospitals, but was later repurposed to also take in COVID-19 patients, thereby playing the role of a field hospital rather than an isolation facility (Thompson et al. 2023). Although facility-based isolation can be more effective than home-based isolation, it may take a heavy toll on the isolated individuals' mental health and may disproportionately burden resource-poor populations, who rely on the work of a family member—who is now isolated in a facility—for their livelihoods or child or elderly care. A cross-sectional study examining individuals infected with COVID-19 in facility-based isolation in Qatar reported high depression and anxiety rates (Reagu et al. 2021). Supportive measures are therefore essential to accompany facility-based isolation. For instance, Fangcang shelter hospitals in China not only provided medical care but also offered emotional and social support for patients (Chen et al. 2020). (Refer to boxes 7.1 through 7.5 for case studies of the use of the various strategies.)

**Table 7.1** Details of Six Targeted Isolation Strategies

| | Advantages | Disadvantages | Where implemented during the COVID-19 pandemic |
|---|---|---|---|
| **VHI** | • Easy to implement economically, socially, and politically.<br>• May better relieve COVID-19-related psychological distress than facility-based isolation. | • Difficult to prevent disease spread and achieve control of the epidemic because of intrafamily transmission.<br>• Nonadherence is a critical barrier. | Brazil (Schuch et al. 2020); France (Patel, Fernandes, and Sridhar 2021); South Africa (National Institute for Communicable Diseases 2020); South Sudan (Waya et al. 2021); United States (Sehgal, Himmelstein, and Woolhandler 2021) |
| **VFI**[a] | • Provides triage to those opting to isolate in a facility.<br>• Offers the option for infected individuals to reduce the risk of disease transmission to their family members and other contacts. | • Costly to implement, particularly with respect to purpose-built facilities (compared to repurposed facilities).<br>• Difficult to predict the degree of use. | — |
| **C-VHI-VFI**[b] | • Provides more choice.<br>• Fulfills different needs of different populations.<br>• Provides triage to those opting to isolate in a facility. | • May be costly to implement, although repurposed facilities may be much more feasible than purpose-built facilities, particularly for LMICs.<br>• May be difficult to ensure epidemic control depending on levels and patterns of use. | Canada (Public Health Agency of Canada 2021); Tokyo, Japan (Yukinori 2020; Akashi et al. 2022) |
| **MHI** | • Fairly easy to implement.<br>• Ensures adherence to home-based isolation. | • Higher transmission rates among family members and other home contacts than in facility-based isolation.<br>• May need supportive measures, such as financial support for infected individuals who cannot afford to stop working, to increase intervention effectiveness and decrease social harms. | Germany (Patel, Fernandes, and Sridhar 2021); Italy (Patel, Fernandes, and Sridhar 2021); Nepal (Government of Nepal Ministry of Health and Population 2020) |
| **MFI** | • Averts intrafamily transmission.<br>• Provides triage. | • Costly to implement in terms of both infrastructure and human resources, particularly in LMICs, and thus may require international support.<br>• Higher risk of social isolation and other negative mental health impacts, and thus may require simultaneous supportive measures.<br>• Social challenges to implementation. | New South Wales, Australia (Shaban et al. 2020); Wuhan, China (S. Chen et al. 2020); Singapore (Patel, Fernandes, and Sridhar 2021); Republic of Korea (Patel, Fernandes, and Sridhar 2021); KwaZulu-Natal, South Africa (Moodley, Obasa, and London 2020) |

*table continues next page*

**Table 7.1** Details of Six Targeted Isolation Strategies *(continued)*

| | Advantages | Disadvantages | Where implemented during the COVID-19 pandemic |
|---|---|---|---|
| | | • May require supportive measures for those who cannot afford to remain in isolation or may need extra assistance (for example, infected individuals with disabilities). | |
| **C-MHI-MFI**[b] | • Provides more flexibility to socially disadvantaged populations and partially compensates for isolation stringency.<br><br>• Ensures complete isolation.<br><br>• Provides triage. | • Costly to implement.<br><br>• Higher risk of social isolation and negative mental health impacts.<br><br>• Requires comprehensive policy guidelines. | Hong Kong SAR, China (The Government of the Hong Kong Special Administrative Region 2022); Jodhpur, India (Bhardwaj et al. 2021) |

*Source:* Original table compiled for this publication.

*Note:* The countries listed are categorized on the basis of the main isolation strategy they employed during the initial stages of the COVID-19 pandemic; however, some cities or regions within a given country may have used a different isolation strategy. C-MHI-MFI = combined mandatory home- and facility-based isolation; C-VHI-VFI = combined voluntary home- and facility-based isolation; LMICs = low- and middle-income countries; MFI = mandatory facility-based isolation; MHI = mandatory home-based isolation; VFI = voluntary facility-based isolation; VHI = voluntary home-based isolation; — means that the corresponding isolation strategy is theoretically plausible and proposed in this chapter but has apparently not yet been implemented in the real world.

a. VFI means that only that strategy was implemented, with no other isolation strategies listed in this chapter implemented simultaneously. Theoretically, VFI may be implemented when policy makers do not see a reason to advise or mandate isolation for the general population, yet certain groups may wish to place themselves in facility-based isolation (for example, an infected individual who does not wish to risk transmitting the virus to an immunocompromised family member).

b. C-VHI-VFI and C-MHI-MFI differ from the other four isolation strategies in that these two strategies offer the choice of whether to isolate at home or in a facility. In some scenarios, individuals could also be asked to enter facility-based isolation for some period (for example, the first seven days following infection) and then remain in home-based isolation for an additional period (for example, the following three days) before exiting isolation.

**Box 7.1**

### Case Study of Voluntary Home-Based Isolation: The United States and South Sudan

Voluntary home-based isolation (VHI) was a common isolation strategy in the US to control the spread of COVID-19 and minimize the impact of the pandemic. The United States recommended self-isolation for COVID-19 around the time when the World Health Organization declared the COVID-19 outbreak a global pandemic.[a] At that time, the US Centers for Disease Control and Prevention advised individuals who were sick with COVID-19 to stay home and stay away from other people and animals in their homes (National Center for Immunization and Respiratory Diseases 2020). The agency initially implemented a test-based strategy to recommend infected individuals isolate until they had two negative test swabs; this guidance was later updated to a time-based strategy that recommended infected individuals isolate for at least 10 days (Stephenson 2020).

VHI is based on the assumption that most households have sufficiently high standards of living and small enough family sizes for home-based isolation to be feasible. This was not the case in many low- and middle-income countries during the COVID-19 pandemic. For example, although South Sudan also employed VHI, David Shearer, Special Representative and Head of the United Nations Mission to the country, explained that few households could adhere to home-based isolation because "the need to earn a living means that people's behavior remains unchanged, as not working today means not eating tomorrow" (United Nations 2020).

a. US Centers for Disease Control and Prevention, "CDC Museum COVID-19 Timeline," https://www.cdc.gov/museum/timeline/covid19.html.

### Case Study of Combined Voluntary Home- and Facility-Based Isolation: Tokyo, Japan

The Tokyo Metropolitan Government implemented a strategy of using care and isolation facilities for COVID-19 patients early in the pandemic. Repurposed from existing hotels and venues with support from the National Center for Global Health and Medicine and the Nippon Foundation (Yukinori 2020), these facilities were designed to provide care and medical treatment to patients who were not seriously ill but needed to be isolated to reduce the spread of the virus (Akashi et al. 2022). The facilities were provided with medical equipment and staffed by medical professionals, including doctors and nurses. In addition, the facilities were designed to be comfortable and to provide patients with basic amenities such as meals and bedding (Yukinori 2020). By using care and isolation facilities, together with other population-wide interventions, such as social distancing measures, Japan was able to prevent hospitals from becoming overwhelmed and limit the spread of COVID-19 within the community. The government did not make home-based isolation and facility-based isolation mandatory, but instead called on the public to exercise self-discipline (Machida et al. 2020; Wang et al. 2021).

### Case Study of Mandatory Home-Based Isolation: Italy

Italy implemented mandatory home-based isolation as part of its COVID-19 response strategy in March 2020, shortly after the country became one of the early epicenters of the pandemic (Wang and Mao 2021). The Italian government issued a decree requiring all individuals who tested positive for COVID-19 to isolate themselves at home (Hofverberg 2020), and violators of the decree were subject to fines or criminal charges. Infected individuals were expected to remain in home-based isolation for a minimum of 14 days, and negative swabs were required for termination of the isolation (Lopes et al. 2020). In addition, general practitioners performed some monitoring of COVID-19 patients' clinical conditions (Bosa et al. 2022; Lopes et al. 2020).

### Case Study of Mandatory Facility-Based Isolation: Wuhan, China

On February 5, 2020, the first Fangcang shelter hospital opened in Wuhan, China. Fangcang shelter hospitals provided the structures for mandatory facility-based isolation as a key measure to control the spread of COVID-19 during the first phase of the pandemic (Li et al. 2020). Fangcang shelter hospitals were created by rapidly repurposing public spaces, such as stadiums and exhibition centers, into temporary health care facilities. They aimed to interrupt transmission between patients (without symptoms or with mild to moderate symptoms) and their families and community members (Chen et al. 2020; China Association for Engineering Construction Standardization 2022). In addition to aiding with isolation, Fangcang shelter hospitals fulfilled several other functions, including triage, monitoring, basic medical care provision, and social engagement (Chen et al. 2020). A total of 16 Fangcang shelter hospitals were implemented between February 5, 2020, and March 10, 2020, accommodating over 12,000 patients (Zhong et al. 2022). The reproduction number dropped sharply after the implementation of Fangcang shelter hospitals (in combination with other interventions including social distancing measures), and this novel isolation approach is estimated to have led to 5,148 fewer confirmed cases between January 16 and March 16, 2020 (Wang, Gao, et al. 2020).

Box 7.5

## Case Study of Combined Mandatory Home- and Facility-Based Isolation: Jodhpur, India

In 2020, the Jodhpur Municipal Corporation managed home-based isolation, and the Office of Medical and Health Services took charge of facility-based isolation in the city. Infected individuals who were asymptomatic or mildly symptomatic were required to isolate in their homes, whereas moderately or severely symptomatic patients were required to isolate in facilities (Bhardwaj et al. 2021). The Indian Ministry of Health and Family Welfare also issued guidelines for home-based isolation of patients who were asymptomatic or suffered from only mild symptoms. According to these guidelines, patients could remain at home but had to stay in continuous contact with their district surveillance officer and a registered hospital. Additionally, these patients were required to sign a formal pledge to remain in telecommunication with physicians and engage in self-monitoring (Murarkar, Mahajan, and Gothankar 2021). Finally, Jodhpur was divided into nine zones, and an incident commander was assigned to monitor patients in each zone daily, either through telephone or video calls (Bhardwaj et al. 2021).

### Supportive Measures for Targeted Isolation Strategies

Supportive measures—often necessary for both people who isolate at home and people who isolate in facilities—can take the form of financial support, practical support, employment benefits, mental health support, social engagement, and effective communication (figure 7.3). During the COVID-19 pandemic, in settings such as Austria and Ireland, infected individuals received lump sum or per diem payments if they isolated at home or in designated facilities (Cardwell et al. 2022; Chung, Marlow, et al. 2021; Patel, Fernandes, and Sridhar 2021). Providing financial support has been found to be an effective means of increasing adherence to isolation guidelines and reducing the number of confirmed cases (Patel, Fernandes, and Sridhar 2021). Very early on in China, the National Healthcare Security Administration and the Ministry of Finance directed that, for confirmed COVID-19 patients, any expenses remaining after coverage by medical insurance would be subsidized through fiscal funds, thereby ensuring that patients were not prevented from receiving treatment due to financial barriers (National Healthcare Security Administration and Ministry of Finance of the People's Republic of China 2020). Practical support in the form of food, testing, medication, or accommodation for infected individuals who could not isolate at home was also provided in some locations (Chung, Marlow, et al. 2021). The French government deployed health teams to carry out home visits to individuals with confirmed cases of COVID-19 and provided practical support for infected individuals and fellow household members (Patel, Fernandes, and Sridhar 2021). Employment benefits, such as guaranteed paid leave or sick pay, were also frequently crucial for incentivizing infected individuals to self-isolate and facilitated pandemic control (Sachs et al. 2022). In the United States, for instance, 1 in 1,300 workers was estimated to be spared from COVID-19 infection per day as a result of the Families First Coronavirus Response Act, which provided 14 days of emergency sick leave at full pay (Pichler, Wen, and Ziebarth 2020). Additionally, information support during COVID-19 was commonly offered through helplines, websites, and mobile phone applications. Research shows that both decision aids and clear information about social and financial support improve adherence (Cardwell et al. 2022).

**Figure 7.3** Supportive Measures for Targeted Isolation

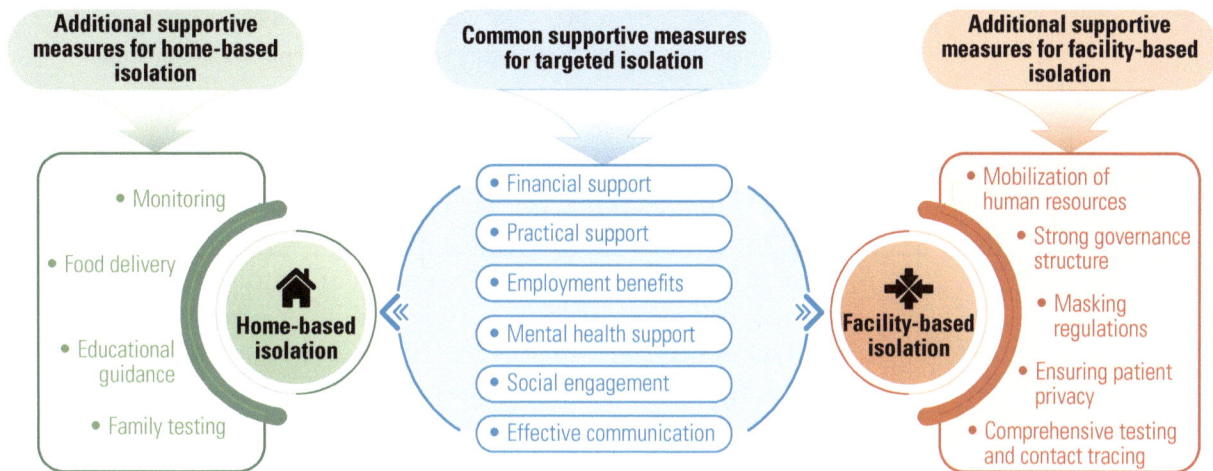

| Additional supportive measures for home-based isolation | Common supportive measures for targeted isolation | Additional supportive measures for facility-based isolation |
|---|---|---|

**Home-based isolation**
- Monitoring
- Food delivery
- Educational guidance
- Family testing

**Common supportive measures for targeted isolation**
- Financial support
- Practical support
- Employment benefits
- Mental health support
- Social engagement
- Effective communication

**Facility-based isolation**
- Mobilization of human resources
- Strong governance structure
- Masking regulations
- Ensuring patient privacy
- Comprehensive testing and contact tracing

*Source:* Original figure created for this publication.

*Note:* The additional supportive measures are intended to highlight specific measures that are particularly important in either home-based or facility-based isolation; however, these measures may be beneficial regardless of the type of targeted isolation strategy employed.

Home-based isolation may require several additional supportive measures, which are less important for facility-based isolation. First, continuous monitoring of biological parameters (for example, oxygen saturation, temperature, and heart rate) can help identify disease progression in infected individuals, particularly among those of advanced age or with preexisting health conditions (Wurzer et al. 2021). Such monitoring can help ensure that patients facing deterioration receive appropriate and timely care. In addition, by preventing unwarranted delays in hospital admissions and improving efficiency, monitoring can help relieve health system strain (Reddy Madhavi et al. 2021). Second, food delivery has been shown to be associated with high acceptance of and adherence to home-based isolation (Patel, Fernandes, and Sridhar 2021). For example, the Singaporean government arranged food deliveries for those in self-isolation through a designated hotline (Chung, Marlow, et al. 2021). Third, providing infected individuals with standard guidance for home-based isolation—such as recommendations pertaining to isolation duration, home zoning, and sanitary guidelines—is essential (Kerkhoff et al. 2020). An internet-based study of a nationally representative sample in Ireland found that decision aids (such as decision trees, online planning tools, and infographics) can help people manage self-isolation at home (Lunn et al. 2021). Fourth, family testing is integral to address intrafamily transmission during home-based isolation. Family members often offer essential support to infected individuals during home-based isolation, and it is essential that family members follow health protocols and engage in frequent testing to mitigate their personal risk (Sirait et al. 2023).

Similarly, facility-based isolation demands additional specific supportive measures for community care centers to operate effectively. According to the existing literature, proposed supportive strategies for future epidemics and pandemics include the following: First, there should be mobilization of human resources across geographic regions to ensure sufficient supply of health workers to control the spread of the pathogen, and mobilized health workers should undergo standardized training for epidemic care and community care center procedures (Chen et al. 2020). Second, a strong governance structure is needed to oversee the planning and regulation of community care centers (Fan et al. 2022). Third, regulations regarding interventions that can prevent pandemic spread, such as masking, should be enforced among both patients and health workers (Chen et al. 2020). Fourth, facility-based isolation should also ensure patient privacy and consider gender differences (Chen et al. 2020). Fifth, comprehensive testing and contact tracing should be employed simultaneously with facility-based isolation to further reduce mortality and transmission (Chen, Chen, et al. 2021). Further empirical evidence is needed on the effectiveness of several of these supportive strategies. Successfully deploying these strategies in LMICs may require international cooperation and financial support, infrastructure, and specifically trained human resources.

Finally, successful implementation of both home- and facility-based targeted isolation strategies may also require adequate provision of mental health support and social engagement to address mental distress and social isolation. Some of the impacts of mandatory isolation include anxiety, depression, felt social isolation and loneliness, and trauma-related stress (Jassim et al. 2021). These impacts may be particularly pronounced among vulnerable groups, including older adults, those who are isolated for prolonged periods of time, and those with preexisting mental health conditions (van Dyck et al. 2020).

Examples of interventions to address mental distress and social isolation include the promotion of healthy behaviors, as well as telephone or video outreach and consultations. By the end of the severe acute respiratory syndrome (SARS) epidemic in 2003, for instance, social support, increased awareness of mental health, and healthy behaviors (for example, regular exercise and reserving adequate time for relaxation and sleep) were all found to be associated with a decrease in perceived stress and incidence of post-traumatic stress disorder (Balanzá-Martínez et al. 2020). In addition, engaging in recreational and leisure activities during extended periods of home-based isolation has been found to confer psychological, sociocultural, and physical benefits (Güzel et al. 2020). Further research should be conducted on the impact of healthy behaviors on infected individuals under home- or facility-based isolation, and related evidence-backed policies and interventions should be designed for local contexts and tested (Balanzá-Martínez et al. 2020). For nursing home residents, one promising supportive strategy is the implementation of telephone outreach programs, under which volunteers engage in weekly phone calls with older adults to address social seclusion and loneliness when isolation protocols are in effect (van Dyck et al. 2020). With respect to formal care provision, telephone or online video consultations are likely a safe and effective option for infected individuals in isolation. Video consultations may be particularly therapeutic for those experiencing anxiety (Razai et al. 2020).

## TARGETED ISOLATION STRATEGIES AND RELATED MEASURES DURING THE INITIAL STAGES OF EPIDEMICS PRIOR TO COVID-19

In 2003, SARS became the first serious and easily transmitted disease to emerge in the twenty-first century (Giesecke 2019; WHO 2003c). In light of the global experience with the SARS outbreak in 2003, the World Health Assembly revised the International Health Regulations (IHR) in 2005 to strengthen information sharing during public health emergencies. The updated IHR require Member States to report accurate information on disease outbreaks that are likely to pose an international public health threat to the World Health Organization (WHO) within a 24-hour assessment period (United Nations 2007). The revised IHR also established a common definition of a public health emergency of international concern (PHEIC) as "an extraordinary event which is determined…(i) to constitute a public health risk to other States through the international spread of disease and (ii) to potentially require a coordinated international response" (WHO 2008, 9). If the WHO declares a PHEIC, states have a legal responsibility to respond through timely action. Since revision of the IHR in 2005, WHO has declared six PHEICs in response to the following viral outbreaks: Influenza A (H1N1), also known as swine flu (2009, worldwide); wild poliovirus (2014, Brazil); Ebola virus (2014, West Africa); Zika virus (2016, worldwide); Ebola virus (2019, Democratic Republic of Congo); and Mpox (2022, worldwide) (Giesecke 2019; WHO 2019).[2]

### Targeted Isolation Strategies and Related Measures

This section summarizes the use of isolation strategies and relevant measures during the initial stages of the PHEICs declared before COVID-19. For the purpose of this analysis, the early stage of an outbreak is considered as the period from when the given pathogen (or disease) was first detected to when WHO declared a PHEIC (with the exception of the COVID-19 pandemic, the early stage of which was defined as spanning roughly from the end of 2019 to the end of 2020, as explained earlier). Table 7.2 gives these dates for each PHEIC, and table 7.3 summarizes the targeted interventions employed in response to each outbreak, as well as relevant epidemiological characteristics of the corresponding diseases.

**Table 7.2** Start and End Points of the Initial Stages of PHEICs

|  | First detection of the pathogen (or disease) | WHO declaration of a PHEIC |
|---|---|---|
| **SARS** | April 16, 2003 (WHO 2003b) | n.a. |
| **Influenza A (H1N1)** | April 15, 2009 (CDC 2019) | April 25, 2009[a] |
| **Poliomyelitis** | March 2014 (WHO 2014b) | May 5, 2014[b] |
| **Ebola virus disease** | West Africa: December 2013 (WHO 2014a); Congo, Dem. Rep.: April 4, 2018 (WHO 2018a, 2018b) | West Africa: August 8, 2014 (WHO 2014a); Congo: July 17, 2019[c] |
| **Zika virus disease** | March 2015[d] | February 1, 2016[e] |

*Sources:* Original table based on sources indicated.

*Note:* PHEIC = public health emergency of international concern; SARS = severe acute respiratory syndrome; WHO = World Health Organization; n.a. = not applicable (that is, when the SARS outbreak occurred in 2003, the PHEIC mechanism had not yet been established).

a. WHO, "H1N1 IHR Emergency Committee," https://www.who.int/groups/h1n1-ihr-emergency-committee.

b. WHO, "Poliovirus IHR Emergency Committee," https://www.who.int/groups/poliovirus-ihr-emergency-committee.

c. WHO, "Ebola Virus Disease in the Democratic Republic of the Congo (Kivu and Ituri) IHR Emergency Committee," https://www.who.int/groups/ebola-virus-disease-in-the-democratic-republic-of-the-congo-kivu-and-ituri-ihr-emergency -committee.

d. WHO, "Zika Virus Disease: Outbreak 2015–2016," https://www.who.int/emergencies/situations/zika-virus-outbreak.

e. WHO, "Zika Virus IHR Emergency Committee," https://www.who.int/groups/zika-virus-ihr-emergency-committee.

**Table 7.3** Summary of Targeted Isolation Strategies Employed during Initial Epidemic Stages, and Relevant Epidemiological Measures

|  | Pathogen | Incubation period | Symptom severity | Infectiousness | Case fatality ratio | Transmission route | Targeted isolation strategies |
|---|---|---|---|---|---|---|---|
| **SARS** | SARS-CoV-1 (Drosten et al. 2003) | Usually 2–7 days[a] | Asymptomatic<br><br>Mildly symptomatic<br><br>Moderately symptomatic<br><br>Severely to critically symptomatic | Data limited<br><br>(WHO 2003a; NAS 2003)<br><br>$R_0 = 2$–$4$<br><br>(Peiris et al. 2003) | 6.6–26.7% (Berber, Sumbria, and Çanakoğlu 2021) | Respiratory transmission; contact transmission | C-MHI-MFI (Le et al. 2004; Liang et al. 2004; WHO 2003c) |
| **COVID-19[b]** | SARS-CoV-2 (Salzberger et al. 2021) | 2–14 days<br><br>Median = 5.7 days (Salzberger et al. 2021) | Asymptomatic<br><br>Mildly symptomatic<br><br>Moderately symptomatic<br><br>Severely to critically symptomatic | $R_0$ (mean) = 3.28<br><br>$R_0$ (median) = 2.79 (Liu, Gayle, et al. 2020) | < 60 years: 1.4% (95% CI: 0.4–3.5%)<br><br>≥ 60 years: 4.5% (95% CI: 1.8–11.1%) (Verity et al. 2020) |  | C-MHI-MFI, C-VHI-VFI, MFI, MHI, VFI, VHI |

*table continues next page*

**Table 7.3** Summary of Targeted Isolation Strategies Employed during Initial Epidemic Stages, and Relevant Epidemiological Measures (continued)

| | Pathogen | Incubation period | Symptom severity | Infectiousness | Case fatality ratio | Transmission route | Targeted isolation strategies |
|---|---|---|---|---|---|---|---|
| **Influenza A (H1N1)** | Influenza A (H1N1) virus (Uyeki 2010) | Mean = 4.3 days (Tuite et al. 2010) | Mostly mildly symptomatic | $R_0$ = 1.31–1.48 (Tuite et al. 2010; Eisenberg 2020) | 0.02% (Van Kerkhove et al. 2013) | | C-VHI-VFI[c] |
| **Poliomyelitis** | Wild poliovirus (Mehndiratta, Mehndiratta, and Pande 2014) | 3–6 days (CDC 2024) | Mostly asymptomatic | $R_0$ = 5–7 (Eisenberg 2020) | Children: 2–5% Adolescents and adults: 15–30% Bulbar involvement:[d] 25–75% (CDC 2021) | Fecal-oral transmission | C-VHI-VFI[e] |
| **Ebola virus disease** | Ebola virus[f] | 2–21 days (Kamorudeen, Adedokun, and Olarinmoye 2020; WHO 2025) | Asymptomatic Symptomatic | None $R_0$ = 1.4–2.0 (Delgado and Simón 2018) | 51% (95% CI: 49–53%) (Kucharski and Edmunds 2014) | Direct contact transmission (blood or other body fluids) | C-VHI-VFI (Mobula et al. 2018; WHO Africa 2020) MFI (Ministry of Health and Social Welfare 2014) |
| **Zika virus disease** | Zika virus[g] | 3–14 days[g] | Mostly asymptomatic | $R_0$ (mean) = 3.02 (Liu, Lillepold, et al. 2020) | None | Bite of Aedes aegypti with virus | None[h] |

*Source:* Original table based on sources indicated.

*Note:* CI = confidence interval; C-MHI-MFI = combined mandatory home- and facility-based isolation; C-VHI-VFI = combined voluntary home- and facility-based isolation; MFI = mandatory facility-based isolation; MHI = mandatory home-based isolation; SARS = severe acute respiratory syndrome; VFI = voluntary facility-based isolation; VHI = voluntary home-based isolation. With respect to epidemics prior to COVID-19, facility-based isolation may also encompass designated isolation wards in hospitals.

a. World Health Organization, "Severe Acute Respiratory Syndrome (SARS)," https://www.who.int/health-topics/severe-acute-respiratory-syndrome#tab=tab_1.

b. For detailed isolation strategies for COVID-19, please refer to the main text of this chapter.

c. US Centers for Disease Control and Prevention, "Interim Guidance on Infection Control Measures for 2009 H1N1 Influenza in Healthcare Settings, Including Protection of Healthcare Personnel," https://archive.cdc.gov/#/details?url=https://www.cdc.gov/h1n1flu/guidelines_infection_control.htm.

d. Bulbar polio presents with weakness of facial, oropharyngeal, and respiratory muscles innervated by cranial nerves. It accounted for 2 percent of cases during this period (CDC 2021).

e. The transmission pathways of poliovirus, which include respiratory droplets and fecal-oral routes, make it essential to implement strict respiratory and intestinal isolation measures. Refer also to New South Wales Government, "Poliomyelitis Control Guideline," https://www.health.nsw.gov.au/Infectious/controlguideline/Pages/polio.aspx.

f. World Health Organization, (2025), "Ebola Virus Disease," https://www.who.int/health-topics/ebola/#tab=tab_1.

g. World Health Organization, "Zika Virus Disease," https://www.who.int/health-topics/zika-virus-disease#tab=tab_1.

h. Neither home- nor facility-based isolation is necessary for Zika because the virus is not airborne and symptoms are mild for most infected individuals. However, Zika virus can spread through mosquito bites and sexual intercourse, so infected individuals are advised to take measures to avoid mosquito bites and either refrain from sexual intercourse or use contraceptives (WHO 2016).

### SARS Epidemic, 2003

The case fatality rate for SARS was estimated at 6.6–26.7 percent, with higher rates among the elderly and those with underlying health conditions (Berber, Sumbria, and Çanakoğlu 2021). About 20–30 percent of patients required admission to intensive care units (ICUs), and most of these individuals required mechanical ventilation (Peiris et al. 2003). Given the high transmissibility and severity of SARS, hospital staff needed to implement strict infection control measures, including wearing masks, gloves, and gowns, and frequent handwashing, to effectively limit transmission (Peiris et al. 2003). Additionally, patients were commonly required to undergo isolation and treatment in hospitals or other facilities until they were no longer contagious (WHO 2003c). In China, the government rapidly implemented strict isolation measures. To address shortages of hospital beds, intensive care facilities, and isolation rooms—and to reduce the risk of hospital-acquired infections—Chinese authorities built a specialized 1,000-bed isolation facility and hospital within eight days (Liang et al. 2004). In Viet Nam, the government quickly implemented mandatory isolation measures in response to local spread of the disease, closing hospitals in affected areas and isolating confirmed cases (Le et al. 2004).

The primary isolation measures recommended by the US Centers for Disease Control and Prevention (CDC) were patient containment and removal of contaminated air from around the patient. The preferred method was to isolate the diagnosed SARS patient in a separate negative-pressure isolation room, with the door closed and only medical personnel allowed to enter (CDC 2003).

### H1N1 Epidemic, 2009

Most H1N1 influenza patients were young, had mild infections, could be cared for at home, and recovered in about a week (Cao et al. 2009; CDC 2019; Tuite et al. 2010).[3] Therefore, the isolation strategy recommended by the US CDC for H1N1-infected patients centered on home-based isolation, cough etiquette, and use of personal protective equipment such as masks (Khazeni et al. 2009). Patients were advised to self-isolate in a separate room with the door closed, with masking urged if the patient had to leave the room (for example, to go to the bathroom or see a doctor). Patients were also encouraged to cover coughing and sneezing with a tissue. In addition, it was recommended that only one family member provide care for the patient and that the air in the isolation room be kept clean by opening windows or using fans.

Elderly individuals were not found to be especially susceptible to infection, but they were more likely to suffer from a severe case if infected, potentially requiring hospitalization (Miller et al. 2008). Because of the need for infection control, hospitalized individuals with H1N1 were isolated from the uninfected patient population (Rello et al. 2009). Isolation precautions for inpatients lasted longer than for those in home-based isolation because the duration of viral shedding was determined to be longer with more severe disease. In addition, to reduce nosocomial infections, infected health care workers were encouraged to isolate at home (US CDC 2009).

### Poliomyelitis Outbreak, 2014

Afghanistan, Nigeria, and Pakistan are the only countries in the world where polio remains a serious threat (Andrade and Hussain 2018). Poliovirus is highly contagious and can be transmitted by both symptomatic and asymptomatic individuals. In symptomatic individuals, transmission occurs before or up to two weeks after symptom onset.[4] Although we could not identify any literature on government isolation responses to this outbreak, standard polio guidelines would have suggested the following procedures. Individuals identified as infected should be isolated in a hospital and should wear masks to prevent the spread of the virus.[5] They should also remain out of school or work for at least 14 days from the onset of illness and until an attending physician confirms full recovery. In communities with adequate modern sewer systems, feces from infected patients can be discharged directly into the sewer without preliminary disinfection.[6] However, in communities lacking such systems, potentially contaminated items require "terminal disinfection," which WHO (2020b) defines as thorough disinfection after the source of infection has left a site.

### Ebola Virus Epidemics, 2013–14 and 2018–19

In areas with limited resources, early isolation of people infected with the Ebola virus was necessary to break the chain of disease transmission in the community. During the Ebola virus disease (EVD) epidemic that started during 2013–14 and extended to 2016 in West Africa, however, inadequate government-mandated isolation measures made it difficult to control the epidemic (Kamorudeen, Adedokun, and Olarinmoye 2020). In addition, infected people often viewed treatment facilities as places of death detached from loved ones and the community, and therefore resisted voluntary admission (Chertow et al. 2014).

Some lessons from the West African EVD epidemic were applied in the response to the subsequent Ebola outbreak in the Democratic Republic of Congo, which started in 2018 (WHO 2020a). For instance, rapid diagnosis through viral RNA detection and Ebola-specific immune antibody detection was used to inform timely isolation and treatment, increasing the chances of survival for infected patients (Kamorudeen, Adedokun, and Olarinmoye 2020; WHO 2020a). Because a person infected with Ebola cannot transmit the disease until symptoms appear,[7] rapid diagnosis also helped reduce the spread of Ebola among the family, friends, and social networks of confirmed patients. In addition, innovative bio-secure emergency care units were used, which made it easier for staff to safely care for patients and enabled safe visits from patients' family members (WHO 2020a).

During the Ebola outbreaks in West Africa and the Democratic Republic of Congo, various voluntary and mandatory isolation measures were implemented to control spread of the virus. In West Africa, to prevent community transmission, confirmed cases were typically mandatorily sent to Ebola treatment units operated by international organizations and government agencies; however, because of insufficient medical facilities, some patients had to be placed in temporary community care centers for isolation and treatment, whereas others were forced to isolate at home with necessary medical and living supplies provided by international and nongovernmental organizations (WHO 2014c). To encourage infected individuals in Beni, Democratic Republic of Congo, to undergo a 21-day isolation period within the community, the government delivered food and medical checkups to homes (WHO Africa 2020).

### Zika Virus Epidemic, 2015–16

Because a high proportion of Zika virus infections are asymptomatic and clinical manifestations are similar to those of other diseases (such as dengue fever), Zika virus often spreads covertly (Sun et al. 2020). Zika virus infection can be confirmed only through a laboratory test of blood or other body fluids (such as urine, saliva, or semen) (Sun et al. 2020).

During the Zika epidemic in the Americas, the Caribbean, and Southeast Asia in 2015–16, WHO supported affected countries in controlling the Zika virus through the actions outlined in the Zika Strategic Response Plan (WHO 2016). Isolation measures were not typically deemed necessary because Zika symptoms are mild for most infected individuals and the virus is not airborne. Infected individuals were advised, however, to take measures to avoid mosquito bites to prevent further vector-based transmission of the virus (WHO 2016). Additionally, because Zika virus can be spread through sexual intercourse, sexually active individuals in areas with ongoing transmission should have been provided with counseling and offered a variety of contraceptive methods to enable them to make informed choices about whether and when to become pregnant to prevent possible adverse pregnancy and fetal outcomes (WHO 2016). Patients were also advised to get plenty of rest, drink enough water, treat any pains or fever with ordinary medicines, and seek medical care and advice if symptoms worsened (WHO 2016).

### Limitations of Facility-Based Isolation

Although implementing facility-based isolation has several advantages, its success is likely very context-dependent and may not be suitable in some settings, for some populations, or for some diseases. For example, during the EVD outbreak in West Africa in 2014, there was a lack of public trust and a common fear among local populations that being taken to a treatment center signified death (Bhatnagar et al. 2016). Given such circumstances, mandatory facility-based isolation may not have been a suitable strategy. More generally, lack of health care infrastructure in low-resource settings poses significant challenges, because many communities in LMICs do not have sufficient medical facilities or resources to support widespread facility-based isolation. Lack or scarcity of mental health resources represents an additional barrier, because facility-based isolation can have a negative impact on mental health, exacerbating feelings of anxiety, loneliness, and stress. During the EVD outbreak in West Africa, the trauma of separating patients from their relatives was intensified by insufficient communication between health workers and the families of those admitted (Brown and Marí Sáez 2021). Cultural factors, such as the importance of family and community support, can make facility-based isolation particularly distressing and impractical. Finally, logistical issues, such as the need for transportation to and from isolation facilities, can further complicate implementation in areas with poor infrastructure.

With respect to diseases, human immunodeficiency virus (HIV) represents a clear example of a pathogen for which facility-based isolation is inappropriate. Although HIV is transmitted via an infectious agent, the long incubation period of the virus means that it would be very difficult and unreasonable to enforce isolation of HIV-infected individuals. Nevertheless, such an isolation strategy has previously been attempted. In 1983, Cuba established a National AIDS program that aimed to prevent the spread of HIV through mass screening and lifelong isolation of people identified as living with HIV in public sanatoriums (Granich et al. 1995). This policy was extremely controversial and has long ago been disbanded.

## IMPACTS OF TARGETED ISOLATION STRATEGIES

The following three sections review the epidemiological and economic impacts of targeted isolation strategies, along with ethical and legal considerations when evaluating those impacts. For this review, we first prioritized evidence from empirical studies, including randomized controlled trials and quasi-experimental studies. To that end, we conducted a literature search across MEDLINE, PubMed, and the Cochrane Library (refer to annex 7A for further details). The search identified only one relevant study. In this study, the authors used interrupted time series analysis to evaluate changes in confirmed COVID-19 cases before and after the implementation of Fangcang shelter hospitals in Wuhan, China. Comparing facility-based isolation with home-based isolation, the authors found that facility-based isolation substantially reduced confirmed cases and the reproduction number (Wang, Gao, et al. 2020). Because of the lack of empirical studies, we further considered modeling studies that examine facility- and home-based isolation in our search. The results of such studies inform much of the discussion in this section and the next. Several limitations to modeling studies merit noting: the lack of empirical validation against real-world outcomes, reliance on assumptions about individual behavior and disease dynamics, and simplifications that may not fully capture the complexity of transmission patterns, health care capacity constraints, or policy enforcement in diverse contexts. Nonetheless, modeling studies are commonly grounded in established theories of disease transmission and are typically informed by observed data from similar or related epidemic settings. As such, they can provide valuable insights, particularly when empirical results are sparse or infeasible to obtain. In the following sections, we will also present findings from observational studies and other types of studies to strengthen our discussion.

**Epidemiological Impact**

The epidemiological impact of home-based isolation and facility-based isolation has been studied extensively. Research has shown that home-based isolation can be an effective tool for reducing COVID-19 transmission among patients with mild to moderate symptoms (Li, Peng, and Lu 2021), particularly in resource-limited settings (Doke et al. 2020). In addition, home-based isolation can control local surges in long-term care facilities by blocking potential transmission from visitors (Moghadas et al. 2020). Residents of long-term care facilities should receive special attention due to their particular susceptibility to infectious diseases and underlying health conditions (Moghadas et al. 2020). Furthermore, home-based isolation has proven effective in managing surges of COVID-19 cases in developing countries, such as India, which face health care infrastructure and funding constraints. A survey conducted in Telangana, India, during August–September 2020 revealed that 94 percent of lab-confirmed COVID-19 patients with mild symptoms recovered well in home-based isolation, and less than 6 percent required hospitalization (Bhardwaj et al. 2021).

Although home-based isolation can be an effective targeted intervention during the initial phases of an outbreak, there is a high degree of variation in people's adherence to isolation protocols. A survey conducted in two counties of North Carolina showed that only 45 percent of households with children under 18 years of age and 65 percent of working adults were able to adhere to home-based isolation during the H1N1 pandemic (Horney et al. 2010). In addition, several published studies have estimated that substantial intrafamily transmission of SARS-CoV-2 occurred during the COVID-19 pandemic (Chen et al. 2020; Denford et al. 2021; Lei et al. 2020; López et al. 2021; Wang, Ma, et al. 2020). Overcrowded homes contributed to a higher risk of transmission among household members (López et al. 2021).

A number of studies have examined the impact of facility-based isolation for patients with mild and moderate COVID-19 symptoms on COVID-19 cases and mortality (Chen, Chen, et al. 2021; Dickens et al. 2020; Hao et al. 2020; Wilasang et al. 2020). For example, a modeling study in Singapore estimated that facility-based isolation could delay an outbreak's peak by 18 days and lead to an overall 57 percent reduction in COVID-19 cases, much higher than the 20 percent reduction in cases using home-based isolation (Dickens et al. 2020). Additionally, facility-based isolation for patients with mild to moderate symptoms in Fangcang shelter hospitals in China reduced the estimated reproduction number from 3.19 to lower than 1 within three to four weeks of implementation (Wilasang et al. 2020). Furthermore, a modeling study found that facility-based isolation with moderate capacity of five beds per 10,000 population could avert 4.17 million new infections and 16,000 deaths, representing 57 percent and 37 percent reductions, respectively, compared to home-based isolation (Chen, Chen, et al. 2021). Increasing facility capacity and expanding testing would further increase the positive impact of facility-based isolation on COVID-19 cases and mortality (Chen, Chen, et al. 2021).

Beyond reducing cases and deaths during the COVID-19 pandemic, facility-based isolation has been found to perform well with respect to other relevant evaluative criteria. A microsimulation modeling study that examined the cost-effectiveness of various COVID-19 control measures in KwaZulu-Natal, South Africa, found that facility-based isolation, used together with testing and contact tracing, is cost-effective compared to testing alone (Reddy et al. 2021). According to a recent study in China, long-term health outcomes among patients isolating in Fangcang shelter hospitals were similar to those who were admitted to designated COVID-19 hospitals (Cui et al. 2022). Studies have also shown that an Ebola outbreak could be effectively slowed and ultimately halted by placing patients in environments that minimize the risk of further transmission (Washington and Meltzer 2015). Such environments include Ebola treatment units, community care centers, or similar community-based settings that encourage behaviors to reduce transmission risk, such as safe burial practices and limited contact with Ebola patients (Washington and Meltzer 2015).

Overall, using the recent COVID-19 pandemic as an example, targeted isolation focusing on infected individuals showed promise as a strategy for achieving containment, suppression, and mitigation, especially when implemented early and complemented by testing, contact tracing, and supportive measures. Nevertheless, countries implementing suppression and mitigation strategies were more likely to opt for population-based interventions in practice (Wu et al. 2021). In the Republic of Korea, the government rapidly scaled up testing and implemented targeted isolation for confirmed cases, supported by digital contact tracing and quarantine monitoring systems, enabling the country to achieve short-term containment and suppression at a national level (Dighe et al. 2020). In addition, findings from a systematic review show that targeted isolation was effective in lowering the reproduction number and achieving mitigation efforts (Ayouni et al. 2021).

Despite the potential of targeted isolation as an effective pandemic response, such interventions are unlikely to achieve global containment if implemented unevenly across countries. The COVID-19 pandemic highlighted how transmission in one region can quickly undermine progress elsewhere if international coordination is lacking. Uncoordinated or delayed implementation allows for continued cross-border transmission, leading to prolonged or repeated interventions. Future pandemic preparedness must prioritize not only national capacity for targeted isolation but also global collaboration, including data sharing, harmonized policies, and support for low-income countries.

## Economic Impact

In addition to assessing the epidemiologic impact of targeted isolation strategies for controlling epidemics, explicating the pathways through which these interventions affect the economy and evaluating their overall economic impact are critical to determining their financial viability and societal utility. Implementation of targeted isolation strategies carries both economic benefits and costs. Economic benefits include the amount of health expenditure saved due to the isolation strategy's impact on cases and mortality as well as other medical and societal resources saved or gained because of epidemic control. Economic costs include those stemming from the initial implementation of isolation strategies, including expenditures for physical and human resources, as well as the opportunity costs of isolation.

### Economic Benefits

The targeted isolation strategies used in the past epidemics and pandemics discussed earlier resulted in an array of economic benefits. First, the reductions in infections and mortality achieved through isolation led to lower health care costs. This is demonstrated indirectly by the substantial health expenditures resulting from the outbreaks, which is equivalent to avoidable costs when targeted isolation strategies were leveraged to reduce cases (discussed in the above section on epidemiological impact). Second, studies show that self-isolation measures can reduce strain on limited medical and social resources and provide time to better control an epidemic.

### Pathway 1: Reduced infections and mortality from targeted isolation strategies, leading to reduced health care costs

#### COVID-19

- The median cost of a single hospitalization for COVID-19 in China was US$2,158.06; total hospitalization costs amounted to US$373.20 million as of May 20, 2020 (An et al. 2022).
- In Massachusetts, providing financial support for infected individuals in home- or facility-based isolation—including salary replacement, essentials, and counseling—was estimated at US$430 per person, considerably lower than the US$2,500 health care cost per patient if transmission was not controlled (Bourdeaux et al. 2021). Early intervention could further reduce overall health expenditures, offsetting the costs of targeted measures (Bourdeaux et al. 2021; De Foo et al. 2022).

#### SARS

- The cost of medical treatment per patient in Beijing was ¥17,150 (US$1,886) (Xiao et al. 2004).

#### H1N1

- During the 2015 H1N1 outbreak in Northern India, mean hospitalization costs were US$1,983 in an H1N1 ward, US$2,554 in single-room isolation, and US$7,172 in ICU—equivalent to 17, 22, and 62 times the monthly per capita income, respectively (Kumar et al. 2015).
- The annual socioeconomic cost of H1N1 in the Republic of Korea was US$1.09 billion (0.14 percent of national gross domestic product). Direct costs

included US$322.6 million in health care costs (29.6 percent of the total costs) (Kim, Yoon, and Oh 2013).

### Polio

- The cost of treating a polio survivor has been estimated to range from US$250,000 to US$1.5 million; annual medical expenses for both paralyzed and nonparalyzed survivors were 20–30 percent higher than those for individuals without a history of polio, according to studies from Denmark and the United States (Nielsen et al. 2016).

### Ebola

- The estimated societal cost (including direct costs and productivity losses) of a recovered EVD case in Guinea, Liberia, and Sierra Leone ranged from US$480 to US$912; the cost of a nonsurviving case ranged from US$5,929 to US$18,929 (Bartsch, Gorham, and Lee 2015).

### Zika

- Hospital costs for newborns with microcephaly following Zika virus infection were approximately one order of magnitude higher than for those without the condition in Texas (US$6,751 vs. US$725) (Shewale et al. 2019).
- Estimates of total direct medical expenses and future productivity losses for children with Zika-related microcephaly in Puerto Rico ranged from US$280 million to US$1.13 billion in 2016 (Alfaro-Murillo et al. 2016).

### Pathway 2: Reduced health care utilization, implying reduced costs

### COVID-19

- Modeling estimated that, if 20 percent of patients with mild COVID-19 symptoms self-isolated within 48 hours of symptom onset, ICU bed use would be reduced by 24.6 percent (Moghadas et al. 2020).
- If 85 percent of mildly symptomatic COVID-19 patients self-isolated within 24 hours, ICU capacity shortages could be completely avoided (Moghadas et al. 2020).
- Facility-based isolation is recommended when hospitals are at capacity, because it allows for triage and reserves traditional hospitals for critically ill patients (Chen et al. 2020; Feng et al. 2020).
- According to projections using COVID-19 cases in Canada, self-isolation of 20 percent of infected individuals resulted in a 23.5 percent reduction in ICU bed usage and shifted the peak of the outbreak by two to four weeks, compared to scenarios without self-isolation (Shoukat et al. 2020).

Based on the above research findings, the economic benefits of isolation strategies in future epidemics will likely depend substantially on the type and timing of the isolation strategy, the current capacity of the health care system, and population adherence to the isolation recommendations.

### Economic costs

In addition to producing benefits, targeted isolation strategies also result in economic costs. First, significant implementation and maintenance expenditures may be required for both home- and facility-based isolation, which may be particularly difficult to mobilize in resource-poor settings. Second, lost labor productivity also contributes to the economic costs of targeted isolation strategies. Third, human resources constitute an additional economic cost of isolation measures.

### Pathway 1: Implementation and maintenance costs

#### COVID-19

- In China, the cost of operating a community care center for facility-based isolation was estimated to be US$543.72 per 1,000 population (An et al. 2022).
- In India's Jodhpur district, the cost of home- and facility-based isolation for mildly symptomatic or asymptomatic COVID-19 patients was estimated at US$7.43 and US$33.02 per person, respectively (Bhardwaj et al. 2021).

#### Ebola

- During the 2014 Ebola outbreak in Nigeria, rapid detection and isolation using existing polio surveillance infrastructure cost a total of US$13 million (Kellerborg, Brouwer, and van Baal 2020).

### Pathway 2: Lost labor productivity

#### COVID-19

- By December 31, 2020, labor force participation in China was reduced by more than 1.6 million person-days because of COVID-19 patient rehabilitation or isolation (Tan et al. 2022).

#### SARS

- During the 2003 SARS epidemic, the value of lost productivity per quarantined individual was estimated at US$1,140 (Gupta, Moyer, and Stern 2005). Although this finding refers to quarantined individuals and not targeted isolated individuals, it sheds light onto potential productivity losses from targeted isolation.

### Pathway 3: Costs for human resources

#### Ebola

- During the 2014 Ebola outbreak in Liberia, large human resources were required to recruit, train, protect, and pay government employees, temporary workers, and international volunteers to implement control and treatment strategies (Paterson, Widner, and Godefroy 2017).

- In March and October 2014, Bomi County in Liberia constructed two isolation wards for Ebola patients. Continuous staffing by local health workers and trained Ebola survivors imposed a substantial human resource burden on Liberia's already overstretched health system, highlighting the intensive personnel demands (and costs) of effective isolation measures (Logan et al. 2014).

## Ethical and Legal Considerations

Ethical and legal perspectives are important when evaluating the health, economic, and social impacts of epidemics, as well as designing epidemic responses, including isolation strategies to control the spread of diseases. In this section, we discuss isolation strategies from three broad ethical perspectives—distributive, procedural, and retributive justice.

"Distributive justice" refers to the normative judgment on the distribution of benefits and burdens across people (for example, in a community, a country, or globally). Isolation strategies targeted at people suffering from an infection will (1) place a burden on those isolating (including the inconvenience of restricted movement, loss of direct contact with loved ones, and income loss) and (2) benefit those at risk of infection because isolation reduces the risk. It is easy to imagine that unequal distributions of benefits and burdens across relevant dimensions could result from targeted isolation. For instance, if resource-poor people face higher or earlier risk of infection than resource-rich people, those asked or mandated to isolate may tend to be resource-poor, while those who benefit from the isolation of others may tend to be resource-rich. During the COVID-19 pandemic, such a scenario was likely, because people in low-paying service jobs faced particularly high risk of infection, such as frontline workers in the retail, social care, and transport industries (Mutambudzi et al. 2022). Whether such a distributional inequality is deemed unjust will depend on whether the dimensions of benefits (protection from infection) and burdens (isolation-associated losses) are deemed relevant for justice. Assuming that these dimensions are indeed relevant, the judgment on whether a particular distribution is unjust will then depend on which basis distributions should be made.

On one such basis—utilitarianism—we would need to measure all losses (for example, due to isolation) and gains (for example, due to protection from infection) across all people and test whether or not the gains outweigh the benefits. Accordingly, from a utilitarian perspective, it is not immediately clear how we would judge the normative goodness of different targeted isolation strategies. On another such basis—prioritarianism, with priority given to resource-poor over resource-rich people—targeted isolation would likely be judged unjust: the resource-poor (people in low-paying jobs) bear the burden of isolation, while everyone else (who will on average be resource-richer) benefits.

Providing the options of either facility- or home-based isolation would likely boost distributive justice, because people would choose the option that is less burdensome to them, given their individual circumstance (Reutskaja and Hogarth 2009). Financial compensation for those in isolation could be another corrective to distributive injustice. Compensation may have the added benefit that it may boost adherence to epidemic control measures, as was observed in Israel (Bodas and Peleg 2020). Finally, distributive injustice may be reduced by making isolation as pleasant as possible, such as by providing opportunities for exercise and social engagement in isolation facilities (Chung, Genoe, et al. 2021; Chen et al. 2020).

"Procedural justice" refers to the fairness of the processes that lead to decisions or outcomes. Following precepts of procedural justice in the design and implementation of isolation strategies may be key to strengthening their legitimacy. People are more likely to follow laws and regulations when they perceive authorities as trustworthy and just (Nagin and Telep 2020). Trust in health authorities can therefore support an effective and efficient health system response during an epidemic (Jiao et al. 2023). Active citizen participation in decision-making processes is particularly critical: all segments of the population, including vulnerable and historically disadvantaged populations, should have a voice in policy and intervention formulation for inclusive and legitimate decisions (Sandrin and Simpson 2022). Such a diversity of voices and participation will likely make decision-making processes on epidemic responses, including isolation strategies, more just; it will make it more likely that the particular needs and wants of all population segments are reflected in the final policy decisions (Kayman and Ablorh-Odjidja 2006).

Two novel and promising approaches are available to foster broad participation in decision-making processes. The first approach emphasizes expanding civic participation and fostering co-governance between citizens and authorities through technological innovations and digital platforms. These tools help overcome geographical and physical barriers that often limit participation (Staykova 2023). However, not all individuals have equal access to digital technologies, putting a limit on the potential of this approach to boost procedural justice through broadening participation. Addressing this situation requires increases in digital literacy and access, such as providing public internet access points and making platforms accessible to those with disabilities. The second approach is deliberative workshops. Deliberative workshops are intended to facilitate informed, public discussions of matters that directly relate to the workshop participants, such as policy making on isolation and social distancing measures in an epidemic (Baum, Jacobson, and Goold 2009). Beyond these two approaches, more traditional participatory mechanisms, such as open forums and community gatherings, can also promote public engagement and contribute to strengthening procedural justice related to decisions on epidemic responses, including isolation strategies (Misuraca 2020).

"Retributive justice" involves fair punishment when wrongful actions have occurred (Walen 2014). Penalties for breaking epidemic control rules (for example, breaches of mandatory isolation) should be enforced fairly and consistently across all segments of society. Comprehensive guidelines on the precise nature of the wrongful actions and the conditions under which penalties are enforced are important conditions for fair and consistent punishment. In addition, the forms of the penalties, such as fines or raised taxes, should be clearly justified and widely communicated to the public. Punishments should not be overly harsh, and opportunities for appeal should be easily and equally available to everyone receiving a penalty.

When considering implementation of mandatory targeted isolation, it is also important to consider legal requirements—in addition to ethical implications. Implementing mandatory isolation during public health emergencies necessitates a careful balance between safeguarding public health and upholding individual rights. This balance hinges on three fundamental legal components: legal authority, due process, and enforcement measures. The following paragraphs discuss each of these components in detail, drawing on the COVID-19 pandemic as an example.

Effective mandatory isolation requires a clearly defined legal framework that specifies who is authorized to issue isolation orders and under which laws. For example, Singapore's main legal basis for isolation is the Infectious Diseases Act (Cap. 137), which explicitly empowers the Director-General of Health to order the isolation and treatment of persons infected with a transmissible disease.[8] In the Republic of Korea, the relevant legal framework is the Infectious Disease Control and Prevention Act. Under this law, the Minister of Health and Welfare, the Korea Disease Control and Prevention Agency, and local authorities may order the compulsory isolation of patients confirmed to have infectious disease.[9] In New Zealand, the Health Act 1956 empowers Medical Officers of Health to require infected individuals to isolate.[10] In addition, the government passed the COVID-19 Public Health Response Act 2020 in May 2020 to provide a specific legal basis for COVID-19 orders.[11] Overall, although legal procedures differ across countries, a firm legal authority to impose targeted isolation on infected individuals existed in most countries that used this measure during the COVID-19 pandemic.

Even in a public health crisis, the rule of law requires regard for individual rights and due process, including legal protections for those subjected to isolation. Although countries varied with respect to due process during the pandemic, most had some mechanism to ensure isolation orders were not unlimited or abusive. For example, in New Zealand, isolation orders were deemed "disallowable instruments," which implied that the House of Representatives could review and overturn these orders.[12] This legislative oversight ensured that targeted isolation orders were subject to checks and balances within the government. Furthermore, individuals required to isolate under these orders had the right to judicial review.[13] Similarly, in the Republic of Korea, if someone believes they are being kept in isolation longer than necessary or without legal justification, they have the right to petition a court for release.[14]

The legal framework for isolation is also likely to affect adherence to isolation orders through the legal enforcement options and perceived legitimacy of the enforcement. During the COVID-19 pandemic, many countries paired isolation mandates with enforcement mechanisms to make sure people stayed isolated, while striving to avoid overly punitive measures. These mechanisms fell into two broad categories: support measures to help isolated individuals adhere to isolation orders and penalties for nonadherence. For example, in China, businesses had to continue paying wages to employees in isolation and employers were explicitly prohibited from taking punitive actions against isolating workers under the Law of the People's Republic of China on Prevention and Treatment of Infectious Diseases.[15] At the same time, Article 330 of the Criminal Law in China stated that those who refused to execute prevention and control measures resulting in the spread, or a serious risk of spread, of an infectious disease could be punished with up to three years imprisonment (Li, Hu, and Liu 2020). Similar mechanisms were employed in Singapore, where nonadherence to epidemic control measures, including isolation, could be prosecuted with imprisonment or fines under the Infectious Diseases Act (Chung, Marlow, et al. 2021).

## RECOMMENDATIONS TO CONTROL EPIDEMICS

Several key lessons can be drawn from recent epidemics, including the COVID-19 pandemic. First, timely targeted isolation strategies during the early stage of an epidemic are likely beneficial to achieve control. As discussed in this chapter, targeted isolation measures are more likely to be useful for short-term containment early in an epidemic than for long-term mitigation. This is particularly likely to be true for epidemic-prone pathogens with features similar to those of COVID-19, especially high transmissibility.

Second, international cooperation is very important, particularly for LMICs. Resource-poor communities often face significant challenges in responding to outbreaks, including limited health care infrastructure, inadequate medical supplies, and lower capacity for rapid response. The international community can provide essential resources, such as medical supplies, financial aid, and technical expertise, which are vital for establishing and maintaining isolation facilities. International partnerships may also be important for funding supportive measures for different isolation strategies, such as ensuring that meals and basic necessities are provided to isolated individuals and their households.

Third, facility-based isolation contributed significantly to achieving COVID-19 pandemic control in some locations. This strategy should be considered when little is known about an emerging pathogen and vaccines are not yet available.

As discussed in this chapter, home-based isolation could be effective in controlling epidemics at a low cost if strictly enforced with clear guidance from health professionals. If infected individuals do not strictly adhere to home-based isolation policies, however, this type of intervention could increase the risk of intrafamily and community transmission (Ilesanmi and Afolabi 2021). Although facility-based isolation may yield better control of disease transmission, it likely also requires more intensive supportive measures for effective, efficient, and ethical implementation. Whether facility-based isolation should be voluntary or mandatory will require careful consideration of cultural, social, and economic factors.

Fourth, with the frequent occurrence of infectious disease outbreaks over the past two decades, it has now become apparent that the global community needs to actively prepare for future epidemics and build a coordinated response system in advance. For example, government officials may wish to consider potential emergency response functions when designing new large public venues in preparation for their future use as repurposed facilities for isolation and quarantining. In addition, it is crucial to establish general clinical triage guidelines, communication strategies, and ethical and legal frameworks in advance of emergency scenarios to ensure rational allocation of limited medical resources under the pressures and uncertainties of an emerging epidemic.

Based on the sum of the available evidence, targeted isolation is likely to be effective, efficient, and ethical in interrupting the spread of an epidemic. The benefits associated with the rapid control that targeted isolation can achieve are likely to outweigh the costs of isolation to societies and individuals. Depending on cultural, social, and economic contexts, either home- or facility-based isolation may be preferable. Offering individuals a choice between these two approaches will likely boost the acceptability and desirability of targeted isolation, particularly when isolation is mandated. Well-designed targeted isolation policies can serve as a cornerstone of future pandemic responses, balancing public health goals with societal costs and individual rights.

## ANNEX 7A. SEARCH STRATEGY FOR EMPIRICAL STUDIES ON THE EPIDEMIOLOGICAL AND ECONOMIC IMPACTS OF TARGETED ISOLATION

To identify empirical studies evaluating the epidemiological and economic effects of targeted isolation interventions during public health emergencies, a literature search was conducted across MEDLINE, PubMed, and the Cochrane Library. We used combinations of search terms related to public health emergencies of international concern, including SARS, COVID-19, Influenza A, H1N1, Polio, Ebola, and Zika. Our literature review focused on terms such as "isolation," "social distancing," and "quarant*" (the asterisk is the truncation symbol, which leads to a search for all words that start with the same initial letters but end with different letters, such as "quarantine," "quarantines," and "quarantining"). Our search excluded terms such as "vaccine" and "vaccination." Although the main focus of the review was targeted isolation, the search included the concept of quarantine because isolation and quarantine are frequently conflated in the literature. "Isolation" refers to restriction of activities and separation of infected individuals from other members of the population, whereas "quarantine" refers to restriction of activities and separation of individuals who may have been exposed to an infectious disease from the rest of the population (Aliyu 2021; Mubayi et al. 2010). However, many studies use these terms interchangeably or without clear definitions. Therefore, to ensure comprehensiveness and avoid missing relevant empirical studies that might have misused or loosely defined the terms, the search included "quarant*." We also included search terms related to epidemiological impacts, such as "epidemic" and "epidemiological," and economic impacts, such as "economic burden," "economic cost," "cost," "economic loss," "willingness to pay," and "economic benefit."

In terms of empirical study designs, the review focused on randomized controlled trials, quasi-experimental studies (for example, regression discontinuity design, instrumental variables, difference in differences, and interrupted time series), and fixed-effects models. Based on this strategy, the search focused on the following three comparisons of specific types of target-intervention: comparison of facility-based isolation and home-based isolation, comparisons of the six strategies identified and discussed in the chapter (MFI, MHI, VFI, VHI, C-MHI-MFI, and C-VHI-VFI), and comparisons of (1) home-based isolation with no isolation or (2) facility-based isolation with no isolation. Few results were found, and after screening, only one study remained as relevant; in that study, the authors used interrupted time series analysis to evaluate changes in confirmed COVID-19 cases before and after the implementation of Fangcang shelter hospitals in Wuhan, China, effectively comparing facility-based isolation with home-based isolation, because home-based isolation was implemented before the establishment of Fangcang shelter hospitals (Wang, Gao, et al. 2020).

## NOTES

Funding for this chapter came from the Chinese Academy of Medical Sciences Innovation Fund for Medical Sciences (2022-I2M-CoV19-003).

1. Other chapters cover pharmaceutical interventions targeted at infected individuals. Targeted isolation strategies involve sequestering individuals who are known to be infected but do not require hospitalization to protect those who remain uninfected, whereas nontargeted isolation encompasses measures applied uniformly regardless of infection status, such as stay-at-home orders or population-wide lockdowns. Targeted and nontargeted isolation both aim to prevent transmission. Targeted isolation does so by removing confirmed cases from the general population, whereas nontargeted isolation does so through widespread reduction in interpersonal contact. In particular, quarantine refers to restriction of activities and separation of potentially exposed individuals from the rest of the population (Aliyu 2021; Mubayi et al. 2010). Targeted isolation is highly precise, focusing only on infected individuals, whereas nontargeted isolation affects all individuals, including those who are uninfected. In terms of resource requirements, targeted isolation requires robust testing capacity and contact tracing (Kucharski et al. 2020), and nontargeted approaches often impose broad restrictions that may result in significant economic and social burdens (Asahi et al. 2021). Targeted isolation typically involves minimal disruption to the uninfected population, although it may cause psychological anxiety among isolated individuals (Ju et al. 2021). By contrast, nontargeted isolation can result in widespread feelings of loneliness and other forms of social instability (Williams et al. 2021).
2. Refer also to WHO, "Mpox," https://www.who.int/news-room/fact-sheets/detail/mpox.
3. Refer also to US CDC, "CDC H1N1 Flu Caring for Someone Sick at Home," https://archive.cdc.gov/#/details?url=https://www.cdc.gov/h1n1flu/homecare/index.htm.
4. US CDC, "About Polio in the United States," https://www.cdc.gov/polio/about/?CDC_AAref_Val=https://www.cdc.gov/polio/what-is-polio/index.htm.
5. NSW [New South Wales] Health, "Poliomyelitis Control Guideline," https://www.health.nsw.gov.au/Infectious/controlguideline/Pages/polio.aspx.
6. NSW [New South Wales] Health, "Poliomyelitis Control Guideline," https://www.health.nsw.gov.au/Infectious/controlguideline/Pages/polio.aspx.
7. WHO, "Ebola Virus Disease," https://www.who.int/health-topics/ebola/#tab=tab_1.
8. Communicable Diseases Agency Singapore, "Infectious Diseases Act" (accessed April 12, 2025), https://www.cda.gov.sg/public/infectious-diseases-act.
9. Korea Legislation Research Institute, "Infectious Disease Control and Prevention Act," https://elaw.klri.re.kr/eng_mobile/viewer.do?hseq=67634&type=part&key=36.
10. Parliamentary Counsel Office, New Zealand, "Health Act 1956," https://www.legislation.govt.nz/act/public/1956/0065/latest/DLM307083.html#DLM307083.
11. Parliamentary Counsel Office, New Zealand, "COVID-19 Public Health Response Act 2020," https://www.legislation.govt.nz/act/public/2020/0012/latest/LMS344134.html.
12. Parliamentary Counsel Office, New Zealand, "COVID-19 Public Health Response Act 2020," https://www.legislation.govt.nz/act/public/2020/0012/latest/LMS344134.html.
13. Parliamentary Counsel Office, New Zealand, "Judicial Review Procedure Act 2016," https://www.legislation.govt.nz/act/public/2016/0050/latest/whole.html#DLM6942108.
14. Korea Legislation Research Institute, "Infectious Disease Control and Prevention Act," https://elaw.klri.re.kr/eng_mobile/viewer.do?hseq=67634&type=part&key=36.
15. Ministry of Human Resources and Social Security of the People's Republic of China, "Notice of the General Office of the Ministry of Human Resources and Social Security on Properly Handling Labor Relations during the Prevention and Control of the Novel Coronavirus-Infected Pneumonia." https://www.mohrss.gov.cn/SYrlzyhshbzb/dongtaixinwen/buneiyaowen/202001/t20200127_357746.html.

## REFERENCES

Note: All references cited in this chapter are used solely for their academic content and should not be interpreted as an endorsement by the authors of the geopolitical positions or other views expressed therein.

Akashi, Hidechika, Haruka Kodoi, Shinichiro Noda, Toyomitsu Tamura, Hiroko Baba, Eiki Chinda, Moe M. Thandar, et al. 2022. "Reporting on the Implementation to Set Up a 'Care and Isolation Facility' for Mild COVID-19 Cases in Tokyo." *Global Health & Medicine* 4 (2): 71–77. https://doi.org/10.35772/ghm.2022.01022.

Alfaro-Murillo, Jorge A., Alyssa S. Parpia, Meagan C. Fitzpatrick, Jules A. Tamagnan, Jan Medlock, Martial L. Ndeffo-Mbah, Durland Fish, et al. 2016. "A Cost-Effectiveness Tool for Informing Policies on Zika Virus Control." *PLOS Neglected Tropical Diseases* 10 (5): e0004743.

Aliyu, Alhaji A. 2021. "Public Health Ethics and the COVID-19 Pandemic." *Annals of African Medicine* 20 (3): 157.

An, X., L. Xiao, X. Yang, X. Tang, F. Lai, and Xiao-Hua Liang. 2022. "Economic Burden of Public Health Care and Hospitalisation Associated with COVID-19 in China." *Public Health* 203: 65–74.

Andrade, Gabriel E., and Azhar Hussain. 2018. "Polio in Pakistan: Political, Sociological, and Epidemiological Factors." *Cureus* 10 (10): e3502. https://doi.org/10.7759/cureus.3502.

ANI/Xinhua. 2020. "Nearly Half of Nepal's COVID-19 Patients Stay in Home Isolation, Says Authority." ANI, September 20, 2020. https://www.aninews.in/news/world/asia/nearly -half-of-nepals-covid-19-patients-stay-in-home-isolation-say-authorites20200920201339/.

Asahi, Kenzo, Eduardo A. Undurraga, Rodrigo Valdés, and Rodrigo Wagner. 2021. "The Effect of COVID-19 on the Economy: Evidence from an Early Adopter of Localized Lockdowns." *Journal of Global Health* 11: 05002.

Ayouni, Imen, Jihen Maatoug, Wafa Dhouib, Nawel Zammit, Sihem Ben Fredj, Rim Ghammam, and Hassen Ghannem. 2021. "Effective Public Health Measures to Mitigate the Spread of COVID-19: A Systematic Review." *BMC Public Health* 21 (1): 1015.

Balanzá-Martínez, V., B. Atienza-Carbonell, F. Kapczinski, and R. B. De Boni. 2020. "Lifestyle Behaviours during the COVID-19—Time to Connect." *Acta Psychiatrica Scandinavica* 141 (5): 399–400. https://doi.org/10.1111/acps.13177.

Bartsch, Sarah M., Katrin Gorham, and Bruce Y. Lee. 2015. "The Cost of an Ebola Case." *Pathogens and Global Health* 109 (1): 4–9.

Baum, Nancy M., Peter D. Jacobson, and Susan D. Goold. 2009. "'Listen to the People': Public Deliberation about Social Distancing Measures in a Pandemic." *American Journal of Bioethics* 9 (11): 4–14.

Berber, Engin, Deepak Sumbria, and Nurettin Çanakoğlu. 2021. "Meta-analysis and Comprehensive Study of Coronavirus Outbreaks: SARS, MERS and COVID-19." *Journal of Infection and Public Health* 14 (8): 1051–64. https://doi.org/10.1016/j.jiph.2021.06.007.

Bhardwaj, Pankaj, Nitin Kumar Joshi, Manoj Kumar Gupta, Akhil Dhanesh Goel, Suman Saurabh, Jaykaran Charan, Prakash Rajpurohit, et al. 2021. "Analysis of Facility and Home Isolation Strategies in COVID 19 Pandemic: Evidences from Jodhpur, India." *Infection and Drug Resistance*: 2233–39.

Bhatnagar, Nidhi, Manoj Grover, Atul Kotwal, and Himanshu Chauhan. 2016. "Study of Recent Ebola Virus Outbreak and Lessons Learned: A Scoping Study." *Annals of Tropical Medicine and Public Health* 9 (3).

Bodas, Moran, and Kobi Peleg. 2020. "Self-Isolation Compliance in the Covid-19 Era Influenced by Compensation: Findings from a Recent Survey in Israel: Public Attitudes toward the Covid-19 Outbreak and Self-Isolation: A Cross Sectional Study of the Adult Population of Israel." *Health Affairs* 39 (6): 936–41.

Bosa, Iris, Adriana Castelli, Michele Castelli, Oriana Ciani, Amelia Compagni, Matteo M. Galizzi, Matteo Garofano, et al. 2022. "Response to COVID-19: Was Italy (Un) Prepared?" *Health Economics, Policy and Law* 17 (1): 1–13.

Bourdeaux, Margaret, Jessica Kaushal, Linda Bilmes, Annmarie Sasdi, Megan Mishra, and Anne Hoyt. 2021. "Estimating the Costs and Benefits of Supported Quarantine and Isolation in Massachusetts: The Missing Link in COVID-19 Response." HKS Working Paper No. RWP21-003, John F. Kennedy School of Government, Cambridge, MA.

Brown, Hannah, and Almudena Marí Sáez. 2021. "Ebola Separations: Trust, Crisis, and 'Social Distancing' in West Africa." *Journal of the Royal Anthropological Institute* 27 (1): 9–29.

Cao, Bin, Xing-Wang Li, Yu Mao, Jian Wang, Hong-Zhou Lu, Yu-Sheng Chen, Zong-An Liang, et al. 2009. "Clinical Features of the Initial Cases of 2009 Pandemic Influenza A (H1N1) Virus Infection in China." *New England Journal of Medicine* 361 (26): 2507–17.

Cardwell, Karen, Sinéad M. O'Neill, Barrie Tyner, Natasha Broderick, Kirsty O'Brien, Susan M. Smith, Patricia Harrington, et al. 2022. "A Rapid Review of Measures to Support People in Isolation or Quarantine during the Covid-19 Pandemic and the Effectiveness of Such Measures." *Reviews in Medical Virology* 32 (1): e2244.

Carvalho, Thiago, Florian Krammer, and Akiko Iwasaki. 2021. "The First 12 Months of COVID-19: A Timeline of Immunological Insights." *Nature Reviews Immunology* 21 (4): 245–56.

CDC (US Centers for Disease Control and Prevention). 2003. "Cluster of Severe Acute Respiratory Syndrome Cases among Protected Health-Care Workers—Toronto, Canada, April 2003." *Morbidity and Mortality Weekly Report* 52 (19): 433–36.

CDC (US Centers for Disease Control and Prevention). 2007. "Interim Pre-pandemic Planning Guidance: Community Strategy for Pandemic Influenza Mitigation in the United States—Early, Targeted, Layered Use of Nonpharmaceutical Interventions." CDC. https://stacks.cdc.gov/view/cdc/11425.

CDC (US Centers for Disease Control and Prevention). 2019. "2009 H1N1 Pandemic Timeline." CDC. https://archive.cdc.gov/#/details?url=https://www.cdc.gov/flu/pandemic-resources/2009-pandemic-timeline.html.

CDC (US Centers for Disease Control and Prevention). 2021. "Chapter 18: Polio; Epidemiology and Prevention of Vaccine-Preventable Diseases." CDC. https://www.cdc.gov/pinkbook/hcp/table-of-contents/chapter-18-poliomyelitis.html.

CDC (US Centers for Disease Control and Prevention). 2024. "Clinical Overview of Poliomyelitis." CDC. https://www.cdc.gov/polio/hcp/clinical-overview/index.html.

Cevik, Muge, Stefan D. Baral, Alex Crozier, and Jackie A. Cassell. 2021. "Support for Self-Isolation Is Critical in COVID-19 Response." *BMJ* 372.

Chen, Qiulan, Lance Rodewald, Shengjie Lai, and George F. Gao. 2021. "Rapid and Sustained Containment of Covid-19 Is Achievable and Worthwhile: Implications for Pandemic Response." *BMJ* 375: e066169.

Chen, Simiao, Qiushi Chen, Juntao Yang, Lin Lin, Linye Li, Lirui Jiao, Pascal Geldsetzer, et al. 2021. "Curbing the COVID-19 Pandemic with Facility-Based Isolation of Mild Cases: A Mathematical Modeling Study." *Journal of Travel Medicine* 28 (2). https://doi.org/10.1093/jtm/taaa226.

Chen, Simiao, Zongjiu Zhang, Juntao Yang, Jian Wang, Xiaohui Zhai, Till Bärnighausen, and Chen Wang. 2020. "Fangcang Shelter Hospitals: A Novel Concept for Responding to Public Health Emergencies." *The Lancet* 395 (10232): 1305–14. https://doi.org/10.1016/s0140-6736(20)30744-3.

Chertow, Daniel S., Christian Kleine, Jeffrey K. Edwards, Roberto Scaini, Ruggero Giuliani, and Armand Sprecher. 2014. "Ebola Virus Disease in West Africa—Clinical Manifestations and Management." *New England Journal of Medicine* 371 (22): 2054–57.

Chia, Ming Li, Dickson Hong Him Chau, Kheng Sit Lim, Christopher Wei Yang Liu, Hiang Khoon Tan, and Yan Ru Tan. 2021. "Managing COVID-19 in a Novel, Rapidly Deployable Community Isolation Quarantine Facility." *Annals of Internal Medicine* 174 (2): 247–51.

China Association for Engineering Construction Standardization. 2022. *Technical Specification for Large Space Building Retrofitted Fangcang Shelter Hospital.* China Architecture and Building Press.

Chung, Sheng-Chia, Sushila Marlow, Nicholas Tobias, Alessio Alogna, Ivano Alogna, San-Lin You, Kamlesh Khunti, et al. 2021. "Lessons from Countries Implementing Find, Test, Trace, Isolation and Support Policies in the Rapid Response of the COVID-19 Pandemic: A Systematic Review." *BMJ Open* 11 (7): e047832. https://doi.org/10.1136/bmjopen-2020-047832.

Chung, Wonock, M. Rebecca Genoe, Pattara Tavilsup, Samara Stearns, and Toni Liechty. 2021. "The Ups and Downs of Older Adults' Leisure during the Pandemic." *World Leisure Journal* 63 (3): 301–15.

Cui, Dan, Simiao Chen, Luzhao Feng, Mengmeng Jia, Yeming Wang, Weijun Xiao, Yanxia Sun, et al. 2022. "Long-Term Outcomes in COVID-19 Patients Who Recovered from the First Wave of the Pandemic." *National Science Review* 9 (11): nwac192.

De Foo, Chuan, Victoria Haldane, Anne-Sophie Jung, Karen A. Grépin, Shishi Wu, Sudhvir Singh, Niranjala Perera, et al. 2022. "Isolation Facilities for Covid-19: Towards a Person Centred Approach." *BMJ* 378: e069558.

Delgado, Rafael, and Fernando Simón. 2018. "Transmission, Human Population, and Pathogenicity: The Ebola Case in Point." *Microbiology Spectrum* 6 (2): 10.

Denford, Sarah, Kate Morton, Jeremy Horwood, Rachel de Garang, and Lucy Yardley. 2021. "Preventing within Household Transmission of Covid-19: Is the Provision of Accommodation to Support Self-Isolation Feasible and Acceptable?" *BMC Public Health* 21 (1): 1–13.

Dickens, Borame L., Joel R. Koo, Annelies Wilder-Smith, and Alex R. Cook. 2020. "Institutional, Not Home-Based, Isolation Could Contain the COVID-19 Outbreak." *The Lancet* 395 (10236): 1541–42.

Dighe, Amy, Lorenzo Cattarino, Gina Cuomo-Dannenburg, Janetta Skarp, Natsuko Imai, Sangeeta Bhatia, Katy A. M. Gaythorpe, et al. 2020. "Response to COVID-19 in South Korea and Implications for Lifting Stringent Interventions." *BMC Medicine* 18: 1–12.

Doke, Purwa, Jitendra S. Oswal, Disha A. Padalkar, and Mohit P. Jain. 2020. "Feasibility of the Home Isolation Programme for Adults and Children with COVID-19." *International Journal of Advances in Medicine* 7 (11): 1647–51.

Drosten, Christian, Stephan Günther, Wolfgang Preiser, Sylvie van der Werf, Hans-Reinhard Brodt, Stephan Becker, Holger Rabenau, et al. 2003. "Identification of a Novel Coronavirus in Patients with Severe Acute Respiratory Syndrome." *New England Journal of Medicine* 348 (20): 1967–76.

Eisenberg, Joseph. 2020. "$R_0$: How Scientists Quantify the Intensity of an Outbreak like Coronavirus and Its Pandemic Potential." *The Pursuit*, February 12, 2020. https://sph.umich.edu/pursuit/2020posts/how-scientists-quantify-outbreaks.html.

Fan, Victoria Y., Craig T. Yamaguchi, Ketan Pal, Stephen M. Geib, Leocadia Conlon, Joshua R. Holmes, Yara Sutton, et al. 2022. "Planning and Implementation of COVID-19 Isolation and Quarantine Facilities in Hawaii: A Public Health Case Report." *International Journal of Environmental Research and Public Health* 19 (15): 9368.

Feng, Z.-H., Y.-R. Cheng, L. Ye, M.-Y. Zhou, M.-W. Wang, and J. Chen. 2020. "Is Home Isolation Appropriate for Preventing the Spread of COVID-19." *Public Health* 183 (June): 4–5. https://doi.org/10.1016/j.puhe.2020.03.008.

Giesecke, Johan. 2019. "The Truth about PHEICs." *The Lancet*. https://www.thelancet.com/journals/lancet/article/PIIS0140-6736(19)31566-1/fulltext.

The Government of the Hong Kong Special Administrative Region. 2022. "LCQ1: Community Isolation Facility Hotel Scheme." Press Releases, https://www.info.gov.hk/gia/general/202205/04/P2022050400452.htm.

Government of Nepal Ministry of Health and Population. 2020. "Health Sector Emergency Response Plan COVID-19 Pandemic." https://www.who.int/docs/default-source/nepal -documents/novel-coronavirus/health-sector-emergency-response-plan-covid-19 -endorsed-may-2020.pdf.

Granich, Reuben, Bradly Jacobs, Jonathan Mermin, and Allan Pont. 1995. "Cuba's National AIDS Program. The First Decade." *Western Journal of Medicine* 163 (2): 139.

Gupta, Anu G., Cheryl A. Moyer, and David T. Stern. 2005. "The Economic Impact of Quarantine: SARS in Toronto as a Case Study." *Journal of Infection* 50 (5): 386–93. https://doi.org/10.1016/j.jinf.2004.08.006.

Güzel, Pınar, Kadir Yildiz, Melike Esentaş, and Devrim Zerengök. 2020. "'Know-How' to Spend Time in Home Isolation during COVID-19; Restrictions and Recreational Activities." *International Journal of Psychology and Educational Studies* 7 (2): 122–31.

Hao, Xingjie, Shanshan Cheng, Degang Wu, Tangchun Wu, Xihong Lin, and Chaolong Wang. 2020. "Reconstruction of the Full Transmission Dynamics of COVID-19 in Wuhan." *Nature* 584 (7821): 420–24. https://doi.org/10.1038/s41586-020-2554-8.

Hofverberg, Elin. 2020. "Recent Legislation Enacted by Italy to Tackle COVID-19." *In Custodia Legis* (blog), March 12, 2020. https://blogs.loc.gov/law/2020/03/recent -legislation-enacted-by-italy-to-tackle-covid-19/.

Horney, Jennifer A., Zack Moore, Meredith Davis, and Pia D. M. MacDonald. 2010. "Intent to Receive Pandemic Influenza A (H1N1) Vaccine, Compliance with Social Distancing and Sources of Information in NC, 2009." *PLOS One* 5 (6): e11226.

Ilesanmi, Olayinka S., and Aanuoluwapo A. Afolabi. 2021. "A Scope Review on Home-Based Care Practices for COVID-19: What Nigeria Can Learn from Other Countries." *Ibom Medical Journal* 14 (1): 1–9.

Jamison, Dean T., Lawrence H. Summers, Angela Y. Chang, Omar Karlsson, Wenhui Mao, Ole F. Norheim, Osondu Ogbuoji, et al. 2024. "Global Health 2050: The Path to Halving Premature Death by Mid-century." *The Lancet* 404 (10462): 1561–614.

Jassim, Ghufran, Mariam Jameel, Edwina Brennan, Manaf Yusuf, Nebras Hasan, and Yusuf Alwatani. 2021. "Psychological Impact of COVID-19, Isolation, and Quarantine: A Cross-Sectional Study." *Neuropsychiatric Disease and Treatment* 17: 1413–21.

Jiao, Lirui, Jonas Wachinger, Selina Dasch, Till Bärnighausen, Shannon A. McMahon, and Simiao Chen. 2023. "Calculation, Knowledge and Identity: Dimensions of Trust When Making COVID-19 Vaccination Choices in China." *SSM-Qualitative Research in Health* 4: 100288.

Ju, Yumeng, Wentao Chen, Jin Liu, Aiping Yang, Kongliang Shu, Yun Zhou, Mi Wang, et al. 2021. "Effects of Centralized Isolation vs. Home Isolation on Psychological Distress in Patients with COVID-19." *Journal of Psychosomatic Research* 143: 110365.

Kamorudeen, Ramat Toyin, Kamoru Ademola Adedokun, and Ayodeji Oluwadare Olarinmoye. 2020. "Ebola Outbreak in West Africa, 2014–2016: Epidemic Timeline, Differential Diagnoses, Determining Factors, and Lessons for Future Response." *Journal of Infection and Public Health* 13 (7): 956–62. https://doi.org/https://doi.org/10.1016/j .jiph.2020.03.014.

Kayman, Harvey, and Angela Ablorh-Odjidja. 2006. "Revisiting Public Health Preparedness: Incorporating Social Justice Principles into Pandemic Preparedness Planning for Influenza." *Journal of Public Health Management and Practice* 12 (4): 373–80.

Kellerborg, Klas, Werner Brouwer, and Pieter van Baal. 2020. "Costs and Benefits of Early Response in the Ebola Virus Disease Outbreak in Sierra Leone." *Cost Effectiveness and Resource Allocation* 18: 1–9.

Kerkhoff, Andrew D., Darpun Sachdev, Sara Mizany, Susy Rojas, Monica Gandhi, James Peng, Douglas Black, et al. 2020. "Evaluation of a Novel Community-Based COVID-19 'Test-to-Care' Model for Low-Income Populations." *PLOS One* 15 (10): e0239400.

Khazeni, Nayer, David W. Hutton, Alan M. Garber, Nathaniel Hupert, and Douglas K. Owens. 2009. "Effectiveness and Cost-Effectiveness of Vaccination against Pandemic Influenza (H1N1) 2009." *Annals of Internal Medicine* 151 (12): 829–39.

Kim, Yang-Woo, Seok-Jun Yoon, and In-Hwan Oh. 2013. "The Economic Burden of the 2009 Pandemic H1N1 Influenza in Korea." *Scandinavian Journal of Infectious Diseases* 45 (5): 390–96. https://doi.org/10.3109/00365548.2012.749423.

Kucharski, Adam J., and W. John Edmunds. 2014. "Case Fatality Rate for Ebola Virus Disease in West Africa." *The Lancet* 384 (9950): 1260. https://doi.org/10.1016/s0140 -6736(14)61706-2.

Kucharski, Adam J., Petra Klepac, Andrew J. K. Conlan, Stephen M. Kissler, Maria L. Tang, Hannah Fry, Julia R. Gog, et al. 2020. "Effectiveness of Isolation, Testing, Contact Tracing, and Physical Distancing on Reducing Transmission of SARS-CoV-2 in Different Settings: A Mathematical Modelling Study." *The Lancet Infectious Diseases* 20 (10): 1151–60.

Kumar, Pratyush, Anurag Sachan, Atul Kakar, and Atul Gogia. 2015. "Socioeconomic Impact of the Recent Outbreak of H1N1." *Current Medicine Research and Practice* 5 (4): 163–67.

Lavecchia, Adam M., Heidi Liu, and Philip Oreopoulos. 2016. "Behavioral Economics of Education: Progress and Possibilities." In *Handbook of the Economics of Education (Volume 5)*, edited by Eric A. Hanushek, Stephen J. Machin, and Ludger Woessmann, 1–74. Elsevier.

Le, Dand Ha, Sharon A. Bloom, Quang Hien Nguyen, Susan A. Maloney, Quynh Mai Le, Katrin C. Leitmeyer, Huy Anh Bach, et al. 2004. "Lack of SARS Transmission among Public Hospital Workers, Vietnam." *Emerging Infectious Diseases* 10 (2): 265–68. https://doi.org/10.3201/eid1002.030707.

Lei, Hao, Xiaolin Xu, Shenglan Xiao, Xifeng Wu, and Yuelong Shu. 2020. "Household Transmission of COVID-19: A Systematic Review and Meta-analysis." *Journal of Infection* 81 (6): 979–97.

Li, Hang, Yuan-Yuan Peng, and Jin-Ping Lu. 2021. "Investigation and Analysis of 108 Cases of Home Isolated Patients with Mild COVID-19." *Disaster Medicine and Public Health Preparedness* 15 (6): e8–e11.

Li, Hao, Mengnan Hu, and Shuang Liu. 2020. "The Need to Improve the Laws and Regulations Relevant to the Outbreak of COVID-19: What Might Be Learned from China?" *Journal of Global Health* 10 (1): 010328.

Li, Juan, Pei Yuan, Jane Heffernan, Tingting Zheng, Nick Ogden, Beate Sander, Jun Li, et al. 2020. "Fangcang Shelter Hospitals during the COVID-19 Epidemic, Wuhan, China." *Bulletin of the World Health Organization* 98 (12): 830–41D. https://apps.who.int/iris /handle/10665/337613.

Liang, Wannian, Zonghan Zhu, Jiyong Guo, Zejun Liu, Xiong He, Weigong Zhou, Daniel P. Chin, and Anne Schuchat. 2004. "Severe Acute Respiratory Syndrome, Beijing, 2003." *Emerging Infectious Diseases* 10 (1): 25–31.

Liu, Ying, Albert A. Gayle, Annelies Wilder-Smith, and Joacim Rocklöv. 2020. "The Reproductive Number of COVID-19 is Higher Compared to SARS Coronavirus." *Journal of Travel Medicine* 27 (2). https://doi.org/10.1093/jtm/taaa021.

Liu, Ying, Kate Lillepold, Jan C. Semenza, Yesim Tozan, Mikkel B. M. Quam, and Joacim Rocklöv. 2020. "Reviewing Estimates of the Basic Reproduction Number for Dengue, Zika and Chikungunya across Global Climate Zones." *Environmental Research* 182: 109114.

Logan, Gorbee, Neil M. Vora, Tolbert G. Nyensuah, Alex Gasasira, Joshua Mott, Henry Walke, Frank Mahoney, et al. 2014. "Establishment of a Community Care Center for Isolation and Management of Ebola Patients—Bomi County, Liberia, October 2014. " *Morbidity and Mortality Weekly Report* 63 (44): 1010–12.

Lopes, Noemi, Federica Vernuccio, Claudio Costantino, Claudia Imburgia, Cesare Gregoretti, Salvatore Salomone, Filippo Drago, and Giuliano Lo Bianco. 2020. "An Italian Guidance Model for the Management of Suspected or Confirmed COVID-19 Patients in the Primary Care Setting." *Frontiers in Public Health* 8: 572042.

López, Mercé, Claudia Gallego, Rafael Abós-Herrándiz, Ana Tobella, Nuria Turmo, Alba Monclús, Alba Martinez, et al. 2021. "Impact of Isolating COVID-19 Patients in a Supervised Community Facility on Transmission Reduction among Household Members." *Journal of Public Health* 43 (3): 499–507. https://doi.org/10.1093/pubmed/fdab002.

Lunn, Peter D., Shane Timmons, Hannah Julienne, Cameron A. Belton, Martina Barjaková, Ciarán Lavin, and Féidhlim P. McGowan. 2021. "Using Decision Aids to Support Self-Isolation during the COVID-19 Pandemic." *Psychology & Health* 36 (2): 195–213.

Machida, Masaki, Itaru Nakamura, Reiko Saito, Tomoki Nakaya, Tomoya Hanibuchi, Tomoko Takamiya, Yuko Odagiri, et al. 2020. "The Actual Implementation Status of Self-Isolation among Japanese Workers during the COVID-19 Outbreak." *Tropical Medicine and Health* 48 (1): 63. https://doi.org/10.1186/s41182-020-00250-7.

Mbunge, Elliot. 2020. "Effects of COVID-19 in South African Health System and Society: An Explanatory Study." *Diabetes & Metabolic Syndrome: Clinical Research & Reviews* 14 (6): 1809–14.

Mehndiratta, Man Mohan, Prachi Mehndiratta, and Renuka Pande. 2014. "Poliomyelitis: Historical Facts, Epidemiology, and Current Challenges in Eradication." *Neurohospitalist* 4 (4): 223–29.

Miller, Mark A., Cecile Viboud, Donal R. Olson, Rebecca F. Grais, Maia A. Rabaa, and Lone Simonsen. 2008. "Prioritization of Influenza Pandemic Vaccination to Minimize Years of Life Lost." *Journal of Infectious Diseases* 198 (3): 305–11.

Ministry of Health and Social Welfare, Republic of Liberia. 2014. "*The Anti-Ebola Regulation (MOHSW/R-001/2014).*" https://ebolacommunicationnetwork.org/ebolacomresource /liberia-the-anti-ebola-regulation/.

Misuraca, Gianluca. 2020. "Rethinking Democracy in the 'Pandemic Society': A Journey in Search of the Governance with, of and by AI." https://ceur-ws.org/Vol-2781/invited1 .pdf.

Mobula, Linda M., Jolene H. Nakao, Sonia Walia, Justin Pendarvis, Peter Morris, and David Townes. 2018. "A Humanitarian Response to the West African Ebola Virus Disease Outbreak." *Journal of International Humanitarian Action* 3 (1): 10. https://doi.org/10.1186 /s41018-018-0039-2.

Moghadas, Seyed M., Affan Shoukat, Meagan C. Fitzpatrick, Chad R. Wells, Pratha Sah, Abhishek Pandey, Jeffrey D. Sachs, et al. 2020. "Projecting Hospital Utilization during the COVID-19 Outbreaks in the United States." *Proceedings of the National Academy of Sciences* 117 (16): 9122–26.

Moodley, Keymanthri, Adetayo Emmanuel Obasa, and Leslie London. 2020. "Isolation and Quarantine in South Africa during COVID-19: Draconian Measures or Proportional Response?" *South African Medical Journal* 110 (6): 1–2.

Mubayi, Anuj, Christopher Kribs Zaleta, Maia Martcheva, and Carlos Castillo-Chávez. 2010. "A Cost-Based Comparison of Quarantine Strategies for New Emerging Diseases." *Mathematical Biosciences & Engineering* 7 (3): 687–717.

Murarkar, Sujata, Sudhanshu Mahajan, and Jayashree Gothankar. 2021. "The Symptoms and Co-morbidities of COVID-19 Patients at Home Isolation in India." *International Journal of Health Services Research and Policy* 6 (2): 182–89.

Mutambudzi, Miriam, Claire Niedzwiedz, Ewan Beaton Macdonald, Alastair Leyland, Frances Mair, Jana Anderson, Carlos Celis-Morales, et al. 2022. "Occupation and Risk of Severe COVID-19: Prospective Cohort Study of 120 075 UK Biobank Participants." *Occupational and Environmental Medicine* 78, (5): 307–14.

Nagin, Daniel S., and Cody W. Telep. 2020. "Procedural Justice and Legal Compliance: A Revisionist Perspective." *Criminology & Public Policy* 19 (3): 761–86.

NAS (National Archives of Singapore). 2003. "Biosafety and SARS Incident in Singapore September 2003: Report of the Review Panel on New SARS Case and Biosafety. September 2003." NAS, Singapore.

National Center for Immunization and Respiratory Diseases (U.S.). Division of Viral Diseases. 2020. Preventing the Spread of Coronavirus Disease 2019 in Homes and Residential Communities: Interim Guidance: February 14, 2020. https://stacks.cdc.gov/view/cdc/85942.

National Healthcare Security Administration and Ministry of Finance of the People's Republic of China. 2020. Notice on Ensuring Medical Security for the Pneumonia Epidemic Caused by the Novel Coronavirus Infection [关于做好新型冠状病毒感染的肺炎疫情医疗保障的通知]. January 22, 2020. https://www.gov.cn/zhengce/zhengceku/2020-01/23/content_5562418.htm.

National Institute for Communicable Diseases. 2020. "Clinical Management of Suspected or Confirmed COVID-19 Disease." https://www.nicd.ac.za/wp-content/uploads/2020/03/Clinical-Management-of-COVID-19-disease_Version-3_27March2020.pdf.

Nielsen, Nete Munk, Lise Kay, Benedikte Wanscher, Rikke Ibsen, Jakob Kjellberg, and Poul Jennum. 2016. "Long-Term Socio-economic Consequences and Health Care Costs of Poliomyelitis: A Historical Cohort Study Involving 3606 Polio Patients." *Journal of Neurology* 263: 1120–28.

Patel, Jay, Genevie Fernandes, and Devi Sridhar. 2021. "How Can We Improve Self-Isolation and Quarantine for Covid-19?" *BMJ* 372: n625.

Paterson, David, Jennifer Widner, and Béatrice Godefroy. 2017. "Filling Skills Gaps: Mobilizing Human Resources in the Fight against Ebola, 2014–2015." Global Challenges: Ebola Outbreak, Innovations for Successful Societies, Princeton University. https://successfulsocieties.princeton.edu/publications/ebola-skills-mobilizing-human-resources-liberia.

Peiris, Joseph S., Kwok Y. Yuen, Albert D. Osterhaus, and Klaus Stöhr. 2003. "The Severe Acute Respiratory Syndrome." *New England Journal of Medicine* 349 (25): 2431–41.

Pichler, Stefan, Katherine Wen, and Nicolas R Ziebarth. 2020. "COVID-19 Emergency Sick Leave Has Helped Flatten the Curve in the United States: Study Examines the Impact of Emergency Sick Leave on the Spread of COVID-19." *Health Affairs* 39 (12): 2197–204.

Public Health Agency of Canada. 2021. "Government of Canada Announces Funding for COVID-19 Safe Voluntary Isolation Sites in British Columbia." News release, November 26, 2021. https://www.canada.ca/en/public-health/news/2021/11/government-of-canada-announces-funding-for-covid-19-safe-voluntary-isolation-sites-in-british-columbia.html.

Razai, Mohammad S., Pippa Oakeshott, Hadyn Kankam, Sandro Galea, and Helen Stokes-Lampard. 2020. "Mitigating the Psychological Effects of Social Isolation during the Covid-19 Pandemic." *BMJ* 369: m1904.

Reagu, Shuja, Ovais Wadoo, Javed Latoo, Deborah Nelson, Sami Ouanes, Naseer Masoodi, Mustafa Abdul Karim, et al. 2021. "Psychological Impact of the COVID-19 Pandemic within Institutional Quarantine and Isolation Centres and Its Sociodemographic Correlates in Qatar: A Cross-Sectional Study." *BMJ Open* 11 (1): e045794.

Reddy, Krishna P., Fatma M. Shebl, Julia H. A. Foote, Guy Harling, Justine A. Scott, Christopher Panella, Kieran P. Fitzmaurice, et al. 2021. "Cost-Effectiveness of Public Health Strategies for COVID-19 Epidemic Control in South Africa: A Microsimulation Modelling Study." *The Lancet Global Health* 9 (2): e120–29.

Reddy Madhavi, K., Y. Vijaya Sambhavi, M. Sudhakara, and K. Srujan Raju. 2021. "COVID-19 Isolation Monitoring System." *Data Engineering and Communication Technology: Proceedings of ICDECT 2020*. https://link.springer.com/chapter/10.1007/978-981-16-0081-4_60.

Rello, Jordi, Alejandro Rodríguez, Pedro Ibanez, Lorenzo Socias, Javier Cebrian, Asunción Marques, José Guerrero, et al. 2009. "Intensive Care Adult Patients with Severe Respiratory Failure Caused by Influenza A (H1N1)v in Spain." *Critical Care* 13 (5): R148.

Reutskaja, Elena, and Robin M. Hogarth. 2009. "Satisfaction in Choice as a Function of the Number of Alternatives: When 'Goods Satiate.'" *Psychology & Marketing* 26 (3): 197–203.

Sachs, Jeffrey D., Salim S. Abdool Karim, Lara Aknin, Joseph Allen, Kirsten Brosbøl, Francesca Colombo, Gabriela Cuevas Barron, et al. 2022. "The *Lancet* Commission on Lessons for the Future from the COVID-19 Pandemic." *The Lancet* 400 (10359): 1224–80.

Salzberger, Bernd, Felix Buder, Benedikt Lampl, Boris Ehrenstein, Florian Hitzenbichler, Thomas Holzmann, Barbara Schmidt, and Frank Hanses. 2021. "Epidemiology of SARS-CoV-2." *Infection* 49 (2): 233–39. https://doi.org/10.1007/s15010-020-01531-3.

Sandrin, Ryan, and Rylan Simpson. 2022. "Public Assessments of Police during the COVID-19 Pandemic: The Effects of Procedural Justice and Personal Protective Equipment." *Policing: An International Journal* 45 (1): 154–68.

Schuch, Felipe B., Rugero A. Bulzing, Jacob Meyer, Davy Vancampfort, Joseph Firth, Brendon Stubbs, Igor Grabovac, et al. 2020. "Associations of Moderate to Vigorous Physical Activity and Sedentary Behavior with Depressive and Anxiety Symptoms in Self-Isolating People during the COVID-19 Pandemic: A Cross-Sectional Survey in Brazil." *Psychiatry Research* 292: 113339.

Sehgal, Ashwini R., David U. Himmelstein, and Steffie Woolhandler. 2021. "Feasibility of Separate Rooms for Home Isolation and Quarantine for COVID-19 in the United States." *Annals of Internal Medicine* 174 (1): 127–29.

Shaban, Ramon Z., Shizar Nahidi, Cristina Sotomayor-Castillo, Cecilia Li, Nicole Gilroy, Matthew V. N. O'Sullivan, Tania C. Sorrell, et al. 2020. "SARS-CoV-2 Infection and COVID-19: The Lived Experience and Perceptions of Patients in Isolation and Care in an Australian Healthcare Setting." *American Journal of Infection Control* 48 (12): 1445–50.

Shewale, Jitesh B., Cecilia M. Ganduglia Cazaban, D. Kim Waller, Laura E. Mitchell, Peter H. Langlois, and A. J. Agopian. 2019. "Microcephaly Inpatient Hospitalization and Potential Zika Outbreak in Texas: A Cost and Predicted Economic Burden Analysis." *Travel Medicine and Infectious Disease* 30: 67–72.

Shoukat, Affan, Chad R. Wells, Joanne M. Langley, Burton H. Singer, Alison P. Galvani, and Seyed M. Moghadas. 2020. "Projecting Demand for Critical Care Beds during COVID-19 Outbreaks in Canada." *CMAJ* 192 (19): E489–96.

Sirait, Reni Aprinawaty, Andani Eka Putra, Adang Bachtiar, Rizanda Machmud, and Putri Chairani Eyanoer. 2023. "A Monitored Self-Isolation Model for Asymptomatic COVID-19 Patients to Prevent the Family-Based Transmission." *Open Public Health Journal* 16 (1).

Smith, Louise E., Richard Amlôt, Helen Lambert, Isabel Oliver, Charlotte Robin, Lucy Yardley, and G. James Rubin. 2020. "Factors Associated with Adherence to Self-Isolation and Lockdown Measures in the UK: A Cross-Sectional Survey." *Public Health* 187: 41–52.

Staykova, Evelina. 2023. "The Digital Transformation of Local Democracy during the Pandemic." In *Participatory and Digital Democracy at the Local Level: European Discourses and Practices*, edited by Gilles Rouet and Thierry Côme, 347–60. Springer.

Stephenson, Joan. 2020. "CDC Revises Guidance on Isolation after Positive COVID-19 Test, Reports Prolonged COVID-19 Illness among Nonhospitalized Patients." *JAMA Health Forum* 1 (8): e200997. https://doi.org/10.1001/jamahealthforum.2020.0997.

Sun, Haoyang, Borame L. Dickens, Mark Jit, Alex R. Cook, and L. Roman Carrasco. 2020. "Mapping the Cryptic Spread of the 2015–2016 Global Zika Virus Epidemic." *BMC Medicine* 18 (1): 399. https://doi.org/10.1186/s12916-020-01845-x.

Tan, Ling, Xianhua Wu, Ji Guo, and Ernesto D. R. Santibanez-Gonzalez. 2022. "Assessing the Impacts of COVID-19 on the Industrial Sectors and Economy of China." *Risk Analysis* 42 (1): 21–39.

Tasker, John Paul, and Ashley Burke. 2020. "Canada Preparing Makeshift Hospitals to House Patients as COVID-19 Pandemic Stretches Capacity." CBC, March 29, 2020. https://www.cbc.ca/news/politics/covid-19-makeshift-hospitals-1.5513846.

Thompson, Chad N., Christopher Mugford, Joel R. Merriman, Mark A. Chen, Joseph D. Hutter, Thomas J. Maruna, Wanza R. Bacon, et al. 2023. "Healthcare Worker Safety

Program in a Coronavirus Disease 2019 (COVID-19) Alternate Care Site: The Javits New York Medical Station Experience." *Infection Control & Hospital Epidemiology* 44 (2): 268–76.

Tuite, Ashleigh R., Amy L. Greer, Michael Whelan, Anne-Luise Winter, Brenda Lee, Ping Yan, Jianhong Wu, et al. 2010. "Estimated Epidemiologic Parameters and Morbidity Associated with Pandemic H1N1 Influenza." *CMAJ* 182 (2): 131–36.

United Nations. 2007. "International Health Regulations Enter into Force." News release, June 14, 2007. https://www.who.int/news/item/14-06-2007-international-health -regulations-enter-into-force.

United Nations. 2020. "COVID-19 Potentially Greatest Threat to South Sudan's Already Fragile Health System, Special Representative Warns Security Council." Press release, June 23, 2020. https://press.un.org/en/2020/sc14221.doc.htm.

US CDC (Centers for Disease Control and Prevention). 2009. "H1N1 Influenza: Risk of Illness among Healthcare Personnel." CDC Archive, October 16, 2009. https://archive.cdc .gov/www_cdc_gov/niosh/topics/h1n1flu/healthcare-risk.html.

Uyeki, Timothy M. 2010. "2009 H1N1 Virus Transmission and Outbreaks." *New England Journal of Medicine* 362 (23): 2221–23.

van Dyck, Laura I., Kirsten M. Wilkins, Jennifer Ouellet, Gregory M. Ouellet, and Michelle L. Conroy. 2020. "Combating Heightened Social Isolation of Nursing Home Elders: The Telephone Outreach in the COVID-19 Outbreak Program." *American Journal of Geriatric Psychiatry* 28 (9): 989–92. https://doi.org/10.1016/j.jagp.2020.05.026.

Van Kerkhove, Maria D., Siddhivinayak Hirve, Artemis Koukounari, and Anthony W. Mounts. 2013. "Estimating Age-Specific Cumulative Incidence for the 2009 Influenza Pandemic: A Meta-analysis of A(H1N1)pdm09 Serological Studies from 19 Countries." *Influenza and Other Respiratory Viruses* 7 (5): 872-86. https://doi.org/10.1111/irv.12074.

Verity, Robert, Lucy C. Okell, Iliaria Dorigatti, Peter Winskill, Charles Whittaker, Natsuko Imai, Gina Cuomo-Dannenburg, et al. 2020. "Estimates of the Severity of Coronavirus Disease 2019: A Model-Based Analysis." *The Lancet Infectious Diseases* 20 (6): 669–77. https://doi.org/10.1016/s1473-3099(20)30243-7.

Walen, Alec. 2014. "Retributive Justice." https://plato.stanford.edu/entries/justice-retributive/.

Wang, Di, and Zhifei Mao. 2021. "A Comparative Study of Public Health and Social Measures of COVID-19 Advocated in Different Countries." *Health Policy* 125 (8): 957–71. https:// doi.org/10.1016/j.healthpol.2021.05.016.

Wang, Ke-Wei, Jie Gao, Xiao-Xiao Song, Jiang Huang, Hua Wang, Xiao-Long Wu, Qin-Fang Yuan, et al. 2020. "Fangcang Shelter Hospitals Are a One Health Approach for Responding to the COVID-19 Outbreak in Wuhan, China." *One Health* 10: 100167.

Wang, Xiaohan, Leiyu Shi, Yuyao Zhang, Haiqian Chen, and Gang Sun. 2021. "Policy Disparities in Fighting COVID-19 among Japan, Italy, Singapore and China." *International Journal for Equity in Health* 20 (1): 33. https://doi.org/10.1186/s12939-020-01374-2.

Wang, Zhongliang, Wanli Ma, Xin Zheng, Gang Wu, and Ruiguang Zhang. 2020. "Household Transmission of SARS-CoV-2." *Journal of Infection* 81 (1): 179–82. https://doi.org/10.1016 /j.jinf.2020.03.040.

Washington, Michael L., and Martin L. Meltzer. 2015. "Effectiveness of Ebola Treatment Units and Community Care Centers—Liberia, September 23–October 31, 2014." *Morbidity and Mortality Weekly Report* 64 (3): 67–69.

Waya, Joy Luba Lomole, David Ameh, Joseph Lou K. Mogga, Joseph F. Wamala, and Olushayo Oluseun Olu. 2021. "COVID-19 Case Management Strategies: What Are the Options for Africa?" *Infectious Diseases of Poverty* 10 (02): 38–43.

WHO (World Health Organization). 2003a. "Consensus Document on the Epidemiology of Severe Acute Respiratory Syndrome (SARS)." Document WHO/CDS/CSR/GAR/2003.11, WHO, Geneva.

WHO (World Health Organization). 2003b. "Coronavirus Never Before Seen in Humans Is the Cause of SARS." News release, April 16, 2003. https://www.who.int/news/item/16-04 -2003-update-31---coronavirus-never-before-seen-in-humans-is-the-cause-of-sars.

WHO (World Health Organization). 2003c. "One Month into the Global SARS Outbreak: Status of the Outbreak and Lessons for the Immediate Future." News release, April 11, 2003. https://www.who.int/emergencies/disease-outbreak-news/item/2003_04_11-en.

WHO (World Health Organization). 2008. "International Health Regulations (2005) Second edition." Geneva: WHO.

WHO (World Health Organization). 2014a. "Statement on the 1st Meeting of the IHR Emergency Committee on the 2014 Ebola Outbreak in West Africa." News release, August 8, 2014. https://www.who.int/news/item/08-08-2014-statement-on-the-1st -meeting-of-the-ihr-emergency-committee-on-the-2014-ebola-outbreak-in-west-africa.

WHO (World Health Organization). 2014b. "WHO Statement on the Second Meeting of the International Health Regulations Emergency Committee Concerning the International Spread of Wild Poliovirus." News release, August 3, 2014. https://www.who.int/news /item/03-08-2014-who-statement-on-the-second-meeting-of-the-international-health -regulations-emergency-committee-concerning-the-international-spread-of-wild -poliovirus.

WHO (World Health Organization). 2014c. "Package and Approaches in Areas of Intense Transmission of Ebola Virus: Ebola Response." WHO, Geneva. https://www.who.int /publications/i/item/who-evd-guidance-strategy-14.2#.

WHO (World Health Organization). 2016. "Zika Strategic Response Plan, Quarterly Update, July–September 2016." WHO, Geneva. https://www.who.int/publications/i/item/zika -strategic-response-plan.

WHO (World Health Organization). 2018a. "Statement on the 1st Meeting of the IHR Emergency Committee Regarding the Ebola Outbreak in 2018." News release, May 18, 2018. https://www.who.int/news/item/18-05-2018-statement-on-the-1st-meeting-of-the -ihr-emergency-committee-regarding-the-ebola-outbreak-in-2018.

WHO (World Health Organization). 2018b. "Statement on the October 2018 Meeting of the IHR Emergency Committee on the Ebola Virus Disease Outbreak in the Democratic Republic of the Congo." News release, October 17, 2018. https://www.who.int/news /item/17-10-2018-statement-on-the-meeting-of-the-ihr-emergency-committee-on-the -ebola-outbreak-in-drc.

WHO (World Health Organization). 2019. "Statement on the Meeting of the International Health Regulations (2005) Emergency Committee for Ebola Virus Disease in the Democratic Republic of the Congo on 18 October 2019." News release, October 18, 2019. https://www.who.int/news/item/18-10-2019-statement-on-the-meeting-of-the -international-health-regulations-(2005)-emergency-committee-for-ebola-virus-disease -in-the-democratic-republic-of-the-congo.

WHO (World Health Organization). 2020a. "Ebola Then and Now: Eight Lessons from West Africa That Were Applied in the Democratic Republic of the Congo." WHO Newsroom, April 10, 2020. https://www.who.int/news-room/feature-stories/detail/ebola-then-and -now.

WHO (World Health Organization). 2020b. "Technical Protocol for Site-Specific Disinfection." WHO, Geneva. https://www.who.int/docs/default-source/wpro ---documents/countries/china/covid-19-briefing-nhc/8-annex-5-guideline-for-site-specific -disinfection.pdf.

WHO (World Health Organization). 2022. "Coronavirus Disease (COVID-19): Home Care for Families and Caregivers." WHO Newsroom, April 12, 2022. https://www.who.int/news -room/questions-and-answers/item/coronavirus-disease-covid-19-home-care-for-families -and-caregivers.

WHO (World Health Organization). 2025. "Ebola Disease." WHO Newsroom, April 24, 2025. https://www.who.int/news-room/fact-sheets/detail/ebola-disease.

WHO Africa (World Health Organization Regional Office for Africa). 2020. "Reducing Ebola Risk through Voluntary Isolation." News release, March 4, 2020. https://www.afro.who.int/news/reducing-ebola-risk-through-voluntary-isolation.

Wilasang, Chaiwat, Chayanin Sararat, Natcha C. Jitsuk, Noppamas Yolai, Panithee Thammawijaya, Prasert Auewarakul, and Charin Modchang. 2020. "Reduction in Effective Reproduction Number of COVID-19 Is Higher in Countries Employing Active Case Detection with Prompt Isolation." *Journal of Travel Medicine* 27 (5): taaa095.

Williams, Christopher Y. K., Adam T. Townson, Milan Kapur, Alice F. Ferreira, Rebecca Nunn, Julieta Galante, Veronica Phillips, Sarah Gentry, and Juliet A. Usher-Smith. 2021. "Interventions to Reduce Social Isolation and Loneliness during COVID-19 Physical Distancing Measures: A Rapid Systematic Review." *PLOS One* 16 (2): e0247139.

Wu, Shishi, Rachel Neill, Chuan De Foo, Alvin Qijia Chua, Anne-Sophie Jung, Victoria Haldane, Salma M. Abdalla, et al. 2021. "Aggressive Containment, Suppression, and Mitigation of Covid-19: Lessons Learnt from Eight Countries." *BMJ* 375.

Wurzer, David, Paul Spielhagen, Adonia Siegmann, Ayca Gercekcioglu, Judith Gorgass, Simone Henze, Yuron Kolar, et al. 2021. "Remote Monitoring of COVID-19 Positive High-Risk Patients in Domestic Isolation: A Feasibility Study." *PLOS One* 16 (9): e0257095.

Xiao, F., B. W. Chen, Y. F. Wu, Y. X. Wang, and D. M. Han. 2004. "Analysis on the Cost and Its Related Factors of Clinically Confirmed Severe Acute Respiratory Syndrome Cases in Beijing." *Zhonghua Liu Xing Bing Xue Za Zhi* 25 (4): 312–16.

Yukinori, Hashino. 2020. "A Look at the New Isolation Facility in Odaiba." *Nippon.com*, August 21, 2020. https://www.nippon.com/en/japan-topics/g00918/.

Zhong, Yaping, Huan Zhao, Tsorng-Yeh Lee, Tianchi Yu, Ming Fang Liu, and Ji Ji. 2022. "Experiences of COVID-19 Patients in a Fangcang Shelter Hospital in China during the First Wave of the COVID-19 Pandemic: A Qualitative Descriptive Study." *BMJ Open* 12 (9): e065799.

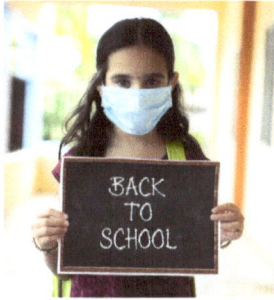

# 8

# The Role of School Closures and the Education System in Pandemic Preparedness and Response

Donald A. P. Bundy, Valentina Baltag, Biniam Bedasso, Carmen Burbano, W. John Edmunds, Ugo Gentilini, Eric Hanushek, Hitoshi Oshitani, Edith Patouillard, Linda Schultz, Anna-Maria Tammi, and Julian Jamison

## ABSTRACT

Reflecting public health experience with managing influenza, countries worldwide closed schools during COVID-19 (coronavirus) as a precautionary measure, even before the availability of direct evidence of the epidemiological role of children and adolescents in transmission. There remains no consensus regarding whether closing schools, or preventive actions in schools that did not close, had meaningful consequences for the transmission of COVID-19 in either the school population or the general population. In contrast, global evidence clearly shows significant negative consequences for human capital formation and well-being of learners, more so in vulnerable populations: school closures in the context of the pandemic led to 6–12 months of lost learning. The closures had additional unforeseen societal consequences, including increased rates of early pregnancy for school-age girls, inappropriate labor for school-age children, and substantial dropout from school. This experience of removing support from schoolchildren and adolescents has spurred national governments to reestablish and strengthen investments in school-based services, especially national school meals programs. Lessons learned can shape evidence-based policies regarding schools in subsequent pandemics, which will again need to weigh any potential trade-offs between protecting public health and ensuring the integrity of the school system.

## INTRODUCTION

In addition to the millions of excess deaths, for many people today among the worst long-term legacies of the COVID-19 pandemic are the social and economic consequences of the countermeasures, particularly the worldwide school closures. Despite continuing evidence on post-COVID-19 condition (long COVID),[1] from a health perspective the pandemic is mostly over. The health focus now, as in most of this volume, is on the lessons learned by the health community. However, for the 1.6 billion children affected by school closures at the peak of the lockdowns, and for their parents and their political representatives, the consequences are still real and present; for many, those consequences are among the most salient and lingering of the pandemic.

The next section of this chapter explains why schools matter, beyond schooling, and explores the mutually positive relationship between health, well-being, and education that existed before the COVID-19 pandemic. The third section examines how the historical role of schools as a social safety net for children became subsumed in the effort to respond urgently to the emerging pandemic. The fourth section tracks the evolution of the decision to close (or sometimes adapt) schools as a contribution to reducing transmission and examines the evidence for health and epidemiological benefits from those choices. The fifth section looks beyond health to explore the wider social and economic consequences of the global school closures, and the subsequent section tells the story, less salient to the health community, of how countries across the world and across income groups have come together to rebuild and enhance the ability of schools to contribute to the well-being and social development of the world's children. Finally, the chapter begins to look at the question of whether closing schools was an appropriate response to COVID-19 and, very important from a health perspective, whether that experience has made it a reasonable expectation that countries will ever again close their schools at the behest of health considerations.

## WHY SCHOOLS MATTER: THE MUTUAL BENEFITS OF SCHOOLS FOR COMMUNITY EDUCATION, HEALTH, AND WELL-BEING

This section explores the importance of the first 20 years of life for the creation of human capital, which includes everything that allows individuals to realize their potential to contribute meaningfully to society. The period of development from conception to adulthood is increasingly called the "first 8,000 days," indicating the importance of continuing support from the crucial "first 1,000 days" to secure early gains, provide opportunities for catch-up, and ensure well-being during later vulnerable phases, such as puberty and the brain rewiring of adolescence. This section examines the role of schools as a platform for delivering both education and well-being more broadly (Bundy et al. 2017; Ross et al. 2020), and sets the scene for the role of schools in health and education before the pandemic.

### The Importance of Well-Being, Education, and Development during the First 8,000 Days

Almost all societies worldwide have adopted compulsory, universal access to education as a guiding principle for the development of children and young people. The concept that health and well-being are essential counterparts to educational achievement is more recent. *Disease Control Priorities, Third Edition* (*DCP3*) and other analyses conclude that the condition of learners is essential to their learning, through direct effects on cognitive engagement and indirect effects such as incentivizing attendance at school (Global Financing Facility 2021; Schultz, Appleby, and Drake 2018; UNESCO, UNICEF, and WFP 2022), and that children and adolescents undergo transformative physical, emotional, and cognitive changes during their school-age years (Bundy et al. 2018; Bundy and Horton 2017). The exceptional success of country efforts to achieve the Millenium Development Goal of universal primary education access by 2015 has brought the world the nearest it has ever been to universal provision. We have also learned, however, that just attending school is not sufficient to get the desired outcomes from education. The Sustainable Development Goals, adopted by the United Nations (UN) in 2015, replaced the Millenium Development Goals and underscored the importance of actual learning. Quality education not only helps determine individual economic success but is also central to the long-run growth of national economies and to achieving other laudable goals in the Sustainable Development Goals, such as poverty reduction and gender equality (Hanushek and Woessmann 2008; Lange, Wodon, and Carey 2018).

Together, these policy considerations help explain why schools and education systems play a key role in creating human capital. School systems provide a platform that allows all-day, daily access to children throughout middle childhood and adolescence, and that can deliver learning while also contributing to good health, well-being, and the development of lifelong healthy behaviors. In this virtuous cycle, health promotes learning, education supports good health, and both together contribute to young people's achieving their human capital potential throughout the life course. For instance, health and nutrition in adolescence show significant associations with adult outcomes, such as health status, employment, violence exposure and perpetration, and education in later life (Banati et al., forthcoming).

Even though human capital—the aggregated skills and knowledge of a population—is now recognized as essential for the growth and development of economies (Hanushek and Woessmann 2008; Lange, Wodon, and Carey 2018), much of the world is unprepared to participate in a modern economy (Gust, Hanushek, and Woessmann 2024). Overall, data from the 2020 World Bank Human Capital Index suggest that 70–80 percent of the wealth of high-income countries is attributable to human capital, but that the share can be as low as 30–40 percent in low-income countries. Most countries with the lowest global rankings in terms of human capital are in Africa, where the median age of the population is as low as 15–16 years and where school enrollment is lowest (Lange, Wodon, and Carey 2018; World Bank 2019). The cost of inaction is high, given that education has numerous other benefits to societies, including playing a vital role in peacebuilding before, during, and after crises; each year, countries may lose up to 7 percent of their projected total gross domestic product (GDP) because of death, illness, or injury (WHO 2024a).

Bringing the skills of populations of all countries up to minimal levels is estimated to result in substantially faster growth of world GDP than now possible. The present value of added growth over the twenty-first century is about five times current world GDP (Gust, Hanushek, and Woessmann 2024). Although developing countries would gain the most, the world's high-income countries would also gain. The COVID-19 pandemic has made this situation more challenging, and the need to improve skills is even greater today.

### Supporting Human Capital with School-Based Health and Nutrition Services

For the health and nutrition conditions prevalent among school-age children and adolescents, schools can provide a cost-effective platform to deliver an integrated package of services. The *DCP3* Child and Adolescent Health and Development volume described an essential school-based package of health services appropriate for school-age children (Fernandes and Aurino 2017), including interventions to improve cognition and learning. Those interventions include the provision of deworming tablets in endemic settings, vision screening and provision of spectacles, promotion of oral health, the use of insecticide-treated bed nets in malaria-endemic areas, nutrition education and nutritious school meals, and tetanus-toxoid and human papillomavirus (HPV) vaccinations. This package was evaluated as (1) good value for money in multiple settings; (2) able to address a significant disease burden; and (3) feasible to implement in a range of low- and lower-middle-income countries, making it suitable for inclusion within essential health benefit packages (Watkins et al. 2018). Depending on the country-specific epidemiological context, guidelines from the World Health Organization (WHO) on school health services discuss a broader package of services that includes mental health, sexual and reproductive health, violence, and substance use prevention services (WHO 2021).

Because learners typically spend some 7,500 hours in the classroom over 8–10 years during primary and lower-secondary school, school-based health and nutrition services can build on existing infrastructure and education systems to support the learners' holistic health and well-being (WHO 2023a; WHO and UNESCO 2021). Schools can encourage health promotion through policies and governance, the physical and social environment, curricula including health literacy, links with parents, and access to school health and nutrition services (Baltag et al. 2022). The evidence for the effectiveness of such approaches is mixed. On the one hand, a Cochrane review in 2015 provided an equivocal assessment (Langford et al. 2015). On the other hand, such whole-school approaches, also called health-promoting schools, may improve education outcomes and can influence students' depressive symptoms, bullying, violence, attitudes about gender, and knowledge of sexual and reproductive health (Langford et al. 2014; WHO 2023a), with a potential for high benefit-cost ratios (Sheehan et al. 2023). Some 72 percent of countries participating in a WHO policy survey in 2023 report having national standards for health-promoting schools, a 7 percent increase from the previous round.[2]

### A Decade of Expansion of School-Based Health and Nutrition Programs and Policy Guidance

The decade leading up to the arrival of the global pandemic in 2020 saw a substantial increase in cross-sectoral policy guidance focused on school-age children and adolescents, including systems approaches to school health at all levels of the educational system (such as the Global Partnership for Education, WHO, and the United Nations Educational, Scientific and Cultural Organization), the role of diets and food systems in schools (such as the Food and Agriculture Organization of the United Nations, UN Nutrition, and the World Food Programme), and the role of the school in human capital development (such as the Global Financing Facility, US Agency for International Development, and World Bank Group) (Schultz et al. 2025).

Globally, the number of children receiving daily school meals increased by 9 percent between 2013 and 2020, reaching 388 million children, equivalent to half of the world's primary school population, with the fastest increase (86 percent) in lower-middle-income countries (WFP 2020). Of these mostly government-owned programs, 98 percent are supported by domestic funds and 87 percent are formally part of national policy. These programs are also increasingly self-reliant even in low-income countries, where the proportion of domestic funding on school meals increased from 17 percent to 28 percent between 2013 and 2020 (WFP 2020).

By January 2020, national school meals programs were clearly established as the world's most extensive social safety net, and nearly every country offered some form of school-based health or nutrition services, with many delivering comprehensive and affordable interventions at scale (WFP 2020). In terms of complementary health interventions, more than 100 countries offered school-based vaccination, nearly all integrated health education in their curriculum, and schoolchildren had received more than 3.3 billion school-based deworming treatments since 2010 (Baltag, Pachyna, and Hall 2015; Montresor et al. 2020; UNESCO, UNICEF, and WFP 2022).

## HOW THE ADVANCING PANDEMIC UNDERMINED THE ROLE OF SCHOOLS AS A SOCIAL SAFETY NET

This section examines why school health and school meals programs became the world's most extensive social safety net during the decade leading to 2020. It also explores the process that led to the closing of schools and the removal of the safety net from schoolchildren and adolescents worldwide during the pandemic. Much of the focus is on national school meals programs as a proxy for school-based health and nutrition interventions generally.

### The 2008 Food, Fuel, and Financial Crisis Relative to School Health and School Meals

Even before the pandemic, governments identified their school meals programs as having multiple objectives across several sectors, going beyond health and education and including social protection. Results of a 2019 questionnaire survey by the Global Child Nutrition Foundation illustrate the wide range of objectives and how they differ across income groups (table 8.1). Although respondents most frequently reported objectives involving education and health, the social safety net and income transfer role comes in a close third and is most popular in low- and lower-middle-income countries. The importance of this social protection role was recognized as an outcome of the 2008 food, fuel, and financial crisis (Bundy et al. 2009).

**Table 8.1** Objectives of School Meals Programs, by Country Income Level, 2021

*Percent of programs*

| Objective | Low-income | Lower-middle-income | Upper-middle-income | High-income | Total |
|---|---|---|---|---|---|
| Agriculture | 62.5 | 48.9 | 30.3 | 30.2 | 42.1 |
| Average number of objectives per program | 3.0 | 2.2 | 1.7 | 2.1 | 2.2 |
| Education | 100 | 91.5 | 78.8 | 69.8 | 83.6 |
| Health and nutrition | 90.0 | 93.6 | 93.9 | 93.7 | 92.9 |
| Income transfer | 85.0 | 78.7 | 69.7 | 63.5 | 73.2 |
| Obesity mitigation | 5.0 | 17.0 | 30.3 | 68.3 | 34.4 |

*Source:* Bundy et al. 2024.

*Note:* Table shows results from 185 respondents of a 2021 questionnaire survey by the Global Child Nutrition Foundation.

The 2008 crisis highlighted the interconnectedness of school-based health and nutrition interventions and social protection objectives, as low-income countries leveraged World Bank emergency agricultural funds to expand the coverage of national school meals programs (Bundy et al. 2024). Although offered the funds as crisis response to make food more affordable, many low-income countries decided instead to expand what for many was their largest extant safety net for their children. The response was seen first in low-income countries; however, as the recession deepened worldwide in 2010, many middle- and high-income countries that may not have previously viewed school meals as a social protection measure—such as Italy, Scotland, and Spain (Bundy et al. 2009)—leveraged school meals programs to reach more children, even during vacations.

In 2009, the World Bank publication *Rethinking School Feeding* explored the origin and structures of that country-led demand, drawing from the education, health, and social protection sectors, as well as from UN and development partners (Bundy et al. 2009). The report marked a sea change in thinking about the role of school meals as a multisectoral intervention and accelerated the introduction and expansion of school meals programs taking a social protection perspective, for countries and for UN agencies. For example, as part of their support for emerging from the global recession, China and the Russian Federation independently launched national school meals programs using *Rethinking School Feeding* as the empirical rationale (Bundy et al. 2024). The World Food Programme, the world's primary source of school meals program support, introduced a new school meals policy in 2013 to support nation building as well as to protect the well-being and education of school-age children and adolescents in low-resource settings (WFP 2020, 2023).

### Factors Early in the Pandemic Leading to School Closures and Loss of Safety Net

In the early days of COVID-19, little was known regarding the extent to which the school environment constituted an engine for broader transmission of the disease. Despite children's relatively high vulnerability to influenza, it was established quite early in the pandemic that children (and young adults) had a low COVID-19 case fatality rate (Levin et al. 2020) and that children were unlikely to suffer severe disease and might be refractory to infection (Davies et al. 2020; Ferguson et al. 2020; Viner et al. 2020). The choice before governments, however, was stark: countries faced a dangerous new epidemic and had very few public health control options open to them. Closing schools was one of the few non-pharmaceutical interventions for which there was good evidence of effectiveness at reducing influenza transmission and that, by implication, might be effective against COVID-19. In response, almost all governments closed their schools within the first couple of months of the pandemic, leaving over 90 percent of students out of school. Lower-income countries in particular struggled with providing continued education at a distance, and children also missed school meals: 370 million in April 2020 alone (WFP 2023).

At least five convergent factors may have contributed to that outcome. First, governments are naturally precautionary (Cronert 2022), preferring to do something rather than nothing and to make the seemingly safe decision, especially given societal expectations regarding the short-term safety and protection of children. This tendency is especially true for electoral democracies. In the United States, for example, most counties were under emergency orders (99.4 percent) and closed schools (98 percent) before reporting a single COVID-19 case (Yan et al. 2021). A study examining county-level differences in closures in the United States explored the importance of local politics, finding that political party affiliation was strongly correlated with the number of days of closure but that COVID-19 case rates were not (Jack and Oster 2023). The study also found that counties with a higher composition of minorities (and lower broadband usage) had more closure, heightening preexisting disparities. Once countries had policies in place, a desire for consistency and an aversion to anything that might resemble admitting being wrong, along with weak evidence-to-policy mechanisms in many countries, led to continuation of initial policy decisions despite shifts and improvements in the understanding of the situation.

Second, the technical side of the pandemic response was, appropriately, informed by health experts, including virologists and modelers, which may have resulted in the downplaying of factors important to other sectors. Relatedly, almost all existing pandemic preparedness plans focused on influenza. Although the public debate on this front often revolved around lives versus the economy, the tension was perhaps even more stark, but less publicly recognized until later, with respect to education and safety nets. Refer also to WHO Regional Office for Europe (2022) for more discussion of some of these trade-offs in the context of Europe in particular.

Third, education sector staff, especially teachers, had understandable concerns about the risks to themselves of in-person schooling. Evidence from the United States, for example, suggests that school reopening decisions were closely tied to the strength of local teachers' unions (Grossmann et al. 2021).

Fourth, the role and perceptions of parents changed over time. At first, parents tended to advocate for school closures in order to protect their children, especially given the early uncertainty about the later recognized strong correlation between age and fatality rates. Regardless of whether schools formally closed, many parents initially kept their children at home, for example in the United Kingdom (Adams, Weale, and Bannock 2020). Later, many parents demanded that schools reopen, especially with the removal of strict lockdowns and with parents' return to work, raising the salience of schools as safe places to spend the day. Furthermore, many countries put in place considerable efforts to try to reduce the risk of transmission in schools. Examples include mask-wearing, ventilation, and increased social distancing. Surveys of US parents revealed that most became increasingly concerned about children's falling behind academically and about negative impacts to their emotional well-being without in-person school attendance (Menasce Horowitz 2022).

Fifth, low-income countries were less prone to reopen schools even with the emergence of data showing that children are less affected by the infection and that safe school reopening is possible. From March 2020 through February 2022, schools worldwide were fully or partially closed for 41 weeks on average (WHO Regional Office for Europe 2022). Although low- and middle-income countries had different circumstances and considerations—including larger class sizes, a higher likelihood of having a parent at home, lower feasibility of hybrid education options, and so on—their children also faced higher costs of closure, suggesting increased importance of the ability to act rapidly in the face of relevant evidence.

Two other contexts may have been important, but we have no specific evidence about them in the case of school closures. First, general evidence shows that, throughout the pandemic and across many geographies, voluntary behavior change was a major driver, above and beyond formal regulations: in many situations people had already acted before any formal lockdown or other mandate (Jamison et al. 2021). This might imply that, for the behavioral reasons related to staff and parents, mentioned earlier, school closures were inevitable, whether mandated or not. Second, despite significant variability in school closure, as with lockdowns (Jamison 2020), low-income countries appeared to follow the lead of high-income nations.

On average, COVID-19 led to 199 days of full or partial school closure (the equivalent of 12 months of learning), affecting 1.6 billion children globally. According to Stacy and Lambrechts (2023), the period of closure was related in a complex way to income level. High-income countries had, on average, 148 days of closure; low-income countries, 158 days; and lower-middle-income countries, 236 days.

## THE ROLE OF SCHOOLS IN THE TRANSMISSION OF COVID-19

Before the COVID-19 pandemic a substantial literature already existed on the role of schools in the transmission of respiratory viruses, as perhaps most clearly demonstrated by the role of the school year cycle as a driver of epidemics.

This history was also supported by the projections of mathematical models and the observational data sets pointing to the role of schools in the transmission of respiratory viruses, and it aligned with the common-sense perceptions of parents. In addition, evidence showed that transmission occurred in school settings where children mixed outside the classroom, such as at sporting events (Boutzoukas et al. 2022). All these reasons appear to have contributed to the closing of schools worldwide as part of the overall global effort to control COVID-19. This section reviews the evidence that led to that decision and the subsequent consequences.

## Previous Knowledge about the Role of School Closures in Managing Viral Disease Transmission

Long before the arrival of the COVID-19 pandemic, an established literature indicated that children, particularly in schools, played an important role in influenza transmission, because of the high incidence of social contact and physical interaction among this age group (Cauchemez et al. 2009; Mossong et al. 2008). Furthermore, mathematical modeling, for example of data from the 2009 avian influenza A (H1N1) pandemic had made a strong case for the potential effectiveness of extensive school closures to mitigate the role of schools as drivers of influenza epidemics (Ferguson et al. 2006; Germann et al. 2006).

Those and similar studies led to the proposition that school closure or other forms of school dismissal that avoided the aggregation of school-age children represented a potentially important part of interventions for mitigating pandemic influenza (Bell et al. 2006; Cauchemez et al. 2009), and perhaps viral epidemics generally. Although some evidence suggested greater effectiveness of school closures implemented in the early phase of any outbreak (Cauchemez et al. 2009; Germann et al. 2006; Haber et al. 2007), others suggested that "heterogeneity in the data available means that the optimum strategy (eg, the ideal length and timing of closure) remains unclear" (Jackson et al. 2013, 1). Nevertheless, countries had an imperative to act quickly because they faced a public health crisis and because early interventions tend to be more effective (Jackson et al. 2014). When the COVID-19 pandemic emerged and countries considered the potential of school closures as a control measure, a key question related to the generalizability of influenza findings to SARS-CoV-2.

## Evolving Understanding of the Impact of School Closures on COVID-19 Transmission

The earliest evidence, from the start of 2020 when most schools remained open but attendance had dropped precipitously, suggested low transmission within schools.[3] A study in Australia of 27 primary cases (56 percent of which were staff) identified only 18 secondary cases when nearly half of 1,448 close contacts were tested virologically or serologically (Macartney et al. 2020); a study of six confirmed cases (50 percent adults) in Ireland identified no secondary cases from the pediatric cases (Heavey et al. 2020). Other studies suggested that the probability of transmission among students was age-dependent. For instance, France had high attack rates in secondary-school students ages 14–18 years and staff (38 percent and 49 percent, respectively) but no convincing evidence of any secondary transmission within primary schools (Fontanet et al. 2021; Fontanet et al. 2020). Household contact tracing in the Republic of Korea suggested that rates were lower when the index case was younger than the age of 10 years (3 of 57, or 5 percent) and higher when the case was over 10 but less than 19 years (43 of 231, or 19 percent) (Park et al. 2020).

As noted earlier, countries needed to make a decision needed before the epidemic became established if their action was to be effective. Although the emerging evidence did not suggest higher attack rates in children than in adults, some 90 percent of countries decided to close their schools beginning in April 2020. Most countries monitored the situation, with plans as early as July 2020 to carefully monitor the impact of reopening schools (for example, refer to Public Health England 2021) and recognition that it was "becoming increasingly clear that governments around the world need to find solutions that allow children and young adults to return to full-time education as safely and as quickly as possible" (Edmunds 2020, 797). A framework for reopening schools, published in June 2020 by UN agencies and the World Bank, advised that the "timing of school reopenings should be guided by the best interest of the child and overall public health considerations, based on an assessment of the associated benefits and risks and informed by cross-sectoral and context-specific evidence, including education, public health and socio-economic factors" (UNESCO et al. 2020, 2).

As the pandemic wore on, the evidence in support of reopening schools did not become more definite. On the one hand, an extensive assessment of the partial reopening of schools in the United Kingdom mid-2020 identified few SARS-CoV-2 outbreaks despite a median of 928,000 children attending and that any secondary cases linked to within-school exposure occurred more frequently among teaching and administrative staff (Ismael et al. 2021). On the other hand, a variety of other sources, mainly based on mathematical modeling projections, suggested that such passive surveillance must have missed or underestimated many outbreaks, and that secondary schools in particular might play a considerable role in transmission between households (Flasche and Edmunds 2021). Although the risk of reopening schools was still evaluated, the substantial risks of keeping them closed were already known before the pandemic started. For the beginning of the new school year, WHO, UNESCO, and UNICEF (2020) recommended therefore that a risk-based approach—considering not only the local epidemiology of COVID-19 but also other social, health, and well-being impacts—should guide the decision to close or open schools.

During 2021, growing reaction to the social, logistical, and economic consequences of continued school closures—as well as rising concerns about the long-term consequences for educational attainment and the generation of human capital—culminated in a global movement focused on the safe reopening of schools. During this phase multiple studies and systematic reviews sought to assess the impact of school closures and in-school mitigation measures on SARS-CoV-2 transmission (Jamison et al. 2021; Li et al. 2021).

Attempts in 2022 and 2023 to undertake analysis of these reviews aimed to clarify the conclusions, but many difficulties in interpretation remained. For instance, a review of 26 systematic reviews found only one of high confidence, the remainder being of low (10) or critically low (15) confidence (Hume, Brown, and Mahtani 2023). That review noted:

> Both school closures and in-school mitigations were associated with reduced COVID-19 transmission, morbidity and mortality in the community. School closures were also associated with reduced learning, increased anxiety and increased obesity in pupils. We found no SRs [systematic reviews] that assessed potential drawbacks of in-school mitigations on pupils. The certainty of evidence according to GRADE [Grading of Recommendations, Assessment, Development, and Evaluations] was mostly very low." (Hume, Brown, and Mahtani 2023, 164)

Most countries implemented school closures as mitigating measures for COVID-19 (Hale et al. 2021), but the literature on effectiveness is still controversial and shows mixed results (Haug et al. 2020; Viner et al. 2020). Available data suggest that in many cases young adults, but not school-age children, were a main driving force for COVID-19 transmission (Monod et al. 2021; Tran Kiem et al. 2021). In some settings where, for example, most adolescents and adults were vaccinated, however, the role of schools may become more important, as suggested by the UK Office of National Statistics Prevalence surveys, which at times showed the highest prevalence of infection among school-age children.

## Effectiveness of School-Based Mitigation Measures Short of Complete Closure

School closure was only one of many school-based or education system interventions that sought to reduce the transmission of SARS-CoV-2. In considering the implications of the lack of clear evidence that widespread school closures had an important impact on transmission, other interventions become more interesting as potential alternatives for addressing future coronavirus epidemics even when schools remain open. Examples include reducing the opportunity for contact (for example, via scheduling), improved ventilation, increased handwashing, and regular screening with isolation as necessary. As technology improves, including artificial intelligence, it may also be increasingly feasible to operate hybrid or part-time systems even in resource-constrained settings.

This topic is the subject of a recently updated Cochrane review of 15 empirical studies of schools, with 12 of those studies from the Americas (Littlecott et al. 2024). The authors of that review conclude in their abstract that, across all bodies of evidence, certainty of evidence ratings limits confidence in the findings. Another Cochrane review looks at the unintended consequences of school measures other than school closures (Kratzer et al. 2022). A set of evidence-based school guidelines during COVID-19 has been developed in Germany, which used the Cochrane results and the WHO-INTEGRATE framework to formally assess all criteria, adopting a whole-of-society, multisectoral perspective. Each recommendation has a multipage assessment, and table 8.2 summarizes the assessment for schools.

**Table 8.2** Evidence-Based Guidelines during COVID-19 for Suspected Cases among Students without Known Risk Contact, Weighing Benefits and Harms of the Measure in German Schools

| Weighing benefits and harms of the measure |
| --- |
| **Benefits** |
| • Prevention of infections and secondary cases of quarantine, which as a result do not occur among students, teachers, in the household, and in the community. |
| **Harms** |
| • Consequences of the quarantine for students and their associated absence from school, interruption of social contacts and social participation. |
| • Consequences for parents and guardians due to the increased need for care and supervision of the students in quarantine, in particular social and financial consequences due to reduced availability to work. |
| • Consequences for society and economy through the frequent and unpredictable absence of employees. |
| **Overall assessment** |
| • While the individual in quarantine is always harmfully affected by the measure, there is only a benefit from the measure if the person is actually infected with SARS-CoV-2 after a risk exposure. |
| • Therefore, the assessment of the probability of an infection depending on the kind of contact is critical. |

*Source:* AWMF 2022.

These analyses illustrate the considerable efforts undertaken to clarify the role of schools, school-based mitigation measures, and school closures in SARS-CoV-2 transmission and health. The main conclusion at the current stage of analysis is that, despite those considerable efforts, the role of schools and school-based interventions in reducing transmission in schools or from schools to the general population remains unclear. Policy analyses suggest that safe reopening is possible, with the creation of safe conditions, and desirable from both the public health and societal perspectives, and that school closures should be a solution of last resort (ECDC 2020).

## THE ECONOMIC AND SOCIAL CONSEQUENCES OF SCHOOL CLOSURES DURING THE PANDEMIC

This section explores what we now understand to have been the "nonhealth" consequences of the pandemic due to school closures. It focuses first on the long-term human capital consequences for the generation of children who lost educational opportunities during the pandemic, and then on the longer-term sociological consequences for the children who were shut out of school.

### Impact on Human Capital Outcomes

Although most countries attempted to continue education through remote learning modalities—whether through digital, TV, radio, or paper-based approaches—those efforts had mixed effectiveness (Andrabi, Daniels, and Das 2023; Munoz-Najar et al. 2021). In high- and middle-income countries, digital instruction frequently substituted for in-person instruction during initial closure periods. In Africa, however, it is estimated that less than 10 percent of children had access to digital sources for distance education (Wang et al. 2021). In some countries, schools reopened relatively quickly, whereas many countries had a disruptive cycle of reopening and reclosing. For some countries, the withdrawal of schooling was long term: for example, schools in the Philippines and Uganda only reopened more than two years later. It is now recognized that generations of children have lost out on educational opportunities—with lifelong consequences. The World Bank estimates that in low-income countries the already poor level of educational achievement has deteriorated further: the proportion of children in Africa unable to read a simple age-appropriate sentence has increased from 53 percent to 70 percent, as compared to before the pandemic (World Bank, UNESCO, and UNICEF 2021). Evidence from Ethiopia shows that because of school closures children in primary school "learned only 30–40% as much in math as they would during a normal year, and the learning gap between urban and rural students increased" (Kim et al. 2021).

Recent cross-country student test data show significant declines in student performance over the pandemic, with larger losses where closures were longer (Jakubowski, Gajderowicz, and Patrinos 2024). Those declines add to the existing low levels of achievement found in low-income countries before the pandemic (Gust, Hanushek, and Woessmann 2024). For example, the latter study provides prepandemic estimates of the percentage of children lacking the basic skills needed to participate in a modern economy (table 8.3). Although one-third of the world's youth are not in secondary education, those in school show considerable skill deficits—deficits worsened by the pandemic.

Substantial international evidence exists that achievement levels strongly influence individuals' lifetime incomes (Hanushek et al. 2015). Although the returns to skills vary across countries, those returns are clearly significant across the range of economic development. Moreover, the long-run growth of nations relates closely to the skills of the population as measured by the international tests (Hanushek and Woessmann 2015). A common rule of thumb is that each additional year of schooling leads to about 10 percent higher annual income in adulthood (Montenegro and Patrinos 2014); therefore, school closures—even if partially offset by versions of remote learning—could likely lead to substantial declines in lifetime earnings for the entire affected cohort. Previous research has found this relationship to hold causally; for instance, teacher strikes in Argentina, which closed schools for an average of 88 days, led to 2–3 percent lower annual labor market earnings (Jaume and Willen 2019). Despite the lack of complete data about the educational impacts of COVID-19 from all countries, much less the ultimate human capital consequences, a clear picture is emerging: learning losses equal somewhere between half and one year of education, with the most disadvantaged students and those affected by longer school closures bearing the worst impacts. In the case of reading scores, students lost more than a year of learning (Jakubowski, Gajderowicz, and Patrinos 2024).

**Table 8.3** Percentage of Children below Basic Skill Levels before COVID-19 Pandemic, by Country Income Level

|  | Low-income | Lower-middle-income | Upper-middle-income | High-income | World total |
|---|---|---|---|---|---|
| % with less than basic skill | 95.6 | 85.8 | 42.3 | 25.5 | 67.2 |

*Source:* Adapted from Gust, Hanushek, and Woessmann 2024, which draws on available data from before the COVID-19 pandemic; this analysis anchors its measure in mastering at least the most basic level of the Programme for International Student Assessment (PISA)—that is, PISA Level 1 skills—using the most recent assessment available for each country from before the pandemic.

Some of the best data on test scores come from the United States, where the National Assessment of Educational Progress tests 13-year-olds every year. Comparing the most recent 2023 data to scores from just before the pandemic, math scores fell by nine points—erasing all gains since 1990—and reading scores by four points—sufficient to erase all gains since 1975 (Hanushek 2023). Given historical patterns, these numbers correspond to 6 percent lower lifetime earnings for the average student in school during the pandemic. One recent analysis, combining estimated learning impacts with the types of virus-control impacts discussed earlier, finds that school closure scored extremely poorly in terms of cost-effectiveness (Irons and Raftery 2024). Meanwhile, estimates from Italy (Carlana, La Ferrara, and Lopez 2023) and elsewhere in Europe similarly suggest large declines in test scores, especially in mathematics (0.14 standard deviation) but also in reading; and preliminary evidence from early-grade reading assessments in five Sub-Saharan African countries suggests learning losses of almost one year (Angrist et al. 2021). Modeling suggests that such early deficits can compound over time, as students who are already behind struggle to catch up when faced with standard curricula; a similar dynamic was observed after the 2005 earthquake in Pakistan (Andrabi, Daniels, and Das 2023).

Another striking empirical regularity is that, in essentially all cases, school closures (whose extent was driven by sociodemographic differences) exacerbated existing sociodemographic inequalities. Both within and across countries, the schools in lower-resource settings were less equipped to provide remote or hybrid learning options, and parents or caregivers were less able to support at-home learning. For instance the same data set from Italy shows larger declines in test scores for low socioeconomic status and immigrant students, whereas a large data set from over 2 million students across the United States exhibited widening achievement gaps by race and income level (Goldhaber et al. 2023). That the poorest children would experience the worst effects from school closures during COVID-19 is consistent with earlier evidence from Ebola. Furthermore, COVID-19 also resulted in bigger learning losses for girls and for children in earlier grades in lower-income countries (World Bank, UNESCO, and UNICEF 2021). Overall, school closures hurt the most vulnerable children most, in terms of educational attainment, future opportunities, and (as discussed in the next subsection) other health and well-being indicators.

Tracking of education sector finance during the pandemic, by the Education Finance Watch, suggests that financing for education has not fully responded to the damage inflicted or adequately addressed the learning crisis (World Bank and UNESCO 2023). The pandemic exacerbated the global learning crisis, and government education spending is insufficient to close the learning gap. Along with a slight rise in annual real spending on education, government per capita education spending increased in 2021. In low- and middle-income countries, even when there were (previously planned) spending increases, they were far from sufficient to make a dent in the large learning gap (World Bank and UNESCO 2023). Now that external support is needed most, official development assistance is falling—and could be spent more efficiently. Aid to education fell by 7 percent, from US$19.3 billion in 2020 to US$17.8 billion in 2021, because of the reduction in general budget support. Since then, responses and finance levels have varied greatly across countries but have not generally been sufficient to overcome the accumulated shortfall in outcomes from the height of the pandemic.

## Impact on School Dropout, Early Pregnancy, and Entrance into the Workforce

The indirect impact of lengthy school closures and travel restrictions altered the educational trajectory and widened gender and health disparities for the most vulnerable school-age children and adolescents. Although adolescents were spared much of the morbidity and mortality caused by the COVID-19 pandemic, school closures largely eliminated access to the broad range of preventive health interventions previously delivered through the school platform, such as immunizations, child protection, and psychosocial support services. The disruption in daily school meals provision was salient, and attempts to mitigate the loss of school meals by alternative means were much more costly and much less efficient (WFP 2023). Those efforts were particularly important because one in three people worldwide did not have access to adequate food in 2020 (FAO et al. 2021). Households in Nigeria, for example, reported a 9 percent higher increase in skipping meals after the interruption in school meals provision (Abay et al. 2021).

As the pandemic wore on, many families lost their livelihoods and 60 million more children lived in monetarily poor households in 2021 than in 2019 (Save the Children and UNICEF 2021). Although not a direct impact of school closure, this poverty resulted in the first increase in child labor in two decades and shows how household poverty can increase the opportunity cost of staying in school. Children ages 5–11 years accounted for just over half of the 160 million child laborers in 2021, with at least half engaging in hazardous work (ILO and UNICEF 2021). In response to economic hardships, an estimated 10 million additional girls entered into early marriage to relieve financial pressure on their families (UNICEF 2021). Despite the lack of data on the increase in gender-based violence due to school closures, programs working closely with girls saw increases in the number of cases reported, for example in East Africa (Girls' Education Challenge and UK Aid 2021).

School dropout rates among older adolescents remained elevated two years later (Moscoviz and Evans 2022). In Malawi, adolescent boys most often cited financial constraints to reenrolling, whereas girls cited marriage and pregnancy (Kadzamira et al. 2021). For adolescent girls, the combination of economic fragility, school closures, and social isolation increased their likelihood of early marriage and unplanned pregnancies. A study in Kenya found that female adolescents who experienced disrupted schooling were more likely than their peers who sat for exams to drop out of school (9.7 percent vs. 3.0 percent), initiate sex (47.4 percent vs. 25.5 percent), and become pregnant (10.9 percent vs. 5.2 percent) (Meherali et al. 2021). Access to reproductive health services, counseling, and commodities was disrupted in nearly 60 percent of countries (WHO 2020b), putting adolescent girls at risk of unintended pregnancies and sexually transmitted infections.

As the education system builds back from the pandemic, increasing evidence indicates the need to consider the mental health status of students. The most recent World Happiness Report included a specific focus on children and adolescents for the first time, showing a global decline in well-being after the pandemic (Marquez et al. 2024). Data from 12 longitudinal studies from across geographies reveal that adolescent depressive symptoms worsened during the pandemic (Barendse et al. 2023), and evidence suggests that symptoms persisted two years later (Thorisdottir et al. 2023). For the most vulnerable children, for whom school-based mental health programs are often the only accessible source of services, school closures have exacerbated the issues (WHO 2020a).

## STRENGTHENING SCHOOL-BASED HEALTH AND NUTRITION AS A LEGACY OF PANDEMIC SCHOOL CLOSURES

The scale and near universality of school closures in response to the COVID-19 pandemic helped highlight to many governments the vital role schools play in protecting the health and well-being of learners and in developing the human capital that is key to national development. The world's first attempt to simultaneously close all its schools has provided convincing counterfactual evidence of what happens when school-based health services are no longer provided. It led to recommendations for continuity of health promotion and school health services when distance or virtual learning is required (for example, in response to a public health emergency and diverse learner needs) as a standard of practice (WHO and UNESCO 2021).

Also as a result of learnings from COVID-19, the updated WHO benchmarks for strengthening health emergency capacities now include new benchmarks related to the continuity of essential health services and education during a health emergency (WHO 2023b). Thus, the benchmark on the protection of livelihoods, business continuity, and continuity of education and learning systems says that a country has a demonstrated capacity to deal with emergencies if it has "integrated emergency preparedness and response strategies into national education policies, to sustain continuous and inclusive learning opportunities during health emergencies, as well as continuity of school-based and school-linked social protection and healthcare services" (WHO 2023b, 325).

As early as July 2020, this experience had begun to strengthen the resolve of countries to reestablish their investment in their school-age children. This resolve included both reopening education systems and strengthening the investment in the well-being of the children, with the objectives of improving education through better access, participation, and learning. Countries sought to achieve these objectives in various ways, and one of the most visible and important health-related initiatives was the creation of a multicountry, multilateral School Meals Coalition at the October 2021 UN Food System Summit. The coalition aims to rebuild the school-based services severely damaged by the pandemic closures and to ensure the well-being of current and future generations of schoolchildren.

Today, 109 countries, comprising more than 67 percent of the world's population have signed onto the coalition (map 8.1). Those countries identified three specific goals: (1) to restore national school meals and complementary school health programs to prepandemic coverage by 2023; (2) to develop new approaches to reach by 2030 an additional 73 million of the most in-need children who had not previously been reached; and (3) to raise the quality of school health and nutrition programs globally by 2030.[4]

Governments and international development organizations are delivering on this response. At the Food Systems Stocktaking +2 event in Rome in July 2023, the School Meals Coalition was recognized as the most substantial coalition to arise from the pandemic. This momentum is also confirmed by the rebound in coverage of programs: today, 418 million children receive a daily meal in school, exceeding levels before the COVID-19 pandemic by 7 percent (WFP 2023). Universal schemes, representing 44 percent of all programs, provide meals to 186 million children daily, with more than half of all national school meals programs anticipated to become universally offered by 2024 (Cohen et al. 2023). This result suggests that the coalition has largely achieved its first goal, but the trend has not been observed consistently across income groups. High-income, upper-middle-income, and lower-middle-income countries show a consistent, modest increase, but low-income countries experienced a net decline in coverage of 4 percent (figure 8.1).

**Map 8.1** Signatories of the Declaration of Commitment to the School Meals Coalition, as of March 2025

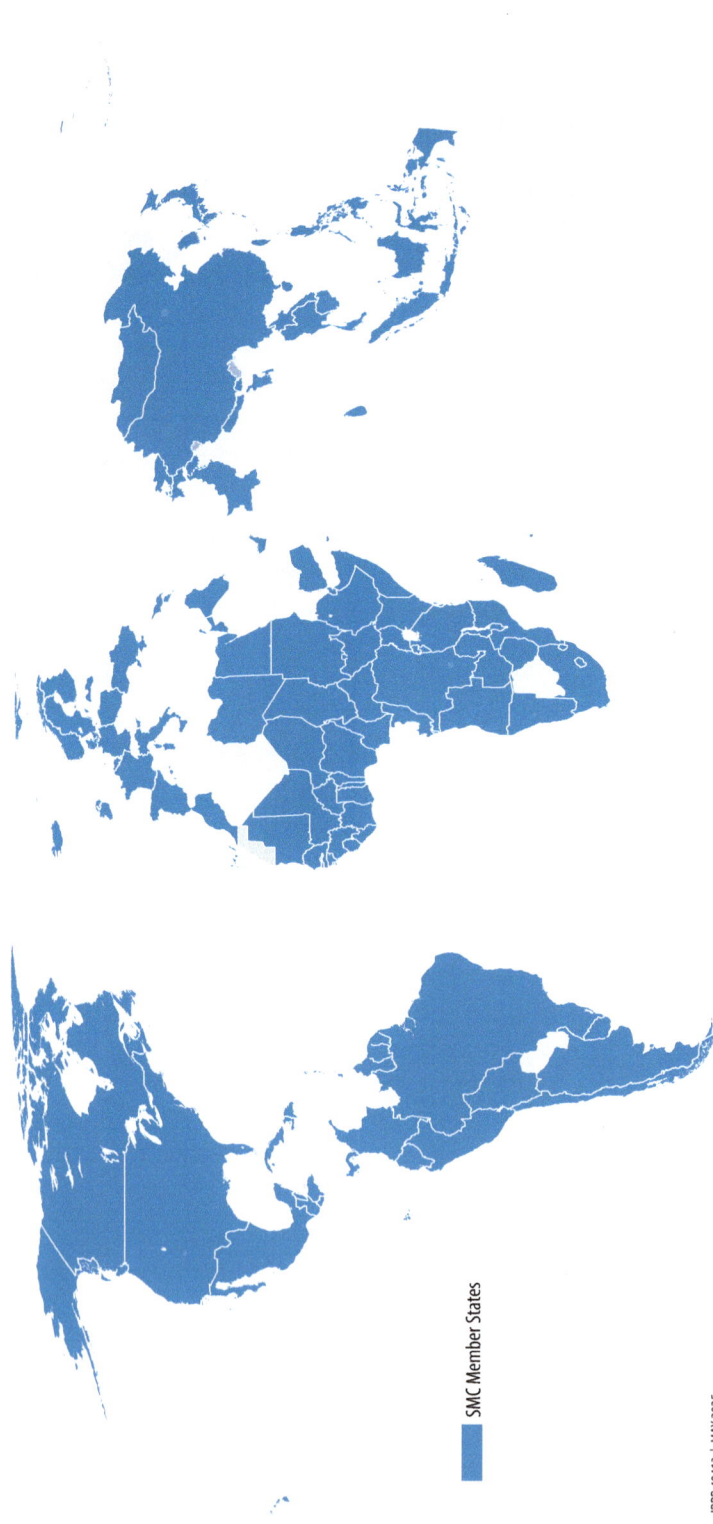

SMC Member States

IBRD 48413 | MAY 2025

*Source:* Original map created for this publication.
*Note:* SMC = School Meals Coalition.

Investing in Pandemic Prevention, Preparedness, and Response  |  Siddhanth Sharma et al.

**Figure 8.1** Change in the Number of Children Receiving School Meals, by Country Income Level, 2020 and 2022

Million children

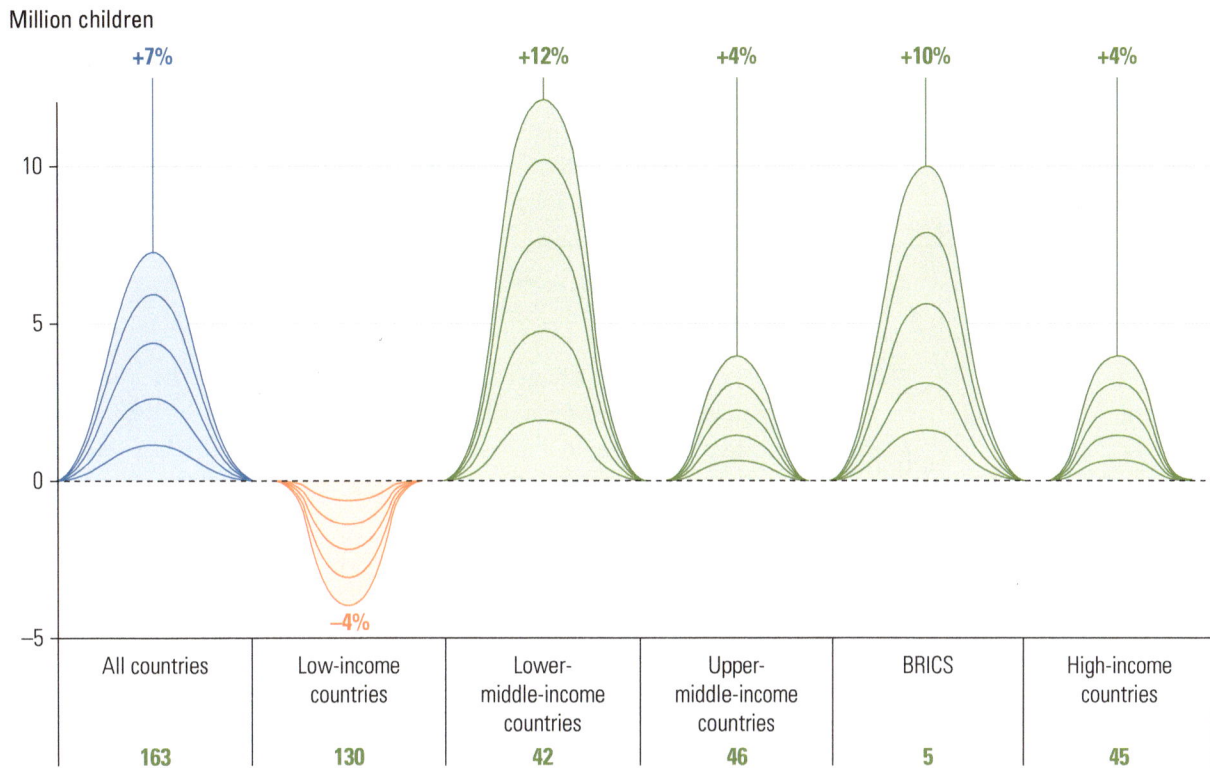

| All countries | Low-income countries | Lower-middle-income countries | Upper-middle-income countries | BRICS | High-income countries |
|---|---|---|---|---|---|
| +7% | −4% | +12% | +4% | +10% | +4% |
| 163 | 130 | 42 | 46 | 5 | 45 |

*Source:* WFP 2023.

*Note:* BRICS = Brazil, Russian Federation, India, China, and South Africa

It was already apparent in 2024 that the School Meals Coalition has helped provide new momentum for rebuilding school-based health services more broadly, including bringing back to school the most vulnerable, reintegration programs, mental health services, and other lines of actions discussed during the Transforming Education Summit. This achievement is particularly impressive because these programs continue to be more than 98 percent supported by domestic funds despite the severe constraints on fiscal space occasioned by the COVID-19 pandemic (WFP 2023). The global investment in school meals has increased by US$5 billion to fund the national programs, rising to US$48 billion in 2022 (WFP 2023). This increase in domestic funding is offset by a 6 percent decrease in aid and multilateral development funding for school meals programming in low-income countries since 2020, following slower GDP growth, reduced revenue collection, and external debt pressures (WFP 2023). Importantly, low-income countries have increased the proportion of the costs of school meals from domestic budgets: up to 45 percent from 30 percent before the pandemic (WFP 2023).

School meals have proved important in elevating school participation and attendance, especially because chronic absenteeism has gone up after the pandemic-driven closures (DiMarco 2023). As noted earlier, however, their economic impact is highly dependent on school quality. The reactions to COVID-19 clearly harmed quality of education during the pandemic, and education systems have been finding it difficult to get back to their prepandemic levels. Importantly, just getting back to prepandemic levels will leave countries permanently worse off because the pandemic cohort of students will be less skilled than other workers and will be a drag on long-term economic growth (Hanushek and Woessmann 2020). Thus, countries must necessarily work to improve school quality and learning for all if they are to fully recover from the pandemic. These actions go well beyond just ensuring student access and attendance, even in the presence of school meals.

## IMPLICATIONS FOR THE ROLE OF SCHOOL CLOSURES IN MANAGING FUTURE PANDEMICS

The COVID-19 pandemic is often framed as a public health issue. The evidence collected for this chapter shows that in the case of school closures there were indeed important public health implications, but also major social, educational, and economic consequences that went far beyond the health outcomes. As shown by the continuing levels of uncertainty in the evidence, these complex interactions have yet to be fully unraveled, but understanding them will again be necessary when the world faces the next pandemic.

It is not the role of the DCP series to make specific recommendations, and normative agencies have since published legal considerations for health emergency measures in schools (WHO 2024b). In concluding this chapter, however, two main areas would especially reward more in-depth analysis: the need to consider consequences beyond public health, and assurance that decisions to close schools are based on sound evidence.

### Understanding the Balance of Consequences across Sectors and Society, beyond Public Health Alone

Even today with benefit of hindsight, and despite systematic reviews, the evidence for the cross-sectoral impact of school closures is mixed and sometimes contradictory. From a public health perspective, there is generally low confidence in the evidence that closing schools, or preventive actions in schools that did not close, had meaningful consequences for the transmission of SARS-CoV-2 infection for either the primary school population or the general population. That belief does not imply that school closure had no effect, or no other implications for public health, but rather that an effect is hard to detect when closing just one of the multiple routes of transmission.

Evidence does show that school closures in the context of the COVID-19 pandemic have had strong and long-lasting negative impacts for education, human capital creation, and the prospects of the "COVID generation." The impacts on learning and education attainment, with implications for employment, lifelong earnings, adult health, and human capital creation, are estimated to have reduced learning by nine points in the standardized US national progress test, corresponding to 6 percent lower lifetime earnings. This impact was associated with major social consequences in some settings, such as increased rates of early marriage and early pregnancy for school-age girls and of inappropriate labor for all school-aged children. The closures have caused substantial and often irreversible dropout from school, reinforcing the cycle of educational underachievement.

For many governments, the counterfactual experience of closing schools, and removing most forms of support to schoolchildren and adolescents, has become the most salient long-term consequence of the COVID-19 pandemic. It has caused national governments to prioritize the reestablishment and strengthening of investments in school-based services to support the well-being of schoolchildren, as seen in the example of the 109 countries participating in the creation of a School Meals Coalition. The combination of the uncertain benefits and significant negative consequences of closing schools contributed to this global momentum for rebuilding, strengthening, and protecting school systems as a safety net and a key contributor to human capital creation.

## Having the Right Information to Make Well-Founded Early Decisions

During the pandemic, the initial thinking about a potential role of school closures in reducing SARS-CoV-2 transmission reflected the public health experience that targeted school closures could reduce influenza transmission. This experience indicated that the effectiveness of school closures depended upon the timeliness of the decision, and this experience in turn led to the recognition that for the SARS-CoV-2 epidemic the decision had to be made at a time of the greatest parameter uncertainty. Adding to the pressures were new political and sociological factors that quickly emerged. The COVID-19 experience showed that in some cases societies reacted more quickly than policy makers to the pandemic, with teachers staying away from schools and parents keeping children at home before formal closures—and before direct evidence of harm or benefits. Evidence also shows a change in the direction of public opinion during the pandemic, with a strong later movement toward reopening schools. In hindsight, it may have been preferable for the original closure decisions to have been simultaneously paired with a clear evidence-based process regarding reopening. In preparing for the next pandemic, understanding the implications of these issues of public policy may be as instrumental as better understanding of the epidemiology.

In conclusion, when faced by the next pandemic, governments will again have to consider taking action in schools while simultaneously balancing public health concerns. The COVID-19 experience shows that it may be considered dangerous and lacking in prudence not to take near immediate precautionary action. Yet that decision will inevitably be made at a time when least is known, especially with regard to the epidemiological role of children and adolescents, and in communities for which the COVID-19 experience has established bodies of opinion that may strongly and negatively shape their reactions to the next event. The experiences described in this chapter show the considerable differences in overall consequences between school closures, which have massive and often unforeseen side effects that often exacerbate existing inequalities, versus protecting the integrity of the school system and introducing specific school-based measures, which are a research topic on their own. Better understanding of the implications of these two options may be crucial to appropriate decision-making when we face the next pandemic.

## NOTES

1. WHO (World Health Organization), "Increasing Recognition, Research and Rehabilitation for Post COVID-19 Condition (long COVID)," https://www.who.int/europe/activities /increasing-recognition-research-and-rehabilitation-for-post-covid-19-condition-long-covid.
2. WHO, "Maternal, Newborn, Child and Adolescent Health and Ageing" (accessed April 22, 2024), https://platform.who.int/data/maternal-newborn-child-adolescent-ageing/national -policies#:~:text=Through%20the%20SRMNCAH%20policy%20survey,that%20are%20 relevant%20to%20SRMNCAH.
3. Finnish Institute for Health and Welfare, "Coronavirus Infections in Schools" (accessed April 22, 2024), https://thl.fi/en/topics/infectious-diseases-and-vaccinations/what-s-new /coronavirus-covid-19-latest-updates/situation-update-on-coronavirus/coronavirus -infections-in-schools.
4. For more on the School Meals Coalition, refer to its website, https://schoolmealscoalition.org.

## REFERENCES

Abay, K. A., M. Amare, L. Tiberti, and K. S. Andam. 2021. "COVID-19-Induced Disruptions of School Feeding Services Exacerbate Food Insecurity in Nigeria." *Journal of Nutrition* 151 (8): 2245–54.

Adams, R., S. Weale, and C. Bannock. 2020. "Schools in England Struggle to Stay Open as Coronavirus Hits Attendance." *The Guardian*, March 17. https://www.theguardian.com /education/2020/mar/17/schools-across-england-struggle-as-coronavirus-hits-attendance.

Andrabi, T., B. Daniels, and J. Das. 2023. "Human Capital Accumulation and Disasters." *Journal of Human Resources* 58 (4): 1057–96.

Angrist, N, A. de Barros, R. Bhula, S. Chakera, C. Cummiskey, J. DeStefano, J. Floretta, et al. 2021. "Building Back Better to Avert a Learning Catastrophe: Estimating Learning Loss from COVID-19 School Shutdowns in Africa and Facilitating Short-Term and Long-Term Learning Recovery." *International Journal of Educational Development* 84: 102397.

AWMF (Arbeitsgemeinschaft der Wissenschaftlichen Medizinischen Fachgesellschaften, Working Group of Scientific Medical Societies). 2022. "S3-Leitlinie Maßnahmen zur Prävention und Kontrolle der SARS-CoV-2-Übertragung in Schulen | Lebende Leitlinie Evidenzgrundlage." AWMF-Registernummer 027-076, Kurzfassung Version 2.0, September 2022, AWMF Online. https://register.awmf.org/assets /guidelines/027-076e_Praevention_und_Kontrolle_SARS-CoV-2-Uebertragung_in _Schulen_2022-10.pdf.

Baltag, V., A. Pachyna, and J. Hall. 2015. "Global Overview of School Health Services: Data from 102 Countries." *Health Behavior and Policy Review* 2 (4): 268–83.

Baltag, V., E. Sidaner, D. Bundy, R. Guthold, C. Nwachukwu, K. Engesveen, D. Sharma, et al. 2022. "Realising the Potential of Schools to Improve Adolescent Nutrition." *BMJ* 379: e067678.

Banati, P., D. A. Ross, B. Weobong, S. Kapiga, H. A. Weiss, V. Baltag, F. Nzvere, et al. 2024. "Adolescent Health and Well-Being Check-up Programme in Three African Cities (Y-Check): Protocol for a Multimethod, Prospective, Hybrid Implementation-Effectiveness Study." BMJ Open14:e077533. https://doi.org/10.1136/bmjopen-2023-077533.

Barendse, M. E. A., J. Flannery, C. Cavanagh, M. Aristizabal, S. P. Becker, E. Berger, R. Breaux, et al. 2023. "Longitudinal Change in Adolescent Depression and Anxiety Symptoms from before to during the COVID-19 Pandemic." *Journal of Research on Adolescence* 33 (1): 74–91.

Bell, D., A. Nicoll, K. Fukuda, P. Horby, A. Monto, F. Hayden, C. Wylks, et al. 2006. "Nonpharmaceutical Interventions for Pandemic Influenza, National and Community Measures." *Emerging Infectious Diseases* 12 (1): 88. https://doi.org/10.3201/eid1201.051371.

Boutzoukas, A. E., K. O. Zimmerman, D. K. Benjamin, G. P. DeMuri, I. C. Kalu, M. J. Smith, K. A. McGann, et al. 2022. "Secondary Transmission of COVID-19 in K–12 Schools: Findings from 2 States." *Pediatrics* 149 (Supplement 2).

Bundy, D. A. P., C. Burbano, M. Grosh, A. Gelli, M. Jukes, and L. Drake. 2009. *Rethinking School Feeding: Social Safety Nets, Child Development, and the Education Sector.* Directions in Development. Washington, DC: World Bank.

Bundy, D. A. P., U. Gentilini, L. Schultz, B. Bedasso, S. Singh, Y. Okamura, H. T. M. M. Iyengar, et al. 2024. "School Meals, Social Protection and Human Development: Revisiting Global Trends, Evidence, and Practices with a Focus on South Asia." Social Protection & Jobs Discussion Paper 2401, World Bank, Washington, DC.

Bundy, D. A. P., N. de Silva, S. Horton, G. Patton, L. Schultz, D. T. Jamison, T. D. Hollingsworth, et al. 2018. "Investment in Child and Adolescent Health and Development: Key Messages from Disease Control Priorities, 3rd Edition." *The Lancet* 391 (10121): 687–99.

Bundy, D. A. P., and S. Horton. 2017. "Impact of Interventions on Health and Development during Childhood and Adolescence: A Conceptual Framework." In *Disease Control Priorities, Third Edition: Child and Adolescent Health and Development,* Volume 8, edited by D. A. P. Bundy, N. de Silva, S. Horton, D. T. Jamison, and G. C. Patton, 73–78. Washington, DC: World Bank.

Bundy, D. A. P., L. Schultz, B. Sarr, L. Banham, P. Colenso, and L. Drake. 2017. "The School as a Platform for Addressing Health in Middle Childhood and Adolescence." In *Disease Control Priorities, Third Edition: Child and Adolescent Health and Development,* Volume 8, edited by D. A. P. Bundy, N. de Silva, S. Horton, D. T. Jamison, and G. C. Patton, 269–85. Washington, DC: World Bank.

Carlana, M., E. La Ferrara, and C. Lopez. 2023. "Exacerbated Inequalities: The Learning Loss from COVID-19 in Italy." *AEA Papers and Proceedings* 113: 489–93.

Cauchemez, S., N. M. Ferguson, C. Wachtel, A. Tegnell, G. Saour, B. Duncan, A. Nicoli, et al. 2009. "Closure of Schools during an Influenza Pandemic." *The Lancet Infectious Diseases* 9 (8): 473–81.

Cohen, J. F. W., S. Verguet, B. B. Giyose, and D. Bundy. 2023. "Universal Free School Meals: The Future of School Meal Programmes?" *The Lancet* 402 (10405): P831–33.

Cronert, A. 2022. "Precaution and Proportionality in Pandemic Politics: Democracy, State Capacity, and COVID-19-Related School Closures around the World." *Journal of Public Policy* 42 (4): 705–29.

Davies, N. G., P. Klepac, Y. Liu, K. Prem, M. Jit, C. A. B. Pearson, et al. 2020. "Age-Dependent Effects in the Transmission and Control of COVID-19 Epidemics." *Nature Medicine* 26 (8): 1205–11.

DiMarco, B. 2023. "Tracking State Trends in Chronic Absenteeism." FutureEd Explainer, October 13 (updated February 7, 2025). https://www.future-ed.org/tracking-state-trends-in-chronic-absenteeism/.

ECDC (European Centre for Disease Prevention and Control). 2020. "COVID-19 in Children and the Role of School Settings in Transmission—First Update." Technical Report, ECDC, Stockholm. https://www.ecdc.europa.eu/sites/default/files/documents/COVID-19-in-children-and-the-role-of-school-settings-in-transmission-first-update_1.pdf.

Edmunds, W. J. 2020. "Finding a Path to Reopen Schools during the COVID-19 Pandemic." *The Lancet Child & Adolescent Health* 4 (11): 796–97.

FAO (Food and Agriculture Organization of the United Nations), IFAD (International Fund for Agricultural Development), UNICEF (United Nations Children's Fund), WFP (World Food Programme), and WHO (World Health Organization). 2021. *The State of Food Security and Nutrition in the World 2021. Transforming Food Systems for Food Security, Improved Nutrition and Affordable Healthy Diets for All.* Rome: FAO. https://doi.org/10.4060/cb4474en.

Ferguson, N. M., D. A. T. Cummings, C. Fraser, J. C. Cajka, P. C. Cooley, and D. S. Burke. 2006. "Strategies for Mitigating an Influenza Pandemic." *Nature* 442 (7101): 448–52. https://www.nature.com/articles/nature04795.

Ferguson, N. M., D. Laydon, G. Nedjati-Gilanti, N. Imai, K. Ainslie, M. Baguelin, S. Bhatia, et al. 2020. "Impact of Non-pharmaceutical Interventions (NPIs) to Reduce COVID-19 Mortality and Healthcare Demand." Imperial College London. https://doi.org/10.25561/77482.

Fernandes, M., and E. Aurino. 2017. "Identifying an Essential Package for School-Age Child Health: Economic Analysis." In *Disease Control Priorities, Third Edition: Child and Adolescent Health and Development,* Volume 8, edited by D. A. P. Bundy, N. de Silva, S. Horton, D. T. Jamison, and G. C. Patton, 355–68. Washington, DC: World Bank.

Flasche, S., and W. J. Edmunds. 2021. "The Role of Schools and School-Aged Children in SARS-CoV-2 Transmission." *The Lancet Infectious Diseases* 21 (3): 298–99.

Fontanet, A., L. Tondeur, R. Grant, S. Temmam, Y. Madec, T. Bigot, L. Grzelak, et al. 2021. "SARS-CoV-2 Infection in Schools in a Northern French City: A Retrospective Serological Cohort Study in an Srea of High Transmission, France, January to April 2020." *Eurosurveillance* 26 (15).

Fontanet, A., L. Tondeur, Y. Madec, R. Grant, C. Besombes, N. Jolly, S. F. Pellerin, et al. 2020. "Cluster of COVID-19 in Northern France: A Retrospective Closed Cohort Study." *Eurosurveillance* 26 (15). https://www.eurosurveillance.org/content/10.2807/1560-7917. ES.2021.26.15.2001695.

Germann, T. C., K. Kadau, I. M. Longini, and C. A. Macken. 2006. "Mitigation Strategies for Pandemic Influenza in the United States." *Proceedings of the National Academy of Sciences* 103 (15): 5935–40. https://www.pnas.org/doi/abs/10.1073/pnas.0601266103.

Girls' Education Challenge and UK Aid. 2021. "Emerging Findings: The Impact of COVID-19 on Girls and the Girls' Education Challenge Response—Focus on East Africa (Ethiopia, Kenya and Somalia)." Girls' Education Challenge. https://girlseducationchallenge.org /media/ka4gkdei/emerging_findings_east-africa.pdf.

Global Financing Facility. 2021. "School Health & Nutrition: Reach and Relevance for Adolescents." World Bank, Washington, DC. https://www.globalfinancingfacility.org /resource/school-health-and-nutrition-reach-and-relevance-adolescents.

Goldhaber, D., T. J. Kane, A. McEachin, E. Morton, T. Patterson, and D. O. Staiger. 2023. "The Educational Consequences of Remote and Hybrid Instruction during the Pandemic." *American Economic Review Insights* 5 (3): 377–92.

Grossmann, M., S. Reckhow, K. O. Strunk, and M. Turner. 2021. "All States Close but Red Districts Reopen: The Politics of In-Person Schooling during the COVID-19 Pandemic." *Educational Researcher* 50 (9): 637–48.

Gust, S., E. A. Hanushek, and L. Woessmann. 2024. "Global Universal Basic Skills: Current Deficits and Implications for World Development." *Journal of Development Economics* 166: 103205.

Haber, M. J., D. K. Shay, X. M. Davis, R. Patel, X. Jin, E. Weintraub, et al. 2007. "Effectiveness of Interventions to Reduce Contact Rates during a Simulated Influenza Pandemic." *Emerging Infectious Diseases* 13 (4): 581–89.

Hale, T., N. Angrist, R. Goldszmidt, B. Kira, A. Petherick, T. Phillips, S. Webster, et al. 2021. "A Global Panel Database of Pandemic Policies (Oxford COVID-19 Government Response Tracker)." *Nature Human Behaviour* 5 (4): 529–38.

Hanushek, E. A. 2023. "Generation Lost: The Pandemic's Lifetime Tax." *Education Next* (blog), October 6, 2023. https://www.educationnext.org/generation-lost-the-pandemics-lifetime -tax/.

Hanushek, E. A., G. Schwerdt, S. Wiederhold, and L. Woessmann. 2015. "Returns to Skills around the World: Evidence from PIAAC." *European Economic Review* 73 (1): 103–30.

Hanushek, E. A., and L. Woessmann. 2008. "The Role of Cognitive Skills in Economic Development." *Journal of Economic Literature* 46 (3): 607–68.

Hanushek, E. A., and L. Woessmann. 2015. *The Knowledge Capital of Nations: Education and the Economics of Growth.* Cambridge, MA: MIT Press.

Hanushek, E. A., and L. Woessmann. 2020. "The Economic Impacts of Learning Losses." OECD Education Working Paper No. 225, OECD Publishing, Paris. https://doi .org/10.1787/21908d74-en.

Haug, N., L. Geyrhofer, A. Londei, E. Dervic, A. Desvars-Larrive, V. Loreto, B. Pinior, et al. 2020. "Ranking the Effectiveness of Worldwide COVID-19 Government Interventions." *Nature Human Behaviour* 4 (12): 1303–12.

Heavey, L., G. Casey, C. Kelly, D. Kelly, and G. McDarby. 2020. "No Evidence of Secondary Transmission of COVID-19 from Children Attending School in Ireland, 2020." *Eurosurveillance* 25 (21): 2000903.

Hume, S., S. R. Brown, and K. R. Mahtani. 2023. "School Closures during COVID-19: An Overview of Systematic Reviews." *BMJ Evidence-Based Medicine* 28 (3): 164–74.

ILO (International Labour Organization) and UNICEF (United Nations Children's Fund). 2021. *Child Labour: Global Estimates 2020, Trends and the Road Forward*. New York: ILO and UNICEF.

Irons, N. J., and A. E. Raftery. 2024. "US COVID-19 School Closure Was Not Cost-Effective, but Other Measures Were." Working Paper. https://arxiv.org/pdf/2411.12016.

Ismail, S. A., V. Saliba, J. Lopez Bernal, M. E. Ramsay, and S. N. Ladhani. 2021. "SARS-CoV-2 Infection and Transmission in Educational Settings: A Prospective, Cross-Sectional Analysis of Infection Clusters and Outbreaks in England." *The Lancet Infectious Diseases* 21 (3): 344–53.

Jack, R., and E. Oster. 2023. "COVID-19, School Closures, and Outcomes." *Journal of Economic Perspectives* 37 (4): 51–70.

Jackson, C., P. Mangtani, J. Hawker, B. Olowokure, and E. Vynnycky. 2014. "The Effects of School Closures on Influenza Outbreaks and Pandemics: Systematic Review of Simulation Studies." *PLOS One* 9 (5): e97297.

Jackson, C., E. Vynnycky, J. Hawker, B. Olowokure, and P. Mangtani. 2013. "School Closures and Influenza: Systematic Review of Epidemiological Studies." *BMJ Open* 3 (2): e002149.

Jakubowski, M., T. Gajderowicz, and H. Patrinos. 2024. "COVID-19, School Closures, and Student Learning Outcomes: New Global Evidence from PISA." Policy Research Working Paper 10666, World Bank, Washington, DC.

Jamison, J. C. 2020. "Lockdowns Will Starve People in Low-Income Countries." *Washington Post*, April 20, 2020. https://www.washingtonpost.com/outlook/2020/04/20/lockdown-developing-world-coronavirus-poverty/.

Jamison, J. C., D. Bundy, D. T. Jamison, J. Spitz, and S. Verguet. 2021. "Comparing the Impact on COVID-19 Mortality of Self-Imposed Behavior Change and of Government Regulations across 13 Countries." *Health Services Research* 56 (5): 874–84.

Jaume, D., and A. Willen. 2019. "The Long-Run Effects of Teacher Strikes: Evidence from Argentina." *Journal of Labor Economics* 37(4).

Kadzamira, E., J. Mazalale, E. Meke, I. V. Mwale, F. Jimu, L. Moscoviz, J. Rossiter, et al. 2021. "What Happened to Student Participation after Two Rounds of School Closures in Malawi—and How Have Schools Responded?" *Center for Global Development* (blog), November 24, 2021. https://www.cgdev.org/blog/what-happened-student-participation-after-two-rounds-school-closures-malawi-and-how-have.

Kim, J., P. Rose, D. Tibebu Tiruneh, R. Sabates, and T. Woldehanna. 2021. "Learning Inequalities Widen Following COVID-19 School Closures in Ethiopia." *RISE* (blog), May 4, 2021. https://riseprogramme.org/blog/learning-inequalities-widen-COVID-19-Ethiopia.html.

Kratzer, S., L. M. Pfadenhauer, R. L. Biallas, R. Featherstone, C. Klinger, A. Movsisyan, J. E. Rabe, et al. 2022. "Unintended Consequences of Measures Implemented in the School Setting to Contain the COVID-19 Pandemic: A Scoping Review." *Cochrane Database of Systematic Reviews* 6 (6): CD015397.

Lange, G. M., Q. Wodon, and K. Carey. 2018. *The Changing Wealth of Nations 2018: Building a Sustainable Future*. Washington, DC: World Bank.

Langford, R., C. Bonell, H. Jones, T. Pouliou, S. Murphy, E. Waters, K. A. Komro, et al. 2014. "The WHO Health Promoting School Framework for Improving the Health and Well-Being of Students and Their Academic Achievement (Review)." *Cochrane Database of Systematic Reviews* 2014 (4): CD008958.

Langford, R., C. Bonell, H. Jones, T. Pouliou, S. Murphy, E. Waters, K. A. Komro, et al. 2015. "The World Health Organization's Health Promoting Schools Framework: A Cochrane Systematic Review and Meta-analysis." *BMC Public Health* 15 (1): 1–15.

Levin, A. T., W. P. Hanage, N. Owusu-Boaitey, K. B. Cochran, S. P. Walsh, and G. Meyerowitz-Katz. 2020. "Assessing the Age Specificity of Infection Fatality Rates for COVID-19: Systematic Review, Meta-analysis, and Public Policy Implications." *European Journal of Epidemiology* 35 (12): 1123–38.

Li, Y., H. Campbell, D. Kulkarni, A. Harpur, M. Nundy, X. Wang, X. Wang, et al. 2021. "The Temporal Association of Introducing and Lifting Non-pharmaceutical Interventions with the Time-Varying Reproduction Number (R) of SARS-CoV-2: A Modelling Study across 131 Countries." *The Lancet Infectious Diseases* 21 (2): 193–202.

Littlecott, H., S. Krishnaratne, J. Burns, E. Rehfuess, K. Sell, C. Klinger, B. Strahwald, et al. 2024. "Measures Implemented in the School Setting to Contain the COVID-19 Pandemic." *Cochrane Database of Systematic Reviews* 2024 (5): 1–100.

Macartney, K., H. E. Quinn, A. J. Pillsbury, A. Koirala, L. Deng, N. Winkler, A. L. Katelaris, et al. 2020. "Transmission of SARS-CoV-2 in Australian Educational Settings: A Prospective Cohort Study." *The Lancet Child & Adolescent Health* 4 (11): 807–16.

Marquez, J., L. Taylor, L. Boyle, W. Zhou, and J. E. De Neve. 2024. "Child and Adolescent Well-Being: Global Trends, Challenges and Opportunities." Chapter 3 in *World Happiness Report 2024*, edited by J. F. Helliwell, R. Layard, J. D. Sachs, J.-E. De Neve, L. B. Aknun, and S. Wang. Oxford: Wellbeing Research Centre.

Meherali, S., B. Adewale, S. Ali, M. Kennedy, B. Salami (Oladunni), S. Richter, P. E. Okeke-Ihejirika, et al. 2021. "Impact of the COVID-19 Pandemic on Adolescents' Sexual and Reproductive Health in Low- and Middle-Income Countries." *International Journal of Environmental Research and Public Health* 18 (24): 13221.

Menasce Horowitz, J. 2022. "Academic, Emotional Concerns Outweigh COVID-19 Risks in Parents' Views about Keeping Schools Open." Pew Research Center Short Reads, February 4, 2022. https://www.pewresearch.org/short-reads/2022/02/04/academic-emotional-concerns-outweigh-covid-19-risks-in-parents-views-about-keeping-schools-open/.

Monod, M., A. Blenkinsop, X. Xi, D. Hebert, S. Bershan, S. Tietze, M. Baguelin, et al. 2021. "Age Groups That Sustain Resurging COVID-19 Epidemics in the United States." *Science* 371 (6536): eabe8372.

Montenegro, C. E., and H. A. Patrinos. 2014. "Comparable Estimates of Returns to Schooling around the World." Policy Research Working Paper 7020, World Bank, Washington, DC.

Montresor, A., D. Mupfasoni, A. Mikhailov, P. Mwinzi, A. Lucianez, M. Jamsheed, E. Gasimov, et al. 2020. "The Global Progress of Soil-Transmitted Helminthiases Control in 2020 and World Health Organization Targets for 2030." *PLOS Neglected Tropical Diseases* 14 (8): 1–17.

Moscoviz, L., and D. K. Evans. 2022. "Learning Loss and Student Dropouts during the COVID-19 Pandemic: A Review of the Evidence Two Years after Schools Shut Down." CGD Working Paper 609, Center for Global Development, Washington, DC. https://www.ungei.org/sites/default/files/2022-04/learning-loss-and-student-dropouts-during-covid-19-pandemic-review-evidence-two-years.pdf.

Mossong, J., N. Hens, M. Jit, P. Beutels, K. Auranen, R. Mikolajczyk, M. Massari, et al. 2008. "Social Contacts and Mixing Patterns Relevant to the Spread of Infectious Diseases." *PLOS Medicine* 5 (3): 0381–91.

Munoz-Najar, A., A. Gilberto, A. Hasan, C. Cobo, J. P. Azevedo, and M. Akmal. 2021. "Remote Learning during COVID-19: Lessons from Today, Principles for Tomorrow." World Bank, Washington, DC.

Park, Y. J., Y. J. Choe, O. Park, S. Y. Park, Y. M. Kim, J. Kim, S. Kweon, et al. 2020. "Contact Tracing during Coronavirus Disease Outbreak, South Korea, 2020." *Emerging Infectious Diseases* 26 (10): 2465–68. http://www.ncbi.nlm.nih.gov/pubmed/32673193.

Public Health England. 2021. "COVID-19 Surveillance in Children Attending Preschool, Primary and Secondary Schools." Public Health England, London. https://assets.publishing.service.gov.uk/media/609178a9e90e076ab07a6de0/sKIDs_protocol_v1.6.pdf.

Ross, D. A., R. Hinton, M. Melles-Brewer, D. Engel, W. Zeck, L. Fagan, J. Herat, et al. 2020. "Adolescent Well-Being: A Definition and Conceptual Framework." *Journal of Adolescent Health* 67 (4): 472–76.

Save the Children and UNICEF (United Nations Children's Fund). 2021. "Impact of COVID-19 on Children Living in Poverty." Technical Note, UNICEF. https://data.unicef .org/resources/impact-of-covid-19-on-children-living-in-poverty/.

Schultz, L., L. Appleby, and L. Drake. 2018. "Maximizing Human Capital by Aligning Investments in Health and Education." Child Rights Resource Centre.

Schultz, L., P. Hangoma, D. T. Jamison, and D. A. P. Bundy. 2025. "Cross-National Experiences on Child Health and Development during School-Age and Adolescence: The Next 7,000 days." In *Disease Control Priorities, Fourth Edition*, edited by A. Alwan, M. K. Mirutse, O. F. Norheim, and P. D. Twea. Washington, DC: World Bank.

Sheehan, P., B. Rasmussen, K. Sweeny, N. Maharaj, J. Symons, M. Kumnick, D. Ross, et al. 2023. *Adolescents in a Changing World: The Case for Urgent Investment—Executive Summary*. Victoria Institute of Strategic Economic Studies, Victoria University, Melbourne.

Stacy, B., and M. Lambrechts. 2023. "Rebuilding Education Systems after COVID-19." In *Atlas of Sustainable Development Goals 2023*, edited by A. F. Pirlea, U. Serajuddin, A. Thudt, D. Wadhwa, and M. Welch. Washington, DC: World Bank. https://datatopics.worldbank .org/sdgatlas/goal-4-quality-education?lang=en.

Thorisdottir, I. E., G. Agustsson, S. Y. Oskarsdottir, A. L. Kristjansson, B. B. Asgeirsdottir, I. D. Sigfusdottir, H. B. Valdimarsdottir, et al. 2023. "Effect of the COVID-19 Pandemic on Adolescent Mental Health and Substance Use up to March, 2022, in Iceland: A Repeated, Cross-Sectional, Population-Based Study." *The Lancet Child & Adolescent Health* 7 (5): 347–57.

Tran Kiem, C., P. Bosetti, J. Paireau, P. Crépey, H. Salje, N. Lefrancq, A. Fontanet, et al. 2021. "SARS-CoV-2 Transmission across Age Groups in France and Implications for Control." *Nature Commununications* 12: 6895.

UNESCO (United Nations Educational, Scientific and Cultural Organization), UNICEF (United Nations Children's Fund), and WFP (World Food Programme). 2022. "Ready to Learn and Thrive: School Health and Nutrition around the World." UNESCO, Paris; UNICEF, New York; WFP, Rome. https://unesdoc.unesco.org/ark:/48223/pf0000381965.

UNESCO (United Nations Educational, Scientific and Cultural Organization), UNICEF (United Nations Children's Fund), World Bank, and WFP (World Food Programme). 2020. "Framework for Reopening Schools." https://www.unicef.org/media/68366/file /Framework-for-reopening-schools-2020.pdf.

UNICEF (United Nations Children's Fund). 2021. COVID-19: "A Threat to Progress against Child Marriage." UNICEF, New York. https://data.unicef.org/resources/covid-19-a-threat -to-progress-against-child-marriage/.

Viner, R. M., S. J. Russell, H. Croker, J. Packer, J. Ward, C. Stansfield, O. Mytton, et al. 2020. "School Closure and Management Practices during Coronavirus Outbreaks Including COVID-19: A Rapid Systematic Review." *The Lancet Child & Adolescent Health* 4 (5): 397–404.

Wang, Y., G. Avanesian, A. Kamei, S. Mishra, and S. Mizunoya. 2021. "Which Children Have Internet Access at Home? Insights from Household Survey Data." *UNICEF Data Blog*, May 21. https://data.unicef.org/data-for-action/where-do-children-have-internet-access-at -home-insights-from-household-survey-data/.

Watkins, D. A., D. T. Jamison, A. Mills, R. Atun, K. Danforth, A. Glassman, S. Horton, et al. 2018. "Universal Health Coverage and Essential Packages of Care." In *Disease Control Priorities, Third Edition, Improving Health and Reducing Poverty*, Volume 9, edited by D. T. Jamison, H. Gelbrand, S. Horton, P. Jha, and R. Laxminarayan, 43–65. Washington, DC: World Bank.

WFP (World Food Programme). 2020. *State of School Feeding Worldwide 2020*. Rome: WFP.

WFP (World Food Programme). 2023. *State of School Feeding Worldwide 2022*. Rome: WFP.

WHO (World Health Organization). 2020a. "Maintaining Essential Health Services: Operational Guidance for the COVID-19 Context." WHO, Geneva.

WHO (World Health Organization). 2020b. "Pulse Survey on Continuity of Essential Health Services during the COVID-19 Pandemic. Interim report." WHO, Geneva.

WHO (World Health Organization). 2021. *WHO Guideline on School Health Services.* Geneva: WHO.

WHO (World Health Organization). 2023a. *Global Accelerated Action for the Health of Adolescents (AA-HA!): Guidance to Support Country Implementation*, Second Edition. Geneva: WHO.

WHO (World Health Organization). 2023b. *WHO Benchmarks for Strengthening Health Emergency Capacities.* Geneva: WHO.

WHO (World Health Organization). 2024a. *Adolescents in a Changing World: The Case for Urgent Investment.* Geneva: WHO.

WHO (World Health Organization). 2024b. *Legal Considerations for Health Emergency Measures in Schools and Education.* Geneva: WHO.

WHO (World Health Organization) and UNESCO (United Nations Educational, Scientific and Cultural Organization). 2021. *Making Every School a Health-Promoting School: Global Standards and Indicators.* Geneva: WHO.

WHO (World Health Organization), UNESCO (United Nations Educational, Scientific and Cultural Organization), and UNICEF (United Nations Children's Fund). 2020. "Considerations for School-Related Public Health Measures in the Context of COVID-19." Annex to "Considerations in Adjusting Public Health and Social Measures in the Context of COVID-19." WHO, Geneva. https://www.who.int/publications/i/item/considerations-for-school-related-public-health-measures-in-the-context-of-covid-19.

WHO (World Health Organization) Regional Office for Europe. 2022. *Ninth Meeting of the Technical Advisory Group on Safe Schooling during the COVID-19 Pandemic.* Copenhagen: WHO. https://www.who.int/europe/publications/i/item/WHO-EURO-2022-5758-45523-65175.

World Bank. 2019. "Africa Human Capital Plan: Powering Africa's Potential through Its People." World Bank, Washington, DC.

World Bank and UNESCO (United Nations Educational, Scientific and Cultural Organization). 2023. *Education Finance Watch 2023.* Washington, DC, and Paris: World Bank and UNESCO. https://www.unesco.org/gem-report/en/2023efw.

World Bank, UNESCO (United Nations Educational, Scientific and Cultural Organization), and UNICEF (United Nations Children's Fund). 2021. *The State of the Global Education Crisis: A Path to Recovery.* Washington, DC, Paris, New York: World Bank, UNESCO, UNICEF.

Yan, Y., A. A. Malik, J. Bayham, E. P. Fenichel, C. Couzens, and S. B. Omer. 2021. "Measuring Voluntary and Policy-Induced Social Distancing Behavior during the COVID-19 Pandemic." *Proceedings of the National Academy of Sciences of the United States of America* 118 (16): e2008814118.

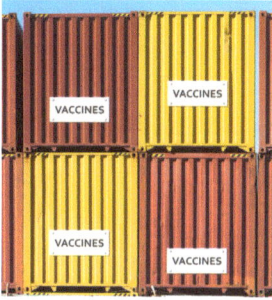

# 9

# Pandemic Preparedness and Prevention: Vaccination

Maddalena Ferranna, David E. Bloom, Nita K. Madhav, Ben Oppenheim, and Nicole Stephenson

## ABSTRACT

This chapter discusses the fundamental role of vaccination in preventing and mitigating future pandemics. It reviews the health, social, and economic benefits of vaccination and discusses strategies to ensure accelerated development, manufacturing, and deployment of vaccines should a future pandemic emerge. The chapter also analyzes the health and economic costs of global vaccine inequity, the existing barriers to vaccine equity, and potential solutions. A simple simulation exercise demonstrates the value of investing in accelerated development, manufacturing, and equitable allocation of vaccines.

## INTRODUCTION

The COVID-19 (coronavirus) pandemic has had staggering health, social, and economic costs. As of October 2023, the official number of COVID-19 deaths worldwide amounted to almost 7 million,[1] with estimates of excess deaths (that is, the number of deaths from all causes attributable to the crisis conditions) at about 27 million (Economist 2022). Globally, school closures affected 1.6 billion students, who lost on average an estimated 35 percent of a year's worth of learning (Betthäuser, Bach-Mortensen, and Engzell 2023). Because of disruptions to routine immunization, one in five children is now undervaccinated, a proportion last seen in 2008 (UNICEF 2023). In 2020, global gross domestic product (GDP) decreased by 3.1 percent. Even though most economies have recovered since then, high inflation and financial instability jeopardized the process (IMF 2023). The health, social, and economic benefits of preparing for future pandemics are indisputable.

The COVID-19 pandemic also highlighted the key role of vaccination in pandemic management and the importance of rapid development and deployment of safe and effective vaccines. COVID-19 vaccines were developed at a historically unprecedented speed (Bloom et al. 2021), with less than 12 months between identification of the genetic sequence of SARS-CoV-2 and vaccine manufacturing and deployment. The mass COVID-19 vaccination campaigns in 2021–22 substantially reduced the numbers of deaths, hospitalizations, and severe illnesses due to COVID-19 (Steele et al. 2022; Watson et al. 2022) and allowed the progressive reopening of the economy and the return to prepandemic patterns of economic activity and socialization (Hansen and Mano 2023).

Vaccine rollout proceeded at widely varying paces throughout the world. As of October 2023, approximately 65 percent of the global population had completed the initial COVID-19 vaccination protocol (that is, two doses for most vaccines). However, whereas in higher-income countries more than 70 percent of the population had completed the initial protocol, among low-income countries only 28 percent had done so (Mathieu et al. 2020). This global inequality has left lower-income countries exposed to significant preventable deaths (Moore et al. 2022), caused an uneven recovery across countries (UN DESA 2021), and been linked to the emergence of new variants (Wagner et al. 2021). Multiple factors explain COVID-19 vaccination inequity, including manufacturing constraints, vaccine nationalism, logistical and infrastructure constraints, and vaccine hesitancy (Larson, Gakidou, and Murray 2022; Wouters et al. 2021).

In light of the COVID-19 pandemic experience, this chapter reflects on the role of vaccination in preparation for the next pandemic. In particular, it covers three related topics. First, it provides an overview of the many health, social, and economic benefits of vaccination should a future pandemic emerge, and argues for a comprehensive assessment of those benefits in the economic evaluation of vaccines. Second, it highlights the benefits of accelerating the development of vaccines against pathogens with pandemic potential. The uncertainty about the timing of the next pandemic and the lengthy process to develop, test, and manufacture vaccines call for moving vaccine development to prepandemic periods as much as possible. Third, it discusses the costs of vaccine inequity and reflects on the optimal allocation of vaccines. To illustrate its arguments, it presents the results of a simulation exercise that estimates the number of deaths and economic costs averted by vaccination in various scenarios. The scenarios differ in terms of characteristics of the next pandemic, timing to develop a vaccine, and equity in the distribution of vaccines. The simulation exercise is based on the model described in chapter 2 of this volume.

Because of space limitations, this chapter will not cover other important vaccination-related topics. Those topics include supply-side issues such as research and development, financing, public-private partnerships, and vaccine patents (refer to chapter 11 of this volume); the optimal stockpiling of vaccines (Carlson et al. 2024); vaccination of animals as a means of preventing human diseases (Monath 2013);

and the complementarity between vaccination and nonpharmaceutical interventions during outbreak responses (refer to chapter 7 of this volume).

## THE VALUE OF VACCINATION AGAINST FUTURE PANDEMICS

This section provides an overview of the literature on the health, social, and economic benefits of vaccination against future pandemics and demonstrates the potential value of accelerated vaccine development through a simple simulation exercise.

### The Benefits of Vaccination

Vaccination is one of the most effective tools for fighting infectious diseases and reducing mortality and morbidity, especially among children. Vaccines have contributed to the worldwide eradication of smallpox and to the substantial reduction in deaths from other major diseases such as polio and measles. More recently, Ebola vaccines have drastically reduced morbidity and mortality during outbreaks, with a recent study finding a 50 percent reduction in deaths (Coulborn et al. 2024). Over the past several decades, coverage rates for basic immunizations have steadily increased, dramatically reducing under-five mortality and overall mortality (Li et al. 2021; McGovern and Canning 2015).

Vaccination typically has direct and indirect effects (Anderson and May 1985). Vaccinated individuals are protected from the risk of infection or severe disease from the targeted pathogens. If the vaccine can reduce the risk of infection or the risk of transmission, vaccination also benefits unvaccinated individuals. Increasing the number of vaccinated people reduces the circulation of the infectious pathogen in the unvaccinated population. If a sufficiently large number of people is vaccinated, further infection spread is unlikely, and the population has effectively reached a level of "herd protection." The proportion of the population that needs to be vaccinated to achieve herd protection depends on the transmissibility of the disease and the characteristics of the vaccine. For example, for measles an estimated 95 percent of the population has to be vaccinated because measles spreads very easily (Pandey and Galvani 2023). For polio, the level is about 80–85 percent (Plans-Rubió 2012). For COVID-19, herd protection is now considered elusive because of the constant emergence of new variants that escape vaccine immunity (Morens, Folkers, and Fauci 2022).

Some vaccines offer long-term immunity, whereas for others immunity wanes over time, requiring booster shots. For example, the measles vaccine is deemed to offer lifelong protection for most individuals (Cohen 2019), whereas protection against mumps wanes on average 27 years after vaccination (Lewnard and Grad 2018). In the case of COVID-19 vaccines, rapidly waning immunity requires repeated shots, much like the yearly flu vaccine (Thompson and Cowling 2022). Effectiveness also varies across vaccines. For instance, two doses of the measles vaccine are about 97 percent effective against measles,[2] whereas the annual flu vaccine is typically less than 50 percent effective. The existing COVID-19 vaccines are very effective at preventing severe disease and death but less effective at preventing mild symptoms and infection (Eyre et al. 2022; Laake et al. 2022). However, even low-effectiveness vaccines are useful. For instance, the US Centers for Disease Control and Prevention estimated that, although only 36 percent effective,[3] the 2021–22 flu vaccine still prevented 1.9 million flu-related illnesses, 26,000 hospitalizations, and 1,500 deaths.[4]

Vaccination has an indisputably positive impact on preventing morbidity and mortality from the targeted disease. Growing empirical research shows that vaccination also provides substantial broad health, social, and economic benefits (Bloom, Fan, and Sevilla 2018). For instance, vaccination can prevent nosocomial infections among hospitalized patients and effectively slow the development of antimicrobial resistance by decreasing the need for antimicrobial treatment (Schueller et al. 2021). Evidence also indicates that some vaccines protect against off-target pathogens; for example, measles vaccination can protect against the loss of acquired immune memory triggered by measles infection (Mina et al. 2019). By improving individuals' health, vaccination also confers sizable socioeconomic benefits. For example, vaccinated adults tend to have higher employment rates and larger earnings than their unvaccinated counterparts (Atwood 2022; Sevilla et al. 2020). Vaccinated children tend to perform better at school and have higher educational attainment (Nandi et al. 2020) and more developed cognitive abilities (Bloom, Canning, and Shenoy 2011). Vaccination protects against catastrophic health care expenditures and the risk of falling into poverty, especially in countries without universal health care (Bloom, Khoury, and Subbaraman 2018), and it reduces the fiscal costs (such as disability subsidies and government assistance for catastrophic medical expenditures) imposed by infectious diseases (Connolly and Kotsopoulos 2020).

The experience with the COVID-19 pandemic highlighted in stark terms the broad benefits of vaccination. Mass COVID-19 vaccination protected the population from the risk of severe health outcomes and death, reduced the pressure on overburdened health care systems, allowed countries to relax the costly nonpharmaceutical interventions (such as social distancing norms, masking, and school and business lockdowns) implemented to control the spread of infections, and revitalized global supply chains (Bloom, Cadarette, and Ferranna 2021).

### Benefits of Accelerated Vaccine Development: A Simulation Exercise

Vaccine development, testing, and manufacturing typically involve a lengthy process. Although COVID-19 vaccines arrived in the market less than one year from the identification of the genetic sequence of the virus, the typical process lasts more than a decade. Several innovations allowed the accelerated development of COVID-19 vaccines, including the use of mRNA technologies that allow fast production, large-scale investment in manufacturing capacity while clinical trials were still ongoing, parallel execution of clinical trial phases, and massive public financial support (Bloom et al. 2021). In preparation for the next pandemic, establishing an infrastructure that will allow fast development, production, and distribution of vaccines is thus essential. The Coalition for Epidemic Preparedness Innovations recently advanced the idea of "100-days vaccines"; that is, countries, pharmaceutical companies, and international donors should aim at vaccine development and large-scale manufacturing within 100 days of the identification of the pathogen responsible for the next pandemic (Saville et al. 2022). Such a strategy requires, among other things, developing a full portfolio of vaccines against pathogens with pandemic potential long before the next pandemic strikes, expanding manufacturing capacity, establishing infrastructures for quickly testing new vaccines at large scale, stockpiling raw materials for vaccine production, and investing in early detection systems globally.

Accelerating the development and manufacturing of vaccines against pathogens with pandemic potential may prevent an outbreak from turning into a pandemic and may shorten the length of a pandemic. A simulation exercise based on the model event catalog described in chapter 2 of this volume illustrates the potential benefits of faster vaccine availability. The catalog was constructed by simulating hundreds of thousands of epidemics caused by respiratory diseases (pandemic influenza and novel/epidemic coronavirus diseases). The simulated events differ in terms of country of origin of the outbreak, efficacy of nonpharmaceutical interventions to control disease transmission, and epidemiological characteristics of the disease (for example, transmissibility, case-fatality ratio, and incubation period). The events were generated using a stochastic, disease-specific, global, metapopulation compartmental model that simulates the daily spatiotemporal progression of disease spread. The model accounts, among other things, for demographics, contact patterns among countries, risk of case underreporting, and differences in preparedness across countries (refer to chapter 2 for further details about the methods).

From the respiratory pathogen model event catalog presented in chapter 2, two pandemic scenarios are considered. For each pandemic scenario, the simulation considers different assumptions concerning the availability and global distribution of vaccines and projects the number of expected deaths in each scenario and for each vaccination assumption. It then determines the overall benefits of vaccination (in 2022 international dollar terms) for each pandemic scenario.

The two pandemic scenarios differ in terms of country of origin of the outbreak and severity of the disease. The country of origin affects the detection threshold (that is, how soon detection of the outbreak occurs) to account for differences in detection capacity and infrastructure across countries (Oppenheim et al. 2019). In both scenarios, nonpharmaceutical interventions begin 30 days after detection in the spark country and 60 days after detection elsewhere. In the absence of vaccination, Pandemic Scenario 1 results in about 38.1 million deaths globally, whereas Pandemic Scenario 2 leads to 145.5 million deaths (table 9.1). Table 9A.1 in annex 9A summarizes the main assumptions underlying the two scenarios.

**Table 9.1** Benefits of Accelerating Vaccine Development

| | Number of deaths | Mortality loss (2022 international $, trillion) | Short-term output loss (2022 international $, trillion) | Total loss (2022 international $, trillion) |
|---|---|---|---|---|
| *Pandemic Scenario 1* | | | | |
| No vaccines | 38,100,000 | 49.7 | 5.1 | 54.8 |
| Vaccines developed in one year (Assumption A) | 12,300,000 | 16.1 | 3.0 | 19.1 |
| Vaccines developed in 100 days (Assumption B) | 387,000 | 0.5 | 0.6 | 1.1 |
| Vaccines developed in 100 days and distributed fairly (Assumption C) | 384,000 | 0.5 | 0.6 | 1.1 |
| *Pandemic Scenario 2* | | | | |
| No vaccines | 145,500,000 | 190.0 | 9.4 | 199.4 |
| Vaccines developed in one year (Assumption A) | 83,400,000 | 108.9 | 7.3 | 116.2 |
| Vaccines developed in 100 days (Assumption B) | 4,500,000 | 5.9 | 1.9 | 7.8 |
| Vaccines developed in 100 days and distributed fairly (Assumption C) | 3,700,000 | 4.8 | 1.7 | 6.5 |

*Source:* Original table compiled for this publication.

Each pandemic scenario considers three assumptions about vaccination. Vaccination Assumption A imagines that vaccines will be available for deployment about one year after the detection of the outbreak (similar to the COVID-19 pandemic). Vaccination Assumption B imagines that vaccines are developed and deployed at accelerated speed (deployment for emergency use 100 days after detection and deployment at scale 140 days after detection). Vaccination Assumption C imagines that vaccines are developed at accelerated speed as in Assumption B; however, unlike Assumption B, vaccines are distributed fairly across countries (proportionally to their population). The vaccine is assumed to be 80 percent effective at preventing both infections and deaths. In Assumptions A and B, vaccination coverage and speed of delivery vary across countries based on their preparedness capacity but are equal across countries in Assumption C. Table 9A.2 in annex 9A reproduces the vaccination assumptions. Figures 9B.1–9B.4 in annex 9B display the weekly number of deaths in the two pandemic scenarios, depending on the vaccination assumptions.

Table 9.1 summarizes the results of the exercise. Compared with the no-vaccination case, the development and deployment of a vaccine in a year (Assumption A) prevent about 25.8 million deaths globally in Pandemic Scenario 1 and 62.1 million deaths in Pandemic Scenario 2. Accelerated development of vaccines in 100 days from detection (Assumption B) leads to more than 37 million deaths averted in Pandemic Scenario 1 (or 99 percent of the death toll) and 141.0 million deaths averted in Pandemic Scenario 2 (or 97 percent of the death toll). Compared with

Assumption B, accelerated development and fairer distribution of vaccines (Assumption C) saves 3,000 additional lives in Pandemic Scenario 1 and 800,000 additional lives in Pandemic Scenario 2.

To quantify the total benefits of vaccination, a measure of pandemic loss is considered that includes the loss of life and the short-term loss of economic output. For a pandemic that causes $D$ deaths, the following expression gives total loss:

$$L = VSL * D + Y * \Delta(D)$$

The first term represents the monetary equivalent of the number of deaths, and the second term represents the reduction in global GDP caused by a pandemic that kills $D$ people, where $Y$ represents global GDP and $\Delta(D)$ is the percentage reduction in GDP as a function of the number of deaths.

The monetary equivalent of the number of deaths is found by multiplying the number of deaths by a global value per statistical life (VSL). The computations use a VSL of $1.3 million (2022 international dollars). This value is extrapolated starting from a VSL of $10 million for the United States and assuming an income elasticity of 1.5 (refer to annex 9C for further details) (Robinson, Hammitt, and O'Keeffe 2019). Such a value for a global VSL is also consistent with recent estimates by Ahuja et al. (2021) and Sweis (2022) and represents a conservative estimate of the value of saving a life.

The expression for the percentage output loss caused by the pandemic, $\Delta(D)$, is derived from Glennerster, Snyder, and Tan (2023), who estimate the relationship between annual output loss and pandemic severity using selected pandemic events in the last century (the 1918 flu pandemic, the SARS outbreak in 2002–03, Ebola in 2013–16, the Zika outbreak in 2015–17, and the COVID-19 pandemic). Note that this measure of economic loss captures only short-term output losses and not the potential impacts of a pandemic on economic growth or human capital accumulation. Annex 9C includes more details on the calibration.

Compared with the no-vaccination scenario, the availability of vaccines one year after the beginning of the pandemic (Assumption A) saves $35.7 trillion in Pandemic Scenario 1 ($54.8 trillion minus $19.1 trillion), which corresponds to 65 percent of the total pandemic burden. However, developing vaccines in 100 days (Assumption B) would save $53.7 trillion ($54.8 trillion minus $1.1 trillion), or 98 percent of the total burden in the absence of vaccination. The benefits of vaccination in Pandemic Scenario 2 are even more pronounced in absolute terms. The benefits of starting vaccination after one year amount to $83.2 trillion ($199.4 trillion minus $116.2 trillion), or 42 percent of the total burden, whereas accelerated vaccine development leads to $191.6 trillion in savings ($199.4 trillion minus $7.8 trillion), or 96 percent of the total burden. In each pandemic scenario, most of the benefits stem from mortality reductions. If vaccines are developed at an accelerated pace and distributed fairly across countries (Assumption C), the total burden decreases by $53.7 trillion in Pandemic Scenario 1 and by $192.9 trillion in Pandemic Scenario 2.

Table 9.1 illustrates the global benefits of accelerated vaccine development. The annexes include additional results on the distribution of the vaccination benefits by geographies (tables 9B.1, 9B.2, 9C.1, and 9C.2). Annex 9C also reports results using different values of the income elasticity of the VSL and different extrapolation methods (tables 9C.3 and 9C.4). Compared with these alternatives, the chosen VSL estimate of $1.3 million leads to a conservative assessment of the overall benefits of vaccination.

The simulation exercise illustrates the sizable benefits of accelerating vaccine development and deployment. The exercise considered two potential pandemic scenarios for illustration purposes. Both pandemic scenarios led to staggering numbers of deaths in the absence of fast vaccination. The probability of those pandemics is not negligible. Under nonaccelerated vaccine development (Assumption A), the two pandemic scenarios correspond to 4 percent (Pandemic Scenario 1) and 1 percent (Pandemic Scenario 2) of the exceedance probability function derived in chapter 2. Thus, there is a 4 percent yearly probability of a pandemic that will cause at least 12.3 million deaths and a 1 percent annual probability of a pandemic that will cause at least 83.4 million deaths. The estimates here indicate that accelerated vaccine development substantially curtails mortality and associated economic losses. A more comprehensive analysis would require estimating the impact of accelerated vaccine development on the entire exceedance probability function: If we invested in pandemic preparedness interventions such that developing and deploying vaccines in 100 days from the beginning of the next pandemic were possible, what would the expected returns of such an investment be?

As with any modeling effort, the scenario analysis is subject to necessary assumptions, limitations, and uncertainty. First, the scenarios are only two illustrative scenarios and do not encompass all plausible scenarios. Second, because the scenarios presented here are for illustration purposes, they are deterministic scenarios that do not include stochastic variation, and uncertainty estimates were not calculated. Third, model parameterization may reflect gaps and biases in historical data. Fourth, additional factors besides those included in the scenarios could affect the availability and effectiveness of vaccines in a future pandemic. Chapter 2 further discusses limitations. The estimation of the output loss caused by pandemics is based on a previous study that uses regression analysis to determine the association between pandemic deaths and output loss (Glennerster, Snyder, and Tan 2023). Although the small sample size (five historic pandemic events) jeopardizes the reliability of the estimates, better studies are lacking.

The exercise sheds new light on the relationship between vaccine inequity and mortality. It finds, for example, that developing and distributing vaccines sufficiently quickly can blunt the damaging effects of inequitable access to vaccines. The incremental benefits of equal vaccine distribution are relatively small compared with the benefits of accelerated development despite unequal global distribution of vaccines (Assumption C versus Assumption B) because, even if lower-income countries are not prioritized in the allocation of vaccines, the accelerated timeline implies that they would likely receive the vaccines much sooner than under nonaccelerated vaccine development. This result underlines the importance of absolute improvements in vaccine development, production, and delivery timelines but does not obviate the ethical imperative of equity in vaccine access (refer to the next section). Clearly, however, this result will not hold if vaccines are developed at typical speed.

The benefits of accelerated vaccine development are indisputable. The issue now is whether such a strategy is feasible and affordable. Uncertainty about the pathogen responsible for the next pandemic requires a large portfolio of investments, including developing multiple vaccines for pathogens with pandemic potential, expanding manufacturing capacity by developing infrastructure that can be easily adjusted to new threats, and improving surveillance systems around the world (Athey et al. 2022). Glennerster, Snyder, and Tan (2023) estimate that a feasible program to expand manufacturing capacity would cost $60 billion up front and $5 billion annually (in 2021 US dollars); the program would ensure capacity to vaccinate 70 percent of the global population in six months. The estimated costs of Operation Warp Speed (the US program to invest in the development and manufacturing of COVID-19 vaccines) amount to $18 billion (Baker and Koons 2020). Historically, the development of a single vaccine, inclusive of failures, costs roughly $1 billion (Plotkin et al. 2017). Although none of these figures represent the full cost of investing in accelerated vaccine development, they suggest that the associated benefits far outweigh the costs.

## VACCINE EQUITY

This section discusses the health, social, and economic costs of global vaccine inequity and the main factors contributing to vaccine inequity.

### Definition and Costs of Global Vaccine Inequity

Mechanisms to foster global vaccine equity are a critical component of pandemic preparedness. Inequitable access to vaccines during a pandemic is costly for countries negatively affected by such inequity and may produce negative global health and economic externalities (Ferranna 2024). As World Health Organization (WHO) Director General Dr. Tedros Adhanom Ghebreyesus said about the COVID-19 pandemic, "The first priority must be to vaccinate some people in all the countries, rather than all the people in some countries" (WHO 2020).

Slow and delayed vaccine rollout leaves countries exposed to high preventable mortality and morbidity risks and to the resulting economic slowdown. For example, in the case of COVID-19, vaccine hoarding by higher-income countries cost more than an estimated 1 million lives in 2021 compared with an alternate scenario in which COVID-19 vaccines were distributed proportionally to the size of the adult population (Moore et al. 2022). Those preventable deaths occurred mostly in low- and middle-income countries. If countries implement costly nonpharmaceutical interventions (such as economic lockdowns, stay-at-home orders, and school closures) to control the spread of infections while waiting for the arrival of vaccines, slow and delayed vaccine rollout means that the population has to endure longer periods of costly containment measures, with resulting negative impacts on consumption spending and GDP (Hansen and Mano 2023). Longer periods of lockdown also translate into higher incidence of mental health problems (Adams-Prassi et al. 2022) and in larger degradation of human capital (Buffie et al. 2023). Even short schooling disruptions can lead to significant learning losses, especially in lower-income settings (Patrinos, Vegas, and Carter-Rau 2023). Slow vaccine rollout during a pandemic increases the risk of school closures, further widening the learning gap between rich and poor countries and compromising the economic future of the latter.

Moreover, enhancing global access to vaccines benefits the whole world. If the vaccine can reduce the risk of disease transmission, increasing vaccination rates in poorer countries reduces the risk of imported infections in higher-income countries, prevents the emergence of new virus variants, and reduces the costs of surveillance (Wagner et al. 2021). Furthermore, equitable access to vaccines reduces the risk of global supply chain disruptions. In particular, prolonged economic lockdowns in lower-income countries may cause shortages of intermediate inputs, higher import prices, and weaker demand for exports of higher-income countries (Çakmaklı et al. 2022; Hafner et al. 2022).

Before discussing barriers to global vaccine equity and possible solutions, providing a more precise definition of global vaccine equity is worthwhile. The United Nations defines global vaccine equity as a situation in which vaccines are "allocated across countries based on needs and regardless of their economic status."[5] Global vaccine equity does not necessarily imply global vaccine equality (that is, the same proportion of people vaccinated in all countries) because countries may have different needs. However, global vaccine equity does imply that countries' ability to pay for vaccines should not affect the global vaccine allocation. For example, if an Ebola outbreak is detected in country X but not in country Y, people in country X have a more urgent need for vaccine doses than people in country Y, and an equitable allocation of Ebola vaccines would require prioritizing country X, regardless of its economic status.

Defining global vaccine equity during a pandemic requires weighing the urgency of needs of different countries and ensuring that vaccine availability across countries matches their needs. Because of the broad health, social, and economic benefits of vaccination, urgency of needs may be evaluated across different dimensions. The first dimension is the expected health burden in the absence of vaccination and the effectiveness of vaccines at reducing it. It includes, for example, the expected numbers of infections, hospitalizations, and pandemic pathogen–related deaths averted by vaccination. If the only concern is to minimize the pandemic health burden, then countries that are predicted to bear the brunt of pandemic morbidity and mortality in the absence of vaccination should have prioritized vaccine access. The geographic distribution of vaccination's expected health benefits is pandemic-specific and depends, among other things, on the characteristics of the pandemic pathogen (for example, the age gradient of mortality risk), the characteristics of the population (for example, the age pyramid), the pandemic transmission patterns (for example, where the outbreak started), the characteristics of the vaccine, and countries' capacity to effectively scale vaccine delivery to the population. Note, however, that we can also consider a broader concept of vaccination's expected health benefits, one that includes not only pandemic pathogen–related deaths and cases but also all-cause mortality and morbidity. For example, the COVID-19 pandemic disrupted routine immunization systems and other health care services. Countries with less resilient health care systems may thus expect a larger overall health burden from a pandemic, all things considered.

The expected social and economic burden in the absence of vaccination is another dimension to consider in evaluating the urgency of needs. The COVID-19 pandemic showed that—because of, for example, labor shortages, economic lockdowns enforced to control the pandemic, and supply chain interruptions—economic disruptions accompany surges of infections and deaths. Overall, by the end of 2021, the COVID-19 pandemic had increased the global poverty rate from 7.8 percent to an estimated 9.1 percent (Mahler, Yonzan, and Lakner 2022). That increase corresponds to 97 million more people living on less than US$1.90 a day because of the pandemic. In addition to income losses, pandemics disrupt the education system. Students in countries with poor online learning infrastructure are thus more exposed to pandemic-induced educational losses. Countries with fewer resources for education or welfare programs (for example, unemployment subsidies) are more likely to bear the social and economic brunt of the pandemic and thus may have a larger claim for prioritized vaccine access.

In defining the equitable global allocation of vaccines, at least two other issues are important to consider: the ability of the vaccine to reduce the transmission risk and the dynamic nature of the problem. The former may call for prioritizing populations that are more likely to infect the rest of the world because of patterns of economic and social interactions. The latter may call for prioritizing populations that have not yet experienced the pandemic burden but may do so in the future (for example, country X has no Ebola outbreak but, because of commercial patterns, is very likely to import the disease from other countries).

A key aspect of pandemic preparedness is establishing guidelines for the equitable allocation of scarce vaccine supplies across countries. Some contributions have proposed frameworks to guide the distribution of vaccines and to judge their reliance on principles of fairness. For COVID-19, a noteworthy proposal is the "fair priority model," which envisions three phases of vaccine allocation, with the goals of reducing premature deaths, reducing serious economic and social deprivation, and reducing community transmission (Emanuel et al. 2020).

**Barriers to Vaccine Equity**

Several factors may contribute to slow and delayed vaccine rollout in some countries. Vaccine supply shortages constitute one of the main barriers to equitable vaccine distribution. WHO's estimates suggest that between 2011 and 2015 one-third of 194 countries ran out of a vaccine for a month or longer (Garrett 2018), mainly because of the limited number of manufacturers able to produce some vaccines (Cernuschi et al. 2022). Recent shortages of products such as human papillomavirus vaccines, Bacillus Calmette-Guérin vaccines, and inactivated polio vaccines point to the constraints in existing manufacturing capacity (du Preez et al. 2019; Garland et al. 2020; Sutter and Zaffran 2019).

Vaccine supply shortages have significant public health consequences. For example, the 2016 yellow fever epidemic in Angola strained the global vaccine supply, prompting WHO to recommend fractional dosing (Wu et al. 2016). Lack of sufficient vaccine supply was partly responsible for the measles outbreak in 2016–17 in Romania (Dascalu 2019). At the beginning of the COVID-19 vaccination campaign, global supply constraints forced countries to set rules to identify the subpopulations to prioritize in allocating vaccine doses within national borders (Ferranna, Cadarette, and Bloom 2021). Countries also implemented dose-sparing strategies—such as the United Kingdom's decision to delay the administration of the second shot of the Oxford-AstraZeneca vaccine to partially protect as many people as possible (Imai et al. 2023). At the global level, vaccine supply constraints meant that lower-income countries started administering vaccine doses several months after higher-income countries.

Vaccine nationalism—that is, the stockpiling of vaccines by high-income countries—has been a major issue since the early phases of COVID-19 vaccine distribution (and was also an issue in the 2009 influenza pandemic). Facing a limited global supply of COVID-19 vaccines and uncertain future needs, countries with manufacturing capacity and other high-income countries prioritized the health of their own people rather than reducing the burden of COVID-19 globally (Katz et al. 2021). Emblematic is the case of Canada, which reserved enough doses to immunize its population six times over (Twohey, Collins, and Thomas 2020). Absent a globally coordinated approach to vaccine allocation, vaccine nationalism will likely be an issue for the next pandemic also.

Unequal global distribution of manufacturing capacity contributes to unequal global access to vaccines (Dzau, Balatbat, and Offodile 2022). With few exceptions (such as the Serum Institute of India), low- and middle-income countries do not maintain substantial manufacturing capacity, must rely on international vaccine supplies, and face the risk and consequences of vaccine-hoarding behaviors (Mukherjee, Kalra, and Phelan 2023). According to WHO (2023), only 10 manufacturers cover 71 percent of the global demand for vaccines. Despite manufacturers' reluctance to provide technology transfers, efforts to enhance global manufacturing capacity are under way. One example is the WHO-supported mRNA vaccine technology hub at Afrigen Biologics and Vaccines (South Africa), which reverse-engineered the Moderna COVID-19 mRNA vaccine in 2022 (Maxmen 2022). The hub's ultimate goal is to build up technological know-how it can apply to other pathogens, including tuberculosis, malaria, and human immunodeficiency virus (HIV) (Bisbas 2023). Transferring fill-and-finish operations of established commercial vaccines to factories in low- and middle-income countries is a pragmatic way to localize manufacturing (Thompson et al. 2023). Other proposals focus on establishing new vaccine production facilities strategically located in "less populous countries with good scientific and training infrastructure, a respect for legal contracts, and a reputation for fair play" (Jha et al. 2021). This production capacity would be export-oriented, and countries housing it would have, by virtue of their small population size, no need to hoard doses for domestic use.

Constraints in health care system capacities further undermine vaccine equity. For example, COVID-19 vaccines based on mRNA technologies require ultra-cold chains, but maintaining ultra-cold chains is difficult in rural areas with unstable electricity supply (Fahrni et al. 2022). Given the seemingly large role that mRNA technologies will play in the future, solving the ultra-cold chain issue is a priority to enhance vaccine equity. Shortages in equipment such as syringes could also threaten vaccination efforts during the next pandemics, especially in lower-income countries (Fritz et al. 2022). The COVID-19 pandemic also highlighted the fundamental role of health care workers in increasing trust and ensuring efficient delivery of vaccines (Ballard et al. 2020). Enabling that role requires constant resources for training and technical support of the health workforce.

Finally, lack of confidence in the government, in the health care system, or in the effectiveness and safety of vaccines can undermine vaccination uptake. Evidence suggests that overall vaccine confidence was decreasing before the COVID-19 pandemic (de Figueiredo et al. 2020), and the COVID-19 pandemic may have exacerbated the lack of vaccine confidence in some populations, despite the successes with the vaccines (Lazarus et al. 2023). Strategies to promote vaccine uptake need to be tailored to the root causes of hesitancy in the various populations. These strategies may include implementing informational campaigns to combat misinformation about the safety and effectiveness of vaccines, such as through the use of personal narratives that emphasize the benefits of vaccination; engaging locally trusted persons, like village elders, to boost confidence; facilitating access to vaccines, for example, with mobile clinics; and providing incentives in the form of cash, prizes, or health insurance premium discounts (Bennett, Bloom, and Ferranna 2022). Countries have also employed vaccine mandates to increase vaccine uptake. For example, school-entry mandates (such as for measles and pertussis) have been effective in improving uptake of childhood vaccines (Lee and Robinson 2016). COVID-19 vaccination mandates spurred vaccine uptake in the countries that implemented them broadly (Karaivanov et al. 2022).

## CONCLUSIONS

The chapter discusses the fundamental role of vaccination in preventing and mitigating future pandemics in light of the COVID-19 experience. The analysis yields several lessons. First, accelerating the global availability of vaccines is key for containing the negative health, social, and economic effects of pandemics. Despite the historically unprecedented pace of COVID-19 vaccine development, one year elapsed between the identification of the virus and the start of the vaccination campaign, and many countries around the world could vaccinate sizable portions of their population only several months later. Accelerated vaccine development, manufacturing, and deployment require, among other things, moving vaccine research and development (R&D) to prepandemic periods as much as possible, for example, by conducting phases 1 and 2 of clinical trials of a large number of vaccines with pandemic potential as the Coalition for Epidemic Preparedness Innovations suggests in its "100-day vaccines" program; investing in manufacturing capacity to quickly produce vaccines once they are developed; strengthening surveillance systems around the world, especially in emergency settings (for example, in countries with conflicts or following natural disasters); and strengthening health care systems for rapid deployment of vaccines.

Collective financing of vaccine R&D and manufacturing capacity can encourage investments in accelerated development and deployment of vaccines (Athey et al. 2022). Vaccines constitute a high-cost, high-risk investment. The process of vaccine R&D, manufacturing, and delivery carries substantial risk of failure, for example, because the product is not as safe or effective as expected, because of competition from other vaccines or therapeutics, or because of growing vaccine hesitancy undermining the demand for vaccines. Cost-sharing across public and private sectors can partially absorb the risk of vaccine development, thereby enhancing pharmaceutical companies' incentives to invest in vaccines. Financing issues have particular relevance for diseases that affect mostly lower-income countries (such as Ebola and Zika) and for which demand is not driven by those with high ability and willingness to pay. Different mechanisms can be used to de-risk vaccine investments, including direct public funding of R&D and manufacturing, advance purchase agreements, bonuses for speed, and social bonds.

Another important lesson from the COVID-19 pandemic concerns the costs of inequitable global allocation of vaccines. Vaccine inequity leaves (mostly) lower-income countries exposed to preventable health, social, and economic burdens caused by pandemics. Global vaccine equity also creates positive externalities. Vaccine equity reduces the risk of vaccine-escape variants and prevents disruptions to global supply chains, thereby yielding benefits for all countries. Protocols to foster fair allocation of vaccines across countries should address barriers on both the supply side (for example, logistical and manufacturing constraints and property rights) and the demand side (for example, vaccine hesitancy). Reinforcing existing health care systems in lower-income settings is also essential to reduce the burden of infectious diseases and accelerate the distribution of vaccines and other health technologies. Developing manufacturing capacity in low- and middle-income countries can ensure a more equitable global distribution of vaccines, because lower-income countries will not have to rely on international donors or manufacturing countries for their vaccine supply. Fill-and-finish agreements for existing vaccines may offer a starting point for developing manufacturing capacity in lower-income countries. An enabling environment is also a strong prerequisite for boosting vaccine manufacturing and achieving vaccine equity. Ensuring such an environment will require, for example, investing in skilled workers—especially those with expertise in pharmaceuticals, chemistry, life sciences, biotechnology, and biochemistry—and boosting regulatory capacity to ensure effective and transparent validation, licensing, and quality assurance of vaccines.

Mitigating vaccine hesitancy is another essential ingredient for effective pandemic prevention and preparedness. Although only 65 percent of the global population completed the initial COVID-19 vaccine protocol, COVID-19 vaccine uptake was overall successful. However, vaccine confidence seems to have declined since the onset of the pandemic (Siani and Tranter 2022; UNICEF 2023). The value of investing in vaccination and the benefits of accelerated vaccine development depend on the demand for those vaccines, underscoring the importance of spending resources to encourage vaccine uptake, such as through targeted, culturally sensitive communication; price mechanisms (vaccine subsidy and elevated insurance prices and deductibles); and nonpecuniary interventions (for example, employer mandates).

Finally, the COVID-19 pandemic shed light on the broad health, social, and economic benefits of vaccination. An accurate appraisal of the overall value of vaccination should include all those benefits. However, traditional evaluation methods of vaccination rely on a narrow set of health-related outcomes (such as deaths and cases averted, or health care cost savings), resulting in an undervaluation of the benefits of vaccination. This undervaluation implies that vaccination programs are often underfunded compared with other programs (Bloom, Cadarette, and Ferranna 2021). To encourage investments in accelerated development, manufacturing, and fair allocation of vaccines, economic evaluation techniques should be updated to incorporate the full value of vaccination.

## NOTES

1. World Health Organization, "WHO COVID-19 Dashboard," https://covid19.who.int/.
2. Centers for Disease Control and Prevention, "Measles Vaccination," https://www.cdc.gov/vaccines/vpd/mmr/public/index.html#what-is-mmr.
3. Centers for Disease Control and Prevention, "CDC Seasonal Flu Vaccine Effectiveness Studies," https://www.cdc.gov/flu-vaccines-work/php/effectiveness-studies/index.html.
4. Centers for Disease Control and Prevention, "Flu Burden Prevented from Vaccination 2021-2022 Flu Season," https://www.cdc.gov/flu-burden/php/data-vis-vac/2021-2022-prevented.html.
5. United Nations Development Programme, 2023, "Global Dashboard for Vaccine Equity," https://data.undp.org/vaccine-equity/.

# REFERENCES

Adams-Prassi, A., T. Boneva, M. Golin, and C. Rauh. 2022. "The Impact of the Coronavirus Lockdown on Mental Health: Evidence from the United States." *Economic Policy* 37 (109): 139–55. https://doi.org/10.1093/epolic/eiac002.

Ahuja, A., S. Athey, A. Baker, E. Budish, J. C. Castillo, R. Glennerster, S. D. Kominers, et al. 2021. "Preparing for a Pandemic: Accelerating Vaccine Availability." *AEA Papers and Proceedings* 111: 331–35. https://doi.org/10.1257/pandp.20211103.

Anderson, R. M., and R. M. May. 1985. "Vaccination and Herd Immunity to Infectious Diseases." *Nature* 318 (6044): 323–29. https://doi.org/10.1038/318323a0.

Athey, S., J. C. Castillo, E. Chaudhuri, M. Kremer, A. Simoes Gomes, and C. M. Snyder. 2022. "Expanding Capacity for Vaccines against Covid-19 and Future Pandemics: A Review of Economic Issues." *Oxford Review of Economic Policy* 38 (4): 742–70. https://doi.org/10.1093/oxrep/grac037.

Atwood, A. 2022. "The Long-Term Effects of Measles Vaccination on Earnings and Employment." *American Economic Journal: Economic Policy* 14: 34–60. https://doi.org/10.1257/pol.20190509.

Baker, S., and C. Koons. 2020. "Inside Operation Warp Speed's $18 Billion Sprint for a Vaccine." *Bloomberg*, October 29, 2020. https://www.bloomberg.com/news/features/2020-10-29/inside-operation-warp-speed-s-18-billion-sprint-for-a-vaccine.

Ballard, M., E. Bancroft, J. Nesbit, A. Johnson, I. Holeman, J. Foth, D. Rogers, et al. 2020. "Prioritising the Role of Community Health Workers in the COVID-19 Response." *BMJ Global Health* 5 (6): e002550. https://doi.org/10.1136/bmjgh-2020-002550.

Bennett, N. G., D. E. Bloom, and M. Ferranna. 2022. "Factors Underlying COVID-19 Vaccine and Booster Hesitancy and Refusal, and Incentivizing Vaccine Adoption." *PLOS One* 17 (9): e0274529. https://doi.org/10.1371/journal.pone.0274529.

Betthäuser, B. A., A. M. Bach-Mortensen, and P. Engzell. 2023. "A Systematic Review and Meta-Analysis of the Evidence on Learning during the COVID-19 Pandemic." *Nature Human Behavior* 7: 375–85. https://doi.org/10.1038/s41562-022-01506-4.

Bisbas, G. 2023. "mRNA Technology Transfer Programme." *The Lancet Microbe* 4 (8): E578. https://doi.org/10.1016/S2666-5247(23)00183-0.

Bloom, D. E., D. Cadarette, and M. Ferranna. 2021. "The Societal Value of Vaccination in the Age of COVID-19." *American Journal of Public Health* 111 (6): 1049–54. https://doi.org/10.2105/AJPH.2020.306114.

Bloom, D. E., D. Cadarette, M. Ferranna, R. N. Hyer, and D. L. Tortorice. 2021. "How New Models of Vaccine Development for COVID-19 Have Helped Address an Epic Public Health Crisis." *Health Affairs* 40 (3): 410–18. https://doi.org/10.1377/hlthaff.2020.02012.

Bloom, D. E., D. Canning, and E. S. Shenoy. 2011. "The Effect of Vaccination on Children's Physical and Cognitive Development in the Philippines." *Applied Economics* 44 (21): 2777–83. https://doi.org/10.1080/00036846.2011.566203.

Bloom, D. E., V. Y. Fan, and J. P. Sevilla. 2018. "The Broad Socioeconomic Benefits of Vaccination." *Science Translational Medicine* 10 (441): eaaj2345. https://doi.org/10.1136/scitranslmed.aaj2345.

Bloom, D. E., A. Khoury, and R. Subbaraman. 2018. "The Promise and Peril of Universal Health Care." *Science* 361 (6404): eaat9644. https://doi.org/10.1126/science.aat9644.

Buffie, E. F., C. Adam, L.-F. Zanna, and K. Kpodar. 2023. "Loss-of-Learning and the Post-COVID Recovery in Low-Income Countries." *Journal of Macroeconomics* 75: 103492. https://doi.org/10.1016/j.jmacro.2022.103492.

Çakmaklı, C., S. Demiralp, S. Kalemli-Özcan, S. Yeşiltaş, and M. A. Yildirim. 2022. "The Economic Case for Global Vaccinations: An Epidemiological Model with International Production Networks." NBER Working Paper 28395, National Bureau of Economic Research, Cambridge, MA. https://doi.org/10.3386/w28395.

Carlson, C. J., R. Garnier, A. Tiu, S. P. Luby, and S. Bansal. 2024. "Strategic Vaccine Stockpiles for Regional Epidemics of Emerging Viruses: A Geospatial Modeling Framework." *Vaccine* 42 (23): 126051. https://doi.org/10.1016/j.vaccine.2024.06.019.

Cernuschi, T., S. Malvolti, S. Hall, L. Debruyne, H. B. Pedersen, H. Rees, and E. Cooke. 2022. "The Quest for More Effective Vaccine Markets—Opportunities, Challenges, and What Has Changed with the SARS-CoV-2 Pandemic." *Vaccine* 42 (Suppl. 1): S64–S72. https://doi.org/10.1016/j.vaccine.2022.07.032.

Cohen, J. 2019. "How Long Do Vaccines Last? The Surprising Answers May Help Protect People Longer." *Science* April 19, 2019. https://doi.org/10.1126/science.aax7364.

Connolly, M. P., and N. Kotsopoulos. 2020. "Estimating the Fiscal Consequences of National Immunization Programs Using a 'Government Perspective' Public Economic Framework." *Vaccines* 8 (3): 495. https://doi.org/10.3390/vaccines8030495.

Coulborn, R. M., M. Bastard, N. Peyraud, E. Gignoux, F. Luquero, B. Guai, S. H. Bateyi Mustafa, E. Mukamba Musenga, and S. Ahuka-Mundeke. 2024. "Case Fatality Risk among Individuals Vaccinated with rVSVΔG-ZEBOV-GP: A Retrospective Cohort Analysis of Patients with Confirmed Ebola Virus Disease in the Democratic Republic of the Congo." *The Lancet Infectious Diseases* 24 (6): 602–10. https://doi.org/10.1016/S1473-3099(23)00819-8.

Dascalu, S. 2019. "Measles Epidemics in Romania: Lessons for Public Health and Future Policy." *Frontiers in Public Health* 7: 98. https://doi.org/10.3389/fpubh.2019.00098.

de Figueiredo, A., C. Simas, E. Karafillakis, P. Paterson, and H. J. Larson. 2020. "Mapping Global Trends in Vaccine Confidence and Investigating Barriers to Vaccine Uptake: A Large-Scale Retrospective Temporal Modelling Study." *The Lancet* 396 (10255): 898–908. https://doi.org/10.1016/S0140-6736(20)31558-0.

du Preez, K., J. A. Seddon, H. S. Schaaf, A. C. Hesseling, J. R. Starke, M. Osman, C. J. Lombard, and R. Solomons. 2019. "Global Shortages of BCG Vaccine and Tuberculosis Meningitis in Children." *The Lancet Global Health* 7 (1): 28–29. https://doi.org/10.1016/S2214-109X(18)30474-1.

Dzau, V. J., C. A. Balatbat, and A. C. Offodile. 2022. "Closing the Global Vaccine Equity Gap: Equitably Distributed Manufacturing." *The Lancet* 399 (10339): 1924–26. https://doi.org/10.1016/S0140-6736(22)00793-0.

Economist. 2022. "The Pandemic's True Death Toll." October 25, 2022. https://www.economist.com/graphic-detail/coronavirus-excess-deaths-estimates. Simulator: https://github.com/TheEconomist/covid-19-the-economist-global-excess-deaths-model.

Emanuel, E. J., G. Persad, A. Kern, A. Buchanan, C. Fabre, D. Halliday, J. Heath, et al. 2020. "An Ethical Framework for Global Vaccine Allocation." *Science* 369 (6509): 1309–12. https://doi.org/10.1126/science.abe2803.

Eyre, D. W., D. Taylor, M. Purver, D. Chapman, T. Fowler, K. B. Pouwels, A. S. Walker, and T. E. A. Peto. 2022. "Effect of Covid-19 Vaccination on Transmission of Alpha and Delta Variants." *New England Journal of Medicine* 386: 744–56. https://doi.org/10.1056/NEJMoa2116597.

Fahrni, M. L., I. A.-N. Ismail, D. M. Refi, A. Almeman, N. C. Yaakob, K. M. Saman, N. F. Mansor, N. Noordin, and Z.-U.-D. Babar. 2022. "Management of COVID-19 Vaccines Cold Chain Logistics: A Scoping Review." *Journal of Pharmaceutical Policy and Practice* 15 (1): 16. https://doi.org/10.1186/s40545-022-00411-5.

Ferranna, M. 2024. "Causes and Costs of Global COVID-19 Vaccine Inequity." *Seminars in Immunopathology* 45 (4–6): 469–80. https://doi.org/10.1007/s00281-023-00998-0.

Ferranna, M., D. Cadarette, and D. E. Bloom. 2021. "COVID-19 Vaccine Allocation: Modeling Health Outcomes and Equity Implications of Alternative Strategies." *Engineering* 7 (7): 924–35. https://doi.org/10.1016/j.eng.2021.03.014.

Fritz, J., E. Griffin, R. Hammack, T. Herrick, and C. Jarrahian. 2022. "Syringes Must Be Prioritized Globally to Ensure Equitable Access to COVID-19 and Other Essential Vaccines and to Sustain Safe Injection Practices." *Human Vaccines & Immunotherapeutics* 18 (7): 2077580. https://doi.org/10.1080/21645515.2022.2077580.

Garland, S. M., M. A. Stanley, A. R. Giuliano, A.-B. Moscicki, A. Kaufmann, N. Bhatla, Y. L. Woo, and IPVS Policy Committee. 2020. "IPVS Statement on 'Temporary HPV

Vaccine Shortage: Implications Globally to Achieve Equity.'" *Papillomavirus Research* 9: 100195. https://doi.org/10.1016/j.pvr.2020.100195.

Garrett, L. 2018. "Inoculate against a Global Vaccine Crisis." *Foreign Policy*, January 16, 2018. https://foreignpolicy.com/2018/01/16/the-answers-are-out-there-natural-disasters-china -north-korea-corruption-economy/#health.

Glennerster, R., C. M. Snyder, and B. J. Tan. 2023. "Calculating the Costs and Benefits of Advance Preparations for Future Pandemics." *IMF Economic Review* 71: 611–48. https:// doi.org/10.1057/s41308-023-00212-z.

Hafner, M., E. Yerushalmi, C. Fays, E. Dufresne, and C. Van Stolk. 2022. "COVID-19 and the Cost of Vaccine Nationalism." *Rand Health Quarterly* 9 (4): 1.

Hansen, N.-J. H., and R. C. Mano. 2023. "COVID-19 Vaccines: A Shot in the Arm for the Economy." *IMF Economic Review* 71: 148 69. https://doi.org/10.1057/s41308-022-00184-6.

Imai, N., T. Rawson, E. S. Knock, R. Sonabend, Y. Elmaci, P. N. Perez-Guzman, L. K. Whittles, al. 2023. "Quantifying the Effect of Delaying the Second COVID-19 Vaccine Dose in England: A Mathematical Modelling Study." *The Lancet Public Health* 8 (3): 174–83. https://doi.org/10.1016/S2468-2667(22)00337-1.

IMF (International Monetary Fund). 2023. *World Economic Outlook Update: Near-Term Resilience, Persistent Challenges.* Washington, DC: IMF. https://www.imf.org/en /Publications/WEO/Issues/2023/07/10/world-economic-outlook-update-july-2023.

Jha, P., D. T. Jamison, D. A. Watkins, and J. Bell. 2021. "A Global Compact to Counter Vaccine Nationalism." *The Lancet* 397 (10289): 2046–47. https://doi.org/10.1016/S0140 -6736(21)01105-3.

Karaivanov, A., D. Kim, S. E. Lu, and H. Shigeoka. 2022. "COVID-19 Vaccination Mandates and Vaccine Uptake." *Nature Human Behavior* 6 (12): 1615–24. https://doi.org/10.1038 /s41562-022-01363-1.

Katz, I. T., R. Weintraub, L.-G. Bekker, and A. M. Brandt. 2021. "From Vaccine Nationalism to Vaccine Equity—Finding a Path Forward." *New England Journal of Medicine* 384 (14): 1281–83. https://doi.org/10.1056/NEJMp2103614.

Laake, I., S. N. Skodvin, K. Blix, I. H. Caspersen, H. K. Gjessing, L. K. Juvet, P. Magnus, et al. 2022. "Effectiveness of mRNA Booster Vaccination against Mild, Moderate, and Severe COVID-19 Caused by the Omicron Variant in a Large, Population-Based, Norwegian Cohort." *Journal of Infectious Diseases* 226 (11): 1924–33. https://doi.org/10.1093/infdis /jiac419.

Larson, H. J., E. Gakidou, and C. L. Murray. 2022. "The Vaccine-Hesitant Moment." *New England Journal of Medicine* 387: 58–65. https://doi.org/10.1056/NEJMra2106441.

Lazarus, J. V., K. Wyka, T. M. White, C. A. Picchio, L. O. Gostin, H. J. Larson, K. Rabin, et al. 2023. "A Survey of COVID-19 Vaccine Acceptance across 23 Countries in 2022." *Nature Medicine* 29 (2): 366–75. https://doi.org/10.1038/s41591-022-02185-4.

Lee, C., and J. L. Robinson. 2016. "Systematic Review of the Effect of Immunization Mandates on Uptake of Routine Childhood Immunizations." *Journal of Infection* 72 (6): 659–66. https://doi.org/10.1016/j.jinf.2016.04.002.

Lewnard, J. A., and Y. H. Grad. 2018. "Vaccine Waning and Mumps Re-Emergence in the United States." *Science Translational Medicine* 10 (433): eaao5945. https://doi.org/10.1126 .scitranslmed.aao5945.

Li, X., C. Mukandavire, Z. M. Cucunubá, S. Echeverria-Londono, K. Abbas, H. Clapham, M. Jit, et al. 2021. "Estimating the Health Impact of Vaccination against Ten Pathogens in 98 Low-Income and Middle-Income Countries from 2000 to 2030: A Modeling Study." *The Lancet* 397 (10272): 398–408. https://doi.org/10.1016/S0140 -6736(20)32657-X.

Mahler, D. G., N. Yonzan, and C. Lakner. 2022. "The Impact of COVID-19 on Global Inequality and Poverty." Policy Research Working Paper 10198. World Bank, Washington, DC. http://hdl.handle.net/10986/38114.

Mathieu, E., H. Ritchie, L. Rodés-Guirao, C. Appel, D. Gavrilov, C. Giattino, J. Hasell, et al. 2020. "Coronavirus Pandemic (COVID-19)." *Our World in Data*. https://ourworldindata.org/covid-vaccinations.

Maxmen, A. 2022. "South African Scientists Copy Moderna's COVID Vaccine." *Nature*, February 3, 2022. https://doi.org/10.1038/d41586-022-00293-2.

McGovern, M. E., and D. Canning. 2015. "Vaccination and All-Cause Child Mortality from 1985 to 2011: Global Evidence from the Demographic and Health Surveys." *American Journal of Epidemiology* 182 (9): 791–98. https://doi.org/10.1093/aje/kwv125.

Mina, M. J., T. Kula, Y. Leng, M. Li, R. D. de Vries, M. Knip, H. Siljander, et al. 2019. "Measles Virus Infection Diminishes Preexisting Antibodies That Offer Protection from Other Pathogens." *Science* 366 (6465): 599–606. https://doi.org/10.1126/science.aay6485.

Monath, T. P. 2013. "Vaccines against Diseases Transmitted from Animals to Humans: A One Health Paradigm." *Vaccine* 31 (46): 5321–38. https://doi.org/10.1016/j.vaccine.2013.09.029.

Moore, S., E. M. Hill, L. Dyson, M. J. Tildesley, and M. J. Keeling. 2022. "Retrospectively Modeling the Effects of Increased Global Vaccine Sharing on the COVID-19 Pandemic." *Nature Medicine* 28: 2416–23. https://doi.org/10.1038/s41591-022-02064-y.

Morens, D. M., G. K. Folkers, and A. S. Fauci. 2022. "The Concept of Classical Herd Immunity May Not Apply to COVID-19." *Journal of Infectious Diseases* 226: 195–98. https://doi.org/10.1093/infdis/jiac109.

Mukherjee, S., K. Kalra, and A. L. Phelan. 2023. "Expanding Global Vaccine Manufacturing Capacity: Strategic Prioritization in Small Countries." *PLOS Global Public Health* 3 (6): e0002098. https://doi.org/10.1371/journal.pgph.0002098.

Nandi, A., S. Kumar, A. Shet, D. E. Bloom, and R. Laxminarayan. 2020. "Childhood Vaccinations and Adult Schooling Attainment: Long-Term Evidence from India's Universal Immunization Programme." *Social Science and Medicine* 250: 112885. https://doi.org/10.1016/j.socscimed.2020.112885.

Oppenheim, B., M. Gallivan, N. K. Madhav, N. Brown, V. Serhiyenko, N. D. Wolfe, and P. Ayscue. 2019. "Assessing Global Preparedness for the Next Pandemic: Development and Application of an Epidemic Preparedness Index." *BMJ Global Health* 4 (1). https://doi.org/10.1136/bmjgh-2018-001157.

Pandey, A., and A. P. Galvani. 2023. "Exacerbation of Measles Mortality by Vaccine Hesitancy Worldwide." *The Lancet Global Health* 11 (4): E478–479. https://doi.org/10.1016/S2214-109X(23)00063-3.

Patrinos, H. A., E. Vegas, and R. Carter-Rau. 2023. "An Analysis of COVID-19 Student Learning Loss." *Economics and Finance*, August 23, 2023. https://doi.org/10.1093/acrefore/9780190625979.013.893.

Plans-Rubió, P. 2012. "Evaluation of the Establishment of Herd Immunity in the Population by Means of Serological Surveys and Vaccination Coverage." *Human Vaccines and Immunotherapeutics* 8 (2): 184–88. https://doi.org/10.4161/hv.18444.

Plotkin, S., J. M. Robinson, G. Cunningham, R. Iqbal, and S. Larsen. 2017. "The Complexity and Cost of Vaccine Manufacturing—An Overview." *Vaccine* 35 (33): 4064–71. https://doi.org/10.1016/j.vaccine.2017.06.003.

Robinson, L. A., J. K. Hammitt, and L. O'Keeffe. 2019. "Valuing Mortality Risk Reductions in Global Benefit-Cost Analysis." *Journal of Benefit-Cost Analysis* 10 (1): 15–50. https://doi.org/10.1017/bca.2018.26.

Saville, M., J. P. Cramer, M. Downham, A. Hacker, N. Lurie, L. Van der Veken, M. Whelan, and R. Hatchett. 2022. "Delivering Pandemic Vaccines in 100 Days—What Will It Take?" *New England Journal of Medicine* 387 (2): e3. https://doi.org/10.1056/NEJMp2202669.

Schueller, E., A. Nandi, J. Joshi, R. Laxminarayan, and E. Y. Klein. 2021. "Associations between Private Vaccine and Antimicrobial Consumption across Indian States, 2009–2017." *Annals of the New York Academy of Sciences* 1494 (1): 31–43. https://doi.org/10.1111/nyas.14571.

Sevilla, J. P., A. Stawasz, D. Burnes, A. Agarwal, B. Hacibedel, K. Helvacioglu, R. Sato, and D. E. Bloom. 2020. "Indirect Costs of Adult Pneumococcal Disease and the Productivity-Based Rate of Return to the 13-Valent Pneumococcal Conjugate Vaccine for Adults in Turkey." *Human Vaccines and Immunotherapeutics* 16 (8): 1923–36. https://doi.org/10.1080/21645515.2019.1708668.

Siani, A., and A. Tranter. 2022. "Is Vaccine Confidence an Unexpected Victim of the COVID-19 Pandemic?" *Vaccine* 40 (50): 7262–69. https://doi.org/10.1016/j.vaccine.2022.10.061.

Steele, M. K., A. Couture, C. Reed, D. Iuliano, M. Whitaker, H. Fast, A. J. Hall, et al. 2022. "Estimated Number of COVID-19 Infections, Hospitalizations, and Deaths Prevented among Vaccinated Persons in the US, December 2020 to September 2021." *JAMA Network Open* 5 (7): e2220385. https://doi.org/10.1001/jamanetworkopen.2022.20385.

Sutter, R. W., and M. Zaffran. 2019. "Addressing the Inactivated Poliovirus Vaccine Shortage." *The Lancet* 393 (10191): 2569–71. https://doi.org/10.1016/S0140-6736(19)30766-4.

Sweis, N. J. 2022. "Revisiting the Value of a Statistical Life: An International Approach during COVID-19." *Risk Management* 24: 259–72. https://doi.org/10.1057/s41283-022-00094-x.

Thompson, L. J. R., M. Grubo, M. Veller, R. H. Badenhorst, J. Nott, L. Debruyne, T. Makadzange, et al. 2023. "Building Global Vaccine Manufacturing Capacity: Spotlight on Africa." *Vaccine* 41 (27): 4050–56. https://doi.org/10.1016/j.vaccine.2023.05.009.

Thompson, M. G., and B. J. Cowling. 2022. "How Repeated Influenza Vaccination Effects Might Apply to COVID-19 Vaccines." *The Lancet Respiratory Medicine* 10 (7): 636–38. https://doi.org/10.1016/S2213-2600(22)00162-X.

Twohey, M., K. Collins, and K. Thomas. 2020. "With First Dibs on Vaccines, Rich Countries Have 'Cleared the Shelves.'" *New York Times*, December 15, 2020. https://www.nytimes.com/2020/12/15/us/coronavirus-vaccine-doses-reserved.html.

UN DESA (United Nations Department of Economic and Social Affairs). 2021. "World Economic Situation and Prospects as of Mid-2021." United Nations, New York. https://www.un.org/development/desa/dpad/publication/world-economic-situation-and-prospects-as-of-mid-2021/.

UNICEF (United Nations Children's Fund). 2023. *The State of World's Children 2023: For Every Child, Vaccination*. Florence: UNICEF Innocenti—Global Office of Research and Foresight. https://www.unicef.org/reports/state-worlds-children-2023#SOWC.

Wagner, C. E., C. M. Saad-Roy, S. E. Morris, R. E. Baker, M. J. Mina, J. Farrar, E. C. Holmes, et al. 2021. "Vaccine Nationalism and the Dynamics and Control of SARS-CoV-2." *Science* 373 (6562). https://doi.org/10.1126/science.abj7364.

Watson, O. J., G. Barnsley, J. Toor, A. B. Hogan, P. Winskill, and A. C. Ghani. 2022. "Global Impact of the First Year of COVID-19 Vaccination: A Mathematical Modelling Study." *The Lancet Infectious Diseases* 22 (9): 1293–302. https://doi.org/10.1016/S1473-3099(22)00320-6.

WHO (World Health Organization). 2020. "WHO Director-General's Opening Remarks at the Media Briefing on COVID-19." Speech, September 4, 2020. https://www.who.int/director-general/speeches/detail/who-director-general-s-opening-remarks-at-the-media-briefing-on-covid-19---4-september-2020.

WHO (World Health Organization). 2023. *Global Vaccine Market Report 2022: A Shared Understanding for Equitable Access to Vaccines*. Geneva: World Health Organization. https://www.who.int/publications/i/item/9789240062726.

Wouters, O. J., K. C. Shadlen, M. Salcher-Konrad, A. J. Pollard, H. J. Larson, Y. Teerawattananon, and M. Jit. 2021. "Challenges in Ensuring Global Access to COVID-19 Vaccines: Production, Affordability, Allocation, and Deployment." *The Lancet* 397 (10278): 1023–34. https://doi.org/10.1016/S0140-6736(21)00306-6.

Wu, J. T., C. M. Peak, G. M. Leung, and M. Lipsitch. 2016. "Fractional Dosing of Yellow Fever Vaccine to Extend Supply: A Modeling Study." *The Lancet* 388 (10062): 2904–11. https://doi.org/10.1016/S0140-6736(16)31838-4.

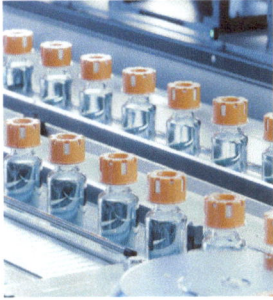

# 10

# Investing in Vaccines to Mitigate Harm from COVID-19 and Future Pandemics

Rachel Glennerster, Catherine Che, Sarrin Chethik, Claire T. McMahon, and
Christopher M. Snyder

## ABSTRACT

This chapter evaluates the social value of investing in vaccine research, development, and manufacturing capacity for pandemic preparedness and response. Rapid vaccination during pandemics can significantly reduce mortality, economic losses, and societal disruptions; however, vaccine manufacturers often lack sufficient incentives for speed and capacity expansion. Governments and international organizations can implement strategic policies to enhance these incentives and improve equitable vaccine distribution. In preparation for future pandemics, governments should make advance investments in vaccine manufacturing capacity as well as in research and development for vaccine prototypes and platforms. Investment to accelerate the research and development for a diverse portfolio of vaccine candidates and at-risk vaccine manufacturing capacity is likely to generate high returns during a pandemic.

## OVERVIEW

By December 2023, COVID-19 (coronavirus) had caused 27 million excess deaths[1] and trillions of dollars in economic output and human capital losses (Azevedo et al. 2021; Walmsley et al. 2023). Madhav et al. (2023) estimate that the world can expect three pandemics at least as severe as COVID-19 each century going forward, with less severe pandemics and regional epidemics occurring more frequently. Since the 1970s, in addition to COVID-19, we have experienced global pandemics due to HIV (human immunodeficiency virus), SARS (severe acute respiratory syndrome), and H1N1 (swine flu) as well as regional Ebola and Zika epidemics.

Vaccines are among the most effective medical countermeasures against pandemic harm. Vaccines protect against severe disease and, for some diseases, can block infection and transmission. Effective vaccines benefit society by reducing mortality and allowing economic activity to resume.

COVID-19 provided important lessons about the global ability to use vaccines as an effective pandemic countermeasure. COVID-19 vaccines were developed at an unprecedented speed thanks to decades of advances in vaccine science, coronavirus research, and mRNA technology development (Dolgin 2021). Supporting multiple vaccine candidates across a range of technologies provided valuable insurance against the risk that some failed. Supply shortages, however, slowed vaccine distribution and contributed to inequitable global access. Nine months after COVID-19 vaccines received regulatory approval, vaccination rates remained below 50 percent worldwide and 8 percent in Africa (Baker, Chaudhuri, and Kremer 2021), in no small part because of insufficient vaccine supply (Mobarak 2023). Such delays in vaccine rollout were responsible for substantial social harm in the form of continued high case counts, excess mortality, and economic losses (Duroseau, Kipshidze, and Limaye 2022). Preparing for future pandemics with advance investments and policies to accelerate vaccine availability can generate substantial social value and be highly cost-effective.

This chapter summarizes recent research on the expected losses from pandemics and the social value of investing in pandemic preparedness and response that can accelerate vaccine availability. It focuses specifically on vaccine research and development (R&D) and manufacturing capacity.

- **Vaccine R&D** encompasses any investments aimed at advancing scientific knowledge and technological capabilities to produce new vaccines, including new vaccines for particular pathogens or research on vaccine platforms (for example, mRNA vaccines). R&D investments can increase the probability of developing a successful vaccine and reduce the time from pathogen identification to authorization.
- **Vaccine capacity** refers to the infrastructure, resources, and processes required to produce and deliver vaccines at scale. Investments in capacity can increase the supply of vaccines, allowing for faster widespread deployment.

Within both domains, preparedness and response are linked. Prepandemic investment can increase the slate of available vaccine technologies, deepen understanding of the pathogen, improve supply chain resiliency, and expand available flexible manufacturing capacity—all of which influence the probability of successful vaccine candidates and accelerate their development and rollout when a pandemic hits.

This chapter discusses the case for investing in pandemic vaccines, but one could make a similar case for investing in other pandemic products, including therapeutics, diagnostics, masks, and health infrastructure. Therapeutics may offer broader efficacy than vaccines, making them potentially useful against a novel pathogen at the start of a pandemic (Karim, Lo, and Einav 2023). However, patients must know they are infected to ask for treatment, which limits the value of therapeutics against pathogens that can spread asymptomatically. Masks can reduce airborne disease transmission even with low compliance and quality. For instance, free surgical masks in Bangladeshi communities reduced symptomatic seroprevalence by over 11 percent (Abaluck et al. 2021). The chapter focuses on vaccines because a large literature supports their substantial benefits and because of the longer time required for development and scaling up manufacturing relative to other countermeasures, leaving more scope for acceleration.

Market and government "failures" have made firms' incentives to supply pandemic vaccines quite low compared to the vaccines' social value. Vaccination of one person benefits others by reducing transmission and helping keep their corner of the economy going, but that person is unlikely to be willing to pay for these broader benefits (refer to Goodkin-Gold et al. 2024 for a full analysis of vaccine externalities). Moreover, selling a treatment to a patient who has contracted a disease can be more lucrative than selling that person a preventive beforehand (Kremer and Snyder 2015). In these various ways, the market "fails" to reflect vaccines' full social value in suppliers' incentives. A pandemic may lead to government "failure," exerting political and social pressures that limit governments' ability to pay a lucrative price for vaccines (Athey et al. 2022). In 2022, COVID-19 vaccines sold for less than US$60 per course, orders of magnitude less than the estimated social value of US$6,200 (Castillo et al. 2021). "Profiting during a pandemic" may be viewed with repugnance (Roth 2007).

Given these constraints, incentivizing socially valuable vaccine investments requires carefully designed policies. This chapter analyzes a suite of such investments and funding options. The next section provides estimates of the enormous expected harm from future pandemics. Subsequent sections analyze the cost-effectiveness of investments in vaccine R&D and capacity, first focusing on prepandemic investments and then on in-pandemic investments.

## FUTURE HARM FROM PANDEMICS

The value of pandemic preparedness hinges on the expected harm from future pandemics to be mitigated. Estimating the expected harm from future pandemics requires forecasting (1) the arrival rate of pandemics of varying sizes and (2) the social harm caused by pandemics of varying sizes. The following subsections discuss each forecasting exercise in turn.

### Pandemic Frequency

Forecasting the arrival of pandemics is difficult because they are driven by highly nonlinear epidemiological forces. Moreover, the rarity of severe global pandemics means that data on such pandemics are sparse. The following surveyed approaches to forecasting expected global pandemic deaths provide a range of estimates, but even the low end is in the hundreds of thousands of lives annually.

One approach used in the literature focuses on a single pathogen—influenza—the most likely pathogen to cause a severe pandemic (Madhav et al. 2023). Forecasting pandemics for influenza is facilitated by the recurrent pattern of outbreaks, which has remained fairly constant over the past 300 years for this pathogen (Potter 2001). Whereas antibiotics successfully curtailed bacterial pandemics, no medical breakthrough has as sharply reduced the risk of future influenza outbreaks. Using historical data on global influenza epidemics since 1700, Fan, Jamison, and Summers (2018) estimate that epidemic influenza will cause 720,000 annual deaths.

A drawback of focusing on influenza is that one pathogen provides only a lower bound on "all-cause" pandemic risk. In addition, advances in treatments and control measures (such as personal protective equipment) have reduced the frequency of influenza pandemics somewhat and may continue to do so. Working in the opposite direction, climate change, habitat fragmentation, population density, and global travel may increase the frequency of pandemics (Madhav et al. 2023). Climate change, for example, may increase viral sharing and thereby the emergence of novel pathogens by bringing mammals into greater contact with each other and with humans (Carlson et al. 2022).

Madhav et al. (2023) expand the set of pathogens included in their forecast of pandemics to include respiratory diseases (for example, pandemic influenza and coronaviruses) and viral hemorrhagic fevers (for example, Ebola and Marburg). Their model of regional disease spread captures the effect of variables, such as global travel, on pandemic frequency. They conclude that a pandemic that matches or exceeds the intensity of COVID-19 can be expected to come along at least once every 50 years and that respiratory diseases will lead to a global annual average of 2.5 million deaths and viral hemorrhagic fevers to a global annual average of 26,000 deaths.

Marani et al. (2021, 2023) further expand the set of pathogens to cover pandemics from any cause. They analyze intensity data on nearly 500 significant epidemics since 1600, more than half of which include detailed information on duration and deaths. Their data contain enough episodes to accurately estimate a power-law distribution for pandemic intensity (deaths per 1,000 people) conditional on arrival. Those authors further estimate the probability of epidemic arrival using the recent 20 years of data. Glennerster, Snyder, and Tan (2023) take the combined estimates from Marani et al. (2023) and translate them into the exceedance probabilities shown in figure 10.1.

**Figure 10.1** Estimated Annual Probability That a Pandemic Will Exceed Specified Intensity

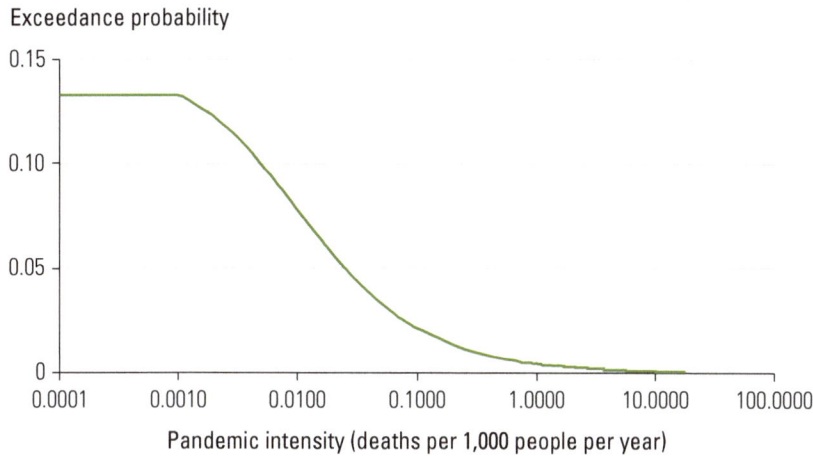

*Source:* Glennerster, Snyder, and Tan 2023, figure 1.

## Social Harm from Pandemics

The next step is to translate forecasts of pandemic frequency into forecasts of total social harm from pandemics, converting losses from different channels (mortality, morbidity, gross domestic product [GDP] reductions, and learning losses) into a common money metric. Maintaining their focus on a single key pathogen, Fan, Jamison, and Summers (2018) estimate social losses from pandemic influenza at about US$500 billion (US$650 billion in 2023 dollars). Their estimate accounts for mortality losses by scaling forecasted deaths by the value of a statistical life, drawn from studies of consumers' willingness to pay for reductions in mortality risk (refer to Viscusi 2014 for a discussion of the value of a statistical life methodology). Mortality constitutes most of their total estimated pandemic losses. GDP losses constitute only about 15 percent, explaining why their estimates exceed earlier assessments focused solely on GDP losses (McKibbin and Sidorenko 2006).

Glennerster, Snyder, and Tan (2023) expand the analysis to pathogens beyond influenza. A search for academic studies providing joint estimates of mortality and GDP losses from historical epidemics and pandemics yielded the five data points graphed in figure 10.2, covering the 1918 flu, SARS, Ebola, Zika, and COVID-19. Glennerster, Snyder, and Tan (2023) use the regression line shown in figure 10.2 to project GDP losses for epidemics of any intensity. They project learning losses for pandemics of any intensity using results from Azevedo et al. (2021) on school closures experienced during COVID-19 combined with estimates of how years of schooling affect future wages. Combining the estimate of the arrival rate of pandemics of varying intensities with estimates of mortality, economic damage, and learning losses, Glennerster, Snyder, and Tan (2023) forecast expected global social losses of about US$700 billion annually (table 10.1).

**Figure 10.2** Relationship between Intensity and GDP Losses Estimated from Studies of Historical Pandemics

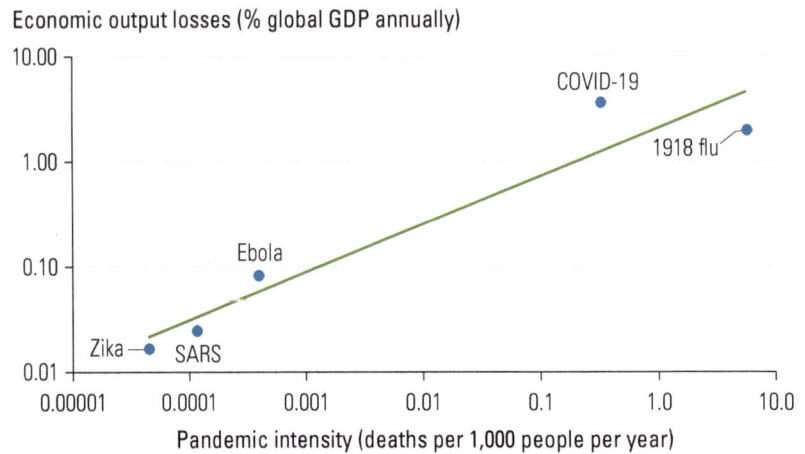

*Source:* Glennerster, Snyder, and Tan 2023, figure 2.

*Note:* GDP = gross domestic product; SARS = severe acute respiratory syndrome.

**Table 10.1** Expected Annual Global Losses from Pandemics Caused by All Pathogens

| Loss category | Expected losses (US$, billion) | Share of total losses (%) |
|---|---|---|
| Mortality | 519 | 73 |
| Economic output | 112 | 16 |
| Learning losses | 81 | 11 |
| Total | 712 | 100 |

*Source:* Glennerster, Snyder, and Tan 2023, table 2.

*Note:* Mortality losses are estimated using the US$1.3 million value of a statistical life estimate from Sweis (2022).

## INVESTMENTS IN PANDEMIC PREPAREDNESS

The forecasted harm from pandemics creates a case for investments to accelerate vaccine availability to mitigate that harm. This section and the next analyze two categories of cost-effective investments: vaccine R&D and vaccine capacity. This section focuses on preparedness investments undertaken in *advance* of future pandemics, whereas the subsequent section focuses on response investments undertaken *during* a pandemic.

### Advance Investments in Vaccine R&D

**Priorities.** No one knows which pathogen will cause the next pandemic, but advance R&D can improve our ability to respond even without perfect foresight. COVID-19 vaccines were developed in record time thanks to decades of advances in vaccine science, coronavirus vaccine research, and mRNA technology (Dolgin 2021). Advance R&D is called for on specific virus families identified as pandemic threats and on technological platforms that apply generally across pathogens (Jain et al. 2021).

Institutions in charge of infectious disease control—including the Coalition for Epidemic Preparedness Innovations (CEPI), World Health Organization, and US National Institute of Allergy and Infectious Disease—have outlined strategic plans prioritizing advance R&D that would enhance our readiness for the next pandemic. The plans include the following priorities.

- **Developing vaccines for pathogens with high epidemic risk.** Notable lists of priority diseases include CEPI[2] and WHO (2018). Lassa fever, MERS (Middle East respiratory syndrome), Nipah, and Rift Valley fever appear on both lists as priorities.
- **Researching prototype vaccines for viral families.** This approach focuses on basic, preclinical, and translational research of the shared characteristics within a viral family to develop generalizable countermeasure strategies. It can accelerate the discovery, development, and evaluation of vaccines against novel pathogens (Cassetti et al. 2022).
- **Advancing technologies that transform vaccine capabilities.** Transformative technologies include universal vaccines against the most likely pandemic threats (influenza and coronavirus), novel routes of administration, and enhancements in immune response. For example, intranasal vaccination could improve the immune response in the respiratory tract at the same time that it reduces hesitancy by eliminating the painful shot (Jabbal-Gill 2010).
- **Innovation in enabling technologies.** Vaccine research, clinical trials, and manufacturing rely on many supporting technologies that could be advanced to accelerate vaccine development. For example, comprehensive antigen-specific and serological assays are critical for evaluating immune response from a vaccine and can enable faster scientific evaluation (CEPI 2021; NIAID 2021).

**Who should pay for advance R&D?** Vaccine R&D that generates broad spillovers across pathogens and advances general purpose technologies is a global public good. The scientific and technological advancements benefit all countries without diminishing the benefit to any single nation. Countries can free ride on others' R&D without paying for it themselves, leading to global underinvestment.

A cooperative global funding agreement might best solve this underinvestment problem. Countries could contribute to the fund in proportion to their GDP, but this requirement may prove overly burdensome to low- and middle-income countries (LMICs). More realistically, high-income countries (HICs) may fund most or all of the R&D for global pandemic threats, coordinated by the Group of Seven or other effective HIC conveners. The benefits to HICs from R&D are likely so much greater than the costs that they should be willing to provide all the funds themselves despite the benefits spillovers to LMICs. For example, the R&D into mRNA technology funded by the US National Institutes of Health was repaid many times by the huge returns for the US economy from accelerating COVID-19 vaccine development. Glennerster, Kelly, et al. (2024) suggest that the United States alone would obtain enough unilateral benefit from a universal COVID-19 vaccine to justify large R&D investments.

R&D for regional epidemic threats or for technologies specific to LMICs may be underfunded if left to HICs' self-interest. LMICs may need to coordinate R&D investments, supplemented by aid (for example, through CEPI), that address regional threats. Multilateral development banks could be well suited to coordinate investments in regional public goods, but new funding facilities may be needed with the flexibility to allow for group lending.

**Funding advance vaccine R&D with push or pull funding.** The general principles laid out in box 10.1 on push versus pull funding provide guidance on how advance vaccine R&D should be funded. General purpose technologies that spill over across products and pathogens, or that are difficult to predict or embody in a technical product profile, may best be funded with push. R&D targeting the production of a tangible vaccine might best be funded with pull. For example, funders could offer a prize for the first firm that gains approval for a Lassa fever vaccine.

When pull funding is feasible, it offers some advantages, incentivizing firms to dynamically reduce their costs and improve their probability of success. It can also help reduce the likelihood that funders pay for innovation approaches with little prospect of succeeding. These advantages can reduce overall program expense and improve the likelihood of developing a successful vaccine candidate (Athey et al. 2022).

**Box 10.1**

### General Principles behind Push versus Pull Funding

Historically, funders have used different mechanisms to incentivize companies, academic researchers, and research institutions to undertake socially valuable research and development. These mechanisms include "push" funding, which pays directly for inputs (for example, grants that pay for developers' materials and labor), and "pull" funding, which links payments to successful achievement of an outcome. Both can play a role in supporting vaccine research and development.

Push funding is well suited to basic research aimed at expanding scientific understanding (Kremer and Glennerster 2004). With such research, many innovations are developed without a clear end-use case. Push funding is compatible with sharing knowledge and intermediate results, awarding grants through competitive research calls.

Pull funding is useful when the funder can specify the needed innovation but does not know who is best placed to develop it or how. Pull funding mechanisms (such as advance market commitments, advance purchase agreements, and prizes) commit to paying developers that successfully produce the specified target (Kremer, Levin, and Snyder 2020). By rewarding firms only if they are successful, pull funding leverages private expertise in identifying promising candidates and incentivizes firms to invest resources in such candidates to improve their probability of success. This mechanism aligns private incentives with public goals. Innovators bear the risk of development failure, whereas funders bear the market risk by committing to pay for an innovation meeting their specifications, even if its value changes over time. This division of risk appropriately accounts for private information held by each party (Kremer 2000).

**Quantifying needed R&D spending.** The next subsection presents estimates from Glennerster, Snyder, and Tan (2023) on determining the optimal amount to spend in advance on pandemic vaccine capacity and the cost-effectiveness of that spending. Those authors are working on using a similar approach to estimate the optimal amount and cost-effectiveness of advance R&D investments. It is reasonable to suppose that the large benefits estimated for accelerating the completion of a pandemic vaccine campaign with more advance capacity will carry over for accelerating the rollout of the first vaccine with more advance R&D.

### Advance Investments in Capacity

**Capacity priorities.** Advance vaccine capacity investments can refer to anything that is needed to produce and deliver vaccines, including manufacturing facilities, workforce readiness, supply-chain resiliency, vaccine distribution infrastructure, and updating regulatory framework.

Supply, rather than lack of demand or delivery capacity, was the major barrier to rapid COVID-19 vaccine deployment in most countries and will likely pose a challenge in future pandemics. Vaccine hesitancy was notably lower in LMICs than in HICs (Mobarak et al. 2022; Solís Arse et al. 2021). Despite initial challenges with vaccine distribution channels and concerns about cold-supply chains, many LMICs quickly and cost-effectively established mobile clinics and other distribution strategies with the help of international aid (Bloxham 2021; Mobarak et al. 2022).[3] Even countries with less developed health infrastructure had experience mobilizing mass immunization campaigns from previous epidemic threats, such as yellow fever, and from childhood vaccination campaigns (Mobarak et al. 2022; WHO 2016). Regulatory agencies achieved record approval times, while maintaining safety, using mechanisms such as the US Food and Drug Administration's Emergency Use Authorization and the World Health Organization's Emergency Use Listing (Kalinke et al. 2022), but manufacturing capacity became the rate-limiting step for vaccine access. This subsection focuses on advance investments in manufacturing capacity as a key limitation to vaccine access in LMICs and the hardest to scale quickly during the pandemic.

Prepandemic investment should create enough contract manufacturing capacity to avoid operating near full capacity during normal times, creating excess capacity available for use during a pandemic. Constructing new plants to sit idle until the next pandemic is not the only or best way to expand pandemic vaccine capacity. Existing facilities can be modified to add production lines quickly, with some of the necessary capital equipment stored on-site. Manufacturers could be paid a retainer or premium on current products to maintain this expansion option. For example, in 2022, Germany contracted with five manufacturers to maintain domestic vaccine production capabilities that could be rapidly activated for multiple vaccine technologies (Paul-Ehrlich-Institut 2022). Routine vaccines could be sourced from rotating facilities to keep excess capacity up-to-date. The platforms used to produce current vaccines can be switched over to more scalable and repurposable alternatives. For example, funders could subsidize mRNA-based seasonal flu vaccines to encourage manufacturers to switch from hard-to-scale egg-based production.

Manufacturing scale-up can also include intellectual property and technology transfer arrangements. A significant literature examines how different intellectual property frameworks—from patent pools to voluntary licensing—affect vaccine access and innovation incentives (refer to, for example, Adekola and Mercurio 2025; Gold 2022; Stevens and Schultz 2022). Successful production requires more than intellectual property rights alone: manufacturers need proper incentives to share technical expertise and coordinate production processes. During COVID-19, Merck and Johnson & Johnson demonstrated the feasibility of voluntary production partnerships when properly incentivized (Merck 2021). Government policies can support these arrangements by helping coordinate supply chains and stockpiling inputs, such as the United States achieved through actions taken under the Defense Production Act (Lupkin 2021).

**Who should pay for advance capacity?** Unlike R&D, manufacturing capacity is a rivalrous private good: capacity tied up in fulfilling one order cannot fulfill another simultaneously. A contract that reserves some capacity for one country without expanding the global total exerts a negative pecuniary externality on other countries, raising the bid needed to secure their place in the vaccine queue. Contracts that expand global capacity, by contrast, exert a positive externality on other countries. Once the contracting country has received the vaccine it needs, the capacity can be used to supply the next countries in line (Athey et al. 2022).

Contracting for advance manufacturing capacity should use competitive and transparent processes to ensure value for money. Procurement officials should consider not only price but also the producer's ability to deliver on supply commitments during crisis. A firm's reputation and its host country's history of respecting the rule of law (for example, by honoring contracts) would bolster confidence in certain producers. Small countries may more credibly promise not to expropriate vaccines intended for export for domestic use because they need less supply to serve their populations. During the second wave of COVID-19, concerns over vaccine nationalism grew when, unable to keep up with domestic demand, India and certain European Union countries restricted vaccine exports (European Commission 2021; Koller et al. 2021). Increased global vaccine manufacturing capacity would have mitigated these disruptions.

Pooling capacity investments via a global compact could help coordinate contracting, reduce supply-chain disruptions, and distribute vaccines to the hardest-hit areas. HICs might be nervous about ceding control in a crisis to a multinational compact, but a world-class compact might still encourage their participation, even if supplemented by unilateral investments. Pooled capacity would have the greatest insurance value in regional epidemics when competition for capacity is less intense, allowing all the capacity to be devoted to serving the countries experiencing outbreaks. Pooling resources would be especially valuable for LMICs, which have less available financing and higher epidemic risk; it would be especially valuable for LMICs with low correlation in epidemic risks (say, countries in Latin America and the Caribbean and Sub-Saharan Africa). Further work is needed to more precisely estimate optimal advance procurement quantities for different regions and countries.

**Cost-effectiveness.** Glennerster, Snyder, and Tan (2023) analyze a program to install advance capacity capable of producing 24 billion annual doses beyond routine vaccination needs. They determine that this capacity level is necessary to vaccinate 70 percent of the global population in six months with a two-dose course, accounting for some wastage of capacity that is not a good match for the ultimately successful vaccines. As ambitious as the size of the advance capacity is, reaching 70 percent coverage in six months requires the world to install substantial additional capacity in-pandemic.

Glennerster, Snyder, and Tan (2023) estimate that the advance capacity program would cost US$60 billion up front and US$5 billion annually for maintenance thereafter. The program has two main benefits. It saves US$32 billion of in-pandemic expenditures by reducing the amount of capacity that the world needs to install in the heat of the pandemic. More important, expanding capacity in advance relaxes the physical limit on rapid in-pandemic expansion. This additional available capacity can accelerate the global vaccination campaign, averting US$539 billion in social losses relative to the status quo of waiting until a pandemic to scale capacity. Based on mortality reductions alone, the advance capacity program would cost US$4,000 per year of life saved. At a third of current global GDP per capita, the program would be judged highly cost-effective according to standard metrics (Marseille et al. 2015).

The precise public health benefits of accelerating vaccinations depend on the nature of the pathogen and the vaccine. A vaccine capable of reducing transmission and maintaining durable protection might push the population over the threshold for herd immunity and end the pandemic sooner. Less capable vaccines can nonetheless generate large benefits. COVID-19 vaccines did not provide the durable protection and transmission prevention that health officials hoped for, leading aspirations for achieving herd immunity to be dropped. Still, these vaccines prevented over 14 million deaths within the first year of their deployment (Watson et al. 2022), and economies were able to reopen. Accelerating the rollout of vaccines can be as important as optimizing their capabilities. According to Castillo et al. (2021), a 70 percent effective COVID-19 vaccine would have the same social value as a 95 percent effective vaccine available two months later.

## IN-PANDEMIC RESPONSE

This section turns to analyzing investments in R&D and capacity made during a pandemic rather than before.

### Investing in Multiple Vaccines and Investing at Risk

Vaccine development is technologically challenging, with low success rates (MacPherson et al. 2020). The high risk of failure calls for supporting multiple vaccine candidates simultaneously to increase the probability that at least one is successful. Early in the COVID-19 pandemic, Baker, Chaudhuri, and Kremer (2021) estimated that obtaining an 80 percent chance of at least one success would require supporting at least 15 vaccine candidates. Even if the marginal vaccine candidate contributes only a few percentage points to the probability of success of the portfolio, the investment to support this candidate may be worthwhile. The over 14 million deaths that Watson et al. (2022) estimated that COVID-19 vaccines averted in the first year of COVID-19 vaccine deployment translate into benefits of over US$18 trillion from reduced mortality alone (using the US$1.3 million value of a statistical life estimate from Sweis [2022]). Increasing the chance of averting such harm by even a percentage point is worth billions.

In-pandemic R&D investments should be complemented with capacity investments to enable rapid vaccine distribution. Waiting until regulatory approval before expanding capacity can result in months of delay during which social harms from the pandemic mount. Expanding capacity "at risk"—that is, concurrently with clinical trials—is essential, even though some expenditures may be for candidates that fail. Ahuja et al. (2021) find that employing this strategy for COVID-19 capacity saved US$1.6 trillion in global harm by accelerating availability by three months. More capacity would have saved more harm: increasing at-risk capacity from the observed level (6 billion annual doses) to the optimal level (14 billion) more than doubles the harm saved in the Ahuja et al. (2021) model. Although the quantitative results are specific to the COVID-19 pandemic, the qualitative principles are relevant for future pandemics.

**Diversifying the Vaccine Portfolio**

When choosing a portfolio of vaccine candidates for R&D and capacity investment during a pandemic, funders should consider the correlation in candidates' prospects to maximize the probability of at least one success. It may be worth passing over candidates that have higher individual probabilities of success to include candidates that have less correlated success with the rest of the portfolio. The point is illustrated in table 10.2, which lists the six COVID-19 vaccine candidates in phase 3 clinical trials by August 2020. Their probabilities of success are derived from the model of Ahuja et al. (2021), reflecting their best estimates of correlated failure risk within technology platforms and declining failure risk for candidates further along in clinical trials.

Table 10.2 Constructing an Optimal Vaccine Portfolio

| Vaccine candidate | Clinical platform | Candidate's stand-alone probability of success (%) | Probability of at least one success in portfolio (%) |
|---|---|---|---|
| A | Inactivated virus | 29 | 29 |
| B | Viral vector | 29 | 48 |
| C | Inactivated virus | 29 | 58 |
| D | Inactivated virus | 29 | 63 |
| E | mRNA | 22 | 70 |
| F | mRNA | 22 | 73 |

*Source:* Original calculations using input from Ahuja et al. 2021 model.

As a thought experiment, consider forming a portfolio of four candidates from the six listed. A portfolio of the four highest-probability candidates (A–D) has a 63 percent success chance. Substituting an mRNA candidate for an inactivated virus candidate increases this chance to 66 percent, because candidates within the same platform share failure risks.

Although the thought experiment assumes equal social benefits for successful candidates, in practice candidates might differ in efficacy, duration of immunity, shelf stability, ease of administration, and so on. Considering these additional factors only strengthens the case for diversifying the candidate portfolio, helping ensure the emergence of a successful candidate that satisfies a variety of criteria. The modeled probabilities come with significant uncertainty, but even a rough understanding of correlations between candidates based on platforms, adjuvants, and antigens can help vaccine buyers make better-calibrated investment decisions.

Moving from thought experiment to formal analysis, Ahuja et al. (2021) construct optimal portfolios of various sizes from the COVID-19 candidates. Figure 10.3 graphs the probability of success generated by those portfolios. The diminishing returns to portfolio size exhibited by the graph arise because incremental candidates are less promising and contribute to the probability of overall success only if other candidates in the portfolio fail.

## Sizing the Optimal Portfolio

How large should a country's at-risk investment portfolio be? To answer that question, Ahuja et al. (2021) scale the probability of a success shown in figure 10.3 by the averted harm from early access to a successful vaccine and weigh the result against the cost of investing in more candidates.

**Figure 10.3** Probability of Success in Optimal Vaccine Portfolio

Probability of at least one success in portfolio (%)

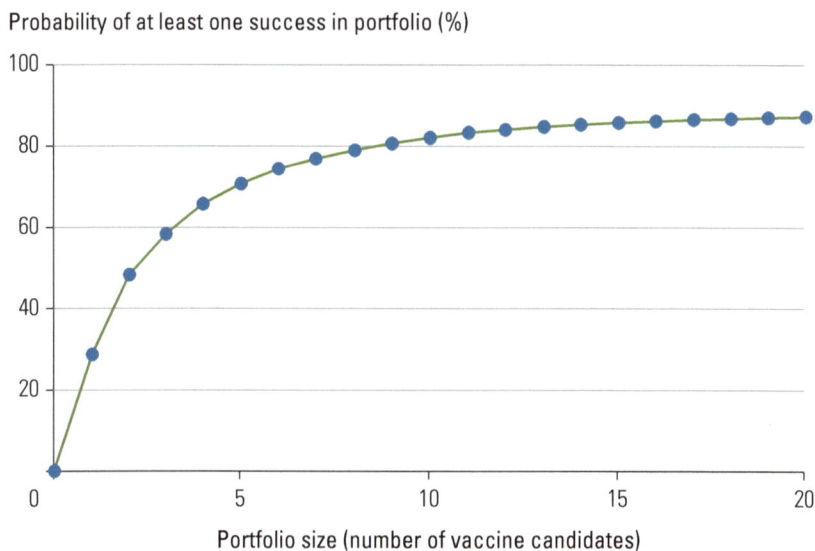

Portfolio size (number of vaccine candidates)

Source: Ahuja et al. 2021, figure A6.

**Table 10.3** Optimal At-Risk Vaccine Capacity, by Country Group

| Country category | Vaccine candidates (per-country mean) | At-risk capacity (annual doses per capita) | Benefit from at-risk investment vs. 3-month delay (US$ per capita) | Cost of at-risk capacity (US$ per capita) |
|---|---|---|---|---|
| High-income | 18.3 | 23.5 | 699.3 | 143.6 |
| Middle-income | 6.7 | 4.1 | 40.7 | 20.4 |
| Low-income | 1.3 | 0.1 | 0.6 | 0.3 |
| All in world | 8.8 | 7.3 | 137.4 | 36.5 |

*Source:* Ahuja et al. 2021, table A2.

The results in table 10.3 show that lower-income countries optimally procure fewer candidates and less capacity per candidate because of their tighter budget constraints. The results may present an overly conservative benefit-cost ratio for at-risk capacity investment by reporting the incremental benefit of accelerating capacity availability by three months, not the benefit of that capacity relative to no capacity. By contrast, this analysis allocates the full cost to the investing country, assuming that waiting allows countries to free ride on others' at-risk capacity expenditures.

The recommended portfolio for the average HIC involves three times the number of candidates funded at risk under Operation Warp Speed, the US program for procuring COVID-19 vaccines, reputedly an aggressive investment program. Mango (2022) suggests that administrative bandwidth was a key constraint on the number of candidates the program could support. Another constraint is the number of large-scale clinical trials that can be conducted simultaneously. Relaxing the constraint on clinical trials by coordinating them more effectively has been suggested as an important investment in pandemic preparation (CEPI 2021).

## Contracting for At-Risk Capacity

Typically, vaccine manufacturers wait until regulatory approval to install substantial capacity, because the investment is wasted if the vaccine fails. As emphasized earlier, the social value of investing in vaccine capacity at risk in a pandemic to reduce the lag in availability can easily justify the "wasted" investment. Bridging the gap between social and commercial incentives to install capacity at risk undoubtedly involves public funding.

Inducing manufacturers to invest at risk can be challenging, even in a pandemic, and therefore requires careful contract design. A fixed price per dose, even if the price is high, provides little incentive to rush production. Penalties for missing delivery deadlines may not work because, if the penalties are set anywhere close to the social cost of delay, they would bankrupt most firms.

A cost-effective approach to get firms to install at-risk capacity is through direct contracts with firms using a combination of push and pull funding (box 10.1). Purchasers can agree to directly fund most of the firm's at-risk capacity costs along with a commitment to buy output at a price that incentivizes the firm to complete the at-risk investment. This scheme transfers most of the risk of failure to the funder but leaves the firm with enough skin in the game to ensure it is a serious entrant and lead it to economize on investment costs. Operation Warp Speed involved hybrid contracts of this form (although some developers opted to participate solely through supply commitments, forgoing push funding) (Congressional Research Service 2021). In contrast, firm-agnostic pull funding may not efficiently incentivize marginal firms with low probabilities of success to scale capacity because a standardized price high enough to attract these developers would overcompensate firms with more promising candidates.

Purchasers should contract for expanded capacity to fulfill procurement orders, not just for delivery of doses at an unspecified date, which might place the purchaser in the middle of a long queue. Such a contract allows the purchaser to secure access to vaccines as soon as they become available and has the external benefit of increasing the global supply of manufacturing capacity. During COVID-19, HICs used advance purchase agreements to secure their place at the front of the vaccine queue. In contrast, LMICs did not have the financing tools to invest at risk, which led to inequitable access to vaccines (Thornton, Wilson, and Gandhi 2022). Agarwal and Reed (2022) attribute more than 60 percent of the delay in vaccine delivery to LMICs to those countries' signing of advance purchase agreements later than HICs.

COVAX (COVID-19 Vaccines Global Access) was established to ensure global equitable access to COVID-19 vaccines but faced several challenges. COVAX had two arms: a self-financing arm whereby HICs and middle-income countries (MICs) could pay for access to a pooled vaccine portfolio and a donation-funded arm providing vaccines to 92 eligible lower-income countries. Unlike sovereign HICs, COVAX lacked the flexibility to act swiftly to contract at risk. COVAX could enter only into contracts equivalent to the cash it had on hand (whether from self-funders or donations), which took months to receive, and it needed to develop novel risk-sharing and mitigation agreements (COVAX 2022). Restrictive lending criteria from multilateral development banks (MDBs) limited the ability of self-funding MICs to purchase vaccines at risk and delayed their contributions to COVAX (Hart, Prizzon, and Pudussery 2021). Consequently, most COVAX commitments occurred after HICs had already signed advance purchase agreements with vaccine developers separate from COVAX.

To address these issues, mechanisms enabling LMICs to borrow for at-risk investment during pandemics should be established through coordination with MDBs. Glennerster, Haria, et al. (2024) detail how MDBs can facilitate greater access to pandemic financing by relaxing restrictive lending criteria, establishing expert advisory panels, creating standardized loan templates and procurement contracts, and developing an optional guarantee mechanism backed by HICs. MDBs or other multilateral organizations such as regional health agencies; Gavi, the Vaccine Alliance; or the World Bank could also help coordinate purchase aggregation, enabling higher-volume capacity expansion contracts, and support a broader portfolio of candidates. This approach would unlock greater up-front financing compared to donor-reliant schemes, enhancing the capabilities of LMICs to make at-risk investments.

### Using Available Capacity Efficiently

During periods of vaccine scarcity, policy makers should optimize allocation strategies to maximize social benefits. Prioritizing high-risk populations, such as those with high mortality and morbidity risks and frontline workers, is essential. Bubar et al. (2021) estimate that vaccinating 20 percent of the population for COVID-19 could reduce mortality by 80 percent. Stretching available supplies through a "first doses first" policy, which involves delaying the second dose of a two-dose sequence to allow more individuals to receive vaccines early, or "fractional dosing," which reduces the active ingredient in each dose, can improve outcomes (Moghadas et al. 2021; Więcek et al. 2022). Cross-country vaccine exchanges can further improve allocation, allowing countries to adjust to their needs and capacities. For example, countries may want to trade vaccines that require substantial cold storage, or trade current orders for more vaccines later if they are facing absorption constraints (Budish et al. 2022).

## CONCLUSION

This chapter emphasizes the enormous social value of investing in vaccine R&D and manufacturing capacity to prepare for and respond to pandemics. Such investments could dramatically reduce the time required to develop and distribute vaccines, mitigating substantial pandemic harm. Given the public good nature of many of these investments, public funding is important for bridging the gap between social and commercial incentives for pandemic preparedness and response. Mechanisms should pool resources from many public actors. The World Bank's Financial Intermediary Fund frameworks offer a proven model for this approach.[4] Examples of such funds include the Pandemic Emergency Financing Facility, which existed before COVID-19, and the Pandemic Fund, which was created in 2023 (Agarwal 2024; John Hopkins Center for Health Security 2020). Looking ahead, stakeholders can apply similar frameworks to implement the strategies outlined in this chapter.

For pandemic preparedness:

- Invest in advance vaccine R&D for priority pathogens and a broad range of vaccine platforms. Consider the use of both push and pull funding.
- Contract advance vaccine manufacturing capacity. Prioritize making this capacity flexible to different technologies.

For pandemic response:

- Invest in a diverse portfolio of vaccine candidates across many platforms. Account for the correlation of probabilities of success between different candidates.

- Directly incentivize vaccine manufacturing firms to build at-risk capacity.
- Use vaccine capacity efficiently. For example, use the "first doses first" strategy, fractional dosing, or cross-country vaccine exchanges. Target vaccines to populations that are more likely to experience high mortality and morbidity if infected.

## ACKNOWLEDGMENTS

The authors thank William Arnesen, Siddhartha Haria, Leah Rosenzweig, and the Market Shaping Accelerator team for support. They also thank editors Dean T. Jamison, Siddhanth Sharma, and Ole F. Norheim for guidance. Christopher M. Snyder thanks the Institute for Progress for funding.

## NOTES

1. Our World in Data, "Estimated Cumulative Excess Deaths During COVID-19," https://ourworldindata.org/grapher/excess-deaths-cumulative-economist.
2. Refer to CEPI's "Priority Diseases" web page, https://cepi.net/priority-pathogens.
3. Refer also to the World Bank's web page, "Eastern and Southern Africa's COVID-19 Vaccination Journey," https://www.worldbank.org/en/news/immersive-story/2022/06/30/unlocking-supply-and-overcoming-hesitancy-eastern-and-southern-africa-s-covid-19-vaccination-journey.
4. World Bank, "Financial Intermediary Funds (FIFs)," https://fiftrustee.worldbank.org/en/about/unit/dfi/fiftrustee/overview.

## REFERENCES

Abaluck, J., L. H. Kwong, A. Styczynski, A. Haque, M. A. Kabir, E. B. Jefferys, E. Crawford, et al. 2021. "Impact of Community Masking on COVID-19: A Cluster-Randomized Trial in Bangladesh." *Science* 375 (6577): eabi9069. https://doi.org/10.1126/science.abi9069.

Adekola, T. A., and B. Mercurio. 2025. "mRNA Technology Transfer Hub and Intellectual Property: Towards a More Equitable and Sustainable Model." *World Trade Review*, January 30, 2025.

Agarwal, R., and T. Reed. 2022. "Financing Vaccine Equity: Funding for Day-Zero of the Next Pandemic." *Oxford Review of Economic Policy* 38 (4): 833–50.

Agarwal, R. 2024. "What Is Day Zero Financing? A Global Security Perspective for Pandemic Response." CGD Note 365, Center for Global Development, Washington, DC. https://www.cgdev.org/publication/what-day-zero-financing-global-security-perspective-pandemic-response.

Ahuja, A., S. Athey, A. Baker, E. Budish, J. C. Castillo, R. Glennerster, S. D. Kominers, et al. 2021. "Preparing for a Pandemic: Accelerating Vaccine Availability." *American Economic Association Papers and Proceedings* 111 (May): 331–35.

Athey, S., J. C. Castillo, E. Chaudhuri, M. Kremer, A. Simoes Gomes, and C. M. Snyder. 2022. "Expanding Capacity for Vaccines against Covid-19 and Future Pandemics: A Review of Economic Issues." *Oxford Review of Economic Policy* 38 (4): 742–70.

Azevedo, J. P. , A. Hasan, D. Goldemberg, K. Geven, and S. A. Iqbal. 2021. "Simulating the Potential Impacts of COVID-19 School Closures on Schooling and Learning Outcomes: A Set of Global Estimates." *World Bank Research Observer* 36 (1): 1–36.

Baker, A., E. Chaudhuri, and M. Kremer. 2021. "Accelerating Vaccinations." *Finance & Development*, December, International Monetary Fund, Washington, DC. https://www.imf.org/en/Publications/fandd/issues/2021/12/Accelerating-Vaccinations-Baker-Chaudhuri-Kremer.

Bloxham, L. 2021. "Covid-19 Vaccine Rollout in Liberia and Sierra Leone Helps Reach Vulnerable People." *Concern Worldwide*, November 30. https://www.concern.org.uk/news/covid-19-vaccine-rollout-liberia-and-sierra-leone-helps-reach-vulnerable-people.

Bubar, K. M., K. Reinholt, S. M. Kissler, M. Lipsitch, S. Cobey, Y. H. Grad, and D. B. Larremore. 2021. "Model-Informed COVID-19 Vaccine Prioritization Strategies by Age and Serostatus." *Science* 371 (6532): 916–21.

Budish, E., H. Kettler, S. D. Kominers, E. Osland, C. Prendergast, and A. A. Torkelson. 2022. "Distributing a Billion Vaccines: COVAX Successes, Challenges, and Opportunities." *Oxford Review of Economic Policy* 38 (4): 941–74.

Carlson, C. J., G. F. Albery, C. Merow, C. H. Trisos, C. M. Zipfel, E. A. Eskew, K. J. Olival, et al. 2022. "Climate Change Increases Cross-Species Viral Transmission Risk." *Nature* 607 (7919): 555–62.

Cassetti. C. M., T. C. Pierson, L. J. Patterson, K. Bok, A. J. DeRocco, A. M. Deschamps, B. S. Graham, et al. 2022. "Prototype Pathogen Approach for Vaccine and Monoclonal Antibody Development: A Critical Component of the NIAID Plan for Pandemic Preparedness." *Journal of Infectious Diseases* 227 (12): 1433–41.

Castillo, J. C., A. Ahuja, S. Athey, A. Baker, E. Budish, T. Chipty, R. Glennerster, et al. 2021. "Market Design to Accelerate COVID-19 Vaccine Supply." *Science* 371 (6534): 1107–09.

CEPI (Coalition for Epidemic Preparedness Innovations). 2021. "2022–2026 Strategy: Objectives and Ambitions for the Second 5-Year Cycle." CEPI, Oslo. https://static.cepi.net/downloads/2023-12/CEPI-2022-2026-Strategy-v3-Jan21_0.pdf.

Congressional Research Service. 2021. "Operation Warp Speed Contracts for COVID 19 Vaccines and Ancillary Vaccination Materials." CRS Insight, updated March 1, 2021. https://crsreports.congress.gov/product/pdf/IN/IN11560.

COVAX. 2022. "COVAX: Key Learnings for Future Pandemic Preparedness and Response." White paper, COVAX. https://www.gavi.org/news-resources/knowledge-products/covax-key-learnings-future-pandemic-preparedness-and-response.

Dolgin, E. 2021. "The Tangled History of mRNA Vaccines." *Nature* 597 (7876): 318–24.

Duroseau, B., N. Kipshidze, and R. J. Limaye. 2023. "The Impact of Delayed Access to COVID-19 Vaccines in Low- and Lower-Middle-Income Countries." *Frontiers in Public Health* 10: 1087138.

European Commission. 2021. "Commission Puts in Place Transparency and Authorisation Mechanism for Exports of COVID-19 Vaccines." Press release, January 28, 2021. https://ec.europa.eu/commission/presscorner/detail/en/ip_21_307.

Fan, V. Y, D. T. Jamison, and L. H. Summers. 2018. "Pandemic Risk: How Large Are the Expected Losses?" *Bulletin of the World Health Organization* 96 (2): 129–34.

Glennerster, R., S. Haria, L. R. Rosenzweig, and L. H. Summers. 2024. "Five Steps MDBs Can Take Now to Unlock Pandemic Financing." *Center for Global Development* (blog), October 23, 2024. https://www.cgdev.org/blog/five-steps-multilateral-development-banks-can-take-now-enable-at-risk-financing-pandemics.

Glennerster, R., T. Kelly, C. T. McMahon, and C. M. Snyder. 2024. "Quantifying the Social Value of a Universal COVID-19 Vaccine and Incentivizing Its Development." *Review of Economic Design* 28: 723–61.

Glennerster, R., C. M. Snyder, and B. J. Tan. 2023. "Calculating the Costs and Benefits of Advance Preparations for Future Pandemics." *IMF Economic Review* 71 (3): 611–48.

Gold, E. R. 2022. "What the COVID-19 Pandemic Revealed about Intellectual Property." *Nature Biotechnology* 40 (10): 1428–30.

Goodkin-Gold, M., M. Kremer, C. M. Snyder, and H. L. Williams. 2024. "Optimal Vaccine Subsidies for Epidemic Diseases." *Review of Economics and Statistics* 106 (4): 895–909.

Hart, T., A. Prizzon, and J. Pudussery. 2021. "What MDBs (and Their Shareholders) Can Do for Vaccine Equity." Briefing Policy Paper, ODI Global. https://odi.org/en/publications /what-mdbs-and-their-shareholders-can-do-for-vaccine-equity/.

Jabbal-Gill, I. 2010. "Nasal Vaccine Innovation." *Journal of Drug Targeting* 18 (10): 771–86.

Jain, S., A. Venkataraman, M. E. Wechsler, and N. A. Peppas. 2021. "Messenger RNA-Based Vaccines: Past, Present, and Future Directions in the Context of the COVID-19 Pandemic." *Advanced Drug Delivery Reviews* 179: 114000.

Johns Hopkins Center for Health Security. 2020. "Financing for Epidemic Response Activities." Fact sheet, Johns Hopkins Center for Health Security, Baltimore. https:// centerforhealthsecurity.org/sites/default/files/2022-11/200129-finance-factsheet.pdf.

Kalinke, U., D. H. Barouch, R. Rizzi, E. Lagkadinou, Ö. Türeci, S. Pather, and P. Neels. 2022. "Clinical Development and Approval of COVID-19 Vaccines." *Expert Review of Vaccines* 14 (March): 1–11.

Karim, M., C.-W. Lo, and S. Einav. 2023. "Preparing for the Next Viral Threat with Broad-Spectrum Antivirals." *Journal of Clinical Investigation* 133 (11): e170236.

Koller, C. N. , C. J. Schwerzmann, A. S. A. Lang, E. Alexiou, and J. Krishnakumar. 2021. "Addressing Different Needs: The Challenges Faced by India as the Largest Vaccine Manufacturer While Conducting the World's Biggest COVID-19 Vaccination Campaign." *Epidemiologia* 2 (3): 454–70.

Kremer, M. 2000. "Creating Markets for New Vaccines. Part I: Rationale." *Innovation Policy and the Economy* 1: 35–72.

Kremer, M., and R. Glennerster. 2004. *Strong Medicine: Creating Incentives for Pharmaceutical Research on Neglected Disease*. Princeton, NJ: Princeton University Press

Kremer, M., and C. M. Snyder. 2015. "Preventives versus Treatments." *Quarterly Journal of Economics* 130 (3): 1167–239.

Kremer, M., J. Levin, and C. M. Snyder. 2020. "Advance Market Commitments: Insights from Theory and Experience." *American Economic Association Papers and Proceedings* 110 (May): 269–73.

Lupkin, S. 2021. "Defense Production Act Speeds Up Vaccine Production." NPR.org, March 13, 2021. https://www.npr.org/sections/health-shots/2021/03/13/976531488/defense -production-act-speeds-up-vaccine-production.

MacPherson, A., N. Hutchinson, O. Schneider, E. Oliviero, E. Feldhake, C. Ouimet, J. Sheng, et al. 2020. "Probability of Success and Timelines for the Development of Vaccines for Emerging and Reemerged Viral Infectious Diseases." *Annals of Internal Medicine* 174 (3): 326–34.

Madhav, N. K, B. Oppenheim, N. Stephenson, R. Badker, D. T Jamison, C. Lam, and A. Meadows. 2023. "Estimated Future Mortality from Pathogens of Epidemic and Pandemic Potential." CGD Working Paper 665, Center for Global Development, Washington, DC.

Mango, P. 2022. *Warp Speed: Inside the Operation That Beat COVID, the Critics, and the Odds*. Washington, DC: Republic Book Publishers.

Marani, M., G. G. Katul, W. K. Pan, and A. J. Parolari. 2021. "Intensity and Frequency of Extreme Novel Epidemics." *Proceedings of the National Academy of Sciences* 118 (35): e2105482118.

Marani, M., G. G. Katul, W. K. Pan, and A. J. Parolari. 2023. "Correction for Marani et al., Intensity and Frequency of Extreme Novel Epidemics." *Proceedings of the National Academy of Sciences* 120 (12): e2302169120.

Marseille, E., B. Larson, D.S. Kazi, J.G. Kahn, and S. Rosen. 2015. "Thresholds for the Cost-Effectiveness of Interventions: Alternative Approaches." *Bulletin of the World Health Organization* 93 (2): 118–24.

McKibbin. W. J., and A. A. Sidorenko. 2006. "Global Macroeconomic Consequences of Pandemic Influenza." Lowy Institute for International Policy, Sydney. https://www .lowyinstitute.org/publications/global-macroeconomic-consequences-pandemic-influenza.

Merck. 2021. "Merck to Help Produce Johnson & Johnson's COVID-19 Vaccine; BARDA to Provide Merck With Funding to Expand Merck's Manufacturing Capacity for COVID-19

Vaccines and Medicines." News release, March 2, 2021. https://www.merck.com/news
/merck-to-help-produce-johnson-barda-to-provide-merck-with-funding-to-expand
-mercks-manufacturing-capacity-for-covid-19-vaccines-and-medicines/.

Mobarak, A.M., E. Miguel, J. Abaluck, A. Ahuja, M. Alsan, A. Banerjee, E. Breza, et al. 2022.
"End COVID-19 in Low- and Middle-Income Countries." *Science* 375 (6585): 1105–10.

Mobarak, A.M. 2023. "Why Did COVID-19 Vaccinations Lag in Low- and Middle-Income
Countries? Lessons from Descriptive and Experimental Data." *American Economic
Association Papers and Proceedings* 113 (May): 637–41.

Moghadas, S. M., T. N. Vilches, K. Zhang, S. Nourbakhsh, P. Sah, M. C. Fitzpatrick, and
A. P. Galvani. 2021. "Evaluation of COVID-19 Vaccination Strategies with a Delayed
Second Dose." *PLOS Biology* 19 (4): e3001211.

NIAID (US National Institute of Allergy and Infectious Disease). 2021. "NIAID Pandemic
Preparedness Plan." NIAID, Bethesda, MD. https://www.niaid.nih.gov/sites/default/files
/pandemic-preparedness-plan.pdf.

Paul-Ehrlich-Institut. 2022."Pandemic Preparedness Contracts Signed for Rapid Availability
of Vaccines." Press Release, July 2022. https://www.pei.de/EN/newsroom/press-releases
/year/2022/07-pandemic-preparedness-contracts-signed-rapid-availability-vaccines.html.

Potter, C. W. 2001. "A History of Influenza." *Journal of Applied Microbiology* 91 (4): 572–79.

Roth, A. E. 2007. "Repugnance as a Constraint on Markets." *Journal of Economic Perspectives*
21 (3): 37–58.

Solís Arce, J. S., S. S. Warren, N. F. Meriggi, A. Scacco, N. McMurry, M. Voors, G. Syunyaev,
et al. 2021. "COVID-19 Vaccine Acceptance and Hesitancy in Low- and Middle-Income
Countries." *Nature Medicine* 27 (8): 1385–94.

Stevens, P., and M. Schultz, 2022. "The Role of Intellectual Property Rights in Preparing for
Future Pandemics." Geneva Network, Fordingbridge, U.K. https://geneva-network.com
/research/the-role-of-intellectual-property-rights-in-preparing-for-future-pandemicss/.

Sweis, N. J. 2022. "Revisiting the Value of a Statistical Life: An International Approach during
COVID-19." *Risk Management* 24 (3): 259–72.

Thornton, I., P. Wilson, and G. Gandhi. 2022. "'No Regrets' Purchasing in a Pandemic:
Making the Most of Advance Purchase Agreements." *Globalization and Health* 18: 62.

Viscusi, W. K. 2014. "The Value of Individual and Societal Risks to Life and Health."
Chapter 7 in *Handbook of the Economics of Risk and Uncertainty*, edited by M. Machina
and W. K. Viscusi. Amsterdam: North-Holland.

Walmsley, T., A. Rose, R. John, D. Wei, J. P. Hlávka, J. Machada, and K. Byrd. 2023.
"Macroeconomic Consequences of the COVID-19 Pandemic." *Economic Modelling*
120 (March): 106147.

Watson, O. J., G. Barnsley, J. Toor, A. B. Hogan, P. Winskill, and A. C. Ghani. 2022.
"Global Impact of the First Year of COVID-19 Vaccination: A Mathematical Modelling
Study." *The Lancet Infectious Diseases* 22 (9): 1293–1302.

Więcek, W., A. Ahuja, E. Chaudhuri, M. Kremer, A. S. Gomes, C. M. Snyder, A. Tabarrok,
and B. J. Tan. 2022. "Testing Fractional Doses of COVID-19 Vaccines." *Proceedings of the
National Academy of Sciences of the United States of America* 119 (8): e2116932119.

WHO (World Health Organization). 2016. "Millions Protected in Africa's Largest-Ever
Emergency Yellow Fever Vaccination Campaign." News, September 2, 2016. https://www
.who.int/news/item/02-09-2016-millions-protected-in-africa-s-largest-ever-emergency
-yellow-fever-vaccination-campaign.

WHO (World Health Organization). 2018. "Annual Review of Diseases Prioritized under
the Research and Development Blueprint." WHO R&D Blueprint, Meeting Report,
February 6–7, Geneva, WHO. https://www.who.int/news-room/events/detail/2018/02/06
/default-calendar/2018-annual-review-of-diseases-prioritized-under-the-research
-anddevelopment-blueprint.

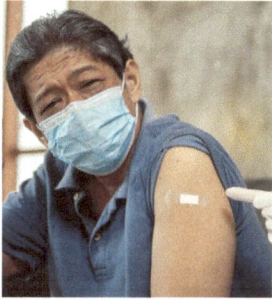

# 11

## An "Always On" Approach to Health Care and Public Health Systems: Building Standing Capabilities That Can Respond to Shocks and Emergencies

Gabriel Seidman, Megan Akodu, Henry Li, Romina Mariano, Kirsten Bell, Helene-Mari van der Westhuizen, Ines Hassan, Ahmad Al-Kasir, Qian Yi Pang, Darcy Ward, Kumeren Govender, Emily Stanger-Sfeile, Tamsin Berry, David Agus,* and John Bell*

### ABSTRACT

"Always On" health systems ensure that routine, quality clinical and public health services can address shocks and health emergencies. Such systems should have dual-use functionality, with utility both for routine care and public health, and for outbreaks and emergencies. That is, they consistently provide quality services in routine settings at the same time that they carry out core prevention, preparedness, and response functions. This chapter describes the health benefits, economic benefits, and policy and research opportunities to develop Always On health systems, with a specific focus on three applications: adult vaccination, clinical research, and pathogen surveillance.

### INTRODUCTION

The COVID-19 (coronavirus) pandemic demonstrated the importance of preparation for health emergencies. A "stop-start approach" of responding to health crises—which created problems initiating ad hoc research and development, vaccine manufacturing, service delivery, and surveillance activities during the pandemic—serves neither public health nor economic interests. As the risk of health emergencies, including from climate change, increases, health systems need to take a different approach to emergency preparedness, prevention, and response (PPR).

*Joint last authors.*

This chapter proposes an Always On approach to health care and public health systems. The description of these systems as "Always On" means that they consistently provide quality clinical and public health services in routine settings while contributing to PPR for shocks and emergencies. Always On systems have dual-use functionality, with utility both for routine care and public health, and for outbreaks and emergencies. This functionality stands in contrast to a more siloed approach (table 11.1).

Although the COVID-19 pandemic catalyzed new investments in global health security, some countries have already started to scale back and shutter key infrastructure. The Pandemic Fund raised only a fraction of its target, and pandemic PPR now takes lower priority on the international political agenda (Rigby 2023). The pandemic also disrupted health care services, led to backlogs of hospital care, and interfered with routine immunization schedules—leading to the largest decline in childhood vaccination coverage in over 30 years (UNICEF 2022). These disruptions to routine services, such as tuberculosis (TB) programs, led to disproportionately higher numbers of deaths in African countries during the COVID-19 pandemic (Soe-Lin, Bowen, and Hecht 2024). As countries build their usual services back up, they must do so in a way that maximizes emergency PPR capabilities.

**Table 11.1** Definitions and Applications of Always On Systems and Dual-Use Functionality

| **Always On systems** | Systems that can consistently provide quality clinical and public health services in routine settings while possessing the ability to respond swiftly to shocks and health emergencies. These routine clinical and public health services should support emergency prevention, preparedness, and response. |
| --- | --- |
| **Dual-use functionality** | Technology and capabilities that can be used for both routine care and public health and during outbreaks and emergencies |

| **Application** | **Always On systems** | **Systems where routine services are siloed from emergency prevention, preparedness, and response activities** |
| --- | --- | --- |
| **Adult vaccination** | Standing infrastructure (comparable to childhood EPI services) used to provide routine vaccinations (and preventive injectables) to key population groups and which can also be used to provide vaccines during an emegency/outbreak | Systems that have not strategically integrated adult vaccinations into routine primary care and only deliver adult vaccinations on an ad hoc basis. Therefore, when emergencies and outbreaks occur, there is a requirement for new infrastructure to be stood up to deliver the appropriate vaccinations. |
| **Clinical research** | Trial-agnostic infrastructure to conduct well-deigned and ethical clinical research and trials. This infrastructure has linkages with routine clinical care and can be used to conduct research and test medical countermeasures at speed during health emergencies. | Clinical research capabilities that are stood up for specific studies, without clear plans for sustainability or use after the specific study. Often, these capabilities are not maintained after the relevant study or research program is completed. During outbreaks and emergencies, there is not sufficient capacity for research using existing capabilities, so new capabilities need to be stood up. |
| **Pathogen surveillance** | Pathogen surveillance systems that leverage, as appropriate, routine clinical diagnostic workflows. As technology develops, these systems will be flexible enough to take a "pathogen-agnostic" approach to surveillance. These systems can also track and monitor the spread of diseases, including novel pathogens, during an outbreak or emergency and results can be shared with relevant stakeholders for emergency response. | A lack of core pathogen surveillance activities, training, and capabilities making the detection of pathogens at the point-of-care level challenging and delaying the Identification, tracking, and response to outbreaks and emergencies. |

*Source:* Original table compiled for this publication.

*Note:* EPI = Expanded Programme on Immunization.

This chapter argues that taking an Always On health approach that has use cases outside the context of emergencies will have more predictable funding, because it will provide reasons to use, and pay for, well-functioning health systems on a continual basis. Continuous funding for strong health systems is essential to guarantee both routine services and emergency PPR capabilities. Investments should support political leaders and the private sector to justify their investments in Always On systems with more predictable and visible utility, rather than providing only "insurance value" against hypothetical catastrophic events. In particular, political leaders can rationalize investments that improve health status, financial risk protection, and citizen satisfaction with the health system (Seidman and Atun 2016).

An Always On approach has relevance at the global, national, and subnational levels across countries of various income levels. It will help embed emergency response capacity in activities that support universal health coverage. Both academic research and strategic planning documents support the theoretical foundation for Always On capabilities. Examples of these frameworks include the World Health Organization (WHO) model for integrating Health Emergency Preparedness, Response, and Resilience, along with frameworks for Health System Strengthening, Pandemic Preparedness and Response, and universal health coverage (FCDO 2021, particularly figure B; Wenham et al. 2019; WHO 2022a, particularly figure 5). Despite that focus, the literature lacks information on how to operationalize such an approach for specific applications.

This chapter demonstrates the benefits and opportunities of applying an Always On approach to three applications of health care and public health: adult vaccination, clinical research, and pathogen surveillance.[1] These three applications highlight essential benefits for both routine health care and emergency PPR, are rapidly evolving because of recent advances in technology, and can have significant value for a country's life sciences industry (for example, research and development, and manufacturing of vaccines, therapeutics, diagnostics, and devices), which can generate sustained commitment from governments interested in economic growth and the private sector. The following sections provide an overview of each application and describe

- Evidence of population health and economic benefits from taking an Always On approach
- Key policy challenges and opportunities to advance the application
- Ethical considerations.

Subsequent sections discuss the importance of digital technology for supporting Always On systems as well as limitations and future directions.

## ADULT VACCINATION

The COVID-19 pandemic not only highlighted inadequate vaccine development, manufacturing, supply chains, and health care delivery systems for adult vaccinations but also showed the far-reaching public health benefits of prioritizing adult vaccination alongside childhood immunization (Williams et al. 2021). The risk now, however, is that these adult vaccine delivery systems are viewed as relevant only for COVID-19 and that the public and private sectors will fail to maintain them. Building robust and adaptable Always On adult vaccination infrastructure could address both endemic diseases and improve response to outbreaks, an approach consistent with WHO's Immunization Agenda 2030 (Wallace et al. 2022).

Critically, the portfolio of vaccines and preventive injectables for both infectious and noncommunicable diseases targeting adults has grown (Alkasir et al. 2022). Strengthening systems that provide routine vaccinations and preventive injectables to adults will be important for maximizing the population health impact of these products. Effectively deploying vaccines in the event of an outbreak will also require Always On adult vaccination systems. The Coalition for Epidemic Preparedness Innovation's 100 Days Mission aims to have vaccines ready for authorization and manufacturing at scale within 100 days of the identification of a pandemic pathogen (CEPI 2022). Despite that commendable target, the world risks having vaccines ready in the event of an outbreak without having the absorption capacity or infrastructure to deliver them, potentially leading to wasted doses similar to the experience of the COVID-19 response (Andersen et al. 2021; Lazarus et al. 2022). For example, in Nigeria, insufficient storage, challenges with health promotion, and accessibility issues resulted in the wastage of over a million doses of COVID-19 vaccines (Musa et al. 2023). Vaccine hesitancy also poses a significant risk to adoption of vaccines. In many countries, the rapid deployment of vaccines during the pandemic led to a missed opportunity to improve long-term service delivery challenges including digital platforms for vaccine tracking, strengthening of the cold chain, implementation of environmentally friendly delivery systems, and the building of public trust (World Bank 2021).

As low- and middle-income countries (LMICs) and the private sector invest in distributed vaccine and biologic manufacturing capacity as a health security measure, keeping manufacturing sites operational and financed will require use cases beyond manufacturing vaccines to respond to outbreaks. Gavi, the Vaccine Alliance, has determined that expanding demand for routine vaccines, both for approved products and those under development that use novel manufacturing platforms, could serve as sustainable business models for novel manufacturing sites (Gavi 2022). Given potentially limited demand for vaccine manufacturing in LMICs, a regionalized vaccine manufacturing approach may help ensure financial sustainability while countering vaccine nationalism. Achieving this expanded demand for vaccines and preventive injectables, including for adults, will require adequate budget, delivery systems, and acceptance of vaccines.

## Population Health and Economic Benefits

More than 10 million adult deaths across the globe are attributable to diseases with existing or forthcoming vaccines and preventive injectables (refer to annex 11A). Vaccinating individuals throughout the course of their life improves population-wide immunity for endemic diseases and improves general health within a population (Privor-Dumm et al. 2021). Vaccination efforts can target the most vulnerable individuals and high-risk groups, for example, by prioritizing the vaccination of health care workers or deploying ring vaccination strategies for those at high risk of disease due to close contact with an infected person (Doherty et al. 2022; Nanni et al. 2017; Swanson et al. 2015).

Importantly, because of the routine nature of select adult vaccinations, such as the seasonal flu vaccine in many countries and potentially COVID-19 or RSV vaccines going forward, adult vaccination systems can provide a point of engagement for individuals to engage with the health care system, often in community and primary care settings, to provide additional preventive services. This delivery infrastructure could bundle the delivery of multiple vaccines and preventive injectables with programs for, among others, high cholesterol, human immunodeficiency virus (HIV), psychiatric conditions, and family planning (Alkasir et al. 2022). These programs could rapidly adapt to incorporate new prevention tools that meet cost-effectiveness and efficacy thresholds (for example, R21/Matrix-M malaria vaccine, potential new TB vaccines, and siRNAs to both PCSK9 and angiotensinogen).

Packaging interventions that have shown cost-effectiveness, and supporting their co-delivery in the context of preventive services at the primary care and community levels, could improve coverage. "Above service delivery" costs (that is, costs to administer health programs not at the points of care) can represent 20–50 percent of all programmatic costs for immunization programs in Africa. Using routine health system capabilities to distribute bundled products would improve the per-unit and per-patient-treated cost of each program. Vaccination programs for working-age adults also minimize absenteeism, promoting a more productive and stable workforce, translating into increased economic output and higher economic resilience in the face of health crises (Quilici, Smith, and Signorelli 2015). (For a summary of cost-effectiveness evidence for specific adult vaccinations, refer to annex 11B.)

Adult vaccination programs also provide significant insurance value in their ability to prevent catastrophic events. Unfortunately classic health economic analyses—which focus only on gains in quality- or disability-adjusted life years and productivity—often miss that insurance value (Lakdawalla et al. 2018). One analysis conducted during the COVID-19 pandemic estimated that an adult vaccination program in the event of another, similar pandemic could save up to US$3.4 trillion in economic losses (Alkasir et al. 2022). However, determining the total value of adult vaccination systems, including insurance value and overall societal benefits, requires further research (Beck et al. 2022).

## Policy Challenges and Opportunities

Developing robust and cost-effective Always On adult vaccination systems will require a coordinated effort from multiple sectors. First, policy makers and researchers must consider broader socioeconomic benefits of adult vaccination, including workforce productivity, social value, and health care system resilience to pandemics (Beck et al. 2022). For example, WHO's Seasonal Influenza Vaccines guide for decision-makers highlights reduced burden of disease, stronger health system, and pandemic preparedness as benefits of such a program (WHO 2020b). Policy makers must also effectively communicate these benefits to the public. Focusing on Always On systems that will have more immediate preventive health benefits against common diseases could help normalize adult vaccination, as done previously for childhood vaccination.

Second, the ability to successfully deliver vaccines relies on patient acceptance and vaccine confidence, which has declined significantly across geographies since the COVID-19 pandemic (UNICEF 2023). Successfully generating demand for adult vaccinations and building sustainable systems that can rapidly pivot to provide vaccinations during outbreaks requires high vaccine confidence and standing systems that can meet demand. For example, the response to the mpox outbreak in the United States in 2022 successfully engaged target populations such as men who have sex with men (World Bank 2021). Unfortunately, supply initially could not meet the demand for vaccines because of insufficient delivery infrastructure, cold chain capacity, vaccine safety systems, and a suitably trained workforce (Dawson and Kates 2023). Encouraging such demand will require engaging with patient acceptance and vaccine confidence—not just during outbreaks but also as part of routine care—with tools such as public education, community engagement, and digital outreach tools.

To remain Always On, health systems will require continuous market access to affordable adult vaccines, particularly in LMICs. Although Gavi has gradually begun to expand its portfolio of vaccines into life course vaccination, most of its products target the under-five population, and Gavi remains rightfully committed to its mission of vaccinating children.[2] As more adult vaccinations and preventive injectables come onto the market, it will be important to ensure market access for target populations without setting prices so low as to jeopardize incentives for pharmaceutical innovation or manufacturing (Gartner 2015). The successful track record of market shaping for essential global health commodities provides a promising template for a similar approach for adult vaccinations. Identified market shaping approaches to support adult vaccinations (and other products, especially for LMICs) include (1) adding adult vaccinations to the WHO Essential Medicines List; (2) harmonizing product registration systems; (3) providing advance market commitments and demand/volume guarantees for manufacturers; (4) subsidizing the cost of manufacturing in LMICs; (5) pooling procurement for adult vaccines, and (6) creating demand among patients for adult vaccines (Berry et al. 2023).

Last, to ensure the financial sustainability of new manufacturing capacity for vaccines and injectables, that capacity should be used to manufacture vaccines for both routine care and outbreaks. It is unclear whether the level of demand for vaccines could sustain regional vaccine manufacturing, especially in Africa. Although investment decisions should remain the purview of individual countries, companies, and institutional investors, more transparent information about potential demand and supply for vaccines and manufacturing capacity could inform investment decisions (Berry et al. 2023).

### Ethical Considerations

Rollout of adult vaccinations must adhere to principles of harm prevention and fairness (Giubilini 2020). Although the ethical issues concerning dual-use adult vaccination systems for routine care and outbreak prevention do not substantively differ from ethical issues concerning vaccinations more broadly, it is important that the public health community reinforce key ethical considerations and principles as adult vaccines gain importance.

## CLINICAL RESEARCH INFRASTRUCTURE

The COVID-19 pandemic not only emphasized the importance of well-designed, randomized clinical trials and new methods to meet public health needs but also highlighted many fundamental issues that exist with the current system (Park et al. 2021). For example, the US Food and Drug Administration found during the pandemic that only 5 percent of 2,895 clinical trial arms were randomized and adequately powered (Bugin and Woodcock 2021). Outside of COVID-19, more than 50 percent of participants annually enter clinical trials with high risk of bias, at a cost of £8 billion (about US$10.35 billion) across 1,659 randomized trials (range: £725 million to £2.1 trillion, or about US$938 million to US$2.7 trillion) (Pirosca et al. 2022). Failure to recruit a sufficient number of patients accounts for one-third of all trial terminations in oncology (Zhang and DuBois 2023).

COVID-19 also demonstrated the power of clinical research infrastructure integrated into routine clinical care. Most notably, the United Kingdom–based RECOVERY trial leveraged such infrastructure to execute the world's largest clinical trial assessing treatment for patients hospitalized with COVID-19, which quickly identified life-saving treatments and those with no effect.[3] Other countries similarly used existing clinical research infrastructure for outbreak response. In Kenya, for example, the established research organization KEMRI led the COVID-19 response for testing (JICA 2021); in South Africa, dedicated HIV and TB research centers pivoted to COVID-19 genomic sequencing and participation in the Oxford-AstraZeneca trial (Nordling 2020).

Clinical research infrastructure, like other essential components of emergency PPR, needs to be Always On and embedded within clinical care. A start-stop approach to clinical research makes it difficult for sites to retain skilled staff and keep equipment operational (Lang et al. 2010). It also leaves sites ill-prepared to rapidly pivot to research during outbreaks and emergencies, a gap that will pose considerable challenges to achieving the Coalition for Epidemic Preparedness Innovation's 100 Days Mission. Africa, in particular, is underrepresented in global clinical research, accounting for approximately 15 percent of the global population and 23 percent of the global burden of disease, but less than 2 percent of all clinical trials globally (figure 11.1).

**Figure 11.1** Population, Disease Burden, and Representation in Clinical Trials, by Region

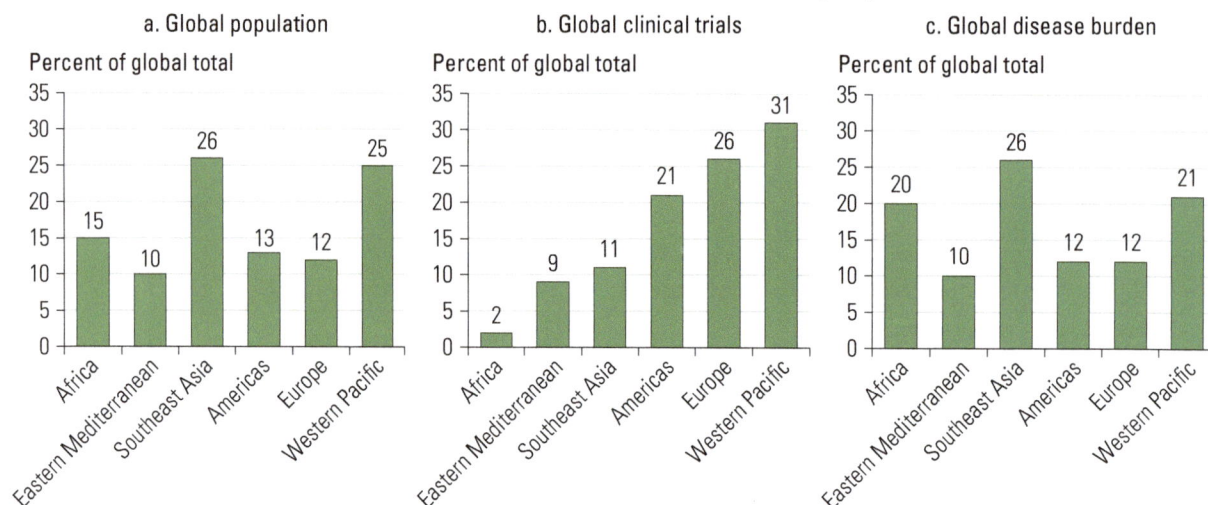

a. Global population

Percent of global total

b. Global clinical trials

Percent of global total

c. Global disease burden

Percent of global total

*Sources:* Original analysis based on Our World in Data, "Global Disease Burden by Region" (https://ourworldindata.org/grapher/disease-burden-by-region); WHO, "Number of Clinical Trials by Year, Country, WHO Region and Income Group (1999–2024)" (https://www.who.int/observatories/global-observatory-on-health-research-and-development/monitoring/number-of-clinical-trials-by-year-country-who-region-and-income-group); WHO 2023.

*Note:* Regions refer to World Health Organization (WHO) regions. Global clinical trials data and global disease burden data reflect 2019 statistics. Global population data reflect 2021 statistics.

Recognizing these challenges, the first WHO Clinical Trials Forum called for an "always on, always busy" clinical trials ecosystem with sufficient volume of research to maintain standing infrastructure between emergencies, and to rapidly pivot to research in an outbreak response (Moorthy et al. 2024). Although supporting that goal, this chapter, consistent with recommendations from the International Vaccines Task Force, emphasizes the importance of strengthening an ecosystem for clinical *research*, not just clinical *trials*. Many of the requirements for Always On clinical trial systems can be built into the context of other clinical research, such as epidemiological studies, real-world evidence and registry-based studies, and pharmacovigilance and surveillance (World Bank 2018).

### Population Health and Economic Benefits

When embedded within health care services, clinical research capacity enables researchers and policy makers to understand the true burden of disease, interpret outcomes, and analyze the impact of interventions. It also builds capacity to deal with diseases of public health concern, such as endemic infectious disease, and offers research experience to frontline staff. Evidence increasingly shows that the health care centers that prioritize clinical research have lower mortality rates and better patient outcomes (Ozdemir et al. 2015). Unfortunately, as noted earlier, certain geographies, especially in Africa and Southeast Asia, and patient population groups have a longstanding history of underrepresentation in clinical trials.

Investments in clinical research also generate strong economic returns for their countries. For example, Ireland, which has invested heavily in building its life sciences sector, received an average of £1.4 trillion (about US$1.8 trillion) in foreign direct investment in life sciences annually from 2012 to 2022, the second-highest level after the United States (DSIT and DHSC 2023). Research indicates that every dollar invested in clinical trials for infectious diseases in Kenya, South Africa, and India would generate a return of US$21, US$33, and US$67, respectively (Schäferhoff et al. 2022).

### Policy Challenges and Opportunities

An Always On approach to clinical research that can support ongoing work and rapidly pivot to address outbreaks and emergencies needs to have strong links with routine clinical care. The WHO Clinical Trials Forum recommends developing a "clinical trial unit maturity framework," which should specifically include Always On principles and capacity (Moorthy et al. 2024). Building on over a decade of investments in networks for clinical care and research, the European Union is investing in a comprehensive research network known as the European Clinical Research Alliance on Infectious Diseases to use perpetual observational studies and platform trials to keep a "warm base" network of clinical research sites operational (European Commission 2022).

Tremendous progress has been made in increasing donor-driven global health investment targeted at building capacity in LMICs, gradually shifting to more locally driven investment in research and development (Olufadewa, Adesina, and Ayorinde 2021). Expansion of the Africa Centres for Disease Control and Prevention and of the Africa Medicines Agency is helping strengthen regulatory and research capacity on the continent via a regional approach (Makoni 2021). As previously mentioned, however, Africa still hosts a disproportionately low percentage of the world's clinical trials. The current structure of global funding for clinical research perpetuates this disparity, limiting the availability of funding for core research infrastructure. For example, of all research and innovation projects funded by the European & Developing Countries Clinical Trials Partnership—a European Union–led effort "funding clinical research for medical tools to detect, treat and prevent poverty-related infectious diseases in sub-Saharan Africa"[4]—more than 60 percent of funding went to coordinating centers in Europe, the United Kingdom, and the United States (figure 11.2).[5] Although much of this funding may eventually have gone to countries in Africa, structuring funding in this way may have implications for the sustainability and coordination of funds reaching research sites.

Moreover, in a recent survey of more than 2,000 African researchers, participants listed institutional support as one of the primary barriers to clinical research (Lang et al., forthcoming; Wellcome Trust and TGHN 2024). Appropriate legal frameworks and institutional support will help overcome other limitations in clinical research capacity in LMICs, such as those identified by the International Vaccines Task Force: experienced clinical trials teams, appropriate space for trials, biobanking, data management systems, regulatory authority, and appropriate administrative functions (World Bank 2018). Overcoming those challenges will

**Figure 11.2** EDCTP2 Funding, by Country

Percent

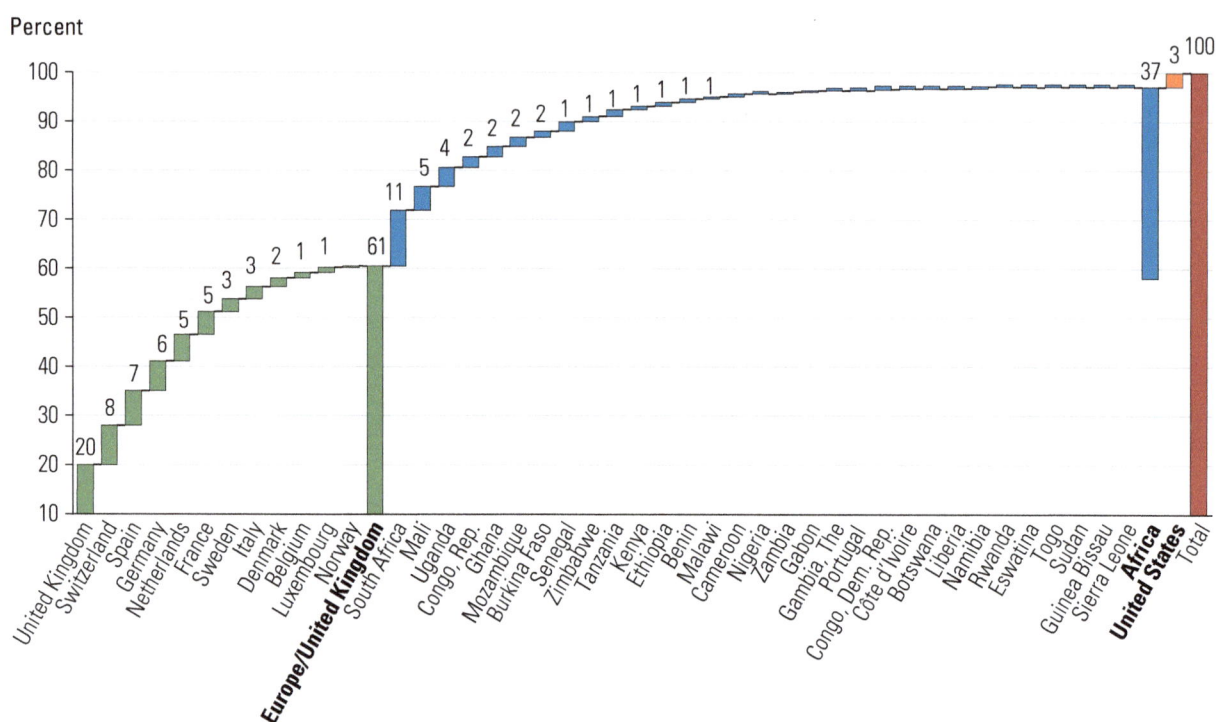

*Source:* Original analysis based on European & Developing Countries Clinical Trials Partnership, "Public Portal of EDCTP2-Funded Projects" (https://www.edctp.org/edctp2-project-portal/).

*Note:* Values rounded to nearest whole number. Values not shown for countries less than 0.5 percent. EDCTP2 = European & Developing Countries Clinical Trials Partnership, Second Programme (2014–24).

require government and institutional leadership, and investments in study-agnostic infrastructure (Lang et al. 2010). Those investments and infrastructure should build upon the strength of existing research sites that can integrate with routine care to recruit patients for research. As multiple sites continue to build capacity, a steadier and more predictable pipeline of clinical research funding to African institutions should help ensure sustainability of this infrastructure. Because of the likely insufficient pipeline to support financially sustainable infrastructure in all LMICs, however, regional coordination could help prioritize investments in clinical research capabilities where they are most likely to succeed, namely in countries with strong existing scientific and regulatory capabilities, and strong existing sites can support development of sites in neighboring countries.

## Ethical Considerations

All research should conform to globally accepted ethical principles and national laws. Establishing Always On clinical research in LMICs raises specific ethical concerns, particularly in LMICs where research frequently involves vulnerable populations and can have severe outcomes or mortality as endpoints (Lang et al. 2010). Substantial gaps exist between where drugs approved by the US Food and Drug Administration are tested and where they ultimately become available to patients, raising concerns about the equitable distribution of research benefits and market access (Miller et al. 2021). Finally, as more research becomes digitized, research sponsors will have to ensure that they have appropriate privacy and security safeguards in place to protect patient data.

## PATHOGEN SURVEILLANCE

The COVID-19 pandemic reinforced the importance of pathogen surveillance systems to provide near real-time information for the detection, tracking, and management of public health events (Ling-Hu et al. 2022; WHO 2022b). Unfortunately, it also revealed significant disparities in countries' abilities to conduct pathogen surveillance, including genomic surveillance, because of varying levels of prepandemic infrastructure, training, and capabilities (Inzaule et al. 2021; refer also to table 11.2 for an overview of relevant surveillance terminology). These issues included data quality, delays in reporting, and an inability to link surveillance data to individual cases (Price et al. 2023).

An Always On system leverages routine diagnosis to support pathogen surveillance when possible, rather than operating in a parallel system. At its most basic level, it involves provider reporting of notifiable conditions, including infectious diseases and cancers, to public health agencies.[6] As diagnostic technologies continue to progress, they have the ability to improve clinical management of patients, reduce oversubscribing of unnecessary antibiotics (potentially helping slow antimicrobial resistance), and contribute data to pathogen programs surveillance (Salami et al. 2020).

In particular, next generation sequencing, which can clearly define pathogen relationships and rapidly identify genetic and functional associations, can support both pathogen surveillance and day-to-day management of certain diseases (Rantsiou et al. 2018; WHO 2022b). The introduction of more affordable genomic sequencing tools and the subsequent decentralization of national platforms have begun to expand countries' surveillance capacities, with the potential to enable sequencing to take place in diverse and remote settings (Price et al. 2023). As clinical applications of genomic sequencing expand—namely, to test drug susceptibility of infectious diseases—the resulting clinical-grade genomic data could also contribute to broader public health surveillance and inform treatments for infectious diseases and cancers (Marquart, Chen, and Prasad 2018).

**Table 11.2** Pathogen Surveillance Definitions

| Pathogen surveillance term | Definition |
|---|---|
| **Next generation sequencing** | Technology able to identify nucleic acid sequence data (DNA and RNA) rapidly and cost-effectively |
| **Whole genome sequencing** | Technique used to establish the full genetic makeup of an organism |
| **Metagenomic sequencing** | Untargeted approach to genomic sequencing directly from an environmental or clinical sample used to identify all present organisms |

*Sources:* Gardy and Loman 2018; Rantsiou et al. 2018.

Investments in genomic infrastructure during the COVID-19 pandemic could be leveraged and pivoted toward more pathogen-agnostic approaches. Metagenomic sequencing involves the reading of all genetic material from a sample, permitting the unbiased detection of both known and unknown pathogens. The technique makes it possible to detect novel pathogen spread early, potentially enabling timely containment of outbreaks and effective suppression of transmission. For example, Liberia successfully used metagenomic capabilities while managing an unexpected outbreak of meningococcal disease in 2017. The country quickly identified the sequence type, linked to a hypervirulent strain with unusual presentation and a high fatality rate (Bozio et al. 2018). Clinical metagenomic sequencing could also aid diagnosis for certain patients with polymicrobial or difficult-to-identify infections (Chiu and Miller 2019).

### Population Health and Economic Benefits

Always On real-time reporting of certain notifiable conditions diagnosed in the clinic to public health agencies will support effective outbreak investigation and response. Building from this approach, genomics data that are routinely collected in clinical care can and should feed into larger data sets that will make it easier to identify novel pathogens or variants of concern, and help understand the spread of a disease within a population (Gardy and Loman 2018). The United Kingdom demonstrated the utility of such a system when it began integrating genomic testing into the routine clinical diagnosis of selected diseases to support outbreak response for gastrointestinal illnesses in 2012 (Grant et al. 2018). In 2022, the United Kingdom's routine sequencing of all presumptive salmonella cases led to the identification of a salmonella disease cluster in children. The quick sharing of genomic data with neighboring countries, which linked to chocolate products originating from a factory in Belgium, led to a comprehensive outbreak response, including product recall to prevent further transmission (UKHSA 2022).

Pathogen surveillance infrastructure, including genomic sequencing, can be flexible enough to support response to outbreaks from multiple pathogens. The Democratic Republic of Congo built up genomic sequencing capacity and infrastructure during the 2018 Ebola outbreak and then maintained the system, allowing a rapid response to the COVID-19 pandemic. It provided COVID-19 surveillance support to surrounding countries and was one of the first countries to share sequencing data on a public database in March 2020, two weeks after its first case was reported. The Democratic Republic of Congo's infrastructure has also been able to pivot to support several other public health emergencies such as malaria, mpox, and polio, emphasizing the flexibility and utility of pathogen-agnostic surveillance (WHO 2022c). Similarly, countries with strong diagnostic infrastructure for TB, such as GeneXpert, could pivot and use their equipment to concurrently test for COVID-19 and other respiratory pathogens—as both Guinea and Nigeria have done successfully (Soe-Lin, Bowen, and Hecht 2024).

These examples show the potential for genomic sequencing infrastructure beyond the borders of a single country, with regional coordination of both equipment and human resources potentially strengthening surveillance capabilities. Regional efforts like the Africa Centres for Disease Control and Prevention's Integrated Genomic Surveillance and Data Sharing Platform, and Integrated Genomic Surveillance for Outbreak Detection show the promise of this approach (Africa CDC 2024). However, regional coordination would also require robust regulatory frameworks for sample sharing and protection of personal health information.

The cost-effectiveness and economic value of pathogen surveillance requires further research, particularly because the total costs of outbreaks and pandemics are difficult to estimate and vary widely (de Vries et al. 2021; Herida, Dervaux, and Desenclos 2016). Additionally, accounting for positive externalities of surveillance systems in cost-effectiveness analyses, and understanding best approaches for implementing novel technologies, will be important to leverage investments in clinical diagnostic infrastructure, especially for applications in LMICs (Price et al. 2023).

Sharma et al. (2023) estimate the costs of metagenomics to detect a novel respiratory pathogen as part of routine surveillance for patients with influenza-like illness across emergency departments in the United States. They estimate that, with 30 percent population coverage, their modeled metagenomic surveillance system has a 95 percent chance of detecting a novel respiratory pathogen with COVID-19 characteristics after approximately 10 emergency department presentations. Despite the considerable costs of implementing such a system (between US$400 million and US$800 million annually for the United States, compared to an annual budget for the US Centers for Disease Control and Prevention's Advanced Molecular Detection program of only US$35 million), it could significantly reduce the expected losses from pandemics.[7]

The application of these genomic systems and their cost-effectiveness needs to be better understood in LMICs. Efforts to reduce the cost of genomic tests through negotiations with manufacturers and multiplexing will play an important role in making this technology more accessible (Marais, Hardie, and Brink 2022). LMICs could adapt and build on existing infectious disease genomic infrastructure to start metagenomic surveillance, and scale coverage as technology and affordability improve.

## Policy Challenges and Opportunities

Sustaining pathogen surveillance systems and adapting to novel technologies will face several challenges. Historically, policy makers have undervalued the importance of pathogen surveillance systems because the benefits of such systems are hidden in insurance value (that is, the avoidance of catastrophic events and costs), which would go unnoticed until the system fails. Undervaluing leads to limited political engagement and financial commitment from governments to maintain systems outside of outbreak contexts (Ling-Hu et al. 2022; WHO 2022b). In LMICs, reliance on external grant-based funding for time- and priority-restricted pathogen surveillance activities can lead to duplication and tends to ignore local disease priorities (Mfuh, Abanda, and Titanji 2023). Researchers and policy makers should better assess the economic case for pathogen surveillance and invest appropriately.

Surveillance systems, including workflows between clinical diagnosis and reporting, are often fragmented, and infrastructure and capacity vary between and within countries, particularly but not only in LMICs (Bentley and Lo 2021). Data collection needs to be interoperable and standardized, with the appropriate governance frameworks in place to allow for the sharing of data nationally, regionally, and globally (Nicholls et al. 2021).

Metagenomics as an emerging approach will be especially important with its broad application to health, but the high cost of the technology may restrict widespread adoption (Chiu and Miller 2019). Governments should invest in and incentivize the development of novel technologies that would reduce the cost and increase the speed of pathogen surveillance, including using metagenomic approaches.

Last, global data sharing platforms must have the appropriate legal and regulatory mechanisms to ensure integrity and transparency, and to guarantee that scientists receive appropriate credit for their work (Lenharo 2023).

### Ethical Considerations

Pathogen surveillance systems that collect individual patient data need to adhere to ethical data sharing principles when analyzing and exchanging information (Crook and Fingerhut 2022). Secure data sharing is of particular importance when dealing with sensitive disease conditions and vulnerable populations. International data sharing should avoid unintended negative consequences such as border closures or trade restrictions, as experienced by South Africa after sharing SARS-CoV-2 Omicron data (Gardy and Loman 2018; Joi 2022). Governing bodies such as WHO should implement incentives to share data, which would encourage countries to collaborate and would prevent withholding of crucial data, as witnessed during the avian influenza A (H5N1) outbreak in 2006, when Indonesia withheld virus information because of controversy around the development of vaccines without consent or assurances for access (Fidler 2008).

## DIGITAL OPPORTUNITIES

Achieving Always On systems, including for the three applications described in this chapter, will require implementation of appropriate digital systems. Given the overlapping and mutually reinforcing value of health data and digital technology, countries should strive to adopt integrated enterprise architecture for Always On systems. That approach is consistent with recommendations from WHO and policy proposals at the Group of Twenty (Seidman et al. 2023; WHO 2020a).

For adult vaccinations, digital tools can offer an integrated ecosystem to optimize vaccination campaigns, including electronic immunization registries, appointment registration, patient communication, clinical trial enrollment, integration of diagnostics and labs data, clinical decision support, population targeting, collection of real-world evidence, and supply chain monitoring (Alkasir et al. 2023).[8]

For clinical research, digital solutions—including linking trial data to electronic health records, electronic data capture, and decentralized trials—can yield 3–13 percent cost savings for a given trial (Sertkaya et al. 2014) (refer to figure 11.3). Digital health has particularly large potential to drive cost savings in health systems in Africa, using digital solutions including virtual interactions, paperless data, workflow automation, decision intelligence systems, patient self-care, and patient self-service. Digital decentralized clinical trials can strengthen community engagement using a digital approach and can enhance equity (McKinsey & Company 2023).

Pathogen surveillance, including for genomics data, requires a well-defined minimum set of data and the ability to electronically report cases (Crook

**Figure 11.3** Cost Saving and Performance Improvements due to Digital Technologies

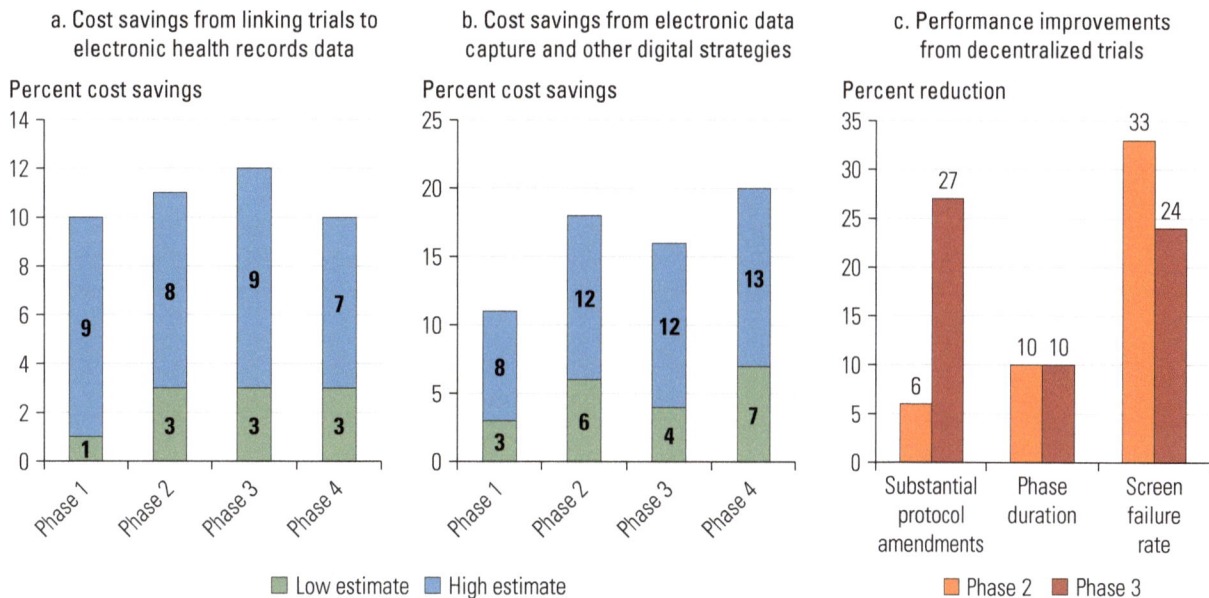

a. Cost savings from linking trials to electronic health records data

b. Cost savings from electronic data capture and other digital strategies

c. Performance improvements from decentralized trials

Low estimate    High estimate

Phase 2    Phase 3

*Sources:* Sertkaya et al. 2014; Tufts Center for the Study of Drug Development 2022.

*Note:* Phases 1–3 refer to clinical drug development phases, and phase 4 refers to postmarket studies.

and Fingerhut 2022). For the data to be actionable, they must be collated in a standardized manner regardless of the surveillance platforms and techniques used to gather the information, with common vocabularies and harmonized processes throughout (Nicholls et al. 2021; WHO 2022b). Interoperability of data sets enables successful harmonization for the analysis and sharing of the metadata at local, national, and global levels. Only with adequate digital systems can researchers and health systems appropriately share data while maintaining privacy and security of personal health information. Various researchers have identified case studies of successful digital applications in global health.[9]

## LIMITATIONS AND FUTURE DIRECTIONS

Always On presents a novel approach that will require practical considerations for implementation. The three applications presented in this chapter share two limitations—resource allocation and political economy.

All countries, particularly LMICs, face resource constraints and limited fiscal space for publicly funded health service delivery and public health. Even high-income countries such as the United States face challenges related to stop-start funding cycles for public health (Bipartisan Policy Center 2021). Cross-sectional analyses have found capability gaps in LMICs for all three of the applications described in this chapter: vaccine deployment, clinical research, and genomic-informed pathogen surveillance (Inzaule et al. 2021; World Bank 2018, 2021).

Despite meaningful and evidence-based means to improve fiscal space for health—including economic growth, budget reprioritization, and efficiency improvements—countries will nonetheless continue to face budget shortfalls for health care. Further, there will always be opportunity costs for public sector investments, and it is difficult, if not impossible, to measure allocative efficiency while considering the insurance value of health systems investments. Often, political priorities, rather than efficiency arguments, drive decisions about resource allocation, financial and otherwise (Seidman and Atun 2016).

Although COVID-19 focused attention on the importance of health systems, and helped justify investments in them, securing additional funding for emergency PPR beyond the pandemic will require elevating other health issues (Fox and Reich 2015). Always On systems with dual-use capabilities will address barriers and allow citizens to benefit outside of emergency contexts, ensuring that the value of investments are maximized to address multiple health problems without requiring a political opening for investment via an outbreak or emergency.

Testing the hypothesis that an Always On approach can help overcome some of the resource allocation and political economy barriers to investing in health systems will require much additional research, implementation science, and country examples. To address these barriers, this chapter proposes the following:

- **Adult vaccination.** Studying the cost-effectiveness of a new delivery models including the "bundling" of vaccines
- **Clinical research.** Investigation into the economic and political benefits of investing in clinical research capabilities to increase funding for research
- **Pathogen surveillance.** Use of implementation science and economic analysis to establish the best pathways to integrate new surveillance technologies into clinical and public health workflows.

Additional implementation considerations cut across all three applications. Although a full treatment of these considerations is beyond the scope of this chapter, researchers and practitioners should consider planning, monitoring, and evaluation with a focus on how Always On systems and dual-use functionality differ from traditional health systems strengthening. They could consider the following relevant questions, among others:

- How should the implementation of functionalities be phased?
- How can available financing be leveraged, and what cost savings are incurred by taking an Always On approach?
- What is the comparative cost-effectiveness of Always On approaches?
- How should capacity building be sequenced to ensure talent and institutions have the full set of capabilities for dual-use functionality?
- How can we ensure that Always On approaches are integrated into existing or novel global health frameworks and with global multilateral organizations, such as the Coalition for Epidemic Preparedness Innovation, Gavi, and WHO?

## CONCLUSION

As we reflect on lessons learned during the COVID-19 pandemic, we must take advantage of the opportunities that event has provided the globe. This chapter has described important health, economic, and political aspects of building Always On health care and public health systems. Always On systems have dual-use functionality; they incorporate emergency and pandemic preparedness into routine health care and public health activities. However, much work remains to define the details of Always On systems, including for applications not described in this chapter (such as climate-resilient health care delivery); to test the best way to implement these systems; and to scale this approach.

# ANNEX 11A. ADULT DEATHS ATTRIBUTABLE TO DISEASES OR RISK FACTORS WITH ADULT VACCINATIONS AND PREVENTIVE INJECTABLES

| Status of vaccine or preventive injectable | Disease | Deaths (thousands) | Year | Notes | Source |
|---|---|---|---|---|---|
| Approved product | Pneumococcal pneumonia | 889 (515–1,316) | 2019 | Assumes 50 percent (29–74 percent) of 1.78 million deaths attributable to lower-respiratory tract infections attributable to pneumococcal pneumonia. | GBD 2016 Lower Respiratory Infections Collaborators 2018 |
| | Influenza | At least 260 (187–333) | 2002–11 (average) | Includes only deaths among population ages 65 and older. Total annual deaths estimated at 389,000 (239,980–518,230). | Paget et al. 2019 |
| | Cervical cancer | 280 | 2019 | | |
| | COVID-19[a] | — | | Age-stratified number of deaths due to COVID-19 not available. Approximately 1.3 million deaths due to COVID-19 in 2022. | IHME[b] |
| | High LDL cholesterol | 4,400 | 2019 | | |
| | Ebola[a] | 3 | 2019 | | |
| | Herpes zoster | 7.8 | 2019 | | |
| | Dengue | 25 | 2019 | | |
| | Meningitis | 101 | 2019 | | |
| | Respiratory syncytial virus | 57 (41–78) | 2019 | Assumes 3.2 percent (2.3–4.4 percent) of 1.78 million deaths attributable to lower-respiratory tract infections attributable to pneumococcal pneumonia. | GBD 2016 Lower Respiratory Infections Collaborators 2018 |
| In clinical development | Tuberculosis | 1,309 | 2019 | Includes HIV/AIDS-related deaths caused by tuberculosis. | |
| | Malaria | 247 | 2019 | | |
| | ETEC and Shigella | 276 | 2015 | Includes all deaths in individuals over five years of age. | Anderson et al. 2019 |
| | Group B streptococcus | 147 | 2015 | Stillbirths and infant deaths. | Seale et al. 2017 |
| | Cholera | — | | Age-stratified number of deaths due to cholera not available. Approximately 117,167 deaths due to cholera in 2019. | Ilic and Ilic 2023 |
| | Leishmaniasis | 2.4 | 2019 | | |
| | Schistomosiasis | 11.1 | 2019 | | |
| | Typhoid | 44 | 2019 | | |
| | Salmonella infections | 15 | 2019 | | |
| | HIV | 594 | 2019 | Excludes tuberculosis-related deaths to avoid double-counting. Includes maternal deaths aggravated by HIV/AIDS. | |
| | Parathyphoid | 11 | 2019 | | |
| | Chikungunya | — | | Age-stratified number of deaths due to chikungunya not available. | |

*table continues next page*

| Status of vaccine or preventive injectable | Disease | Deaths (thousands) | Year | Notes | Source |
|---|---|---|---|---|---|
| In clinical development | Zika[a] | Limited number of deaths | 2019 | | |
| | MERS[a] | Limited number of deaths | 2022 | | WHO Regional Office for the Eastern Mediterranean 2022 |
| | Hepatitis C | 541 | 2019 | | |
| | Rheumatic fever | 300 | 2019 | | |
| | Lassa fever[a] | — | | Age-stratified number of deaths due to Lassa fever not available. About 5,000 deaths due to Lassa fever occur annually. | US Centers for Disease Control and Prevention[c] |

*Source:* All statistics for deaths come from the Institute for Health Metrics and Evaluation (IHME) Global Burden of Disease database ("GBD Results," https://vizhub.healthdata.org/gbd-results/) and include deaths for individuals aged 15 and older, unless otherwise specified in the notes and references.

*Note:* ETEC = Enterotoxigenic *Escherichia coli;* HIV/AIDS = human immunodeficiency virus and acquired immune deficiency syndrome; LDL = low-density lipoprotein; MERS = Middle East respiratory syndrome; — = not available.

a. Indicates World Health Organization (WHO) priority diseases that have epidemic potential or the unavailability of sufficient medical countermeasures; refer to WHO, "Prioritizing Diseases for Research and Development in Emergency Contexts" (accessed August 29, 2023). https://www.who.int/activities/prioritizing-diseases-for-research-and-development-in-emergency-contexts.

b. IHME, "COVID-19 Projections" (accessed August 29, 2023), https://covid19.healthdata.org/global?view=cumulative-deaths&tab=trend.

c. US Centers for Disease Control and Prevention, "About Lassa Fever," https://www.cdc.gov/lassa-fever/about/index.html.

# ANNEX 11B. SUMMARY OF COST-EFFECTIVENESS RESEARCH FOR SELECT ADULT VACCINES

**Table 11B.1** Approved Vaccines

| Disease | Geography | Main outcome metric | Findings and source |
|---|---|---|---|
| Influenza | Multiple LMICs | Systematic review | "Influenza vaccination provided value for money for elderly, infants, adults and children with high-risk conditions. Vaccination was cost-effective and cost-saving for COPD patients and elderly above 65 years from model-based evaluations, but conclusions from RCTs on elderly varied" (Ott et al. 2013). |
| Pneumococcal pneumonia | Multiple LMICs, primarily South America | Systematic review | "Compared with no vaccination, either PPSV23 or PCV13 was economically favorable, highly cost-effective, and in many cases, cost-saving for older adults" (Shao and Stoecker 2020). |
| Pertussis (one component of DTaP vaccine) | Bangladesh, Brazil, and Nigeria | Cost per DALY | "Maternal aP immunization would be cost-effective in Brazil, a middle-income country, under the base-case assumptions, but would be very expensive at infant vaccination coverage in and above the threshold range necessary to eliminate the disease (90–95%). Scenarios representing low-income countries showed that maternal aP immunization could be cost-saving in countries with low infant coverage, such as Nigeria, but very expensive in countries, such as Bangladesh, with high infant coverage" (Kim et al. 2021). |
| Herpes zoster | HICs only | Systematic review | "A majority of studies of ZVL found it to be cost-effective compared with no vaccine using the authors' chosen willingness-to-pay thresholds" [Chiyaka et al. 2019). The high prices observed in HICs mean that these findings are likely not generalizable to LMICs. |
| HPV | Multiple HICs and LMICs | Mean cost per FIG | Cost-effectiveness of the HPV vaccine is widely accepted, and various service delivery strategies can reduce the cost per FIG (Akumbom et al. 2022). |
| RSV | Gavi-eligible countries | Effectiveness and cost-effectiveness of maternal vaccination | "Maternal vaccination would prevent 1.2 million cases [95% PI 0.6–1.9 million], 104 thousand hospital admissions [95% PI 19–309 thousand], and 3 thousand deaths [95% PI 1–11 thousand] in those countries. It can avert 98 thousand discounted DALYs [95% PI 16–308 thousand] and 186 million USD [95% PI 144–206 million]. The mAb strategy would prevent more cases and avert more discounted DALYs and treatment costs). However, the mAb strategy would also result in higher discounted net costs compared to the maternal strategy due to the assumed higher intervention costs (6 USD vs. 3 USD)" (Li et al. 2020). |

*Source:* Original table for this report compiled using the sources cited in the table.

*Note:* COPD = chronic obstructive pulmonary disease; DALY = disability-adjusted life year; FIG = fully immunized girl; HIC = high-income country; HIV = human immunodeficiency virus; HPV = human papillomavirus; LMICs = low- and middle-income countries; RCT = randomized controlled trial; RSV = Respiratory syncytial virus.

**Table 11B.2** Vaccines Currently under Development

| Disease | Country studies | Main outcome metric | Findings and sources |
|---|---|---|---|
| HIV | LMICs | Cost per QALY | An HIV/AIDS vaccine would need to cost below US$20–US$40 per regimen, depending on scale-up and other scenarios (Harmon et al. 2016). |
| Group B streptococcus | 37 countries in Sub-Saharan Africa | Cost per DALY for maternal vaccination | "Maternal GBS immunization could be a cost-effective intervention in low-income sub-Saharan Africa, with cost-effectiveness ratios similar to other recently introduced vaccines. The vaccination cost at which introduction is cost-effective depends on disease incidence and vaccine efficacy" (Russell et al. 2017). |
| Tuberculosis | LMICs | DALY | Depending on the efficacy of the vaccine, a tuberculosis vaccine "targeted at adolescents/adults could be cost-effective at $4, $9, and $20 per dose in low-, lower-middle–, and upper-middle– income countries, respectively" (Knight et al. 2014). |

*Source:* Original table for this report compiled using the sources cited in the table.

*Note:* DALY = disability-adjusted life year; GBS = Group B streptococcus; HIV/AIDS = human immunodeficiency virus and acquired immune deficiency syndrome; LMICs = low- and middle-income countries; QALY = quality-adjusted life year.

## NOTES

1. Refer also to the Tony Blair Institute for Global Change's "Global Health Security Consortium" web page, https://institute.global/tags/global-health-security-consortium.
2. Gavi, "Vaccine Investment Strategy 2024" (accessed August 24, 2023), https://www.gavi .org/our-alliance/strategy/vaccine-investment-strategy-2024.
3. UK Research and Innovation, "The RECOVERY Trial" (accessed October 8, 2023), https:// www.ukri.org/who-we-are/how-we-are-doing/research-outcomes-and-impact/mrc/recovery -trial-identifies-covid-19-treatments/.
4. From the European & Developing Countries Clinical Trials Partnership's home page, https://www.edctp.org.
5. European & Developing Countries Clinical Trials Partnership, "Public Portal of EDCTP2- Funded Projects" (accessed August 24, 2023), https://www.edctp.org/edctp2-project-portal/.
6. Refer to US Centers for Disease Control and Prevention, "Elecronic Case Reporting (eCR)," https://www.cdc.gov/ecr/php/about/?CDC_AAref_Val=https://www.cdc.gov/ecr /what-is-ecr.html.
7. US Centers for Disease Control and Prevention, "National Investment Maps" (accessed August 24, 2023), https://www.cdc.gov/advanced-molecular-detection/php/investments /maps.html?CDC_AAref_Val=https://www.cdc.gov/amd/investments/maps.html.
8. For additional sources, refer to Gavi, "Gavi Digital Health Information Strategy Technical Brief Series," https://www.gavi.org/programmes-impact/our-impact/evaluation-studies /gavi-digital-health-information-strategy-technical-brief-series.
9. For one set of case studies on best practices in digital health applications, refer to Exemplars in Global Health, "Digital Health Tools," https://www.exemplars.health /emerging-topics/epidemic-preparedness-and-response/digital-health-tools.

## REFERENCES

Africa CDC (Africa Centres for Disease Control and Prevention). 2024. "Africa CDC Launches Initiatives to Advance Molecular Diagnostics and Genomic Surveillance in Africa." Press release, April 24, 2024. https://africacdc.org/news-item/africa-cdc-launches -initiatives-to-advance-molecular-diagnostics-and-genomic-surveillance-in-africa/.

Akumbom, Alvine M., Jennifer J. Lee, Nancy R. Reynolds, Winter Thayer, Jinglu Wang, and Eric Slade. 2022. "Cost and Effectiveness of HPV Vaccine Delivery Strategies: A Systematic Review." *Preventive Medicine Reports* 26 (April): 101734. https://doi.org/10.1016/j.pmedr .2022.101734.

Alkasir, Ahmad, Tamsin Berry, Paul Blakeley, Henry Lishi Li, Gabriel Seidman, and Emily Stanger Sfeile. 2023. "A Vision for Global Health: The Digital Toolbox Needed to Deliver One Shot." Global Health Security Consortium. https://assets.ctfassets.net /75ila1cntaeh/3Ha8OUugohTodgSJ6yv5Tj/2a1f56f575c373b3016087b4f86c1bfa/GHSC _One_Shot__Digital_Tools__January_2023_0.pdf.

Alkasir, Ahmad, Tamsin Berry, David Britto, James Browne, Romina Mariano, Gabriel Seidmanm, Daniel Sleat, et al. 2022. "A Global Opportunity to Combat Preventable Disease: How to Use Covid-19 Infrastructure to Transform Public Health Worldwide." Tony Blair Institute for Global Change, Lawrence J. Ellison Institute for Transformative Medicine of USC, and University of Oxford. https://assets.ctfassets .net/75ila1cntaeh/6NUfXY4ghKx5YtPuaSefJl/67d49c718d2ccb36b778fa3aa8347293 /GHSC__A_Global_Opportunity_to_Combat_Preventable_Disease__January_2022.pdf.

Andersen, Hayley, Tamsin Berry, David Britto, Joanna de Boer, Romina Mariano, Brianna Miller, Gabriel Seidman, et al. 2021. "The Absorption-Capacity Challenge." Tony Blair Institute for Global Change and Lawrence J. Ellison Institute for Transformative Medicine of USC. https://assets.ctfassets.net/75ila1cntaeh/2s0aLIDguBTeA0KUxxDfde /e4fb567fde7d6e5053628fe800de9f07/Global_Health_Security_Consortium__The _Absorption-Capacity_Challenge__August_2021.pdf.

Anderson, John D., Karoun H. Bagamian, Farzana Muhib, Mirna P. Amaya, Lindsey A. Laytner, Thomas Wierzba, and Richard Rheingans. 2019. "Burden of Enterotoxigenic Escherichia coli and Shigella Non-fatal Diarrhoeal Infections in 79 Low-Income and Lower Middle-Income Countries: A Modelling Analysis." *The Lancet Global Health* 7 (3): e321–30.

Beck, Ekkehard, Eliana Biundo, Nancy Devlin, T. Mark Doherty, Antonio J. Garcia-Ruiz, Maarten Postma, Shazia Sheikh, et al. 2022. "Capturing the Value of Vaccination within Health Technology Assessment and Health Economics: Literature Review and Novel Conceptual Framework." *Vaccine* 40 (30): 4008–16.

Bentley, Stephen D., and Stephanie W. Lo. 2021. "Global Genomic Pathogen Surveillance to Inform Vaccine Strategies: A Decade-Long Expedition in Pneumococcal Genomics." *Genome Medicine* 13 (1): 84.

Berry, Tamsin, Paul Blakeley, Adam Bradshaw, Henry Lishi Li, Gabriel Seidman, Emily Stanger Sfeile, and Chema Triki. 2023. "A Vision for Global Health: How Demand Forecasting, Supply Planning and Market Shaping Can Deliver a New Model for Global Vaccine Manufacturing." Tony Blair Institute for Global Change, Lawrence J. Ellison Institute for Transformative Medicine of USC, and University of Oxford. https://assets.ctfassets .net/75ila1cntaeh/5JYzbOPJMQbZ3wZmquUB7A/0538bc7e3e75c8431c625119e0262273 /Tony_Blair_Institute_GHSC_One_Shot_Vaccine_Manufacturing_May_2023.pdf.

Bipartisan Policy Center. 2021. "Positioning America's Public Health System for the Next Pandemic." Bipartisan Policy Center, Washington, DC. https://bipartisanpolicy.org/report /preparing-for-the-next-pandemic/.

Bozio, Catherine H., Jeni Vuong, E. Kainne Dokubo, Mosoka P. Fallah, Lucy A. McNamara, Caelin C. Potts, John Doedeh, et al. 2018. "Outbreak of Neisseria Meningitidis Serogroup C outside the Meningitis Belt–Liberia, 2017: An Epidemiological and Laboratory Investigation." *The Lancet Infectious Diseases* 18 (12): 1360–67. https://doi.org/10.1016 /s1473-3099(18)30476-6.

Bugin, Kevin, and Janet Woodcock. 2021. "Trends in COVID-19 Therapeutic Clinical Trials." *Nature Reviews Drug Discovery*, Biobusiness Brief, February 25, 2021. https://www.nature .com/articles/d41573-021-00037-3.

CEPI (Coalition for Epidemic Preparedness Innovations). 2022. "Delivering Pandemic Vaccines in 100 Days: What Will It Take?" CEPI, Washington, DC. https://static.cepi.net /downloads/2024-02/CEPI-100-Days-Report-Digital-Version_29-11-22.pdf.

Chiu, Charles Y., and Steven A. Miller. 2019. "Clinical Metagenomics." *Nature Reviews Genetics* 20 (6): 341–55.

Chiyaka, Edward T., Van T. Nghiem, Lu Zhang, Abhishek Deshpande, Patricia Dolan Mullen, and Phuc Le. 2019. "Cost-Effectiveness of Herpes Zoster Vaccination: A Systematic Review." *Pharmacoeconomics* 37: 169–200.

Crook, Derrick, and Henry Fingerhut 2022. "Global Governance of Genomic Pathogen Surveillance Opportunities and Challenges." Tony Blair Institute for Global Change, London. https://assets .ctfassets.net/75ila1cntaeh/6SQyBJPNAKwQGpCoXS34qz/8c734f522305de9eac0e687c8be1f9d3 /Global_Health_Security_Consortium__Global_Governance_of_Genomic_Pathogen _Surveillance__June_2022.pdf.

Dawson, Lindsey, and Jennifer Kates. 2023. "Mpox One Year Later: Where Is the U.S. Today?" Kaiser Family Foundation, Global Health Policy, May 17, 2023. https://www.kff.org/global -health-policy/issue-brief/mpox-one-year-later-where-is-the-u-s-today/.

de Vries, Linda, Marion Koopmans, Alec Morton, and Pieter van Baal. 2021. "The Economics of Improving Global Infectious Disease Surveillance." *BMJ Global Health* 6 (9). https://doi .org/10.1136/bmjgh-2021-006597.

Doherty, Mark T., Emmanuel Aris, Nathalie Servotte, and Ekkehard Beck. 2022. "Capturing the Value of Vaccination: Impact of Vaccine-Preventable Disease on Hospitalization." *Aging Clinical and Experimental Research* 34 (7): 1551–61. https://doi.org/10.1007/s40520 -022-02110-2.

DSIT (UK Department for Science, Innovation and Technology) and DHSC (UK Department of Health & Social Care). 2023. "Life Sciences Competitiveness Indicators, 2023." UK Government. https://www.gov.uk/government/publications/life-sciences-sector-data-2023 /life-sciences-competitiveness-indicators-2023.

European Commission. 2022. "European Clinical Research Alliance on Infectious Diseases (ECRAID): Business Plan." European Commission. https://cordis.europa.eu/project /id/825715/results.

FCDO (Foreign, Commonwealth & Development Office). 2021. "Health Systems Strengthening for Global Health Security and Universal Health Coverage." FCDO Position Paper, FCDO, London. https://assets.publishing.service.gov.uk/government/uploads /system/uploads/attachment_data/file/1039209/Health-Systems-Strengthening-Position -Paper.pdf.

Fidler, David P. 2008. "Influenza Virus Samples, International Law, and Global Health Diplomacy." Emerging Infectious Diseases 14 (1). https://doi.org/10.3201/eid1401.070700.

Fox, Ashley, and Michael Reich. 2015. "The Politics of Universal Health Coverage in Low- and Middle-Income Countries: A Framework for Evaluation and Action." *Journal of Health Politics, Policy and Law* 40 (5): 1023–60. https://doi.org/10.1215/03616878-3161198.

Gardy, Jennifer L., and Nicholas J. Loman. 2018. "Towards a Genomics-Informed, Real-Time, Global Pathogen Surveillance System." *Nature Reviews Genetics* 19 (1): 9–20. https://doi .org/10.1038/nrg.2017.88.

Gartner, David. 2015. "Innovative Financing and Sustainable Development: Lessons from Global Health." *Washington International Law Journal* 24 (3): 495.

Gavi (Gavi, the Vaccine Alliance). 2022. "Expanding Sustainable Vaccine Manufacturing in Africa: Priorities for Support." White Paper, Gavi. https://www.gavi.org/news-resources /knowledge-products/expanding-sustainable-vaccine-manufacturing-africa-priorities -support.

GBD 2016 Lower Respiratory Infections Collaborators. 2018. "Estimates of the Global, Regional, and National Morbidity, Mortality, and Aetiologies of Lower Respiratory Infections in 195 Countries, 1990–2016: A Systematic Analysis for the Global Burden of Disease Study 2016." *The Lancet Infectious Diseases* 18 (11): 1191–210. https://doi .org/10.1016/s1473-3099(18)30310-4.

Giubilini, Alberto. 2020. "Vaccination Ethics." *British Medical Bulletin* 137 (1): 4–12. https:// doi.org/10.1093/bmb/ldaa036.

Grant, Kathie, Claire Jenkins, Cath Arnold, Jonathan Green, and Maria Zambon. 2018. "Implementing Pathogen Genomics." Case Study, Public Health England. https://assets .publishing.service.gov.uk/government/uploads/system/uploads/attachment_data /file/731057/implementing_pathogen_genomics_a_case_study.pdf.

Harmon, Thomas M., Kevin A. Fisher, Margaret G. McGlynn, John Stover, Mitchell J. Warren, Yu Teng, and Arne Näveke. 2016. "Exploring the Potential Health Impact and Cost-Effectiveness of AIDS Vaccine within a Comprehensive HIV/AIDS Response in Low-and Middle-Income Countries." *PLOS One* 11 (1): e0146387.

Herida, Magid, Benoit Dervaux, and Jean-Claude Desenclos. 2016. "Economic Evaluations of Public Health Surveillance Systems: A Systematic Review." *European Journal of Public Health* 26 (4): 674–80. https://doi.org/10.1093/eurpub/ckv250.

Ilic, Irena, and Milena Ilic. 2023. "Global Patterns of Trends in Cholera Mortality." *Tropical Medicine and Infectious Disease* 8 (3): 169. https://doi.org/10.3390/tropicalmed8030169.

Inzaule, Seth C., Sofonias K. Tessema, Yenew Kebede, Ahmed E. Ogwell Ouma, and John N. Nkengasong. 2021. "Genomic-Informed Pathogen Surveillance in Africa: Opportunities and Challenges." *The Lancet Infectious Diseases* 21 (9): e281–89.

JICA (Japan International Cooperation Agency). 2021. "Boosting COVID-19 Testing Capacity at KEMRI for the National Emergency Response in Kenya." Topics & Events, June 3, 2021. https://www.jica.go.jp/Resource/kenya/english/office/topics/210603.html.

Joi, Priya 2022. "Data-Sharing in a Pandemic: Even Though Scientists Shared More Than Ever, It Still Wasn't Enough." Gavi, the Vaccine Alliance, April 5, 2022. https://www.gavi .org/vaccineswork/data-sharing-pandemic-even-though-scientists-shared-more-ever-it -still-wasnt-enough.

Kim, Sun-Young, Kyung-Duk Min, Sung-mok Jung, Louise B. Russell, Cristiana Toscano, Ruth Minamisava, Ana Lucia S. Andrade, et al. 2021. "Cost-Effectiveness of Maternal Pertussis Immunization: Implications of a Dynamic Transmission Model for Low- and Middle-Income Countries." *Vaccine* 39 (1): 147–57.

Knight, Gwenan M., Ulla K. Griffiths, Tom Sumner, Yoko V. Laurence, Adrian Gheorghe, Anna Vassall, Philippe Glaziou, and Richard G. White. 2014. "Impact and Cost-Effectiveness of New Tuberculosis Vaccines in Low- and Middle-Income Countries." *Proceedings of the National Academy of Sciences* 111 (43): 15520–25.

Lakdawalla, Darius N., Jalpa A. Doshi, Louis P. Garrison Jr., Charles E. Phelps, Anirban Basu, and Patricia Danzon. 2018. "Defining Elements of Value in Health Care—A Health Economics Approach: An ISPOR Special Task Force Report [3]." *Value Health* 21 (2): 131–39. https://doi.org/10.1016/j.jval.2017.12.007.

Lang, Trudie, Ryan J. Walker, Paul Kingpriest, Javier Roberti, Molly Naisanga, Hamsadvani Kuganantham, Wei Zhang, and Vasee Moorthy. Forthcoming. "Equitable Strengthening of Global Clinical Research Infrastructure: Perspectives from the Global Research Community by Professor Trudie Lang." *The Lancet Global Health*.

Lang, Trudie, Nicholas J. White, Tran Tinh Hien, Jeremy J. Farrar, Nicholas P. J. Day, Raymond Fitzpatrick, Brian J. Angus, et al. 2010. "Clinical Research in Resource-Limited Settings: Enhancing Research Capacity and Working Together to Make Trials Less Complicated." *PLOS Neglected Tropical Diseases* 4 (6): e619.

Lazarus, Jeffrey V., Salim S. Abdool Karim, Lena van Selm, Jason Doran, Carolina Batista, Yanis Ben Amor, Margaret Hellard, et al. 2022. "COVID-19 Vaccine Wastage in the Midst of Vaccine Inequity: Causes, Types and Practical Steps." *BMJ Global Health* 7 (4): e009010. https://doi.org/10.1136/bmjgh-2022-009010.

Lenharo, Mariana. 2023. "GISAID in Crisis: Can the Controversial COVID Genome Database Survive?" *Nature* 617 (7961): 455–57.

Li, Xiao, Lander Willem, Marina Antillon, Joke Bilcke, Mark Jit, and Philippe Beutels. 2020. "Health and Economic Burden of Respiratory Syncytial Virus (RSV) Disease and the Cost-Effectiveness of Potential Interventions against RSV among Children under 5 Years in 72 Gavi-Eligible Countries." *BMC Medicine* 18: 1–16.

Ling-Hu, Ted, Estafany Rios-Guzman, Ramon Lorenzo-Redondo, Egon A. Ozer, and Judd F. Hultquist. 2022. "Challenges and Opportunities for Global Genomic Surveillance Strategies in the COVID-19 Era." *Viruses* 14 (11): 2532. https://doi.org/10.3390/v14112532.

Makoni, Munyaradzi. 2021. "Africa's Need for More COVID-19 Clinical Trials." *The Lancet* 397 (10289): 2037.

Marais, Gert, Diana Hardie, and Adrian Brink. 2022. "A Case for Investment in Clinical Metagenomics in Low-Income and Middle-Income Countries." *The Lancet Microbe* 4 (3): e192–99. https://www.thelancet.com/journals/lanmic/article/PIIS2666-5247(22)00328-7 /fulltext.

Marquart, John, Emerson Y. Chen, and Vinay Prasad. 2018. "Estimation of the Percentage of US Patients with Cancer Who Benefit from Genome-Driven Oncology." *JAMA Oncology* 4 (8): 1093–98. https://doi.org/10.1001/jamaoncol.2018.1660.

McKinsey & Company. 2023. "How Digital Tools Could Boost Efficiency in African Health Systems." *Our Insights*, March 10, 2023. https://www.mckinsey.com/industries/healthcare /our-insights/how-digital-tools-could-boost-efficiency-in-african-health-systems.

Mfuh, Kenji O., Ngu Njei Abanda, and Boghuma K. Titanji. 2023. "Strengthening Diagnostic Capacity in Africa as a Key Pillar of Public Health and Pandemic Preparedness." *PLOS Global Public Health* 3 (6): e0001998.

Miller, Jennifer E., Michelle M. Mello, Joshua D. Wallach, Emily M. Gudbranson, Blake Bohlig, Joseph S. Ross, Cary P. Gross, and Peter B. Bach. 2021. "Evaluation of Drug Trials in High-, Middle-, and Low-Income Countries and Local Commercial Availability of Newly Approved Drugs." *JAMA Network Open* 4 (5): e217075. https://doi.org/10.1001/jamanetworkopen.2021.7075.

Moorthy, Vasee, Ibrahim Abubakar, Firdausi Qadri, Bernhards Ogutu, Wei Zhang, John Reeder, and Jeremy Farrar. 2024. "The Future of the Global Clinical Trial Ecosystem: A Vision from the First WHO Global Clinical Trials Forum." *The Lancet* 403 (10422): 124–26.

Musa, Muhammad K., Abdullateef Abdulsalam, Usman A. Haruna, Farida Zakariya, Sanusi M. Salisu, Bisola Onajin-Obembe, Suleman H. Idris, and Don Eliseo Lucero-Prisno. 2023. "COVID-19 Vaccine Wastage in Africa: A Case of Nigeria." *International Journal of Health Planning and Management* 39 (2): 229–36. https://doi.org/10.1002/hpm.3749.

Nanni, Angeline, Stefanie Meredith, Stephanie Gati, Karin Holm, Tom Harmon, and Ann Ginsberg. 2017. "Strengthening Global Vaccine Access for Adolescents and Adults." *Vaccine* 35 (49): 6823–27.

Nicholls, Samuel M., Radoslaw Poplawski, Matthew J. Bull, Anthony Underwood, Michael Chapman, Khalil Abu-Dahab, Ben Taylor, et al. 2021. "CLIMB-COVID: Continuous Integration Supporting Decentralised Sequencing for SARS-CoV-2 Genomic Surveillance." *Genome Biology* 22: 196. https://genomebiology.biomedcentral.com/articles/10.1186/s13059-021-02395-y.

Nordling, Linda. 2020. "South Africa Hopes Its Battle with HIV and TB Helped Prepare It for COVID-19." *Science*, April 7, 2020. https://www.science.org/content/article/south-africa-hopes-its-battle-hiv-and-tb-helped-prepare-it-covid-19.

Olufadewa, Isaac, Miracle Adesina, and Toluwase Ayorinde. 2021. "Global Health in Low-Income and Middle-Income Countries: A Framework for Action." *The Lancet Global Health* 9 (7): e899–900.

Ott, Jördis J., Janna Klein Breteler, John S. Tam, Raymond C. W. Hutubessy, Mark Jit, and Michiel R. de Boer. 2013. "Influenza Vaccines in Low and Middle Income Countries: A Systematic Review of Economic Evaluations." *Human Vaccines & Immunotherapeutics* 9 (7): 1500–11.

Ozdemir, Baris A., Alan Karthikesalingam, Sidhartha Sinha, Jan D. Poloniecki, Robert J. Hinchliffe, Matt M. Thompson, Jonathan D. Gower, et al. 2015. "Research Activity and the Association with Mortality." *PLOS One* 10 (2): e0118253. https://doi.org/10.1371/journal.pone.0118253.

Paget, John, Peter Spreeuwenberg, Vivek Charu, Robert J. Taylor, A. Danielle Iuliano, Joseph Bresee, Lone Simonsen, and Cecile Viboud. 2019. "Global Mortality Associated with Seasonal Influenza Epidemics: New Burden Estimates and Predictors from the GLaMOR Project." *Journal of Global Health* 9 (2): 020421. https://doi.org/10.7189/jogh.09.020421.

Park, Jay J. H., Robin Mogg, Gerald E. Smith, Etheldreda Nakimuli-Mpungu, Fyezah Jehan, Craig R. Rayner, Jeanine Condo, et al. 2021. "How COVID-19 Has Fundamentally Changed Clinical Research in Global Health." *The Lancet Global Health* 9 (5): e711–20. https://doi.org/10.1016/s2214-109x(20)30542-8.

Pirosca, Stefania, Frances Shiely, Mike Clarke, and Shaun Treweek. 2022. "Tolerating Bad Health Research: The Continuing Scandal." *Trials* 23 (1): 458. https://doi.org/10.1186/s13063-022-06415-5.

Price, Vivien, Lucky Gift Ngwira, Joseph M. Lewis, Kate S. Baker, Sharon J. Peacock, Elita Jauneikaite, and Nicholas Feasey. 2023. "A Systematic Review of Economic Evaluations of Whole-Genome Sequencing for the Surveillance of Bacterial Pathogens." *Microbial Genomics* 9 (2).

Privor-Dumm, Lois A., Gregory A. Poland, Jane Barratt, David N. Durrheim, Maria Deloria Knoll, Prarthana Vasudevan, Mark Jit, et al. 2021. "A Global Agenda for Older Adult Immunization in the COVID-19 Era: A Roadmap for Action." *Vaccine* 39 (37): 5240–50. https://doi.org/10.1016/j.vaccine.2020.06.082.

Quilici, Sibilia, Richard Smith, and Carlo Signorelli. 2015. "Role of Vaccination in Economic Growth." *Journal of Market Access & Health Policy* 3 (1): 27044. https://doi.org/10.3402/jmahp.v3.27044.

Rantsiou, Kalliopi, Sophia Kathariou, Annet Winkler, Panos Skandamis, Manuel Jimmy Saint-Cyr, Katia Rouzeau-Szynalski, and Alejandro Amézquita. 2018. "Next Generation Microbiological Risk Assessment: Opportunities of Whole Genome Sequencing (WGS) for Foodborne Pathogen Surveillance, Source Tracking and Risk Assessment." *International Journal of Food Microbiology* 287: 3–9. https://doi.org/10.1016/j.ijfoodmicro.2017.11.007.

Rigby, Jennifer. 2023. "Pandemic Fund Vastly Oversubscribed, More Money Needed – World Bank." *Reuters*, March 7, 2023. https://www.reuters.com/world/pandemic-fund-vastly-oversubscribed-more-money-needed-world-bank-2023-03-07/.

Russell, Louise B., Sun-Young Kim, Ben Cosgriff, Sri Ram Pentakota, Stephanie J. Schrag, Ajoke Sobanjo-Ter Meulen, Jennifer R. Verani, and Anushua Sinha. 2017. "Cost-Effectiveness of Maternal GBS Immunization in Low-Income Sub-Saharan Africa." *Vaccine* 35 (49 Part B): 6905–14. https://doi.org/10.1016/j.vaccine.2017.07.108.

Salami, Olawale, Philip Horgan, Catrin E. Moore, Abhishek Giri, Asadu Sserwanga, Ashish Pathak, Buddha Basnyat, et al. 2020. "Impact of a Package of Diagnostic Tools, Clinical Algorithm, and Training and Communication on Outpatient Acute Fever Case Management in Low- and Middle-Income Countries: Protocol for a Randomized Controlled Trial." *Trials* 21 (1): 974. https://doi.org/10.1186/s13063-020-04897-9.

Schäferhoff, Marco, Armand Zimmerman, Mohamed M. Diab, Wenhui Mao, Vipul Chowdhary, Davinder Gill, Robert Karanja, et al. 2022. "Investing in Late-Stage Clinical Trials and Manufacturing of Product Candidates for Five Major Infectious Diseases: A Modelling Study of the Benefits and Costs of Investment in Three Middle-Income Countries." *The Lancet Global Health* 10 (7): e1045–52. https://doi.org/10.1016/s2214-109x(22)00206-6.

Seale, Anna C., Fiorella Bianchi-Jassir, Neal J. Russell, Maya Kohli-Lynch, Cally J. Tann, Jenny Hall, Lola Madrid, et al. 2017. "Estimates of the Burden of Group B Streptococcal Disease Worldwide for Pregnant Women, Stillbirths, and Children." *Clinical Infectious Diseases* 65 (Suppl. 2): S200–19. https://doi.org/10.1093/cid/cix664.

Seidman, Gabriel, and Ritaf Atun. 2016. "Aligning Values and Outcomes in Priority-Setting for Health." *Journal of Global Health* 6 (2): 020308. https://doi.org/10.7189/jogh.06.020308.

Seidman, Gabriel, Ahmad Alkasir, Megan Akodu, Srinidhi Soundararajan, Paul Blakeley, and Vladimir Choi. 2023. "Strengthening Digital Public Infrastructure for Health." T20 Policy Brief. https://www.orfonline.org/wp-content/uploads/2023/07/T20_PolicyBrief_TF2_DPI-Health.pdf.

Sertkaya, Aylin, Anna Birkenbach, Ayesha Berlind, and John Eyraud. 2014. "Examination of Clinical Trial Costs and Barriers for Drug Development." Report submitted to the US Department of Health and Human Services by Eastern Research Group, Lexington, MA. https://aspe.hhs.gov/reports/examination-clinical-trial-costs-barriers-drug-development-0.

Shao, Yixue, and Charles Stoecker. 2020. "Cost-Effectiveness of Pneumococcal Vaccines among Adults over 50 Years Old in Low- and Middle-Income Countries: A Systematic Review." *Expert Review of Vaccines* 19 (12): 1141–51.

Sharma, Siddanth, Jaspreet Pannu, Sam Chorlton, Jacob L. Swett, and David J. Ecker. 2023. "Threat Net: A Metagenomic Surveillance Network for Biothreat Detection and Early Warning." *Health Security* 21 (5). https://doi.org/10.1089/hs.2022.0160.

Soe-Lin, Shan, Whitney Bowen, and Robert Hecht. 2024. "To Prepare for the Next Pandemic, We Must Spend Now on TB and Other Major Diseases." *Health Affairs Forefront*, January 11, 2024. https://www.healthaffairs.org/content/forefront/prepare-next-pandemic-we-must-spend-now-tb-and-other-major-diseases.

Swanson, Kena A., H. Josef Schmitt, Kathrin U. Jansen, and Annaliesa S. Anderson. 2015. "Adult Vaccination." *Human Vaccines & Immunotherapeutics* 11 (1): 150–55. https://doi.org/10.4161/hv.35858.

Tufts Center for the Study of Drug Development. 2022. "DCTs Substantially Increase Financial Value Based on Key Performance Indicators." *Impact Report* 24 (5). https://assets .website-files.com/63f6c0d2675ee198a17d310a/64498cda6705859c54f258d6_SEP-OCT _IMPACT%20Report_2022-08-26_R-3.pdf.

UKHSA (UK Health Security Agency). 2022. "UKHSA Update on Salmonella Cases Linked to Confectionary Products." GOV.UK, April 13, 2022 (updated May 6, 2022). https://www.gov .uk/government/news/ukhsa-update-on-salmonella-cases-linked-to-confectionary-products.

UNICEF (United Nations Children's Fund). 2022. "COVID-19 Pandemic Fuels Largest Continued Backslide in Vaccinations in Three Decades." Press release, July 15, 2022. https://www.unicef.org/rosa/press-releases/covid-19-pandemic-fuels-largest-continued -backslide-vaccinations-three-decades.

UNICEF (United Nations Children's Fund). 2023. *The State of World's Children 2023: For Every Child, Vaccination.* Florence: UNICEF Innocenti—Global Office of Research and Foresight.

Wallace, A. S., T. K. Ryman, L. Privor-Dumm, C. Morgan, R. Fields, C. Garcia, S. V. Sodha, et al. 2022. "Leaving No One Behind: Defining and Implementing an Integrated Life Course Approach to Vaccination across the Next Decade as Part of the Immunization Agenda 2030." *Vaccine* 8 (42, Suppl 1): S54–63.

Wellcome Trust and TGHN (The Global Health Network). 2024. "Microbial Reservoirs and Transmission Dynamics of Escalating Infectious Diseases." Wellcome Trust and TGHN. https://media.tghn.org/medialibrary/2024/03/Microbial_Reservoirs_Report_Final_1st _March_2024.pdf.

Wenham, Clare, Rebecca Katz, Charles Birungi, Lisa Boden, Mark Eccleston-Turner, Lawrence Gostin, Renzo Guinto, et al. 2019. "Global Health Security and Universal Health Coverage: From a Marriage of Convenience to a Strategic, Effective Partnership." *BMJ Global Health* 4 (1): e001145.

WHO (World Health Organization). 2020a. *Digital Implementation Investment Guide (DIIG): Integrating Digital Interventions into Health Programmes.* Geneva: WHO. https://www.who .int/publications/i/item/9789240010567.

WHO (World Health Organization). 2020b. *Seasonal Influenza Vaccines: An Overview for Decision-Makers.* Geneva: WHO. https://apps.who.int/iris/bitstream/handle/10665 /336951/9789240010154-eng.pdf.

WHO (World Health Organization). 2022a. *10 Proposals to Build a Safer World Together: Strengthening the Global Architecture for Health Emergency Preparedness, Response and Resilience.* Geneva: WHO. https://www.who.int/publications/m/item/10-proposals-to-build -a-safer-world-together---strengthening-the-global-architecture-for-health-emergency -preparedness--response-andresilience--white-paper-for-consultation--june-2022.

WHO (World Health Organization). 2022b. *Global Genomic Surveillance Strategy for Pathogens with Pandemic and Epidemic Potential, 2022–2032.* Geneva: WHO. https://www .who.int/publications/i/item/9789240046979.

WHO (World Health Organization). 2022c. "Reflecting on the Implementation of Genomic Surveillance for COVID-19 and Beyond in the African Region." News, September 16, 2022. https://www.who.int/news/item/16-09-2022-reflecting-on-the-implementation-of -genomic-surveillance-for-COVID-19-and-beyond-in-the-african-region.

WHO (World Health Organization). 2023. *World Health Statistics 2023: Monitoring Health for the SDGs, Sustainable Development Goals.* Geneva: WHO. https://www.who.int /publications/i/item/9789240074323.

WHO (World Health Organization) Regional Office for the Eastern Mediterranean. 2022. "MERS Situation Update December 2022." Fact sheet, Document WHO-EM/CSR/630/E, WHO, Cairo. https://applications.emro.who.int/docs/WHOEMCSR630E-eng.pdf?ua=1.

Williams, Sarah R., Amanda J. Driscoll, Hanna M. LeBuhn, Wilbur H. Chen, Kathleen M. Neuzil, and Justin R. Ortiz. 2021. "National Routine Adult Immunisation Programmes among World Health Organization Member States: An Assessment of Health Systems to Deploy COVID-19 Vaccines." *Eurosurveillance* 26 (17). https://doi.org/10.2807/1560-7917 .Es.2021.26.17.2001195.

World Bank. 2018. "Money and Microbes: Strengthening Clinical Research Capacity to Prevent Epidemics." World Bank, Washington, DC. https://documents.worldbank.org/en /publication/documents-reports/documentdetail/120551526675250202.

World Bank. 2021. "Assessing Country Readiness for COVID-19 Vaccines: First Insights from the Assessment Rollout." World Bank, Washington, DC.

Zhang, Ellen, and Steven G. DuBois. 2023. "Early Termination of Oncology Clinical Trials in the United States." *Cancer Medicine* 12 (5): 5517–25. https://doi.org/10.1002/cam4.5385.

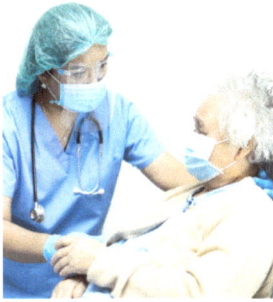

# 12

# Priorities for Acute Care Systems during Pandemics: Lessons from COVID-19

John Rose, Greta Davis, Sharmila Paul, Sri Harshavardhan Malapati, Puspanjali Adhikari, Patrick Amoth, Bin Cao, Lúcia Chambal, Matchecane Cossa, Gabriel Assis Lopes do Carmo, Dipesh Tamrakar, Jiuyang Xu, and David A. Watkins

## ABSTRACT

Health care systems across the world struggled to treat patients during the COVID-19 (coronavirus) pandemic. Treatment narratives from low- and middle-income countries (LMICs) demonstrate that effective emergency, critical, and operative care during a pandemic involves the following: centralized governance, supplemental financing, locally adaptive capacity in physical resources, supply chain management, interfacility triage, workforce deployment, and community engagement within existing public health frameworks. The comprehensive review in this chapter also identifies an essential package of cost-effective clinical interventions for priority investment at district-level hospitals in LMICs that harmonizes with essential care from the Universal Health Coverage Compendium. The scarcity of oxygen during the pandemic reinforced the need for a core package of clinical services with the dual purpose of health systems strengthening and pandemic preparedness. Resilient health care systems should prepare to treat patients affected by future pandemics while avoiding disruptions in routine nonpandemic care.

## INTRODUCTION

The treatment of patients with COVID-19 (coronavirus) posed numerous challenges for health care systems around the world. On December 31, 2019, China's World Health Organization (WHO) Country Office received notification of the first case of a novel coronavirus. Seventy days later, global cases of this novel coronavirus had surpassed 118,000 in 114 countries and claimed 4,291 lives, prompting the WHO Director General to declare a global pandemic.[1] The spread of the virus outpaced emergency, critical, and surgical care (ECSC) capacity to anticipate and prepare for impact in real time, precipitating an unprecedented crisis in the care of patients (Grasselli, Pesenti, and Ceccone 2020; Guan et al. 2020; Huang et al. 2020; Wang, Hu, et al. 2020; Wu et al. 2020; Zhou et al. 2020). For example, as local supplies of oxygen were depleted, deficiencies in global supply chains led to critical shortages with far-reaching effects on patient care (Graham, Kamuntu, et al. 2022; Kayambankadzanja et al. 2021). As patients flooded hospitals, pandemic surges revealed weaknesses in the architecture of health care systems, pushing them beyond their breaking points and exacerbating existing health inequities (El Bcheraoui et al. 2020; Siow et al. 2020) As the international community reflects on COVID-19, policy makers are eager to apply the lessons learned.[2]

## Clinical Interventions and Systems-Level Strategy

Clinical interventions are often underemphasized in discussions of pandemic preparedness (WHA 2005, 2021, 2022). Whereas public health agencies have a duty to control the spread of pathogens, clinicians and the systems they work in have a duty to provide care to those who are suffering. As the medical community adapted to successive waves of COVID-19 variants, innovation was forced upon health care institutions to keep up with demand for clinical services (Haldane et al. 2021). From a policy standpoint, prevention cannot be presented as an alternative to treatment, because individuals who are ill will inevitably seek medical care. The important consideration is how to balance investments in health systems against preparedness and prevention efforts, and what the priorities should be for health system investment in the context of limited resources and a need to maximize value for money.

## Gaps in the Literature

WHO now reports that the pandemic caused such severe disruptions to health care systems that more lives were lost indirectly because of the diversion of resources away from non-COVID-19 health services than because of the pandemic itself (COVID-19 Excess Mortality Collaborators 2022; Knutson et al. 2022; WHO 2022a; Woolf et al. 2020). In retrospect, this finding calls into question the knee-jerk reaction of prioritizing pandemic care at the expense of routine (nonpandemic) health care. During pandemic surges, many health care facilities canceled routine care such as screening, elective surgeries, and follow-up for noncommunicable diseases.

A critical gap in the literature (and in practice) is evident between the competing demands of clinical care during pandemic surges and clinical care for quotidian health needs (WHO 2020c, 2020e, 2021a). This chapter addresses that gap as a fundamental premise by embedding recommendations for cost-effective pandemic preparedness into the framework for overall health systems strengthening from the Universal Health Coverage (UHC) Compendium. In doing so, it aims to reconcile the false dichotomy between pandemic preparedness and systems strengthening and promote a package of essential services that carry the dual purpose of developing resilient health care systems capable of adapting to surges without suspending routine health care (Haldane et al. 2021).

## Goals and Objectives of This Chapter

This chapter aims to define pandemic preparedness for acute care systems, with an emphasis on emergency, critical, and operative services, to optimize the treatment of patients. In three sections this chapter discusses (1) treatment narratives from five countries; (2) an essential cost-effective package of emergency, critical, and surgical interventions (ECSC); and (3) management strategies for district hospitals in low- and middle-income countries (LMICs). This effort builds on the previous edition of *Disease Control Priorities, third edition* (*DCP3*) in which chapters on pandemics, emergency care, and essential surgery outlined synergistic frameworks for implementation (Madhav et al. 2017; Mock et al. 2015; Reynolds et al. 2017). Although this chapter draws on lessons from COVID-19, it also recognizes the possibility that future pandemics may have different characteristics. Issues of transmissibility, physical manifestations of disease, mortality rates, and host-pathogen interaction may vary significantly with the next pandemic. This chapter's recommendations are sufficiently broad to cover the possibility that a nonrespiratory pandemic occurs in the future.

This chapter also lends special focus to the importance of strengthening underdeveloped health care systems in LMICs. It is true that the COVID-19 pandemic created challenges in high-income countries as well, but the profound disparities in health care workforce, physical infrastructure, and quality of care create especially brittle circumstances in LMICs. In 2016, WHO's Global Strategy on Human Resources for Health Workforce 2030 highlighted a shortage of 18 million health workers, and recent updates via National Health Workforce Accounts show slow progress—with 47 LMICs bearing two-thirds of the global workforce shortage (Boniol et al. 2022; WHO 2013, 2016). The *Lancet* Commission on High Quality Health Systems reports that patients in LMICs are less likely to receive appropriate care in general: mothers and children receive less than half of recommended clinical actions during a typical visit, and less than half of suspected tuberculosis cases are correctly managed (Kruk et al. 2015). The *Lancet* Commission on Medical Oxygen Security reports that in LMICs only 30 percent of people in need of medical oxygen receive it (Graham et al. 2025).

The pandemic also exacerbated existing backlogs for elective surgery in a context where 70 percent of the world's population already lacked access to safe surgery before the pandemic began (Alkire et al. 2015; Jain, Dai, and Myers 2020; Klazura et al. 2022; Park et al. 2022). Longstanding disparities in health care infrastructures are further exacerbated during pandemics when vaccine access lags in LMICs. Two years into the pandemic, disparities in vaccinated individuals between countries ranged from 0 to 95 percent, with LMICs consistently falling behind the COVID-19 Vaccines Global Access targets (McIntyre et al. 2022; PLOS Medicine Editors 2022; Privor-Dumm et al. 2023). The achievement of global health equity will require dedicated attention to strengthening health care systems in LMICs.

**Not Covered in This Chapter**

This chapter also dovetails with various other chapters from *Disease Control Priorities, fourth edition* (*DCP4*), which focus on nonclinical domains of the COVID-19 pandemic. Those other chapters cover topics as broad as prevention, detection, biosecurity, early outbreak control, transmission reduction, immunization, financial protection, community engagement, research and development priorities (including pathogen-directed treatments), and historical lessons from past pandemics. The recent *Lancet* Commission on Medical Oxygen Security describes global oxygen need and strategies for service coverage in more detail. Consequently, this chapter does not cover various topics salient to population health despite their obvious overlap with clinical care, such as social distancing, vaccine policy, lab testing, social determinants, community engagement, and travel quarantines. This chapter's narrow focus on health care allows a more granular lens on the health care delivery system included in resilience frameworks (Haldane et al. 2017; Haldane et al. 2021; Kruk et al. 2015).

## REVIEW OF TREATMENT NARRATIVES IN FIVE COUNTRIES

During surges, health care providers and administrators adopted novel strategies across various domains and in diverse clinical settings (Haldane et al. 2021; Kuppalli et al. 2021; Siow et al. 2020). Consider the case of India. In May 2021, India reported more than 400,000 new cases of COVID-19 daily. Oxygen and personal protective equipment (PPE) supplies were rapidly exhausted. Early lessons from overwhelmed hospitals underscored the importance of supply chain management to accommodate clinical needs, equitable training and deployment of medical providers, links between primary care infrastructure and referral hospitals, and real-time data collection to predict clinical demand (Kuppalli et al. 2021; *The Lancet* COVID-19 Commission India Task Force 2021). As the global volume of infections rose, the grim prospect of learning in real time to manage patients became an urgent reality (Siow et al. 2020).

A semistructured survey of health care providers from five countries was performed to better appreciate variations in COVID-19 response globally and gather qualitative information regarding adaptations in clinical care. It aims to better understand the challenges and opportunities providers faced in domains pertinent to patient care, such as staffing, communications, physical space, governance, financing, supply chain management, care of at-risk populations, and post-acute case management (ASPR TRACIE 2020; refer to annex 12A for a description of the data collection instrument). Surveyed providers were senior individuals who had expertise in policy and management and could serve as "key informants" for their unique settings. The survey engaged experts from five countries (Brazil, China, Kenya, Mozambique, and Nepal), covering a variety of health care contexts and geographies across LMIC settings. Providers were encouraged to consider transitions into and out of pandemic surges and responses implemented across all domains of clinical care, from acute to intensive care and from initial triage to recovery.

## Highlights from Health Care Intervention Narratives during the COVID-19 Pandemic

The following paragraphs present concise summaries of the strategies and interventions for each country (designated as a low-income or a middle-income country). For more detailed responses from the survey respondents, refer to annex 12B.

### Brazil (Middle-Income Country)

By *Gabriel Assis Lopes do Carmo*, MD, PhD, Serviço de Cardiologia e Cirurgia Cardiovascular, Faculdade de Medicina da Universidade Federal de Minas Gerais, Belo Horizonte, Brasil

Local governing bodies and individual hospital systems primarily led the COVID-19 response in Brazil. The Ministry of Health assisted with designation of COVID-19-specific facilities and dissemination of protocols for patient care. State and local health secretaries supported intersystem coordination; however, individual hospitals determined acceptance and transfer criteria for COVID-19 patients, supply chain management, and implementation of strategies such as telehealth to permit continuation of routine health services. Of note, telehealth was not previously permitted, but university health systems developed protocols to implement and then expand the reach of clinical services through telehealth visits. This approach, largely guided by individual hospital interest, presented challenges with uniformity of COVID-19-related care, variability in staffing, access to critical supplies (such as PPE), and inconsistencies with interhospital coordination, which ultimately required greater involvement from the Ministry of Health as subsequent pandemic surges exacerbated these issues. During surges, elective surgeries were canceled in several cities where bed shortages required conversion of operating theaters to intensive care unit (ICU) beds. After surges, existing long-term care facilities without dedicated programs managed patients with long COVID. Staff burnout became an issue during subsequent surges, and task-sharing protocols were key, including transitions between clinical, administrative, and clerical roles.

### China (Middle-Income Country)

By *Bin Cao*, MD, Vice President and Director, Department of Pulmonary and Critical Care Medicine, China-Japan Friendship Hospital, National Clinical Research Center for Respiratory Diseases, Clinical Center for Pulmonary Infections, Capital Medical University, Beijing, China; *Jiuyang Xu*, MD, Department of Pulmonary and Critical Care Medicine, China-Japan Friendship Hospital, Beijing, China

The first outbreak of COVID-19 in Wuhan, China, resulted in severe shortages of hospital resources and medical staff, requiring widespread recruitment and dispatch of national medical teams from other parts of the country. The National Health Commission in China drew from prior experience with the SARS-1 pandemic in 2003 and annual influenza outbreaks to rapidly redesignate and expand existing infrastructure. Fever Clinics served the dual purpose of triage and isolation of sick individuals from main hospital campuses. Large-scale public venues were converted temporarily to health care facilities (Fangcang shelter hospitals) for individuals with mild to moderate disease in regions affected by the SARS-CoV-2 virus (Chen et al. 2020). All patients with severe disease were transferred to designated hospitals, and a "dynamic zero" policy allowed continuation of routine medical care in facilities unaffected by COVID-19. Following the initial pandemic surge, widespread screening and contact tracing kept case volumes at a manageable level, which enabled widespread vaccination before native infection. Laboratory testing was initially performed centrally and then expanded peripherally to boost local capacity for testing. This systematic approach based on prior pandemic experience enabled rapid expansion of testing and treatment facilities, early containment of outbreaks, and advanced approaches to studying the virus, its variants, and its long-term effects amid surges.

### Kenya (Middle-Income Country)
By **Patrick Amoth**, MMEd, EBS, Director General of Health, Ministry of Health, Republic of Kenya

Kenya adopted a largely centralized approach to patient care and management during COVID-19. A national task force was created to oversee health care implementation and policy. Financing from the World Bank through the COVID-19 Health Emergency Response Project supported the national task force in disseminating guidelines and providing training for health care workers. This central planning established COVID-19 facilities in each county, expanded critical care units, reassigned staffing between sites, managed supply chains, and more. Individual hospital needs were communicated through designation of key contact personnel, who provided regular updates on staff and patient care metrics to inform regional and national surveillance strategies. High-risk groups—including pregnant women, immunocompromised individuals, and the elderly—received priority immunization. This top-down approach resulted in a largely uniform pandemic response throughout Kenya with little disruption to essential nonpandemic care.

### Mozambique (Low-Income Country)
By **Lúcia Chambal**, MsC, MD, Infectious Disease Specialist, Medicine Department, Maputo Central Hospital, Maputo, Mozambique; **Matchecane Cossa**, MD, Director of National Surgery Program, Ministry of Health, Mozambique; Department of Surgery, University Eduardo Mondlane, Thoracic Surgery, Surgical Department, Maputo Central Hospital, Maputo, Mozambique

The Ministry of Health directed the COVID-19 response in Mozambique. Historically, Maputo City served as a centralized destination for all specialty care and maintained this role throughout most of the pandemic. Initially, smaller hospitals designated isolation units for triage of patients to a single, primary referral center in Maputo City (Maputo Central Hospital) that managed all COVID-19 cases. Isolation units were supplied with oxygen tanks and PPE, and this response adequately met early case needs. Because of the relatively low early case volume, anticipatory planning was not undertaken to guide expansion for subsequent surges. As case volume increased exponentially with new variants (especially the Delta variant), units across other facilities were retrofitted and staff were reassigned to care for COVID-19 patients. Facilities included isolation and triage units within tents in order to accommodate 10-fold increases in capacity. A designated COVID-19 treatment facility (such as a hospital) was identified in a major city within each of 11 provinces, where patients ultimately underwent complex care, including an independent pharmacy exclusively for COVID-19 patients. All testing for COVID-19 was performed in a single lab with three- to five-day turnaround of results. Notably, the supply of oxygen cylinders, ventilators, blood gas analyzers, radiography equipment, and PPE was depleted. With the lack of available staff and resources, all non-COVID-19 care and elective surgeries were halted during subsequent surges. Expanding isolation units and staffing required rapid mobilization of finances, including trainees and foreign assistance from the Cuba Cooperation. Recovery from each surge was enhanced by telehealth visits whereby providers could triage patients without exposing them to risks of infection from travel to facilities.

### Nepal (Low-Income Country)

By *Puspanjali Adhikari*, MBBS, MD, Dhulikhel Hospital Kathmandu University Hospital, Dhulikhel, Nepal; *Dipesh Tamrakar*, MBBS, MD, Department of Community Medicine, Kathmandu University School of Medical Sciences, Dhulikhel, Nepal

Nepal's COVID-19 response evolved as case volume increased. The national governing body activated committees with key players to coordinate the initial response mechanism in a centralized, top-down manner. Clinical guidelines were prepared nationally with support from the WHO Country Office. Provinces established isolation and testing centers in response to increasing case numbers, managed medications, and oversaw supply chains while local governments managed isolation centers and provided services. For purposes of the pandemic, hospitals were designated as "primary" for COVID-19 treatment or "secondary" for non-COVID-19 care. Hospitals rapidly implemented innovations, including retrofitting for negative-pressure air ventilation systems and color-coded isolation levels to differentiate patients at increased risk of transmission. In some provinces, public spaces (such as vacant factories) were converted to COVID-19 treatment hospitals with acute and intensive care capacity. Testing was expanded early from one central site to public and private labs in all provinces to accelerate case finding. Scarcity of oxygen led to a centralized approach for designated domestic supply. This as-needed approach presented initial challenges because of the lack of existing mechanisms to accommodate large-scale funding and resource diversion, yet the flexibility inherent in this strategy ultimately expedited the response to and containment of future surges through swift innovation.

**Lessons Learned**

Multiple themes emerged from the collective responses to this semistructured survey in Brazil, China, Kenya, Mozambique, and Nepal. The following subsections briefly summarize the key messages in the categories of general strategies, supply chain management, and essential (nonpandemic) patient care.

### General Strategies

Initial pandemic responses coordinated at the national level were most rapidly adopted and efficient. Most countries in the preceding case narratives from the countries surveyed assumed a top-down approach, with national governing bodies overseeing the development and dissemination of guidelines and regional or local bodies responsible for implementation and monitoring of outcomes. Countries that adopted a centralized approach reported a more efficient response to COVID-19 and rapid containment of outbreaks. Early designation of isolation and testing centers was performed, either through creation of COVID-19 units or distinct facilities, with varying complexity that appeared to correlate with the size of outbreak in each country. Telehealth options, where implemented, accelerated triage, reduced risk of transmission to patients and providers, and expedited recovery of essential nonpandemic care after surges. In each setting, real-time data from clinical sites were transmitted back to national command centers for active decision-making and coordination. No sites conducted active trials for novel pathogen-directed treatments.

### Supply Chain Management

Responding countries universally experienced supply chain deficiencies. Consumable supplies depleted by surges included PPE, lab testing materials, oxygen, medicines, radiography equipment, and airway support equipment. Innovative maneuvers to maintain adequate supplies at the point of care included cancellation of elective services (for example, surgical care in Mozambique) to repurpose physical resources outside of their original clinical setting; novel sterilization approaches (for example, use of ultraviolet ray in Nepal) for reuse of consumables; novel internal financing mechanisms (for example, through local and national governmental budgets in Mozambique and Nepal); and external support through multinational financers (for example, the World Bank's COVID-19 Health Emergency Response Project program in Kenya) to offset programmatic costs.

Some innovations require greater investment and were not within reach during the pandemic. For example, despite the desire to develop oxygen plants in Nepal, lack of human resources with technical expertise impeded progress. Stockpiling supplies was generally not performed before the first wave, but it was of some utility in planning for subsequent surges. However, utility of stockpiling was limited by multiple uncertainties, such as variation in transmissibility of COVID-19 variants, effectiveness of vaccine campaigns to reduce hospitalizations for severe illness, and fluctuation in budgets restricting discretionary spending. In all settings from this series, supply chain issues were accompanied by hospital overcrowding, staff shortages, and suspension of nonpandemic care during surges.

### Essential (Nonpandemic) Patient Care

High-risk populations received prioritization for pandemic-related care and vaccination in some contexts, but not for routine health care during surges. Essential, non-COVID-19 care was largely deferred during peak surges among surveyed countries but reintroduced later in parallel to—and likely permitted by—improvements in supply chain, workforce, and overall resource management. Strategies to systematically improve priority investments for essential health care can improve patient outcomes in future pandemics. Post-acute care was a low-priority focus during active surges, and few countries adopted a systematic approach to the study and management of COVID-19-related conditions, which remains an issue to this day. By developing strategic health plans for future pandemics, countries can more rapidly implement isolation, testing, and treatment strategies while preserving resources to maintain core functions and support research during outbreaks.

The COVID-19 pandemic challenged health systems worldwide and exposed limitations across both high- and low-performing systems. Standardized anticipatory planning, including supply chain redundancy and stockpiles, facilitates rapid expansion of clinical services and overall health system resilience, especially if based on prior pandemic experience. The paucity of oxygen, in particular, demonstrated the need to bolster public-private partnerships to improve local production of supplies in addition to fostering international collaboration to facilitate rapid procurement and transportation of oxygen during surges. Health system management initially benefits from a top-down approach with built-in flexibility for local emergencies. Emergency financing mechanisms can be deployed to ensure facilities and providers maintain operations. Policies and investments should align across the continuum of care, including post-acute care. National strategies for testing, containment, treatment, and investigation of disease outbreaks are needed alongside strategies that permit continuation of essential health care services.

## ESSENTIAL PACKAGE OF CLINICAL INTERVENTIONS DURING EPIDEMICS AND PANDEMICS

The COVID-19 pandemic provides a unique opportunity to review clinical interventions that underpin the successful treatment of patients during pandemics and harmonize them with the goals of health systems strengthening (WHO 2020c, 2021a). *DCP3* highlighted essential clinical interventions for ECSC to support the achievement of UHC (Madhav et al. 2017; Mock et al. 2015; Reynolds et al. 2017). Without a focus on the unique challenges inherent to pandemic response, however, these recommendations may not be implementable during surges. Although WHO has also published numerous guidelines for clinical management of COVID-19 (WHO 2020d, 2020g, 2022b, 2023), distinct guidelines and interventions for pandemic preparedness and UHC may promote a false dichotomy between preparing for the next pandemic and more general strengthening of health systems. In reality the two goals overlap significantly because UHC and health security are complementary goals (WHO 2020c, 2021a). Passage by the World Health Assembly of Resolution 76/2 in 2023 shows the momentum around these issues. That resolutions calls for "integrated emergency, critical, and operative care for universal health coverage and protection from health emergencies," and acknowledges that "COVID-19 revealed pervasive gaps in capacity of emergency, critical, and operative care services that resulted in significant avoidable mortality and morbidity globally"(WHA 2023, 1).

## Methodology

This chapter presents a concise framework for strategic investments in ECSC systems to improve outcomes during epidemics and pandemics while simultaneously strengthening routine care delivery. Building on the previous section of treatment narratives, this essential package of services was designed around feasibility and cost-effectiveness, with special consideration given for management of surge conditions in LMICs where deficiencies in staffing, supplies, and infrastructure are known to exist. The methodology was designed to promote the resiliency of health care systems as capable of absorbing shock and adapting to dynamic situations during future pandemics while concurrently maintaining critical core (nonpandemic) functions (Kruk et al. 2015; Nuzzo et al. 2019; United Nations 2017; WHO 2020c, 2021a).

First, a list of ECSC interventions for pandemics was created from a structured review of novel scientific research (such as Pubmed), gray literature, and guidance documents from DCP3 and WHO. Publicly available resources from WHO address operational considerations for case management of COVID-19 in a health facility, severe acute respiratory infections treatment centers, clinical care for severe acute respiratory infection, and clinical management of COVID-19 (WHO 2020d, 2020g, 2022b, 2023). Of note, the literature review encountered significant attention to pathogen-directed treatments such as chloroquine, remdesivir, favipiravir, nirmatrelvir/ritonavir, convalescent serum, and others in the scientific literature. However, regardless of their efficacy in treating COVID-19, it is not possible to confirm any single treatment's utility in future pandemics so these specific interventions were underemphasized. This approach was also consistent with identifying dual-purpose interventions that were common to pandemic preparedness and more general health systems strengthening according to the conceptual model in figure 12.1.

**Figure 12.1** Conceptual Model Highlighting Dual-Purpose Interventions at the Intersection of Pandemic Preparedness and Universal Health Coverage

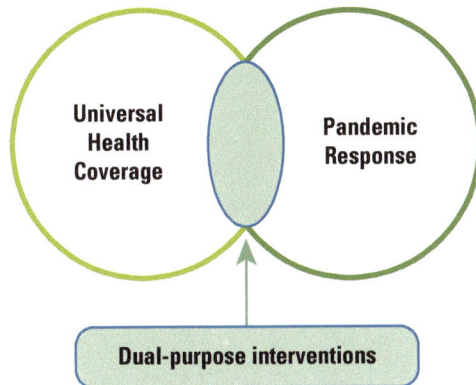

*Source:* Original figure created for this publication.

Second, this list of ECSC interventions for pandemics was vetted with international experts according to the criteria of cost-effectiveness and feasibility from available scientific literature (table 12.1). An important aspect of identifying what interventions are "essential" for treatment of patients during pandemics is determining how much health they generate for a given amount of money spent. The DCP project has always taken the position that cost-effectiveness analysis is a critical tool that becomes even more important in times and places where resources are especially scarce. A structured literature review identified economic evaluations related to treatments for pandemic infections, with a focus on viral respiratory pathogens (such as COVID-19 and influenza) and viral hemorrhagic fevers (such as Ebola). Table 12.1 provides highlights from the original studies identified. Six systematic reviews of cost-effectiveness in ECSC interventions outside of the context of a pandemic also contributed to the understanding of cost-effectiveness for ECSC: two manuscripts for emergency and critical care bundles (Vandepitte et al. 2021; Wilcox et al. 2019) and four for surgical interventions (Chao et al. 2014; Grimes et al. 2014; Ifeanyichi et al. 2024; Saxton et al. 2016).

Third, this list of essential ECSC interventions was cross-referenced with the UHC Compendium (annex 12C). Each intervention was labeled broadly as diagnostic, therapeutic, or population or systems level. Therapeutic categories were also subdivided into groups of procedures, respiratory support, and cardiac support, with those groups subsequently organized according to the broad function of disease management—diagnosis/triage, core management of critical illness, management of complications of critical illness, and systems-level interventions (refer to table 12.2 later in the chapter). Interventions were then assigned to domains of the health care system according to the WHO Building Blocks framework (WHO 2010). These domains initially included all spaces where patients underwent treatment for COVID-19 (such as home, ambulatory clinic, emergency department, hospital ward, and ICU), and were subsequently collapsed into discrete clinical categories of primary health center, first-level (district) hospital, second- or third-level hospital, and postdischarge.

**Table 12.1** Highlights from Literature Review to Identify Economic Evaluations Related to Acute Care Services for Pandemic Infections

| Author | Intervention | Cost-effectiveness data | Comments |
|---|---|---|---|
| Kairu et al. 2021 | (1) EC <br> (2) EC + ACC <br> (3) Status quo | (1) EC-cost/DALY averted (US$, % GDP per capita): 719.61, 0.35 <br><br> (2) EC + ACC-cost/DALY averted (US$, % GDP per capita): 1,711.52, 0.822 <br><br> (3) Status quo-cost/DALY averted (US$, % GDP per capita): 225.11, 0.11 <br><br> ICER cost/DALY averted (Status quo–EC) (US$, % GDP per capita): −23.16, −0.01 <br><br> ICER cost/DALY averted (EC + ACC − EC) (US$, % GDP per capita): 1,378.21, 0.66 | EC = essential care for COVID-19 managed on hospital wards, including supplemental oxygen and IV fluids, according to WHO Living guidance for clinical management of COVID-19 (2021) <br><br> ACC = advanced critical care for critical COVID-19 patients typically provided in ICUs, such as mechanical ventilation, ARDS, thromboembolism, shock management <br><br> Location: Kenya, 2021 GDP per capita = US$2,081.80 |
| Beshah et al. 2023 | (1) Noninvasive management <br> (2) Invasive management | (1) Noninvasive ACER cost/DALY averted (US$, % GDP per capita): 1,991, 2.15 <br><br> (2) Invasive ACER cost/DALY averted (US$, % GDP per capita): 3,998, 4.32 <br><br> ICER cost/DALY averted (invasive–noninvasive): 4,948, 5.35 | Noninvasive management-oxygen without intubation <br> Invasive management-intubation <br><br> Location: Ethiopia, 2021 GDP per capita = US$925.0 |
| Cleary et al. 2021 | (1) GW <br> (2) GW + ICU | ICER cost/DALY averted (GW + ICU − GW) (R, US$, % GDP per capita): 73,091, 3,835.12, 0.54 | GW = general wards management only <br><br> GW + ICU = general wards + ICU management <br><br> Location: South Africa, 2021 GDP per capita = US$7,055.04 |
| Risko et al. 2020 | (1) Constrained PPE supply/status quo <br><br> (2) Investment in PPE | ICER cost/case averted (PPE investment − constrained PPE) (US$): 59 <br><br> ICER cost/death averted (PPE investment − constrained PPE) (US$): 4,309 | Modeling study, locations considered: LMICs aggregate, East Asia and Pacific, Europe and Central Asia, Latin America and the Caribbean, Middle East and North Africa, South Asia, Sub-Saharan Africa |
| Kazungu et al. 2021 | (1) Inadequate supply of PPE <br><br> (2) Adequate/full PPE utilization | ICER cost/case averted (full PPE − inadequate PPE) (US$, % GDP per capita): 51, 0.024 <br><br> ICER cost/death averted (full PPE − inadequate PPE) (US$, % GDP per capita): 3,716, 1.78 | Location Kenya, 2021 GDP per capita = US$2,081.80 |
| Sheinson et al. 2021 | (1) Treatment (no oxygen support; oxygen support without ventilation; oxygen support with ventilation) <br><br> (2) Best supportive care | ICER cost/QALY, payer perspective (treatment − supportive care) (US$, % GDP per capita): 22,933, 0.33 <br><br> ICER cost/QALY, societal perspective (treatment − supportive care) (US$, % GDP per capita): 8,028, 0.11 | Hospitalized patients with COVID-19 <br><br> Location: United States, 2021 GDP per capita = US$70,248.63 |
| Gandjour 2021 | (1) Maintain current ICU bed capacity (no change) <br><br> (2) Expand ICU bed capacity | MCER of last bed added to existing ICU capacity, cost/life year gained (euro, US$, % GDP per capita): 21,958, 23,558.85, 0.46 | Hospitalized patients with COVID-19 <br><br> Location: Germany, 2021 GDP per capita = US$51,203.55 |

*Sources:* As cited in the table.

*Note:* ACER = average cost-effectiveness ratio; ARDS = acute respiratory distress syndrome; DALY = disability-adjusted life year; GDP = gross domestic product; ICER = incremental cost-effectiveness ratio; ICU = intensive care unit; IV = intravenous; LMICs = low- and middle-income countries; MCER = marginal cost-effectiveness ratio; PPE = personal protective equipment; QALY = quality-adjusted life year; R = South African rand; WHO = World Health Organization.

## Economic Evaluation of Essential ECSC during Pandemics

As the intervention under consideration becomes more complex and resource-intensive and uses higher-priced commodities or more skilled labor, it tends to become less cost-effective. For example, two studies that looked at investment in PPE supply both found that these investments would be very cost-effective, because they would prevent many infections and deaths associated with health care; these findings would apply across a range of LMIC contexts (Guinness et al. 2023; Kazungu et al. 2021; Risko et al. 2020). A South African study looking at ICU plus general ward management of persons with COVID-19, compared to general ward management alone, concluded that the latter was cost-effective, albeit in the context of a relatively mature health care system (Cleary et al. 2021). However, although neither noninvasive management nor invasive management of COVID-19 was found to be cost-effective in an Ethiopian context, similarly intensive interventions were found to be cost-effective in Kenya, underscoring that local context, cost drivers, and epidemiology greatly influence the overall value for money in this kind of care (Beshah et al. 2023; Kairu et al. 2021; Kazibwe et al. 2022; Memirie et al. 2022). The seemingly contradictory findings underscore the role that local budgets and implicit cost-effectiveness thresholds can have on cost-effectiveness analysis.

The study from Kenya provides a few additional insights into the spectrum of cost-effectiveness findings (Kairu et al. 2021). That study looked separately at "essential care" (including supplemental oxygen and intravenous fluids) and "advanced critical care" (including invasive management of respiratory failure and shock) as compared to a status quo scenario. Essential care was more cost-effective (that is, cost-saving) than the status quo; when advanced critical care was added to essential care, the combined strategy would be cost-effective compared to the status quo, at local willingness-to-pay thresholds.

Triangulating the findings from these studies leads to the conclusion that basic supportive care in a non-ICU setting is likely to be cost-effective (compared to doing nothing) in many or nearly all countries; however, advanced ICU-level services may or may not be cost-effective, depending on the local health system context and specific intervention components. Finally, regardless of the specific pandemic interventions offered, all countries can and should invest in maintaining basic hospital infection control procedures, oxygen infrastructure, anesthesia capacity, and adequate supplies of PPE to reduce harm to patients (with or without pandemic infection) and health workers.

## A Novel Framework for Essential ECSC during Pandemics

All clinical interventions were grouped to emphasize their place within the system of interrelated health care settings. Clinical interventions can be broadly classified as follows: those that should be available in all settings, those that are core to the function of a strong first-level (district) hospital under nonpandemic conditions, those that should be available selectively in the district hospital during pandemic surge conditions, and those that are better reserved for second- or third-level hospitals because they are either not feasible or not cost-effective (table 12.2). These groupings allow for a concise overview of the salient care in the areas of diagnosis, triage, stabilization, basic and advanced treatment, and rehabilitation. This chapter emphasizes capacity in the district hospital.

The district hospital should be a hub where each community can access safe acute care services. The backbone of clinical care at the district hospital is a healthy, flexible workforce of competent providers who are protected with PPE and trained in basic life support and advanced cardiac life support. Core functionalities at the district hospital level include clinical monitoring, detection of physiologic deterioration, and triage to the appropriate level of care. These functionalities typically will require basic diagnostic studies such as imaging, laboratories, electrocardiogram, and pathology and basic supportive care such as electrolyte repletion, insulin, and anticoagulation. Once admitted to a district hospital, patients should have available to them additional support for acute respiratory failure and shock, including supplemental oxygen, suction, noninvasive ventilatory support, intravenous fluids, antimicrobials, blood product transfusion, and epinephrine. At select district hospitals, advanced care should also be available during pandemic surges to provide timely access in the event of rapid clinical decompensation and to prevent overcrowding in secondary or tertiary facilities. Advanced care for respiratory failure and shock includes mechanical ventilation, central catheters for vasopressive and inotropic medications, and surgical procedures such as surgical airway and gastrostomy tubes and associated anesthesia. In a context of severe or critical illness, management of complications is imperative to treat associated pain with analgesia or sedation, distress with anxiolytics, and basic surgical procedures such as laparotomy, thoracostomy tube, amputation, and wound care or coverage. After treatment and in preparation for discharging a patient from the district hospital, rehabilitation services such as physical therapy and occupational therapy will facilitate transfer to post-acute care. These cost-effective interventions at the district hospital level will allow for treatment of patients during acute pandemic surges and nonpandemic essential care.

Multiple components of clinical care pertinent to pandemic preparedness and UHC are recommended only for higher-level facilities. These components include interventions that are not feasible or not cost-effective at the district level and that require significant investment for acquisition, maintenance, and use. Advanced diagnostic studies in this category are computed tomography (CT) scans and magnetic resonance imaging (MRI) studies, among others. Advanced interventions for organ failure include renal replacement therapy for acute kidney failure and extracorporeal membrane oxygenation for complete respiratory collapse. When available, these services may play a role in select patients' care but should be considered only after first meeting the core functions for district hospitals.

**Table 12.2** Essential ECSC Interventions Relevant to Pandemics Mapped to the UHC Compendium for Implementation at First-Level (District) Hospitals

| | Primary health center | First-level hospital | Second- or third-level hospital | After discharge |
|---|---|---|---|---|
| **Diagnosis/ triage** | | **Basic life support** | | |
| | surge ≪ | **Advanced cardiac life support** | | |
| | surge ≪≪ | **Monitoring, identification, and triage of patients with clinical deterioration** | | |
| | | **Basic supportive care** of patients requiring hospitalization and management of complications of inpatient hospitalization (for example, electrolyte repletion, insulin, and anticoagulation) | | |
| | | **Basic diagnostic studies** including laboratory, pathology, and imaging studies (for example, POC to tier 2 labs, X-ray, ultrasound, and EKG) | | |
| | | | **Advanced diagnostic studies** (laboratory, pathology, and imaging studies including tier 3 labs, CT, and MRI) | |
| **Core management of critical illness** | surge ≪ | **Basic support for acute respiratory failure** with supplemental oxygen, suction, and noninvasive ventilatory support as needed | | |
| | | **Basic management of shock** according to etiology with basic hemodynamic support (for example, IV fluids, blood product transfusions, norepinephrine) and basic interventions (for example, antibiotics, IM epinephrine) | | |
| | | surge ≪ | **Advanced management of shock** with hemodynamic support and etiology-specific interventions (for example, central catheters, multiple pressors, thrombolytics, and inotropy) | |
| | | surge ≪ | **Advanced support for acute respiratory failure** with advanced ventilatory support as needed (for example, mechanical ventilation for ARDS, surgical airway, and gastrostomy tubes) | |
| **Management of complications of critical illness** | | **Management of pain, distress, and other symptoms** (for example, sedation, analgesia, and agitation management) | | |
| | | **Basic surgical procedures and associated anesthesia** (for example, thoracostomy tube, laparotomy, amputation, and wound care/coverage) | | |
| | | | **Specialized interventions for organ failure** (for example, renal replacement therapy for acute kidney failure and extracorporeal membrane oxygenation, including central catheters/cannulations) | |
| | | **Rehabilitation services** to address complications of severe illness and assist with recovery to baseline (for example, PT, OT, SLP, and discharge options) | | |
| **Systems-level interventions** | **Flexible workforce** that can be repurposed to meet surge capacity | | | |
| | **Supply chain reforms** to ensure surge capacity for key commodities | | | |
| | Ensure adequate supply of **PPE** in surges | | | |

*Sources:* Albutt et al. 2020; Aljishi et al. 2022; Bertini et al. 2022; Biswas 2015; Budinger and Mutlu 2014; Chen et al. 2020; Chmielewska et al. 2021; Festic et al. 2017; Inglis, Ayebale, and Schultz 2019; Kassirian, Taneja, and Mehta 2020; Maximous et al. 2021; Mohapatra and Mohan 2020; Palazzuoli, Beltrami, and McCullough 2023; Perez et al. 2023; Santana, Fontana, and Pitta 2021; Schell et al. 2021; Sheth et al. 2020; Thomas, Abdulateef, and Godard 2022; von Zweck et al. 2023; Watkins et al. 2018; Wong et al. 2020; Zahedi et al. 2023; Zainab, Gooch, and Tuazon 2023. Refer also to World Health Organization, "WHO Compendium: Health Interventions for Universal Health Coverage," (accessed June 20, 2023), https://www.who.int/universal-health-coverage/compendium.

*Note:* ARDS = acute respiratory distress syndrome; CT = computed tomography; ECSC = emergency, critical, and surgical care; EKG = electrocardiogram; IM = intramuscular; IV = intravenous; MRI = magnetic resonance imaging; OT = occupational therapy; POC = point of care; PPE = personal protective equipment; PT = physical therapy; SLP = speech language pathology; UHC = Universal Health Coverage.

## IMPLEMENTATION AND MANAGEMENT IN DISTRICT-LEVEL HEALTH CARE SYSTEMS

Global agencies have taken steps to translate lessons learned from COVID-19 into pragmatic policy for the future—for example, WHO's Preparedness and Resilience for Emerging Threats initiative and the World Bank's Health Emergency Preparedness and Response Umbrella Program.[3] Many of these (and other) programs aim to provide special assistance to LMICs, where strain from the pandemic exacerbated chronic deficiencies in care capacity, resulting in significant mortality.[4] The following subsections synthesize care packaging and management strategies from these and other initiatives with a focus on value and efficiency for health care facilities in LMICs. Management strategies are summarized according to the building blocks framework of health care delivery, which has been applied to models of health care resiliency during the pandemic (Haldane et al. 2021).

### Adaptations in Infrastructure: Physical Space

Pandemic surges often require rapid adaptation in local health care infrastructure. Narratives from earlier in the chapter are consistent with the literature that it is critical to secure adequate physical space for clinical care of patients with COVID-19. Future pandemics may require building new facilities, altering existing facilities, or repurposing secular structures for clinical care. In LMICs, it may not be possible to perform construction in every geographic district, but facilities in central locations can be designated as hot spots exclusively for pandemic care and others can be reserved for routine (nonpandemic) health care (ASPR TRACIE 2020; Haldane et al. 2021; Siow et al. 2020). Historically, this approach reinforces the role of pandemic emergency facilities developed by WHO for the Ebola epidemic (Kruk et al. 2015).

### Health Workforce

In most settings, health care workers had a high risk for infection, creating absences of key personnel during surges when care was needed most (Bandyopadhyay et al. 2020; WHO 2020a). Successful strategies to ensure coverage of essential services in LMICs include aggressive implementation of PPE, realignment of duty hours to accommodate staff illness, support to avoid burnout, and incentivized reallocation. Staffing shortages in district hospitals may be addressed by emphasizing key clinical competencies over concrete titles. Educational tools now exist to assess competency and learn skills for a broad spectrum of health care activities, from clinical tasks (such as vaccination, acute stabilization, infection control, charting, and ventilator management) to health care management (such as provider well-being and infodemic strategy) (AHA 2020; CDC 2021; WHO 2021b).[5] During surges, medical and paramedical staff may cover functions outside their job description in order to avoid gaps in key capacities of the health care facility. Accomplishing continuity requires coordinating rapid dissemination of educational modules between medical and nursing societies, facility managers, local and regional centers for disease control, and ministry of health leadership.

Biomedical engineers and technicians are often overlooked in the landscape of critical hospital personnel. These technicians of biomedical devices and supplies proved to be an essential component of the health care team during COVID-19 surges, because they oversee the procurement, maintenance, handling, repair, safety, and preparation of key resources, including but not limited to medical oxygen. A critical lesson from the pandemic is that the mere presence of oxygen in a hospital does not translate inherently into oxygen availability at the point of care with patients (Graham et al. 2025). The expertise of biomedical engineers extends to oxygen-related technologies, such as oxygen delivery devices (for example, nasal cannula, noninvasive ventilatory support machines, and ventilators), oxygen storage devices and safety protocols, oxygen concentrators, and pulse oximetry. Given the obvious need to deliver oxygen across multiple platforms and settings, biomedical engineers are essential members of the pandemic treatment team. In fact, biomedical engineers play key roles in numerous hospital processes—such as sterile processing of biomedical instruments, maintenance of hospital technology, and blood banks—highlighting the importance of such personnel whether or not future pandemics are linked to respiratory collapse.

### Investments in Essential ECSC Interventions at the District Hospital Level

Despite the necessity of investing in core ECSC capacities in district hospitals in LMICs, advanced critical care capacity in many of those countries is restricted to centrally located tertiary centers that become easily overwhelmed during surges. In order to provide rapid, local access at the population level and avoid overcrowding of tertiary facilities, countries can explore strategies to decentralize some care to district hospitals (table 12.2). Ideally, basic management available at the district hospital level includes treatment of shock and acute respiratory failure with intravenous fluids, blood product transfusions, norepinephrine, antibiotics, intramuscular epinephrine, supplemental oxygen, suction, and noninvasive ventilatory support, including anesthesia. In select district hospitals, elements of advanced critical and surgical care capacities—such as acute respiratory distress syndrome, surgical airway, gastrostomy tubes, central catheters, sedation, anesthesia, and analgesia—may also be decentralized. To preserve capacity at the district hospitals themselves, various countries expanded access to supplemental oxygen at home (Haldane et al. 2021; WHO 2020b). When patients require higher levels of care (such as for kidney failure or to undergo extracorporeal membrane oxygenation), urgent referrals and transfer to tertiary centers should be expedited. Of note, pathogen-directed treatments (such as antivirals) may be implementable across multiple levels of care but should be rigorously studied in real time within acute care settings with necessary regulatory oversite for appropriate allocation of resources but sufficient flexibility and adaptability for surge conditions.

## Management of Supply Chains

During pandemic surges, scarcity of medical technologies and supplies undermines the successful treatment of patients, calling attention to supply chain coordination at local, national, and international levels (Best and Williams 2021; Bhaskar et al. 2020; Dai et al. 2021; Miller et al. 2021; Patel et al. 2017). Critical supplies include, but are not limited to, essential medicines, vaccines, PPE, oxygen, pulse oximetry, and ventilators (Cohen and van der Meulen Rodgers 2020). As the pandemic unfolded, the world clearly did not have sufficient supplies for the demands placed on health care systems in high- and low-income settings alike (Kuppalli et al. 2021; Rowen and Laffey 2020; Sharma et al. 2020).

Strategies in supply chain management rest on the pillars of preparedness and responsiveness (Bryce et al. 2020; Day 2014; Hohenstein et al. 2015). *Preparedness* strategy occurs before a shock hits the health system and has a long-term view of solutions. These solutions may include stockpiling resources, increasing domestic production, and supporting innovations in the supply of relevant goods (Plans-Rubió 2020). *Responsiveness* strategy occurs after the crisis strikes and has a short-term view of real-time solutions. These solutions may include emergency procurement through purchase of supplies from the global market of goods or loans of supplies between facilities within a country (Adelman 2020). From a policy and health systems management perspective, countries often engage in both preparedness and responsiveness strategies simultaneously between pandemic surges (Handfield et al. 2020; Jiang, Rigobon, and Rigobon 2022).

Despite the availability of modeling exercises from systems dynamics and game theory approaches, dialing in the appropriate procurement of supplies remains a challenge in pandemic preparedness (Abedrabboh et al. 2021; FalagaraSigala et al. 2022; Gotz, Auping, and Hinrichs-Krapels 2024). For example, in considering stockpiles of PPE, anticipatory procurement can undoubtedly be cost-effective and stockpiling reduces acute deficiencies in supplies when demand increases during peak surge conditions (Dow, Lee, and Lucia 2020; Folkers 2019). Advance stockpiling, however, increases the likelihood that some supplies may expire on the shelf or go unused if the next surge is delayed or never comes. Experts in supply chain management recommend consideration of such uncertainties and discourage overreliance on a single strategy. Other uncertainties include global disruptions in transportation networks, production times, and delivery times; competition for scarce goods; variable pricing; and export restrictions. Most of these factors are outside the control of policy makers and health care administrators, but efforts should be taken to at least reduce the effect of these uncertainties on procurement of critical supplies.

The global experience with medical oxygen highlights the need to coordinate supply chains for emergency situations characterized by soaring demand (Graham, Bakare, et al. 2022; Graham, Kamuntu, et al. 2022; Graham et al. 2025; Kitutu et al. 2022). WHO's recent list of essential medicines included medical oxygen, but in the anesthesia section, which shows an underestimation of oxygen's utility during pandemics. Oxygen plays a foundational role in the treatment of COVID-19 across various stages of disease pathology, across various health care settings, and even in patients' homes. Ensuring availability of a consistent supply for patient care throughout all levels of a health care system, however, presents challenges when considering the various methods of oxygen production (liquid oxygen, pressure swing adsorption, and oxygen concentrators) and matching supply to demand. In addition to production, the transportation, storage, and delivery of oxygen require specialized equipment (such as cylinders and pipes) and experienced biomedical engineers to implement protocols safely. Globally, the supply chain of oxygen depended on limited manufacturing capacity in select countries, underscoring the need for fair market regulation, financial risk protection against catastrophic expenditures for patients, and boosting public-private collaboration for local production. The *Lancet* Commission on Medical Oxygen Security discusses these and other issues as a cautionary tale for future public health emergencies. (Graham et al. 2025; Kitutu et al. 2022).

Principles of successful supply chain management are most effective when considered as a package of interventions that are highly contextualized and systematically deployed to optimize coordination between suppliers and the health system (FalagaraSigala et al. 2022; Gotz, Auping, and Hinrichs-Krapels 2024; van Hoek 2020). First steps for stockpiling include maintaining a national database of available supplies, a crisis plan to calculate additional needs, and storing raw materials for future manufacturing. Other cost-effective tactics include dedicating storage space for PPE and combining with strategies, such as social distancing, to prolong the time between surges (Abedrabboh et al. 2021). In anticipation of the need to urgently purchase goods from the global market, a diversified supplier network can reduce reliance on single-site production and any regional or global transportation disruptions. No one-size-fits-all approach to supply chain management exists; however, by selectively adopting these measures, countries can mitigate the effects of pandemic crises.

## The Need to Maintain Nonpandemic Care during Pandemic Surges

The blanket policy of suspending non-COVID-19 clinical care during surges came into question throughout the pandemic (Haldane et al. 2021; Siow et al. 2020; WHO 2020c, 2021a). During initial surges many health care systems preserved critical resources by canceling clinical services not directly related to COVID-19, including essential diagnostic and therapeutic interventions (refer to annex 12B). This strategy resulted in significant deficiencies in essential care (Caldeira et al. 2020; Schell et al. 2021). For example, patients seeking care for cancer experienced restricted access to screening, such as mammograms and colonoscopies, and vital medications, including cycles of chemotherapy (Jazieh et al. 2020; Le Bihan-Bengamin et al. 2023; Puricelli Perin et al. 2021). Cancellations of elective surgery also led to significant delays, adding an estimated 28 million surgeries to existing backlogs (COVIDSurg Collaborative 2020; Jain, Dai, and Myers 2020; Klazura et al. 2022; Park et al. 2022; Rubenstein et al. 2022; Søreide et al. 2020; Wang, Vahid, et al. 2020). WHO estimates that the pandemic disrupted health care systems so severely that 8 million excess lives were lost indirectly because of diversion of resources away from essential health services (COVID-19 Excess Mortality Collaborators 2022; Knutson et al. 2022; WHO 2022a; Woolf et al. 2020). Consequently, health system resilience literature focuses not only on absorbing shocks during health emergencies but also on maintaining continuity of high-quality care (Haldane et al. 2021; Legido-Quigley and Asgari 2018; Legido-Quigley et al. 2020). Strategies for LMICs include investing in district-level capacity to deliver essential ECSC interventions (from table 12.2) that support both pandemic response and UHC.

### Fair Rationing in Pandemic Surges

Bedside clinicians in LMICs often face rationing decisions when resources for interventions are scarce. As we learned during the COVID-19 pandemic, surges exacerbate resource scarcity and require especially difficult decisions (WHO 2020f). The following principles from medical ethics can be used in tandem with cost-effectiveness evidence to ensure these decisions are made fairly. Emanuel et al. (2020) lay out several recommendations for fair rationing during pandemic surges, summarized here. Because it is possible to conceive of clinical scenarios in which the application of ethical principles fails to identify a clear choice, the process of implementing these principles should be transparent, consistent, and preferably not at bedside in order for the decision-making process to maintain its face validity with the public. Although maximizing health benefits aligns generally with the goals of utilitarianism, policy makers and administrators should adapt these principles to local values before implementing them.

First, the principle of maximizing health benefits is paramount and aligns with the goal of health economic evaluation (for example, to identify interventions with the greatest value for money). Thus, interventions that offer the greatest chance of saving lives or generating healthy life years (that is, providing treatments to those persons who have the most to gain from them) should have priority. Second, frontline health workers and caregivers should—in the event they fall ill—be given priority for interventions. Third, when multiple patients with similar prognoses require a scarce intervention, that intervention should be allocated on a random selection–based (lottery) system, rather than on a first-come, first-served basis. Fourth, people who participate in pandemic-related research studies should receive priority because of their assumption of additional risk. Fifth, the principles for rationing differ by intervention. For preventive interventions like vaccines, higher-risk groups (such as the elderly) should be prioritized because they have the most to gain from not being infected in the first place; by contrast, for curative interventions like ventilators, those with the best prognosis (such as younger individuals with no comorbidities) should be prioritized.

Finally, all patients who need a particular nonspecific intervention (such as mechanical ventilation) should be treated equally: there is no reason to prioritize these interventions for infected persons as compared to persons with other conditions (for example, acute asthma exacerbation or intraoperative respiratory support). This last recommendation is especially salient for health care systems that postponed nonemergent care for non-COVID-19 conditions and experienced excess mortality from delayed care and budget deficits because of, for example, canceled elective procedures.

## Final Recommendations

The COVID-19 pandemic levied a devastating impact on health care systems worldwide. The dual strain of providing routine essential care and managing episodic pandemic surges crippled health care facilities. Successful systems-level adaptations to optimize the treatment of patients include centralized governance, supply chain management (including stockpiling critical resources), interfacility triage, workforce (re)deployment, repurposing physical infrastructure, and community engagement. Urgent investment is necessary in LMICs to support an essential package of ECSC interventions that promote preparedness for surges while bolstering capacity to achieve UHC. These interventions, including medical oxygen, are spread across the continuum of clinical care with the goal of optimizing the utility of the district hospital and avoiding clinical backlogs during surges. The clinical experience of caring for patients during the COVID-19 pandemic provides a cautionary tale of the need to develop resiliency in health care systems for future pandemics.

## NOTES

1. WHO, "WHO Director-General's Opening Remarks at the Media Briefing on COVID-19—11 March 2020," https://www.who.int/dg/speeches/detail/who-director-general-s-opening-remarks-at-the-media-briefing-on-covid-19---11-march-2020; refer also to WHO, "WHO COVID-19 Dashboard" (accessed June 20, 2023), https://covid19.who.int/;
2. WHO, "Initiatives: Preparedness and Resilience for Emerging Threats (PRET)" (accessed June 20, 2023), https://www.who.int/initiatives/preparedness-and-resilience-for-emerging-threats#.
3. Refer also to WHO, "Initiatives: Preparedness and Resilience for Emerging Threats (PRET)"; World Bank Group, "Health Emergency and Preparedness Response (HEPR) Umbrella Program" (accessed June 20, 2023), https://www.healthemergencies.org/.
4. WHO, "WHO COVID-19 Dashboard."
5. Refer also to American Association for Respiratory Care (AARC), "AARC University: Adult Critical Care: COVID-19: Lessons Learned" (accessed June 20, 2023), https://www.aarc.org/education/covid-19-lessons-learned/; National Health Service England, "Education and Training Framework" (accessed June 20, 2023), https://www.england.nhs.uk/coronavirus/documents/c0237-education-and-training-framework/; Open Critical Care, "Suggested COVID-19 Trainings" (accessed June 20, 2023), https://opencriticalcare.org/suggested-trainings/; Oxford Policy Management, "Designing a Learning Tool to Assess the Competencies of Public Health Managers" (accessed June 20, 2023), https://www.opml.co.uk/projects/designing-a-learning-tool-to-assess-the-competencies-of-public-health-managers.

## REFERENCES

Abedrabboh, K., M. Pilz, Z. Al-Fagih, O. Al-Fagih, J.-C. Nebel, and L. Al-Fagih. 2021. "Game Theory to Enhance Stock Management of Personal Protective Equipment (PPE) during the COVID-19 Outbreak." *PLOS One* 16 (2): e0246110.

Adelman, D. 2020. "Thousands of Lives Could Be Saved in the US during the COVID-19 Pandemic If States Exchanged Ventilators." *Health Affairs* 39 (7): 1247–52.

AHA (American Heart Association). 2020. "Oxygenation and Ventilation of COVID-19 Patients—Module 4: Ventilation Management." AHA. https://cpr.heart.org /-/media/cpr-files/resources/covid-19-resources-for-cpr-training/oxygenation -and-ventilation-of-covid-19-patients/ovcovid_mod4_vntmgmt_200401_ed .pdf?la=en&hash=DC07E68C015549A42991BC67BA674DB196D7EDC8.

Albutt, K., C. M. Luckhurst, G. A. Alba, M. El Hechi, A. Mokhtari, K. Breen, J. Wing, et al. 2020. "Design and Impact of a COVID-19 Multidisciplinary Bundled Procedure Team." *Annals of Surgery* 272 (2): E72–73. https://doi.org/10.1097/SLA.0000000000004089.

Aljishi, R. S., A. H. Alkuaibi, F. A. al Zayer, and A. H. al Matouq. 2022. "Extracorporeal Membrane Oxygenation for COVID-19: A Systematic Review." *Cureus* 14 (7). https://doi.org/10.7759/CUREUS.27522.

Alkire, B. C., N. P. Raykar, M. G. Shrime, T. G. Weiser, S. W. Bickler, J. A. Rose, C. T. Nutt, et al. 2015. "Global Access to Surgical Care: A Modelling Study." *The Lancet Global Health* 3 (6): e316–23.

ASPR TRACIE (Assistant Secretary for Preparedness and Response, Healthcare Emergency Preparedness Information Gateway). 2020. "Designated COVID-19 Hospitals: Case Studies and Lessons Learned." US Department of Health and Human Services. https://files .asprtracie.hhs.gov/documents/creating-a-covid-19-specialty-hospital-508.pdf.

Bandyopadhyay, S., R. E. Baticulon, M. Kadhum, M. Alser, D. K. Ojuka, Y. Badereddin, A. Kamath, et al. 2020. "Infection and Mortality of Healthcare Workers Worldwide from COVID-19: A Systematic Review." *BMJ Global Health* 5 (12): e003097.

Bertini, P., F. Guarracino, M. Falcone, P. Nardelli, G. Landoni, M. Nocci, and G. Paternoster. 2022. "ECMO in COVID-19 Patients: A Systematic Review and Meta-analysis." *Journal of Cardiothoracic and Vascular Anesthesia* 36 (8 Pt A): 2700–06. https://doi.org/10.1053/J .JVCA.2021.11.006.

Beshah, S. A., A. Zeru, W. Tadele, A. Defar, T. Getachew, and L. Fekadu Assebe. 2023. "A Cost-Effectiveness Analysis of COVID-19 Critical Care Interventions in Addis Ababa, Ethiopia: A Modeling Study." *Cost Effectiveness and Resource Allocation* 21 (1): 1–11.

Best, S., and S. J. Williams. 2021. "What Have We Learnt about the Sourcing of Personal Protective Equipment during Pandemics? Leadership and Management in Healthcare Supply Chain Management: A Scoping Review." *Frontiers in Public Health* 9: 765501. https://doi.org/10.3389/fpubh.2021.765501.

Bhaskar, S., J. Tan, M. L. A. M. Bogers, T. Minssen, H. Badaruddin, S. Israeli-Korn, and H. Chesbrough. 2020. "At the Epicenter of COVID-19—The Tragic Failure of the Global Supply Chain for Medical Supplies." *Frontiers in Public Health* 8: 562882.

Biswas, A. 2015. "Right Heart Failure in Acute Respiratory Distress Syndrome: An Unappreciated Albeit a Potential Target for Intervention in the Management of the Disease." *Indian Journal of Critical Care Medicine* 19 (10): 606. https://doi.org/10.4103 /0972-5229.167039.

Boniol, M., T. Kunjumen, T. S. Nair, A. Siyam, J. Campbell, and K. Diallo. 2022. "The Global Health Workforce Stock and Distribution in 2020 and 2030: A Threat to Equity and 'Universal' Health Coverage?" *BMJ Global Health* 7 (6): e009316.

Bryce, C., P. Ring, S. Ashby, and J. K. Wardman. 2020. "Resilience in the Face of Uncertainty: Early Lessons from the COVID-19 Pandemic." *Journal of Risk Research* 23 (7–8): 880–87.

Budinger, G. R. S., and G. M. Mutlu. 2014. "β2-Agonists and Acute Respiratory Distress Syndrome." *American Journal of Respiratory and Critical Care Medicine* 189 (6): 624–25. https://doi.org/10.1164/RCCM.201401-0170ED.

Caldeira Brant, L. C., B. Ramos Nascimento, R. Azzeredo Teixeira, M. A. C. Queiroga Lopes, D. Carvalho Malta, G. M. Moraes Oliveira, and A. L. Pinho Ribeiro. 2020. "Excess of Cardiovascular Deaths during the COVID-19 Pandemic in Brazilian Capital Cities." *Heart* 106 (24): 1898–905.

CDC (United States Centers for Disease Control). 2021. "COVID-19 Vaccination Training Programs and Reference Materials for Healthcare Professionals." CDC. https://www.cdc.gov/vaccines/covid-19/downloads/COVID-19-Clinical-Training-and-Resources-for-HCPs.pdf.

Chao, T. E., K. Sharma, M. Mandigo, L. Hagander, S. C. Resch, T. G. Weiser, and J. G. Meara. 2014. "Cost-Effectiveness of Surgery and Its Policy Implications for Global Health: A Systematic Review and Analysis." *The Lancet Global Health* 2 (6): e334–45.

Chen, S., Z. Zhang, J. Yang, J. Wang, X. Zhai, T. Bärnighausen, and C. Wang. 2020. "Fangcang Shelter Hospitals: A Novel Concept for Responding to Public Health Emergencies." *The Lancet* 395 (10232): 1305–14.

Chmielewska, B., I. Barratt, R. Townsend, E. Kalafat, J. van der Meulen, I. Gurol-Urganci, P. O'Brien, et al. 2021. "Effects of the COVID-19 Pandemic on Maternal and Perinatal Outcomes: A Systematic Review and Meta-analysis." *The Lancet Global Health* 9 (6): e759–72.

Cleary, S. M., T. Wilkinson, C. R. Tamandjou Tchuem, S. Docrat, and G. C. Solanki. 2021. "Cost-Effectiveness of Intensive Care for Hospitalized COVID-19 Patients: Experience from South Africa." *BMC Health Services Research* 21: 82.

Cohen, J., and Y. van der Meulen Rodgers. 2020. "Contributing Factors to Personal Protective Equipment Shortages during the COVID-19 Pandemic." *Preventive Medicine* 141: 106263.

COVID-19 Excess Mortality Collaborators. 2022. "Estimating Excess Mortality due to the COVID-19 Pandemic: A Systematic Analysis of COVID-19-Related Mortality, 2020–21." *The Lancet* 399 (10334): 1513–36.

COVIDSurg Collaborative. 2020. "Elective Surgery Cancellations due to the COVID-19 Pandemic: Global Predictive Modelling to Inform Surgical Recovery Plans." *British Journal of Surgery* 107 (11): 1440–49.

Dai, T., M. H. Zaman, W. V. Padula, and P. M. Davidson. 2021. "Supply Chain Failures amid Covid-19 Signal a New Pillar for Global Health Preparedness." *Journal of Clinical Nursing* 30 (1–2): e1–e3.

Day, J. M. 2014. "Fostering Emergent Resilience: The Complex Adaptive Supply Network of Disaster Relief." *International Journal of Production Research* 52 (7): 1970–88.

Dow, W., K. Lee, and L. Lucia. 2020. "Economic and Health Benefits of a PPE Stockpile." UC Berkeley School of Public Health and UC Berkeley Labor Center. https://laborcenter.berkeley.edu/economic-and-health-benefits-of-a-ppe-stockpile/.

El Bcheraoui, C., H. Weishaar, F. Pozo-Martin, and J. Hanefeld. 2020. "Assessing COVID-19 through the Lens of Health Systems' Preparedness: Time for a Change." *Global Health* 16: 112.

Emanuel, E. J., G. Persad, R. Upshur, B. Thome, M. Parker, A. Glickman, C. Zhang, et al. 2020. "Fair Allocation of Scarce Medical Resources in the Time of COVID-19." *New England Journal of Medicine* 382 (21): 2049–55.

FalagaraSigala, I., M. Sirenko, T. Comes, and G. Kovacs. 2022. "Mitigating Personal Protective Equipment (PPE) Supply Chain Disruptions in Pandemics – A System Dynamics Approach." *International Journal of Operations & Production Management* 42 (13): 128–54.

Festic, E., G. E. Carr, R. Cartin-Ceba, R. F. Hinds, V. Banner-Goodspeed, V. Bansal, A. T. Asuni, et al. 2017. "Randomized Clinical Trial of a Combination of an Inhaled Corticosteroid and Beta Agonist in Patients at Risk of Developing the Acute Respiratory Distress Syndrome." *Critical Care Medicine* 45 (5): 798. https://doi.org/10.1097/CCM.0000000000002284.

Folkers, A. 2019. "Freezing Time, Preparing for the Future: The Stockpile as a Temporal Matter of Security." *Security Dialogue* 50 (6): 493–511.

Gandjour, A. 2021. "How Many Intensive Care Beds Are Justifiable for Hospital Pandemic Preparedness? A Cost-Effectiveness Analysis for COVID-19 in Germany." *Applied Health Economics and Health Policy* 19: 181–90.

Gotz, P., W. L. Auping, and S. Hinrichs-Krapels. 2024. "Contributing to Health System Resilience during Pandemics via Purchasing and Supply Strategies: An Exploratory System Dynamics Approach." *BMC Health Services Research* 24: 130.

Graham, H. R., A. A. Bakare, A. I. Ayede, J. Eleyinmi, O. Olatunde, O. R. Bakare, B. Edunwale, et al. 2022. "Cost-Effectiveness and Sustainability of Improved Hospital Oxygen Systems in Nigeria." *BMJ Global Health* 7 (8): e009278.

Graham, H. R., Y. Kamuntu, J. Miller, A. Barrett, B. Kunihira, S. Engol, L. Kabunga, et al. 2022. "Hypoxaemia Prevalence and Management among Children and Adults Presenting to Primary Care Facilities in Uganda: A Prospective Cohort Study." *PLOS Global Public Health* 2: e0000352.

Graham, H. R., C. King, A. E. Rahman, F. E. Kitutu, L. Greenslade, M. Aqeel, T. Baker, et al. 2025. "Reducing Global Inequities in Medical Oxygen Access: The *Lancet* Global Health Commission on Medical Oxygen Security." *The Lancet Global Health* 13: e528–84.

Grasselli, G., A. Pesenti, and M. Cecconi. 2020. "Critical Care Utilization for the COVID-19 Outbreak in Lombardy, Italy: Early Experience and Forecast during an Emergency Response." *JAMA* 323 (16): 1545–46.

Grimes, C. E., J. A. Henry, J. Maraka, N. C. Mkandawire, and M. Cotton. 2014. "Cost-Effectiveness of Surgery in Low- and Middle-Income Countries: A Systematic Review." *World Journal of Surgery* 38 (1): 252–63.

Guan, W.-J., Z.-Y. Ni, Y. Hu, W.-H. Liang, C.-Q. Ou, J.-X. He, L. Liu, et al. 2020. "Clinical Characteristics of Coronavirus Disease 2019 in China." *New England Journal of Medicine* 382 (18): 1708–20.

Guinness, L., A. Kairu, A. Kuwawenaruwa, K. Khalid, K. Awadh, V. Were, E. Barasa, et al. 2023. "Essential Emergency and Critical Care as a Health System Response to Critical Illness and the COVID19 Pandemic: What Does It Cost?" *Cost Effectiveness and Resource Allocation* 21 (1): 15.

Haldane, V., C. D. Foo, S. M. Abdalla, A.-S. Jung, M. Tan, S. Wu, A. Chua, et al. 2021. "Health Systems Resilience in Managing the COVID-19 Pandemic: Lessons from 28 Countries." *Nature Medicine* 27: 964–80.

Haldane, V., S. E. Ong, F. L. Chuah, and H. Legido-Quigley. 2017. "Health Systems Resilience: Meaningful Construct or Catchphrase?" *The Lancet* 389 (10078): 1513.

Handfield, R., D. J. Finkenstadt, E. S. Schneller, A. B. Godfrey, and P. Guinto. 2020. "A Commons for a Supply Chain in the Post-COVID-19 Era: The Case for a Reformed Strategic National Stockpile." *Milbank Quarterly* 98 (4): 1058–90.

Hohenstein, N. O., E. Feisel, E. Hartmann, and L. Giunipero. 2015. "Research on the Phenomenon of Supply Chain Resilience: A Systematic Review and Paths for Further Investigation." *International Journal of Physical Distribution & Logistics Management* 45 (1/2): 90–117.

Huang, C., Y. Wang, X. Li, L. Ren, J. Zhao, Y. Hu, L. Zhang, et al. 2020, "Clinical Features of Patients Infected with 2019 Novel Coronavirus in Wuhan, China." *The Lancet* 395 (10223): 497–506.

Ifeanyichi, M., J. L. Mosso Lara, P. Tenkorang, M. A. Kebede, M. Bognini, A. N. Abdelhabeeb, U. Amaechina, et al. 2024. "Cost-Effectiveness of Surgical Interventions in Low-Income and Middle-Income Countries: A Systematic Review and Critical Analysis of Recent Evidence." *BMJ Global Health* 9 (10): e016439.

Inglis, R., E. Ayebale, and M. J. Schultz. 2019. "Optimizing Respiratory Management in Resource-Limited Settings." *Current Opinion in Critical Care* 25 (1): 45–53. https://doi.org/10.1097/MCC.0000000000000568.

Jain, A., T. B. K. Dai, and C. Myers. 2020. "Covid-19 Created an Elective Surgery Backlog: How Can Hospitals Get Back on track?" *Harvard Business Review*, August 10, 2020. https://hbr.org/2020/08/covid-19-created-an-elective-surgery-backlog-how-can-hospitals-get-back-on-track.

Jazieh, A. R., H. Akbulut, G. Curigliano, A. Rogado, A. A. Alsharm, E. D. Razis, L. Mula-Hussain, et al. 2020. "Impact of the COVID-19 Pandemic on Cancer Care: A Global Collaborative Study." *JCO Global Oncology* 6: 1428–38. https://doi.org/10.1200/GO.20.00351.

Jiang, B., D. Rigobon, and R. Rigobon. 2022. "From Just-in-Time, to Just-in-Case, to Just-in-Worst-Case: Simple Models of a Global Supply Chain under Uncertain Aggregate Shocks." *IMF Economic Review* 70 (1): 141–84.

Kairu, A., V. Were, L. Isaaka, A. Agweyu, S. Aketch, and E. Barasa. 2021. "Modelling the Cost-Effectiveness of Essential and Advanced Critical Care for COVID-19 Patients in Kenya." *BMJ Global Health* 6 (12): e007168.

Kassirian, S., R. Taneja, and S. Mehta. 2020. "Diagnosis and Management of Acute Respiratory Distress Syndrome in a Time of COVID-19. Diagnostics." 10 (12): 1053. https://doi.org/10.3390/diagnostics10121053.

Kayambankadzanja, R. K., C. O. Schell, I. Mbingwani, S. K. Mndolo, M. Castegren, and T. Baker. 2021. "Unmet Need of Essential Treatments for Critical Illness in Malawi." *PLOS One* 16 (9): e0256361. https://doi.org/10.1371/journal.pone.0256361.

Kazibwe, J., H. A. Shah, A. Kuwawenaruwa, C. O. Schell, K. Khalid, P. B. Tran, S. Ghosh, T. Baker, and L. Guinness. 2022. "Resource Use, Availability and Cost in the Provision of Critical Care in Tanzania: A Systematic Review." *BMJ Open* 12 (11): e060422.

Kazungu, J., K. Munge, K. Werner, N. Risko, A. I. Vecino-Ortiz, and V. Were. 2021. "Examining the Cost-Effectiveness of Personal Protective Equipment for Formal Healthcare Workers in Kenya during the COVID-19 Pandemic." *BMC Health Services Research* 21: 992. https://doi.org/10.1186/s12913-021-07015-w.

Kitutu, F. E., A. E. Rahman, H. Graham, C. King, S. El Arifeen, F. Ssengooba, L. Greenslade, and Z. Mullan. 2022. "Announcing the *Lancet* Global Health Commission on Medical Oxygen Security." *The Lancet Global Health* 10 (11): e1551–52.

Klazura, G., P. Kisa, A. Wesonga, M. Nabukenya, N. Kakembo, S. Nimanya, R. Nalumyimbazi, et al. 2022. "Pediatric Surgery Backlog at a Ugandan Tertiary Care Facility: COVID-19 Makes a Chronic Problem Acutely Worse." *Pediatric Surgery International* 38: 1391–97.

Knutson, V., S. Aleshin-Guendel, A. Karlinsky, W. Msemburi, and J. Wakefield. 2022. "Estimating Global and Country-Specific Excess Mortality during the COVID-19 Pandemic." Submitted to the *Annals of Applied Statistics*. https://www.who.int/publications/i/item/estimating-global-and-country-specific-excess-mortality-during-the-covid-19-pandemic.

Kruk, M. E., M. Myers, S. T. Varpilah, and B. T. Dahn. 2015. "What Is a Resilient Health System? Lessons from Ebola." *The Lancet* 385 (9980): 1910–12.

Kuppalli, K., P. Gala, K. Cherabuddi, S. P. Kalantri, M. Mohanan, B. Mukherjee, L. Pinto, et al. 2021. "India's COVID-19 Crisis: A Call for International Action." *The Lancet* 397 (10290): 2132–25.

Le Bihan-Bengamin, C., M. Rocchi, M. Putton, J. B. Meric, and P. J. Bousquet. 2023. "Estimation of Oncologic Surgery Case Volume before and after the COVID-19 Pandemic in France." *JAMA Network Open* 6 (1): e2253204.

Legido-Quigley, H., and N. Asgari, eds. 2018. *Resilient and People-Centred Health Systems: Progress, Challenges and Future Directions in Asia*. Comparative Country Studies, Volume 3, Number 1. New Delhi: World Health Organization, Regional Office for South-East Asia.

Legido-Quigley, H., N. Asgari, Y. Y. Teo, G. M. Leung, H. Oshitani, K. Fukuda, A. R. Cook, et al. 2020. "Are High-Performing Health Systems Resilient against the COVID-19 Epidemic?" *The Lancet* 395 (10227): 848–850.

Madhav, N., B. Oppenheim, M. Gallivan, P. Mulembakani, E. Rubin, and N. Wolfe. 2017. "Pandemics: Risks, Impacts, and Mitigation." Chapter 17 in *Disease Control Priorities* (third edition), Volume 9, *Improving Health and Reducing Poverty*, edited by D. T. Jamison, H. Gelband, S. Horton, P. Jha, R. Laxminarayan, C. N. Mock, and R. Nugent. Washington, DC: World Bank. http://www.ncbi.nlm.nih.gov/books/NBK525302/.

Maximous, S., B. J. Brotherton, A. Achilleos, K. M. Akrami, L. M. Barros, N. Cobb, D. Misango, et al. 2021. "Pragmatic Recommendations for the Management of COVID-19 Patients with Shock in Low- and Middle-Income Countries." *American Journal of Tropical Medicine and Hygiene* 104 (3 Suppl): 72. https://doi.org/10.4269/AJTMH.20-1105.

McIntyre, P. B., R. Aggarwal, I. Jani, J. Jawad, S. Kocchar, N. MacDonald, S. A. Madhi, et al. 2022. "COVID-19 Vaccine Strategies Must Focus on Severe Disease and Global Equity." *The Lancet* 399 (10322): 406–10.

Memirie, S. T., A. Yigezu, S. A. Zewdie, A. H. Mirkuzie, S. Bolongaita, and S. Verguet. 2022. "Hospitalization Costs for COVID-19 in Ethiopia: Empirical Data and Analysis from Addis Ababa's Largest Dedicated Treatment Center." *PLOS One* 17 (1): e0260930.

Miller, F. A., S. B. Young, M. Dobrow, and K. G. Shojania. 2021. "Vulnerability of the Medical Product Supply Chain: The Wake-Up Call of COVID-19." *BMJ Quality & Safety* 30 (4): 331–35.

Mock, C. N., P. Donkor, A. Gawande, D. T. Jamison, M. E. Kruk, and H. T. Debas. 2015. "Essential Surgery: Key Messages of This Volume." Chapter 1 in *Disease Control Priorities* (third edition), Volume 1, *Essential Surgery*, edited by H. T. Debas, P. Donkor, A. Gawande, D. T. Jamison, M. E. Kruk, and C. N. Mock. Washington, DC: World Bank.

Mohapatra, B., and R. Mohan. 2020. "Speech-Language Pathologists' Role in the Multi-Disciplinary Management and Rehabilitation of Patients with COVID-19." *Journal of Rehabilitation Medicine - Clinical Communications* 3 (1): 1000037. https://doi.org/10.2340/20030711-1000037.

Nuzzo, J. B., D. Meyer, M. Snyder, S. J. Ravi, A. Lapascu, J. Souleles, C. I. Andrada, and D. Bishai. 2019. "What Makes Health Systems Resilient against Infectious Disease Outbreaks and Natural Hazards? Results from a Scoping Review." *BMC Public Health* 19: 1310.

Palazzuoli, A., M. Beltrami, and P. A. McCullough. 2023. "Acute COVID-19 Management in Heart Failure Patients: A Specific Setting Requiring Detailed Inpatient and Outpatient Hospital Care." *Biomedicines* 11 (3): 79. https://doi.org/10.3390/BIOMEDICINES11030790.

Park, P., R. Laverde, G. Klazura, A. Yap, B. Bvulani, B. Ki, T. W. Tabsoba, et al. 2022. "Impact of the COVID-19 Pandemic on Pediatric Surgical Volume in Four Low- and Middle-Income Country Hospitals: Insights from an Interrupted Time Series Analysis." *World Journal of Surgery* 46 (5): 984–93.

Patel, A., M. M. D'Alessandro, K. J. Ireland, W. G. Burel, E. B. Wencil, and S. A. Rasmussen. 2017. "Personal Protective Equipment Supply Chain: Lessons Learned from Recent Public Health Emergency Responses." *Health Security* 15 (3): 244–52.

Perez, A. M. C., M. B. C. Silva, L. P. G. Macêdo, A. C. Chaves Filho, R. A. F. Dutra, and M. A. B. Rodrigues. 2023. "Physical Therapy Rehabilitation after Hospital Discharge in Patients Affected by COVID-19: A Systematic Review." *BMC Infectious Diseases* 23 (1): 1–9. https://doi.org/10.1186/s12879-023-08313-w.

Plans-Rubió, P. 2020. "The Cost Effectiveness of Stockpiling Drugs, Vaccines and Other Health Resources for Pandemic Preparedness." *PharmacoEconomics Open* 4 (3): 393–95.

PLOS Medicine Editors. 2022. "Vaccine Equity: A Fundamental Imperative in the Fight against COVID-19." *PLOS Medicine* 19 (2): e1003948.

Privor-Dumm, L., J.-L. Excler, S. Gilbert, Salim S. Abdool Karim, Peter J. Hotez, Didi Thompson, and Jerome H. Kim. 2023. "Vaccine Access, Equity, and Justice: COVID-19 Vaccines and Vaccination." *BMJ Global Health* 8 (6): e011881.

Puricelli Perin, D. M., T. Christensen, A. Burón, J. S. Haas, A. Kamineni, N. Pashayan, L. Rabeneck, et al. 2021. "Interruption of Cancer Screening Services due to COVID-19 Pandemic: Lessons from Previous Disasters." *Preventive Medicine Reports* 23 (September): 101399. https://doi.org/10.1016/j.pmedr.2021.101399

Reynolds, T. A., H. Sawe, A. M. Rubiano, S. D. Shin, L. Wallace, C. N. Mock, D. T. Jamison, et al. 2017. "Strengthening Health Systems to Provide Emergency Care." Chapter 13 in *Disease Control Priorities* (third edition), Volume 9, *Improving Health and Reducing Poverty*, edited by D. T. Jamison, H. Gelband, S. Horton, P. Jha, R. Laxminarayan, C. N. Mock, and R. Nugent. Washington, DC: World Bank.

Risko, N., K. Werner, O. A. Offorjebe, A. I. Vecino-Ortiz, L. A. Wallis, and J. Razzak. 2020. "Cost-Effectiveness and Return on Investment of Protecting Health Workers in Low- and Middle-Income Countries during the COVID-19 Pandemic." *PLOS One* 15 (10): e0240503.

Rowan, N. J., and J. G. Laffey. 2020. "Challenges and Solutions for Addressing Critical Shortage of Supply Chain for Personal and Protective Equipment (PPE) Arising from Coronavirus Disease (COVID19) Pandemic—Case Study from the Republic of Ireland." *Science of the Total Environment* 725: 138532.

Rubenstein, R. N., C. S. Stern, E. L. Plotsker, K. Haglich, A. B. Tadros, B. J. Mehrara, E. Matros, and J. A. Nelson. 2022. "Effects of COVID-19 on Mastectomy and Breast Reconstruction Rates: A National Surgical Sample." *Journal of Surgical Oncology* 126 (2): 205–13. https://doi.org/10.1002/jso.26889.

Santana, A. V., A. D. Fontana, and F. Pitta. 2021. "Pulmonary Rehabilitation after COVID-19." *Jornal Brasileiro de Pneumologia* 47 (1): 1–3. https://doi.org/10.36416/1806-3756 /E20210034.

Saxton, A. T., D. Poenaru, D. Ozgediz, E. A. Ameh, D. Farmer, E. R. Smith, and H. E. Rice. 2016. "Economic Analysis of Children's Surgical Care in Low- and Middle-Income Countries: A Systematic Review and Analysis." *PLOS One* 11 (10): e0165480.

Schell, C. O., K. Khalid, A. Wharton-Smith, J. Oliwa, H. R. Sawe, N. Roy, A. Sanga, et al. 2021. "Essential Emergency and Critical Care: A Consensus among Global Clinical Experts." *BMJ Global Health* 6 (9): e006585.

Sharma, N., Z. Hasan, A. Velayudhan, E. Emil, D. K. Mangal, and S. D. Gupta. 2020. "Personal Protective Equipment: Challenges and Strategies to Combat COVID-19 in India: A Narrative Review." *Journal of Health Management* 22 (2): 157–68.

Sheinson, D., J. Dang. A. Shah, Y. Meng, D. Elsea, and S. Kowal. 2021. "A Cost-Effectiveness Framework for COVID-19 Treatments for Hospitalized Patients in the United States." *Advances in Therapy* 38 (4): 1811–31.

Sheth, P. D., J. P. Simons, D. I. Robichaud, A. L. Ciaranello, and A. Schanzer. 2020. "Development of a Surgical Workforce Access Team in the Battle against COVID-19." *Journal of Vascular Surgery* 72 (2): 414–17. https://doi.org/10.1016/j.jvs.2020.04.493.

Siow, W. T., M. F. Liew, B. R. Shrestha, F. Muchtar, and K. C. See. 2020. "Managing COVID-19 in Resource-Limited Settings: Critical Care Considerations." *Critical Care* 24: 167.

Søreide, K., J. Hallet, J. B. Matthews, A. A. Schnitzbauer, P. D. Line, P., B. S. Lai, J. Otero, et al. 2020. "Immediate and Long-Term Impact of the COVID-19 Pandemic on Delivery of Surgical Services." *Br J Surg* 107 (10):1250–61. https://doi.org/10.1002/bjs.11670.

The *Lancet* COVID-19 Commission India Task Force. 2021. "Country-Wide Containment Strategies for Reducing COVID-19 Cases in India." The *Lancet* COVID-19 Commission, April. https://files.unsdsn.org/Country-wide%20Containment%20Strategies%20for%20 Reducing%20COVID-19%20Cases%20in%20India.pdf.

Thomas, R., M. Abdulateef, and A. Godard. 2022. "A Review of the Role of Non-invasive Ventilation in Critical Care Responses to COVID-19 in Low- and Middle-Income Countries: Lessons Learnt from Baghdad." *Transactions of The Royal Society of Tropical Medicine and Hygiene* 116 (5): 386–89.

United Nations. 2017. "United Nations Plan of Action on Disaster Risk Reduction for Resilience." United Nations. https://www.preventionweb.net/files/49076_unplanofaction.pdf.

Vandepitte, S., T. Alleman, I. Nopens, J. Baetens, S. Coenen, and D. De Smedt. 2021. "Cost-Effectiveness of COVID-19 Policy Measures: A Systematic Review." *Value in Health* 24 (11): 1551–69.

van Hoek, R. 2020. "Research Opportunities for a More Resilient Post-COVID-19 Supply Chain – Closing the Gap between Research Findings and Industry Practice." *International Journal of Operations & Production Management* 40 (4): 341–55.

von Zweck, C., D. Naidoo, P. Govender, and R. Ledgerd. 2023. "Current Practice in Occupational Therapy for COVID-19 and Post-COVID-19 Conditions." *Occupational Therapy International*, May 19, 2023. https://doi.org/10.1155/2023/5886581.

Wang, D., B. Hu, C. Hu, F. Zhu, X. Liu, J. Zhang, B. Wang, et al. 2020. "Clinical Characteristics of 138 Hospitalized Patients with 2019 Novel Coronavirus-Infected Pneumonia in Wuhan, China." *JAMA* 323 (11): 1061–69.

Wang, J., S. Vahid, M. Eberg, S. Milroy, J. Milkovich, F. C. Wright, A Hunter, et al. 2020. "Clearing the Surgical Backlog Caused by COVID-19 in Ontario: A Time Series Modelling Study." *CMAJ* 192 (44): E1347–56. https://doi.org/10.1503/cmaj.201521.

Watkins, D. A., D. T. Jamison, A. Mills, R. Atun, K. Danforth, A. Glassman, S. Horton, et al. 2018. "Universal Health Coverage and Essential Packages of Care." Chapter 3 in *Disease Control Priorities* (third edition), Volume 9, *Improving Health and Reducing Poverty*. Washington, DC: World Bank. https://doi.org/10.1596/978-1-4648-0527-1_CH3.

WHA (World Health Assembly). 2005. "Resolution 58.5 Strengthening Pandemic-Influenza Preparedness and Response." Fifty-Eighth World Health Assembly, May 23. https://apps .who.int/gb/ebwha/pdf_files/WHA58/WHA58_5-en.pdf.

WHA (World Health Assembly). 2021. "Resolution 74.7 Strengthening WHO Preparedness for and Response to Health Emergencies." Seventy-Fourth World Health Assembly, Agenda Item 17.3, May 31. https://apps.who.int/gb/ebwha/pdf_files/WHA74/A74_R7-en.pdf.

WHA (World Health Assembly). 2022. "Resolution 75.7 Strengthening Health Emergency Preparedness and Response in Cities and Urban Settings." Seventy-Fifth World Health Assembly, Agenda Item 16.2, May 24. https://apps.who.int/gb/ebwha/pdf_files/WHA75 /A75_ACONF2-en.pdf.

WHA (World Health Assembly). 2023. "Resolution 76/2 Integrated Emergency, Critical and Operative Care for Universal Health Coverage and Protection from Health Emergencies." Seventy-Sixth World Health Assembly, Agenda Item 13.1, May 30. https://apps.who.int/gb /ebwha/pdf_files/WHA76/A76_R2-en.pdf.

WHO (World Health Organization). 2010. *Monitoring the Building Blocks of Health Systems: A Handbook of Indicators and Their Measurement Strategies*. Geneva: WHO. https://apps .who.int/iris/bitstream/handle/10665/258734/9789241564052-eng.pdf.

WHO (World Health Organization). 2013. "A Universal Truth: No Health without a Workforce." WHO, Geneva.

WHO (World Health Organization). 2016. *Global Strategy on Human Resources for Health: Workforce 2030*. Geneva: WHO.

WHO (World Health Organization). 2020a. "Health Workforce Policy and Management in the Context of the COVID-19 Pandemic Response: Interim Guidance, 3 December 2020." WHO, Geneva. https://www.who.int/publications/i/item/WHO-2019-nCoV-health _workforce-2020.1.

WHO (World Health Organization). 2020b. "Home Care for Patients with Suspected or Confirmed COVID-19 and Management of Their Contacts: Interim Guidance, 12 August 2020." WHO, Geneva. https://www.who.int/publications/i/item/home-care-for-patients -with-suspected-novel-coronavirus-(ncov)-infection-presenting-with-mild-symptoms -and-management-of-contacts.

WHO (World Health Organization). 2020c. "Maintaining Essential Health Services: Operational Guidance for the COVID-19 Context: Interim Guidance, 1 June 2020." WHO, Geneva. https://www.who.int/publications/i/item/WHO-2019-nCoV-essential_health _services-2020.2.

WHO (World Health Organization). 2020d. "Operational Considerations for Case Management of COVID-19 in Health Facility and Community: Interim Guidance, 18 March 2020." WHO, Geneva. https://www.who.int/publications/i/item/10665-331492.

WHO (World Health Organization). 2020e. "Pulse Survey on Continuity of Essential Health Services during the COVID-19 Pandemic: Interim Report, 27 August 2020." WHO, Geneva. https://www.who.int/publications/i/item/WHO-2019-nCoV-EHS_continuity-survey-2020.1.

WHO (World Health Organization). 2020f. "Rational Use of Personal Protective Equipment for Coronavirus Disease (COVID-19) and Considerations during Severe Shortages: Interim Guidance, 23 December 2020." WHO, Geneva. https://www.who.int/publications/i/item/rational-use-of-personal-protective-equipment-for-coronavirus-disease-(covid-19)-and-considerations-during-severe-shortages.

WHO (World Health Organization). 2020g. "Severe Acute Respiratory Infections Treatment Centre: Practical Manual to Set Up and Manage a SARI Treatment Centre and SARI Screening Facility in Health Care Facilities." WHO, Geneva. https://www.who.int/publications/i/item/10665-331603.

WHO (World Health Organization). 2021a. "Building Health Systems Resilience for Universal Health Coverage and Health Security during the COVID-19 Pandemic and Beyond." WHO position paper, WHO, Geneva. https://www.who.int/publications/i/item/WHO-UHL-PHC-SP-2021.01.

WHO (World Health Organization). 2021b. *WHO Competency Framework: Building a Response Workforce to Manage Infodemics*. Geneva: World Health Organization; 2021. https://iris.who.int/bitstream/handle/10665/345207/9789240035287-eng.pdf?sequence=1.

WHO (World Health Organization). 2022a. "14.9 Million Excess Deaths Associated with the COVID-19 Pandemic in 2020 and 2021." News Release, May 5, 2022. https://www.who.int/news/item/05-05-2022-14.9-million-excess-deaths-were-associated-with-the-covid-19-pandemic-in-2020-and-2021.

WHO (World Health Organization). 2022b. "Clinical Care for Severe Acute Respiratory Infection: Toolkit, Update 2022." WHO, Geneva. https://www.who.int/publications/i/item/clinical-care-of-severe-acute-respiratory-infections-tool-kit.

WHO (World Health Organization). 2023. "Clinical Management of COVID-19: Living Guideline, 18 August 2023." WHO, Geneva. https://www.who.int/publications/i/item/WHO-2019-nCoV-clinical-2023.2.

Wilcox, M. E., K. Vaughan, C. A. K. Y. Chong, P. J. Neumann, and C. M. Bell. 2019. "Cost-Effectiveness Studies in the ICU: A Systematic Review." *Critical Care Medicine* 47 (8): 1011–17.

Wong, A. H., L. P. Roppolo, B. P. Chang, K. A. Yonkers, M. P. Wilson, S. Powsner, and J. S. Rozel. 2020. "Management of Agitation during the COVID-19 Pandemic." *Western Journal of Emergency Medicine* 21 (4): 795. https://doi.org/10.5811/WESTJEM.2020.5.47789.

Woolf, S. H., D. A. Chapman, R. T. Sabo, D. M. Weinberger, L. Hill, and D. D. H. Taylor. 2020. "Excess Deaths from COVID-19 and Other Causes, March–July 2020." *JAMA* 324 (15): 1562–64.

Wu, C., X. Chen, Y. Cai Y, J. Xia, X. Zhou, S. Xu, H. Huang, et al. 2020. "Risk Factors Associated with Acute Respiratory Distress Syndrome and Death in Patients with Coronavirus Disease 2019 Pneumonia in Wuhan, China." *JAMA Internal Medicine* 180 (7): 934–43.

Zahedi, M., S. Kordrostami, M. Kalantarhormozi, and M. Bagheri. 2023. "A Review of Hyperglycemia in COVID-19." *Cureus* 15 (4): e37487. https://doi.org/10.7759/CUREUS.37487.

Zainab, A., M. Gooch, and D. M. Tuazon. 2023. "Acute Respiratory Distress Syndrome in Patients with Cardiovascular Disease." *Methodist DeBakey Cardiovascular Journal* 19 (4): 58. https://doi.org/10.14797/MDCVJ.1244.

Zhou, F., T. Yu, R. Du, G. Fan, Y. Liu, Z. Liu, J. Xiang, et al. 2020. "Clinical Course and Risk Factors for Mortality of Adult Inpatients with COVID-19 in Wuhan, China: A Retrospective Cohort Study." *The Lancet* 395 (10229): 1054–62.

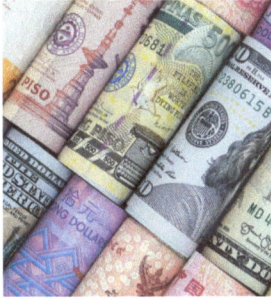

# 13

# Financing the Pandemic Cycle: Prevention, Preparedness, Response, and Recovery and Reconstruction

Victoria Y. Fan, Sun Kim, Diego Pineda, and Stefano M. Bertozzi

## ABSTRACT

The COVID-19 (coronavirus) pandemic exposed critical gaps in the global response to health crises, particularly in the financing of pandemic prevention, preparedness, response, and recovery and reconstruction. This chapter presents a comprehensive framework for pandemic financing that spans the entire pandemic cycle, emphasizing the need for timely, adequate, and effective financial resources. The framework is designed to support policy makers in low- and middle-income countries and in high-income nations, providing a guide to appropriate financing tools for each stage of a pandemic, from prevention and preparedness to response and recovery. To underscore the complexities of pandemic financing, the chapter explores key economic concepts such as global public goods, time preference, and incentives. It also highlights the importance of timely, accessible, and sustainable financial instruments. The chapter lists the pandemic financing instruments used for health during the COVID-19 pandemic, identifying 23 different tools. It uses the Institute for Health Metrics and Evaluation's 2024 Financing Global Health database to estimate that US$91.6 billion was spent for COVID-19 health support, primarily for response financing, over 2020 to 2023. The COVID-19 pandemic wrought significant economic impacts on the order of trillions of dollars, even as investment in pandemic preparedness to mitigate future risks is relatively small, on the order of US$10 billion annually. The chapter concludes with policy recommendations, calling for the establishment of a rapid-response financing mechanism, tailored to the unique challenges of pandemics, and a redesign of global health governance to better address these threats.

## INTRODUCTION

The COVID-19 (coronavirus) pandemic revealed significant weaknesses in the international response and action (Sachs et al. 2022). Countries and multilateral entities faced a major challenge in how to adequately pay for the response. To pay for pandemic response alone, however, is to neglect the entire scope and cycle of pandemic prevention and preparedness before the response as well as the recovery and reconstruction after the response. Financial resources can create a critical bottleneck for addressing many of the challenges faced during a pandemic, including human resources such as health workers and physical resources such as medical supplies and countermeasures. Financing for pandemics is paramount—in terms not just of the adequate amount or volume but also of timeliness, relevance, and usefulness to countries in the pandemic cycle, from prevention to recovery (Agarwal and Reed 2022). Moreover, it is important to recognize that investing in pandemic preparedness is intrinsically linked to strengthening the overall health care system. A robust health care system creates the synergies for effective pandemic response measures.

This chapter presents a comprehensive framework for pandemic financing that spans the entire pandemic cycle, designed to serve both governments and international funding bodies, with applicability beyond low- and middle-income countries (LMICs) to include high-income nations as well. This framework is structured to assist policy makers in differentiating among various financial instruments and strategies, each tailored to specific phases within the pandemic timeline. It focuses on identifying appropriate financing tools—ranging from immediate emergency funding to long-term recovery investments—and the actions these tools are intended to support at different stages of a pandemic. Moreover, it delineates key considerations and characteristics of pandemic financing, such as sustainability, accessibility, and adaptability to changing circumstances.

In framing this discussion, it is crucial to understand the economic principles that underpin pandemic financing. The following key concepts are particularly relevant: global public goods, time preference, incentives, market failures, and political economy. The prevention and containment of pandemics are considered *global public goods* because their benefits extend beyond individual countries, requiring collective international investment and cooperation. *Time preference* refers to the tendency of individuals and countries to prioritize immediate rewards over future benefits, often leading to underinvestment in pandemic preparedness. This issue is particularly acute in countries where immediate needs overshadow the need to prepare for long-term risks. *Incentives* shape government behavior and financial decision-making. For example, financial instruments such as insurance mechanisms have incentives to encourage countries to act now, by offering lower premiums for countries that invest in preventive measures. *Market failures* refers to when the free market fails to distribute goods and services efficiently, which can occur during a pandemic. *Political economy*, which refers to the study of how politics and economics interact, may help explain why governments fail to allocate sufficient resources toward preparedness. These concepts provide a basic framework for understanding the complexities and challenges of pandemic financing, as detailed throughout this chapter.

The structure of the chapter is as follows: First, it introduces the pandemic cycle, delineating its different phases along with categorizing actions. Next, it delves into the interplay between basic epidemiologic and economic concepts, such as public goods and time preference. Following that discussion, it provides a formal definition of pandemic financing and the range of financing instruments available to countries and international funding agencies. Afterward, it presents a case study that examines the financial flows during the COVID-19 pandemic. Building upon those sections, the next section proposes funding schemes tailored to each phase of a pandemic. Finally, it summarizes the chapter's primary recommendations, emphasizing the imperative for establishing a rapid-response mechanism.

## Definition of the Pandemic Cycle

For the purpose of this chapter on financing the pandemic cycle, this section first introduces and defines the pandemic cycle, encompassing four distinct phases of pandemic prevention, preparedness, response, and recovery and reconstruction (figure 13.1). The overall pandemic cycle emphasizes the recurrent nature of pandemics and the corresponding strategies and actions required. Each phase reflects both aspects of timing and types of actions relative to the occurrence of a pandemic, with the prevention, preparedness, and recovery phases considered as

**Figure 13.1** Framework for the Phases of the Pandemic Cycle

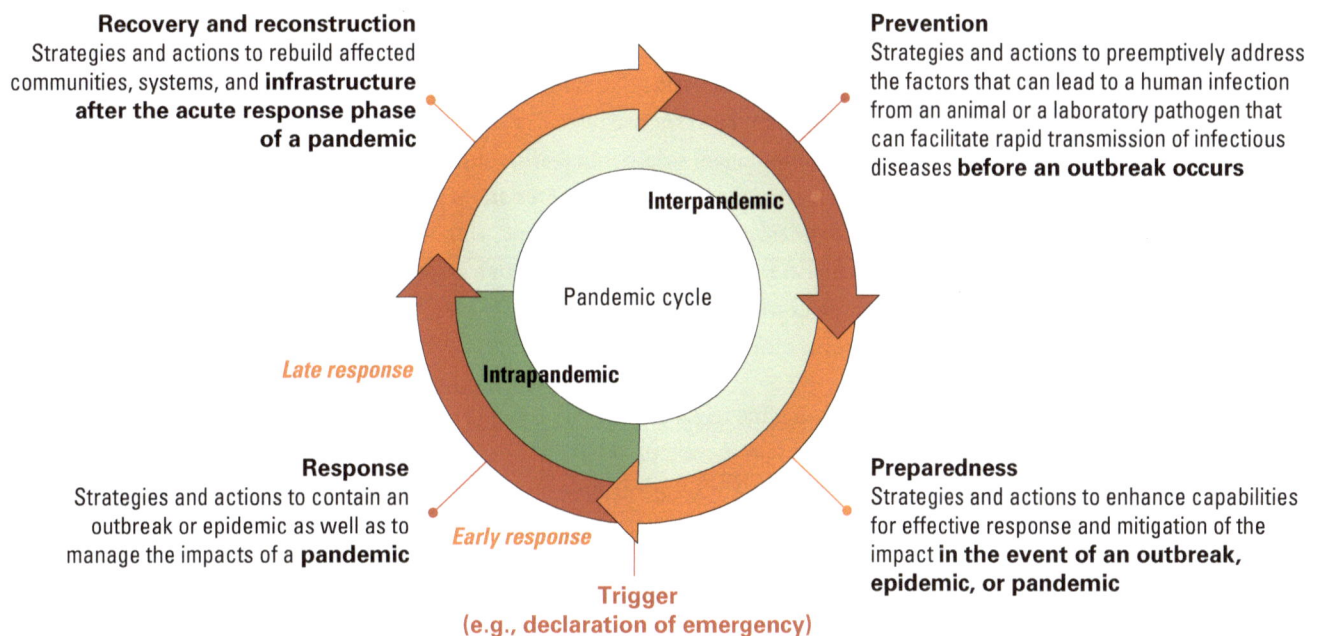

**Recovery and reconstruction**
Strategies and actions to rebuild affected communities, systems, and **infrastructure after the acute response phase of a pandemic**

**Prevention**
Strategies and actions to preemptively address the factors that can lead to a human infection from an animal or a laboratory pathogen that can facilitate rapid transmission of infectious diseases **before an outbreak occurs**

Interpandemic

Pandemic cycle

*Late response*

Intrapandemic

**Response**
Strategies and actions to contain an outbreak or epidemic as well as to manage the impacts of a **pandemic**

*Early response*

**Preparedness**
Strategies and actions to enhance capabilities for effective response and mitigation of the impact **in the event of an outbreak, epidemic, or pandemic**

**Trigger**
**(e.g., declaration of emergency)**

*Source:* Original figure created for this publication.

"interpandemic" or between pandemics, and the response phase as "intrapandemic" or during the pandemic. Further, prevention and preparedness often occur simultaneously—that is, before a pandemic—but the two phases entail different types of actions. Similarly, recovery commonly overlaps with response.

This chapter aims to inclusively address pandemic financing in a manner that is applicable across various health systems and countries, with a special emphasis on the unique challenges and opportunities present in LMICs. However, the principles and frameworks discussed herein hold relevance for all nations, underscoring the universal challenges pandemics pose and the collective efforts required for effective prevention, preparedness, response, and recovery.

First, the *prevention phase* refers to the strategies and actions that preemptively address the factors that can lead to a human infection from an animal or a laboratory pathogen, or that can facilitate rapid transmission of infectious diseases before an outbreak occurs. The foundation of prevention lies in the initial event that leads to the spread to humans, such as the initial crossover event from animals to human (for example, as governed by a ministry of agriculture or land) or the spread from a laboratory to humans, as well as measures to lower the natural $R_0$ (the basic reproduction number, or the average number of secondary cases generated by one infected individual in a fully susceptible population), such as the use of universal precautions in health care settings and improved ventilation in public transportation (for example, defined by a ministry of transportation).

Second, the *preparedness phase* also refers to the strategies and actions taken before an outbreak occurs but that focus on enhancing capabilities for effective response and mitigation of the impact in the event of a potential outbreak, epidemic, or pandemic.

The *trigger* is the critical juncture that separates the prevention and preparedness phases from the response phase (refer to chapter 14 in this volume). The trigger is an action taken by a public health authority for a given geographic jurisdiction, which officially labels and declares an incident using an alert system, such as an outbreak, epidemic, or pandemic, with a pandemic typically involving a formal emergency declaration and in accordance with relevant jurisdictional law, and which can benefit from having a tiered scale of alerts for improving communication (Fan, Cash, et al. 2023).

Following the trigger, the *response phase* refers to the strategies and actions to respond to and contain or mitigate the impacts of the labeled incident in a given jurisdiction. The *early response* is characterized by efforts to prevent an outbreak from becoming an epidemic or an epidemic from becoming a pandemic. The goal is to stop all transmission of the pathogen—that is, "to put the genie back into the bottle." The *late response* occurs if the early response does not stop all transmission, and it aims at reducing death and disease through public health measures as well as the development and application of treatments and vaccines. The response phase includes the period of surge or exponential growth of a given disease as well as its decline following an epidemic curve. The response phase is demarcated by the trigger, indicating the start of the pandemic, and a declaration by the same public health authority that the response phase of the labeled incident has ended. Further, the end of the intrapandemic period or response phase is conceptually simpler for diseases that can be controlled or eliminated, but the ending is less obvious for conditions that persist as naturally occurring in a seasonal fashion or that continue to spread even after an acute response phase, such as with HIV/AIDS or COVID-19.

Next, the *recovery and reconstruction phase* refers to the strategies and actions to rebuild affected communities, systems, and infrastructure following the shocks and traumas of the pandemic period. Arguably, this phase overlaps with the prevention and preparedness phases (for future pandemics), but it is labeled as a distinct postpandemic phase for which the strategies and actions address the societal changes and impacts that resulted from the pandemic.

## Categorization of Pandemic Actions

The considerations outlined in the previous subsection guide the systematic identification and categorization of pandemic actions into the four crucial phases of the pandemic cycle (table 13.1), drawing from multiple lists such as the Pandemic Influenza Preparedness framework and Joint External Evaluation tool of the World Health Organization (WHO), Group of Twenty High Level Independent Panel Report, Oxford COVID-19 Government Response Tracker, International Monetary Fund's COVID-19 Policy Tracker,[1] and others (G20 HLIP 2021; Hale et al. 2021; WHO 2022, 2024). This categorization serves as a road map or playbook of possible pandemic actions for which strategic financial planning is necessary to allocate funds at pandemic phase. This approach ensures a methodical, comprehensive, and coordinated strategy for responding to global health crises, addressing the challenges at the global, regional, national, and local levels. Identifying and classifying actions can help improve coordination, collaboration, and assignment of responsibilities, particularly across ministries and sectors as well as between different authorities and agencies, and thus can better address the control of a pandemic.

This categorization aligns with WHO's new framework on Health Emergency Prevention, Preparedness, Response, and Resilience, which emphasizes comprehensive strategies for managing health emergencies (WHO 2023). It differs, however, by incorporating a stronger focus on international governance and regional capacity development, ensuring that both global coordination and local self-sufficiency are emphasized to enhance overall resilience. Although this chapter's list of pandemic actions—or interventions—does not include all the interventions identified in the WHO 2023 report, having a common vocabulary and a consolidated list or playbook of pandemic actions can help policy makers better understand the decision space and the range of available options.

**Table 13.1** Pandemic Actions Categorization through the Pandemic Cycle

| Category | Strategies and actions |
|---|---|
| **Policies, guidelines, and legal instruments** | *Development and dissemination.* Creation of distribution of global and regional policies, guidelines, and recommendations for pandemic prevention, preparedness, response, and reconstruction, including the establishment of a National IHR Focal Point and sharing of national policies |
| | *Regulatory frameworks.* Development of regulatory frameworks to expedite the review and approval of products (such as PPE) during emergencies |
| | *Guidelines for points of entry.* Establishment of guidelines for international travel, transportation, and points of entry to prevent the spread of disease |
| | *Implementation of national policies.* Enforcing national policies, guidelines, and laws regarding case management, testing strategies, health care facility management, and the continuity of essential health services |
| | *Travel and border control.* Implementation of travel restrictions, quarantine measures, and health screening at borders to limit the importation of cases |
| **International collaboration, coordination, and initiatives** | *Global funding and aid.* Mobilization of international aid and funding to support pandemic prevention, preparedness, response, and reconstruction efforts |
| | *Investment incentives.* Encouraging investments from countries and partners to strengthen pandemic response capacities |
| | *Coordination mechanisms.* Establishment of clear coordination mechanisms across sectors and levels of government for effective emergency response |
| | *Strengthening global health governance.* Enhancing the role of international organizations in coordinating pandemic response, ensuring compliance with international health regulations, and fostering global collaboration |
| | *Accountability mechanisms.* Implementing mechanisms for monitoring and evaluating the performance of countries and international bodies in pandemic prevention, preparedness, and response |
| | *Regional capacity development.* Supporting the development of regional capacities, including the establishment of regional health centers, strengthening local health systems, and enhancing regional manufacturing capabilities for medical supplies and vaccines |
| | *Global initiatives.* Establishment of global initiatives, such as those to address socioeconomic impacts and inequalities exacerbated by the pandemic |
| **Surveillance systems (early detection, monitoring, and reporting)** | *Biosafety and biosecurity systems.* Establishment and strengthening of national biosafety and biosecurity systems |
| | *Global surveillance networks.* Development of global networks for early detection and monitoring of outbreaks, including genome sequencing and real-time data-sharing platforms |
| | *One-Health surveillance.* Routine surveillance to identify new or rare infections in humans (for example, surveillance of fevers of unknown origin) and any zoonotic links of such infections |
| | *National laboratory systems.* Strengthening national laboratories by enhancing testing capacities, integrating digital surveillance tools, and improving real-time data reporting and analysis |
| | *Contact tracing and monitoring.* Tracking cases, conducting contact tracing, and monitoring disease trends to inform response strategies |
| **Health system capacity and resources** | *Pandemic simulation exercises.* Design and implementation of simulation exercises to test and improve pandemic preparedness |
| | *Health care infrastructure.* Strengthening of health care infrastructure, including the expansion of hospital beds, critical care units, medical equipment, laboratory capacity, and health care workforce capacities |
| | *Essential health services.* Ensuring the continuity of essential health services during a pandemic |
| | *Capacity building for regional manufacturing.* Developing regional capacities for the production of medical supplies, including training local workforce, technology transfer, and establishing supply chains |

*table continues next page*

**Table 13.1** Pandemic Actions Categorization through the Pandemic Cycle (continued)

| Category | Strategies and actions |
|---|---|
| **Health system capacity and resources** | *Supply allocation and distribution.* Planning and managing the allocation and distribution of essential medical supplies (such as PPE and ventilators), vaccines, and other critical resources, including cold chain management, stockpiling, and developing vaccine distribution plans |
| | *Resource mobilization.* Deployment of resources, including medical supplies and health care personnel, to regions heavily affected by an epidemic or pandemic |
| **Research and development (vaccines, therapeutics, diagnostics, and PPE)** | *Market shaping.* Using mechanisms such as advance market commitments and pooled purchasing to incentivize the development of vaccines and therapeutics |
| | *Fast-track R&D.* Accelerating research and development processes for new countermeasures, including diagnostics, drugs, monoclonal antibodies, and vaccines |
| | *Regulatory approval.* Streamlining regulatory approval processes to ensure timely access to critical medical interventions, especially in the context of an epidemic |
| | *Technology transfer and IP.* Facilitating technology transfer, managing IP rights, and ensuring equitable access to pandemic countermeasures |
| | *Manufacturing and production.* Scaling up manufacturing and production capacities to meet global demand |
| | *Supply chain management.* Ensuring robust supply chain and logistics management for the delivery and administration of pandemic countermeasures |
| | *Knowledge sharing.* Promoting global collaboration and sharing of research findings, best practices, and lessons learned |
| **Risk communication and community engagement** | *Public awareness campaigns.* Global campaigns to raise public awareness and trust as well as to counter mistrust and promote preventive behaviors |
| | *Situation updates and misinformation.* Regular provision of updates on the pandemic situation, preventive measures, and treatment options while addressing misinformation |
| | *Community-driven assessments.* Development of community-driven risk assessments and capacity mapping to tailor responses to local needs |
| **Epidemic control and mitigation measures** | *Infection prevention and control.* Implementation of control measures to reduce transmission in research laboratories, health care settings, public spaces, and communities |
| | *Testing and diagnosis.* Ensuring access to testing supplies, laboratory services, and information about the most effective and cost-effective diagnostic protocols and tools |
| | *Tier-specific strategies.* Development and execution of tier-specific diagnostic testing strategies, treatment plans, and care protocols based on the severity and spread of the pandemic |
| **Reconstruction efforts (throughout the entire cycle)** | *Economic recovery.* Implementation of economic recovery measures, including stimulus packages and support for affected industries and businesses |
| | *Social support.* Provision of financial assistance, unemployment benefits, food security measures, and support for vulnerable populations |
| | *Mental health services.* Establishment of mental health support and counseling services for populations affected by the pandemic |

*Source:* Original table created for this publication.

*Note:* Green refers to prevention, yellow to preparedness, red to response, and purple to multiple pandemic phases. IHR = International Health Regulations; IP = intellectual property; PPE = personal protective equipment; R&D = research and development.

## KEY EPIDEMIOLOGIC AND ECONOMIC CONCEPTS

Understanding the financing of pandemics requires a grasp of epidemiologic and economic principles that can shape how resources are allocated and used. This section delves into the critical concepts of pandemic epidemiology, including the unique characteristics of infectious diseases that differentiate them from other types of disasters. It also explores essential economic concepts such as public goods, time preference, incentives, market failures, and political economy, which underpin the strategies for effective pandemic preparedness and response.

### Infectious Disease Epidemiology

Epidemics and pandemics, the latter classified as disasters, possess distinct characteristics that set them apart from other types of disasters such as floods, hurricanes, volcanic eruptions, earthquakes, and tsunamis. They also differ among themselves, including in terms of their time frames, growth patterns, detectability, and transboundary natures.

The time frames differ greatly between natural disasters and epidemics. Whereas natural disasters such as hurricanes can occur over the period of a day, the unfolding impact of an epidemic can be longer, even as cases spread to many people (that is, with a high $R_0$), but epidemic detection may take weeks depending on the specific biology of the pathogens, the symptoms, or the lack thereof.

Unlike disasters, which generally have an acute phase followed by diminishing impact, infectious diseases unfold in a manner characterized by exponential growth, which can result in surging and widespread transmission. In the case of respiratory pathogens, such epidemics have the potential to eventually reach the entire population unless contained. Infectious diseases invariably follow an epidemic curve in which cases (as well as hospitalizations and deaths) surge, peak, and then decline; however, compared to physical disasters such as earthquakes or hurricanes with peak intensity in a short period of time, such as a day, epidemics are slow. They are also less visible and in some cases invisible, especially if an extended period of asymptomatic infection occurs or if some infections are completely asymptomatic. The most important difference is that, as they grow exponentially, they become exponentially more difficult to contain. Finally, if containment is not possible, then the death and disability they cause does not abruptly end, unlike with a hurricane, tsunami, or flood. Thus, addressing epidemics both early and effectively while considering the potential for sustained efforts over time for mitigation makes infectious diseases quite different from natural disasters.

The transmissible nature of infectious diseases implies that a disease can originate locally but has the potential to escalate into global crises if not contained. Unlike some natural disasters, which are constrained in their cross-border effects, pandemics, particularly of respiratory pathogens, have global reach. A failure to detect and contain an outbreak in one region can eventually trigger devastating consequences worldwide.

## Infectious Disease Economics

Four economic concepts are especially important to pandemic financing: public goods, time preference, incentives, market failures, and political economy.

### *Public Goods*

A *public good* is one that benefits everyone, from which nobody can be excluded, and whose consumption does not reduce availability for subsequent consumption. For example, if the use of personal protective equipment by bat guano harvesters in one cave in Liberia makes a pandemic less likely to occur, it will benefit people in the Arab Republic of Egypt, Japan, and Uruguay—and the benefit for someone in Japan is no less because it also benefits Egyptians. Conversely, failure to contain an outbreak does not affect just the community or country that failed to contain it but can have repercussions for every country, as demonstrated by the COVID-19 pandemic (Schäferhoff et al. 2019).

The prevention and control of infectious diseases as public goods are challenging because, once infected, an individual will underinvest in the control and spread to others. At the same time, those who are not yet infected may also underinvest in protection because they can free ride on others protecting themselves individually—for example, through immunization and adequate herd immunity.

Public goods have a characteristic of geographic scale or scope: local (for example, fire protection), national (for example, national defense), regional (for example, regional epidemics), and global (for example, pandemics and mitigation of climate change). The control and prevention of pathogens may vary in their local, national, regional, or global spread and thus their geographic scope as a public good. For example, the control of respiratory pathogens arguably has greater scope to be a global public good, whereas the control of bloodborne diseases may be mostly limited to a regional public good (Fan, Cash, et al. 2023).

Public goods become more challenging as scale increases, because the involved entities increase in their number, diversity, and type beyond individuals. In the case of global public goods, entities are no longer individuals alone but countries, with countries able to free ride on the levels of preparedness of other countries. Consequently, according to this logic, individual countries would underinvest in preparedness if most of the benefits accrue to those in other nations. Standard economic theory would justify government or at least collective intervention to address public goods. Adequate funding of global public goods would require that countries everywhere contribute proportionately so that each country can benefit.

Pandemic preparedness has often been framed as a public good, but it may also be characterized as a merit good with positive externalities. Unlike pure public goods, which are both nonexcludable and nonrivalrous, many core capacities for prevention and preparedness—such as surveillance systems, laboratory networks, and health workforce training—confer substantial direct benefits to the countries that invest in them, in addition to providing spillover benefits to others. Countries with strong prevention, preparedness, and response (PPR) systems are better equipped to detect and contain outbreaks early, reducing domestic health and economic disruptions while simultaneously lowering the risk of cross-border spread.

### Time Preference

The economic concept of *time preference* or time discounting refers to the differential valuation that individuals or countries place on receiving a good now compared to later, or at an earlier date compared to a later date, with a tendency to discount rewards in the future compared to the present. Time preference or discounting may explain the much lower investment in preparing for pandemics for which benefits would be observed at an unknown future date, compared to more investment in responding to a pandemic when the benefits are immediately observed (even if, as noted earlier, the immediacy of epidemics is less immediate than other natural disasters). Countries with greater resource constraints, such as LMICs, may have more significant time preference, especially countries addressing immediate or basic needs such as food security. Political cycles also affect time preference, because leaders tend to focus on short-term gains that can be seen during their time in office.

Adopting a long-term perspective can counter the tendency for large time discounting compounded by short-term preferences of political cycles. A long-term view would imply not only a smaller discount rate but also the role of contracts and agreements, such as through international cooperation, that can create long-term commitments for countries to persist in their investments in pandemic preparedness over time, irrespective of changes in leadership and political priorities, or as a deterrent if they fail to do so. Such a long-term perspective may also be interpreted as sustainability, previously defined by the United Nations Brundtland Commission as meeting "the needs of the present without compromising the ability of future generations to meet their own needs" (United Nations Brundtland Commission 1987, section I, para. 27).

### Incentives

The theory of *incentives* and the principal-agent problem are essential to understanding any payment of financial resources and the risks of moral hazard (Laffont 1993; Laffont and Martimort 2002). Paying a country to be prepared involves different incentives compared to a country investing its own resources to be prepared. Given the potential global impact of local preparedness or lack thereof, neighboring areas and beyond may be concerned that the lack of preparedness in another locale can spread and affect their locale. In contrast, purchase of insurance by a country, on the expectation that the insurer will provide assistance, may result in moral hazard, that is, engaging in risky behavior that may necessitate a payout from the insurer. Thus, any discussion of pandemic financing should recognize the ways in which funding flows and recognize that associated agreements and contracts have incentives in shaping behavior, particularly of governments.

The relationship between an international funding agency and a country can be formally defined as a contract and interpreted formally as a principal-agent relationship, with its associated challenges of incentives. A financing flow thus has two aspects: (1) its role of mobilizing revenues and resources to a country (from the perspective of the receiving country), and (2) the aspect of purchasing and payment, in which an international agency pays a receiving country for a contractually agreed set of services or goods. From the perspective of external financing as resource mobilization, external financing represents one of multiple sources of revenues as a government policy maker decides how to spend its resources. Past research on the consequences of foreign assistance to countries indicates the potential for aid fungibility; that is, an increase in foreign assistance for health may be associated with a decrease by the country in domestic government health spending, with implications for sustainability (Dieleman, Graves, and Hanlon 2013).

### Market Failures

During a pandemic, *market failures*—when the free market fails to distribute goods and services efficiently—become evident in the allocation of scarce inputs such as diagnostic tests, antimicrobial drugs, and vaccines. For instance, countries with resources or production capacity may hoard or ban the export of supplies instead of distributing them to populations in greater need or lacking the ability to pay.

The market failures in this context arise from several factors. First, the global inequality in incomes underpins stark differences in ability to pay for supplies and medical countermeasures during a pandemic, not least of which are vaccines. Compounding this inequality is the lack of timely sharing of financial resources between high-income nations and lower-income nations that lack resources to purchase needed supplies or put down deposits to get in the queue for the purchase of such supplies. The sharing of those resources requires a coordinated international mechanism involving timely, respected, and authoritative resource allocation. Second, intellectual property rights create time-bound monopolies to encourage the private sector to invest in developing new products. International agreements provide for the suspension of such monopolies when needed to confront a public health emergency. However, the mechanisms to do so are so slow, cumbersome, and restrictive that they have not successfully accelerated access to products in the event of an emergency such as the COVID-19 pandemic—not even for products developed with a large proportion of public funding. Third, national governments have exacerbated the problem by restricting export of key products until fully satisfying local demand (even enabling stockpiling) before meeting the needs of people at greater risk in other countries. During the COVID-19 pandemic, short supply and individual hoarding behaviors among those who could pay led to temporary shortages of key products such as face masks.

### Political Economy Factors

Although externalities justify some level of international financing and coordination, the significant internalized benefits may suggest that underinvestment in PPR cannot be attributed solely to the public good dilemma. The other microeconomic concepts such as time preference and incentives provide useful insights into decision-making, but their application to pandemic preparedness must be complemented by a broader political economy and institutional design perspective. *Political economy* refers to the study of how politics and economics interact and how they shape each other. A broader set of political economy factors may play a larger role in explaining why many governments fail to allocate sufficient resources for preparedness.

Unlike individuals or firms, national governments operate within political, bureaucratic, and fiscal constraints that shape their willingness and ability to invest in preparedness. Political leaders, for instance, may prioritize short-term electoral gains over long-term resilience, particularly in democratic systems with frequent election cycles. Institutional fragmentation—both within governments and across international actors—can further limit coordinated action, leading to underinvestment in preparedness despite clear long-term benefits.

Moreover, despite their relevance in shaping the production and allocation of medical countermeasures, market failures interact with geopolitical competition, industrial policy, and national security concerns, which influence decisions on research and development, manufacturing, and distribution. Consequently, financing mechanisms for pandemic preparedness cannot be framed solely as correcting market failures but must also account for political incentives, institutional coordination challenges, and the strategic interests of key players. Thus, an approach that may be more pragmatic or feasible relative to a proportional allocation system may be to align preparedness financing with equity-driven investments in lower-income countries, recognizing the political and economic motivations of wealthier nations while leveraging their potential spillover benefits.

### Policy Implications

Together these economic concepts force us to consider how the allocation of resources and responsibilities should vary throughout different phases of a pandemic, including considerations on whether funding should be withheld from countries that opt out of global efforts.

In an ideal scenario, all countries would contribute to funding for pandemic prevention, preparedness, and early response—at least for regional or global public goods—under a fair and agreed-upon funding formula. Such a formula could rely solely on countries' ability to pay, akin to assessed contributions to the regular budgets of international organizations like the United Nations Secretariat or WHO. Alternatively, it could be refined to account for the fact that larger countries derive a substantial portion of the global benefits, whereas smaller countries benefit less, thus implying consideration of gross domestic product or population in aggregate. This approach would acknowledge that smaller countries might require a more favorable cost of participation because they have fewer incentives for engagement in global prevention and preparedness efforts.

In practice, however, existing multilateral institutions of the United Nations, and WHO specifically, remain the only global mechanism to which all countries will contribute, regardless of their level of preparedness or ability to respond. Proposals to use standard measures of preparedness as the basis for allocation funds to countries have not advanced because the COVID-19 pandemic demonstrated that such scores did not predict preparedness and health performance. The presumption that countries with higher incomes or even higher preparedness scores would necessarily be better able to respond to a pandemic did not bear out during the COVID-19 pandemic (Pablos-Méndez et al. 2022). Thus, it follows that developing an acceptable formula for allocation funding for pandemic preparedness and response remains elusive.

If an outbreak or an epidemic occurs anywhere on the planet, every country, regardless of preparedness status or contribution to a multilateral institution, should be fully eligible for global assistance—financial, human, informational, and material—as needed to contain the outbreak or epidemic. Besides obvious humanitarian reasons, not trying to contain outbreaks or epidemics in a country would not be in the enlightened self-interest of neighboring countries and the global community, because of the global public good nature of controlling the pathogen (or disease), which helps reduce the risk of cross-border spread.

Once a pandemic takes hold and containment becomes infeasible, however, the dynamic shifts. The country will primarily retain most of the benefits from country-level efforts to slow transmission or reduce the case fatality rate through treatment. In the context of a pathogen with high potential for mutation, such as COVID-19, country-level efforts to reduce transmission may have some global benefits, but even that outcome is uncertain.

A commonly understood public good, fire protection, serves as an illustrative analogy for infectious disease. It would be illogical to deny assistance from the fire department to a house lacking fire insurance. Doing so would put neighboring houses at risk. If the homeowner lacks insurance or engages in fire-prone risks, however, the community may not feel obligated to rebuild or provide temporary housing. Similarly, although the global community may opt to provide humanitarian assistance to countries whose leaders previously declined to participate in global pandemic financing mechanisms, it does not have the same global imperative to aid those that abstained from prior engagement or actively engaged in risky behavior. In this regard, the International Health Regulations could be seen as an indication of participation, good faith, and compliance with agreed-upon prevention and preparedness efforts.

### Addressing Market Failures in Medical Countermeasures and Manufacturing

Among the alternatives to address these market failures, two approaches stand out and are not mutually exclusive: (1) implementing binding international agreements to ensure equitable distribution of supplies (for example, streamlining the Agreement on Trade-Related Aspects of Intellectual Property Rights (TRIPS) waiver process during emergencies like pandemics) and (2) establishing distributed manufacturing capacity to ensure availability across all regions, not just in a select few producing or high-income countries (coupled with, for example, implementing a robust and swift protocol for technology transfer pools), and assuming that regional manufacturing improves equitable distribution.

Setting up manufacturing in different parts of the world is a strategic move to improve resiliency in pandemic response and offers several advantages. First, it allows for quicker and more accessible distribution of medical supplies and vaccines, because products can be made closer to where they are urgently needed. Regional manufacturing reduces the time and complexity involved in shipping goods across long distances, especially in crisis situations when time is of the essence.

Second, it enhances the resilience of global supply chains by diversifying the locations of manufacturing. Such diversification helps avoid the severe disruptions that occur when a key production area is hit by an outbreak or other crises, or imposes (often temporary) export bans as a result of "vaccine nationalism" to ensure national stockpiles and adequacy (Wagner et al. 2021). Decentralization also promotes equity in access to essential health products. During the COVID-19 pandemic, countries hosting manufacturing facilities—such as China, India, the Russian Federation, and the United States—had prioritized access to vaccines and supplies, leaving other countries at a disadvantage in terms of timely and affordable access. Distributed manufacturing capabilities can help address the principle of fair access to the tools needed to combat a pandemic.

Third, local manufacturing can drive economic, technological, and scientific development and capabilities in different regions. Such development and capabilities can empower regions to become more self-sufficient and less reliant on imports for critical health supplies, allowing them to serve as potential industrial producers, and with potential spillovers in other technological domains. Overall, regionalized manufacturing prepares us better for future health emergencies, making our response more resilient, rapid, equitable, and effective.

## DEFINITION OF PANDEMIC FINANCING

This section moves on from an examination of epidemiologic and economic concepts to defining pandemic financing as inclusive of three aspects: health financing and two of its subcategories (official development finance and non-flow financial instruments), official development finance pertaining to a pandemic, and non-flow financial instruments[2] relevant to ministries of finance in addressing a pandemic or disaster.

## Health Financing Frameworks

Definitions of *health financing* vary. WHO defines it from a national perspective as revenue raising, pooling of funds, and purchasing of services related to health, typically the remit of a ministry or department of health. Roberts et al. (2008) emphasize the revenue mobilization and pooling functions of financing, classified into six categories: general revenues, social insurance, private insurance, community financing, out-of-pocket financing, and external flows. That framework distinguishes between financing and payment. *Payment* is defined as the methods and incentives associated with transferring funds between the principal and the agent in a contractual relationship, often conditional on the delivery of a given service or good and with incentives as noted earlier. In contrast, the WHO framework places the purchasing function as part of financing[3] (Fan, Sharma, and Hou 2023).

Of the six different sources of financing identified by Roberts et al. (2008), external flows generally refer to the varieties of official development finance (ODF), for which the ODF addressing pandemics is the next component of this chapter's definition of pandemic financing. The Organisation for Economic Co-operation and Development formally defines external flows as inclusive of ODF, which comprises official development assistance (ODA) of a concessional nature and other official flows (OOF), which are nonconcessional. Within the ODA category, it further distinguishes between health ODA and other ODA (for example, for other sectors such as education), with an additional distinction between health ODA for pandemics compared to health ODA not explicitly for addressing pandemics (figure 13.2). The same classification can also be applied to other ODA, with some portion of other ODA addressing pandemics and the rest not, and similarly parsed for OOF (health and pandemics). Despite the necessity of considering flows for other sectors, for the purpose of quantitative analyses in this chapter, discussion is restricted primarily to external flows related to health and, within that, for pandemics. This chapter presents analyses of external flows based on this definition, supplemented by international spending on research and development for COVID-19. Note also that this analysis does not capture non-flow instruments, namely international insurance contracts, discussed later in the chapter.

### *Implications of Organizational Design and Structures on Pandemic Financing*

The characteristics of governance and organizational structures largely determine pandemic financing rather than the other way around. The authorized ministry or agency (of a particular sector) responsible for the funds often categorizes and classifies these funds, at both the national and the international level. These sectoral or ministerial silos define who has the resources and who does the implementation—consequently, different incentives exist depending on differences in the principal-agent relationship across ministries (Das Gupta et al. 2009). The organizational design, structure, and governance within a country and between countries and agencies for international cooperation have great implications for pandemic financing. Silos remain a major, if not inevitable, challenge in ensuring synergistic coordination of resources and avoidance of duplication of efforts (or even working at cross-purposes).

**Figure 13.2** Classification of Official Development Finance for Health ODA

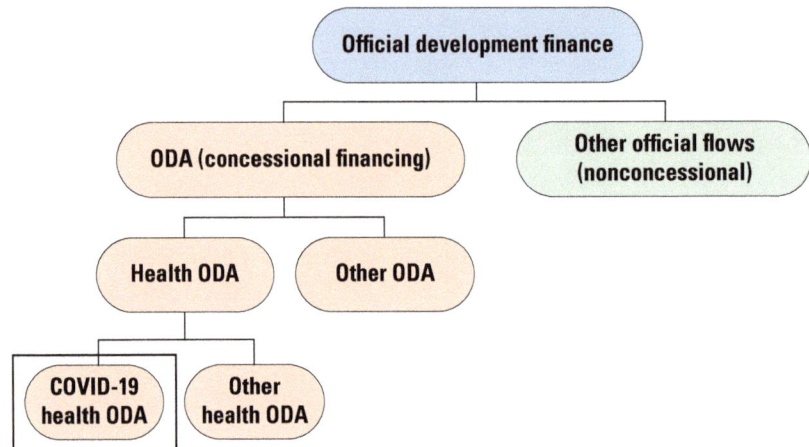

*Source:* Original figure created for this publication.

*Note:* ODA = official development assistance. The box around "COVID-19 health ODA" highlights it as a subset of health ODA that was separately tracked because of its relevance during the pandemic response.

From a national perspective, professionals in the health sector continue to view health as the primary sector responsible for preparing, responding, and recovering from a pandemic, even though a pandemic affects all sectors and several sectors may contribute to increasing pandemic risks, such as land use and environmental planning, agriculture, animal husbandry, and One Health considerations. The organizational design and structure in which ministries relate to each other, such as hierarchically or laterally, all have implications for how financing incentives affect different ministries (Das Gupta et al. 2009; Fan 2022).

From an international perspective, different international agencies are responsible for different functions in the pandemic cycle. International financial institutions function within governance frameworks shaped by member states, shareholders, and their own internal mechanisms. These governance structures influence how decisions are made and resources are allocated. Rather than a single entity determining the course of action, pandemic response governance emerges from the interactions among multiple institutions, each operating within its own mandate, priorities, and constraints. The fragmentation in international governance reveals a fundamental tension and unresolved question about which agency should decide what happens and how—for example, should it be WHO as the leading United Nations entity on health matters or the Bretton Woods institutions that currently have the lion's share of the multilateral resources?

This chapter argues that sectoral silos are both necessary and a potential hindrance during a pandemic. During the pandemic response phase, all sectors—not only health—are stressed and responding to dynamical changes because of the pandemic; thus, a large proportion of financing in all sectors could be labeled as pandemic financing. Before and after a pandemic or health emergency, however, most countries clearly do not use most ODF and government financing to address pandemic prevention, preparedness, response, or recovery. An overly broad notion of pandemic financing will not be pragmatic, but an overly narrow one will miss significant expenditures, especially outside of the health sector. Whereas sectors are necessary for implementation, their creation of silos also risks poor coordination, duplication of effort, and confusion in terms of authority and responsibilities—a pattern arguably seen regularly at both national and international levels during the COVID-19 response.

## Definition of Pandemic Financing

A definition of pandemic financing restricted to domestic and external financing for health and specifically for pandemic-related health, adopted for this chapter, is admittedly too narrow. Unfortunately, because of data limitations, the chapter presents data only on health ODA for COVID-19. Excluded from the analysis of funding flows is a complete listing of OOF for COVID-19 including health OOF as well as other COVID-19 ODA not focused on health (refer to figure 13.2).

Despite the limitations of this quantitative analysis of flows, this chapter's definition of pandemic financing goes beyond health financing and health ODA for COVID-19. As noted by others, ODF is a concept limited to actual flows, rather than promises or contractual agreements or arrangements for payment, such as guarantees or insurance payouts. Such contractual agreements may not require immediate payment from one actor to another but set the conditions under which payments can be rapidly made or in some cases be suspended, in the case of debt suspension clauses that suspend debt servicing payments in the context of an emergency.

Many health financing mechanisms, including for ODF—such as ODA and OOF—also have contractual arrangements or terms and conditions of what is required for a country to be eligible to receive such flows (so-called eligibility policies), how much the country should contribute (so-called domestic financing policies), and how much risk a country is responsible for (which can refer to repayment or debt servicing in the case of loans, whether concessional or nonconcessional). Non-flow tools often refer to contractual arrangements between a payer and payee, which would reflect the purchasing or payment function rather than the revenue mobilization or pooling function of financing.

## Instruments for Pandemic Financing

Multiple instruments are available for external pandemic financing, each serving different purposes across the pandemic cycle (figure 13.3). These financial instruments can be categorized by their terms and conditions, including whether they are concessional or at market rate, and whether they are contingent or noncontingent. Such classifications help policy makers and stakeholders identify the most appropriate financing mechanisms to address the various stages of the pandemic cycle.

**Figure 13.3** Classification of External Pandemic Financing Tools, by Key Characteristics

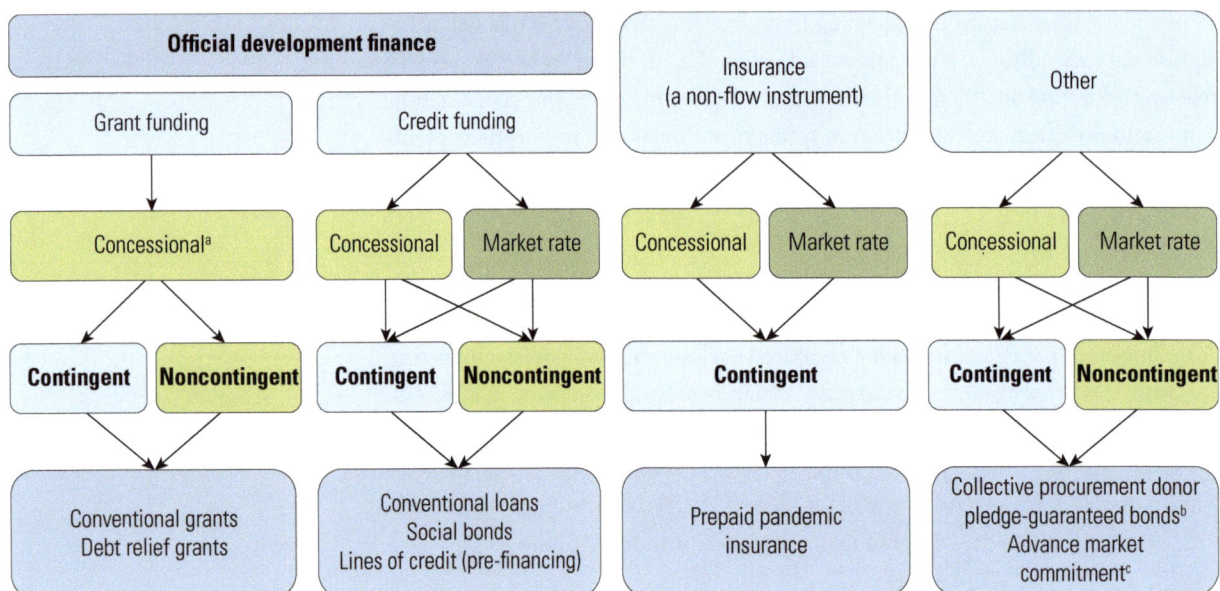

*Source:* Original figure created for this publication.

a. *Concessional* refers to various forms of subsidies by donors. Grants are typically fully subsidized but can require national cofinancing. Concessional credit usually has interest rates that are below market rates. Concessional insurance reduces the premium paid by the insured. Concessional collective procurement uses subsidies to reduce the prices paid by some purchasers.

b. For example, under the International Finance Facility for Immunisation, donor pledges guarantee private bonds that enable immediate expenditures.

c. A mechanism like an advance market commitment could be nonconcessional if the agreed minimum demand for a product is met but could trigger a donor-funded payment if the demand is not met (similar to a concessional insurance policy). The quantitative analysis used here does not capture non-flow instruments.

This chapter defines *contingent* as referring to funding that is prenegotiated but released or activated only when specific trigger conditions are met. These trigger conditions—such as a pandemic, a natural disaster, or financial crisis—are typically possible, but not likely, in any given year. Such contingent financing refers to a specific type of conditionality on financing, but other kinds of financing conditionalities exist, such as conditions on whether the recipient complies with the terms of the financing (for example, ensuring financial controls and reporting requirements, using the funding for designated purposes, and demonstrating cofinancing), common to development financing.

Figure 13.3 categorizes instruments for pandemic financing into four primary types: official development finance (subdivided into grant funding and credit funding), insurance, and other.

- Grant funding includes conventional grants and financial mechanisms such as debt relief, which can be either contingent or noncontingent in nature. Whereas conventional grants are nonrepayable funds, debt relief involves modifying or reducing existing debt obligations to alleviate financial burdens.

- Credit funding includes concessional loans (offered at lower-than-market interest rates), market-rate loans, social bonds, and lines of credit (preagreed financing). The loans can be contingent or noncontingent, depending on whether they are activated only when specific conditions are met.

- Insurance represents a non-flow instrument such as prepaid pandemic insurance, which is inherently contingent, activating upon the occurrence of specific events or conditions and with regular premium payments, which can be market rate or concessional (subsidized).

- The "other" category refers to purchasing arrangements and market-shaping instruments, as distinct from the first three instruments that function primarily for revenue mobilization and pooling (Dissanayake and Camps Adrogué 2022, 2023). Collective or pooled procurement can both reduce required outlays by reducing prices and increase access because producers prioritize large buyers (Dubois, Lefouili, and Straub 2021). The instruments can be concessional if donor subsidies reduce effective prices for some purchasers. Advance market commitments (AMCs) are binding commitments to purchase a specified product at a preset price as an incentive for producers to allocate their resources for developing the desired product (Kremer, Levin, and Snyder 2020). The AMC for a pneumococcal vaccine arranged by Gavi, the Vaccine Alliance was donor funded (concessional) with country financing. AMCs do not necessarily require pooled procurement but can benefit from pooled procurement—that is, pooling demand from multiple countries. Pooled procurement and the pneumococcal AMC have not been contingent on an epidemic or pandemic. A prenegotiated mechanism that pools country demand could be triggered in a future pandemic to collectively purchase vaccines, for example, and would be an example of a contingent collective purchase instrument. If linked to a contingent financing mechanism, it could enable LMICs to compete more effectively for scarce products with high-income countries on both volume and price.

Box 13.1 provides an overview of the types of external financing instruments, which exclude domestic revenue mobilization involving government revenue, primarily derived from taxation.

### Box 13.1

### Overview of the Types of External Financing Instruments

**Grants** do not have repayment requirements. Two broad categories of grants exist: those that fall within the on-budget framework and those that operate off-budget. On-budget grants are funds directed through the recipient country's government budget and financial system, whereas off-budget grants do not follow the recipient country's official budget and financial management systems. In the on-budget framework, the recipient government assumes ownership of the financing and is responsible for fund use. Conversely, in the off-budget framework, donors retain more control over fund allocation, enabling them to target specific projects or sectors inside or outside of government institutions.

*box continues next page*

## Box 13.1 Overview of the Types of External Financing Instruments (continued)

**Debt relief** instruments are measures creditors take, often in coordination with international financial institutions, to reduce or restructure the debt burden of debtor countries. These initiatives can include forgiveness of a portion of the debt, extension of payment periods, reduction of interest rates, or conversion of debt into grants. The goal is to alleviate the financial stress on nations struggling to meet their debt obligations, enabling them to direct more resources to critical needs such as health care and social programs, particularly during economic hardship. Debt relief programs often span several years, with gradual reductions in debt burdens. Debt relief can be triggered by prespecified conditions (contingent).

**Concessional loans** typically have below-market interest rates because the negotiated interest rate is below market or because the loans have interest-free grace periods. The lending institution or a third party may subsidize the interest rate. The loans may also offer the option to repay in the borrower's local currency or provide other terms that reduce the exchange rate risk.

**Nonconcessional loans** are financial credits provided at terms and interest rates closer to market rates. They typically have shorter grace periods and repayment schedules than concessional loans. Such loans are usually used by middle-income and high-income countries for larger-scale projects with the capacity to generate economic returns.

**Emergency or contingent loans** are specific types of loans that have expedited approval processes to ensure rapid access to funds during emergencies requiring immediate financial intervention. To facilitate rapid disbursement, these loans often come with prenegotiated terms activated in an emergency, with interest rates and repayment schedules that reflect the situation's urgency and the borrower's repayment capacity. The preset terms allow for quick action when conventional loan procedures might be too slow to address the pressing needs of the situation. Although designed for rapid disbursement, emergency loans can be limited by the availability of emergency financing facilities and the prenegotiated terms. Similar to a contingent loan is a line of credit that can be activated by the borrower, perhaps with conditions that limit what the funds can be used for.

**Insurance mechanisms** are financial arrangements designed to manage risk and provide compensation in the event of specific losses or damages. They collect regular payments, or premiums, from a large group of policyholders. When a covered event occurs, the mechanism disburses funds from the collective pool to the affected parties per the terms outlined in their insurance policies. In global health, insurance can play a crucial role by offering countries a way to mitigate financial risks associated with large-scale health crises like epidemics and pandemics. Despite offering quick access to funds in the event of an incident, international insurance mechanisms are limited by the coverage scope and the ability to accurately predict and quantify risks. Concessional insurance products typically involve a donor paying a portion of the premiums.

**Guarantees** are commitments by a guarantor, usually an international financial institution, to assume responsibility for a debt obligation in the event that the borrower country defaults. Guarantees are often used to secure a loan, reduce the risk for lenders, and improve the borrower's credit terms. Because they mitigate the risk to the lender by providing a promise of repayment from a financially stable guarantor, guarantees can enable developing countries to access capital markets or secure loans for development projects at better rates. The timeline for guarantees depends on the underlying financial arrangements and agreements, typically aligned with the project. Guarantees may be associated with either conventional loans or contingent loans.

## Mapping Instruments to External Stakeholders

Table 13.2 presents a mapping of the existing external financing instruments by the different stakeholders. It categorizes each instrument by source, type of instrument, purpose, trigger/eligibility criteria, and repayment terms. Because of time and effort limitations, 15 funding agencies were purposively selected, with a focus on the largest agencies involved in COVID-19, those with a history of substantial contributions to global health, and organizations actively adapting their instruments in response to lessons learned from the pandemic. Additionally, agencies representing diverse funding mechanisms and geographic regions were considered to ensure a comprehensive overview of the global financing landscape. For each agency, review of a number of information sources, including financial reports, funding announcements, and press releases, resulted in a catalog of 31 different instruments. Although not comprehensive, the list captures many of the primary external instruments in use or under active consideration for pandemic prevention, preparedness, response, and recovery and reconstruction.

Different types of stakeholders were examined for this chapter: international multilateral organizations (such as WHO, the United Nations Children's Fund, and the United Nations Development Programme); multilateral regional organizations such as the Africa Centres for Disease Control and Prevention, and Pan American Health Organization; international financial institutions such as the African Development Bank, Asian Development Bank, Inter-American Development Bank, International Monetary Fund, and World Bank; bilateral donor agencies (such as the German Agency for International Cooperation, Japan International Cooperation Agency, and US Agency for International Development); global health initiatives (such as the Coalition for Epidemic Preparedness Innovations; Gavi, the Vaccine Alliance; and the Global Fund to Fight AIDS, Tuberculosis and Malaria); philanthropic organizations (such as the Gates Foundation); and research institutes (such as Institut Pasteur).

Box 13.2 presents an overview of the external organizational stakeholders. Excluded from the landscaping exercise was financing for national security or defense purposes. Importantly, although the broader stakeholder list for this chapter includes some regional organizations—such as the Africa Centres for Disease Control and Prevention—box 13.2 focuses only on global and multilateral external organizations, and therefore does not include regional entities or domestic financing arrangements.

The landscaping exercise found most of the financial instruments in the response phase of the pandemic cycle, with 23 identified tools representing most of the available resources. Those instruments, primarily contingent loans, were crucial for providing immediate financial liquidity in a crisis. The emergence of several tools in the aftermath of the COVID-19 pandemic indicated a strategic pivot to developing new financial mechanisms to address health crises. The landscaping exercise revealed that reactive financing strategies are more prevalent than proactive ones that address pandemic prevention and preparedness.

**Table 13.2** Pandemic Financing Instruments Matched to Pandemic Phases

| Source | Facility | Instrument type | Pandemic phase(s) | Purpose | Trigger/Eligibility | Repayment terms |
|--------|----------|-----------------|-------------------|---------|---------------------|-----------------|
| World Bank | Pandemic Fund | Grant | Prevention, Preparedness | A multilateral financing mechanism dedicated to providing multiyear grants for enhancing pandemic preparedness in LMICs. | Prioritize high-impact investments in (1) early warning and disease surveillance systems, (2) laboratory systems, and (3) strengthening human resources/public health and community workforce capacity. | Does not apply. |
| World Bank | IDA19 Scale-Up Window | Concessional loan | Prevention, Preparedness | Designed to scale up IDA financing to support high-quality, transformational, country-specific or regional or both, with a strong development impact. | Countries must have a low or moderate risk of debt problems. | Different choices of repayment schedules. |
| World Bank | IBRD Flexible Loan | Market-based loan | Prevention, Preparedness | Leading loan product of the World Bank for public sector borrowers of middle-income countries. Allows to customize repayment terms (that is, grace period, repayment period, and amortization profile) to meet debt management or project needs. | IBRD general lending terms. | Long maturities, up to 35 years. Market-based interest rates. |
| IMF | Resilience and Sustainability Facility (RSF) | Concessional loan | Prevention, Preparedness | Provides affordable long-term financing to countries undertaking reforms to reduce risks to prospective balance of payments stability, including those related to climate change and pandemic preparedness. | Linked to reform progress. Each measure is connected to one RSF disbursement. A reform measure can be a single policy action or a set of very closely related actions constituting a single reform. | 20-year maturity and a 10½-year grace period during which no principal is repaid. |
| ADB | Ordinary Capital Resources (OCR) | Concessional or market-based loan | Prevention, Preparedness | General ADB financial mechanisms for member countries seeking to strengthen their health systems and enhance preparedness for future pandemics. | Market-based OCR loans are usually given to middle-income countries with stronger economies, whereas concessional OCR loans are for those with lower per-capita GNI. | Depending on group categorization: A, B, and C. |
| PAHO | Revolving Fund for Procurement | Collective procurement | Prevention, Preparedness | Designed to facilitate the procurement of essential medicines and health supplies for member countries by leveraging collective purchasing power. Operates on a revolving basis whereby member countries are expected to repay the funds they use for the procurement of health supplies. | Membership, commitment to repay; health product needs; financial integrity. | Varies per case. |
| World Bank | Development Policy Loan with Deferred Drawdown Options for Catastrophe Risks | Concessional or market-based loan | (Early) Response | A contingent financing line that provides immediate liquidity following a natural disaster or health-related event. Concessional for IDA members, market-based for IBRD members. | The member country's declaration of a state of emergency. Recipients must (1) have an adequate macroeconomic policy framework; and (2) be preparing, or already have, a satisfactory disaster risk management program. | Standard IDA or IBRD repayment terms. |

*table continues next page*

**Table 13.2** Pandemic Financing Instruments Matched to Pandemic Phases (continued)

| Source | Facility | Instrument type | Pandemic phase(s) | Purpose | Trigger/Eligibility | Repayment terms |
|---|---|---|---|---|---|---|
| World Bank | Immediate Response Mechanism (IRM) | Concessional loan | (Early) Response | Allows participating IDA countries to have immediate access to up to 5 percent of the undisbursed balances of their IDA project portfolio in the event of an eligible crisis or emergency and thus shorten IDA's response time. It complements longer-term emergency response tools available to IDA countries, such as the Crisis Response Window. | In crises like natural disasters and economic shocks, it offers immediate financing for recovery efforts, including scaling up safety nets for vulnerable groups, restoring basic assets, and protecting essential spending on health. The IRM also facilitates crisis planning and disaster risk mitigation dialogue with IDA clients. | Standard IDA repayment terms. |
| IMF | Rapid Financing Instrument | Concessional or market-based loan | (Early) Response | Provides rapid, low-access financial assistance to countries facing urgent balance of payments that, if not addressed, would result in an immediate and severe economic disruption. Optimal for transitory situations when a full-fledged economic program is not necessary or feasible. | All member countries. For those eligible for the Poverty Reduction and Growth Trust, there is the concessional Rapid Credit Facility. | Single disbursement. Repayment within 3¼ to 5 years. |
| WHO | Contingency Fund for Emergencies | Grant | (Early) Response | Ensures that WHO can respond quickly and effectively to health crises and emergencies without having to wait for external funding. Supported by voluntary contributions from countries, organizations, and individuals. | Urgency and scale of the emergency; potential for international spread; insufficient local or national resources | Does not apply. |
| World Bank | Crisis Response Window (CRW) | Concessional loan | (Late) Response | Provides funding to help IDA countries respond to exceptionally severe crises, including public health emergencies. The CRW offers Early Response Financing to address slower-onset crises that are at an early stage. | The member country has declared a national public health emergency, and/or WHO has declared that the outbreak is a public health emergency of international concern | Standard IDA repayment terms. |
| World Bank | Contingency Emergency Response Component (CERC) | Concessional loan | Response | Designed to provide an immediate response to a national or regional emergency, enhancing the capacity for disaster risk management and crisis response. CERC allows for the rapid reallocation of funds or the mobilization of additional financing to address emergency response needs after a crisis or disaster has been declared. | The member country has declared a national public health emergency, and/or the WHO has declared that the outbreak is a public health emergency of international concern. | Standard IDA repayment terms. |
| IMF | Flexible Credit Line | Market-based loan | Response | Designed to meet the demand for crisis-prevention and crisis-mitigation lending for countries with very strong policy frameworks and track records in economic performance. Although not specifically created for pandemic financing, it serves as a valuable tool in providing rapid and unconditional support to countries facing external shocks. | The member country or international system has declared a public health emergency. Limited to countries with very strong economic fundamentals and institutional policy frameworks. | Renewable credit line, initially for 1 or 2 years. Repayment within 3¼ to 5 years. |

*table continues next page*

**Table 13.2** Pandemic Financing Instruments Matched to Pandemic Phases *(continued)*

| Source | Facility | Instrument type | Pandemic phase(s) | Purpose | Trigger/Eligibility | Repayment terms |
|--------|----------|-----------------|-------------------|---------|---------------------|-----------------|
| ADB | Countercyclical Support Facility (CSF) COVID-19 Pandemic Response Option (CPRO) | Concessional or market-based loan | Response | The CSF is a part of ADB's strategy for addressing economic challenges, especially during crises. Specifically designed under the CSF umbrella, the CPRO was created to swiftly address the unique challenges posed by the COVID-19 pandemic. | Eligibility based on (1) emergency status, (2) per capita income, and 3) credit worthiness. | Varies per case. |
| AfDB | COVID-19 Rapid Response Facility | Concessional or market-based loan | Response | Ensures rapid disbursement of funds to address immediate challenges, implement emergency measures, and strengthen health care systems. | Severity of the impact on the economy and fiscal stress. Degree to which denying assistance would threaten to reverse gains and undermine degree of resilience achieved in recent years. | Varies per case. |
| IDB | Contingent Credit Facility for Natural Disaster Emergencies | Concessional or market-based loan | Response | Includes both a one-time temporary coverage of COVID-19 given the unprecedented magnitude of the present outbreak, and a longer-term ex ante coverage for future pandemics and epidemics. | A natural disaster or health crisis of unexpected, sudden, and unusual proportions, until other sources of funding can be accessed. | Varies per case. |
| IsDB | COVID-19 project-specific funding | Market-based project loan | Response | IsDB focused on specific project-based interventions per country to mitigate the impact of the pandemic. | Not specified. | Varies per case; a variety of Shariah-compliant financial instruments. |
| UNOCHA | Central Emergency Response Fund (CERF) | Grant | Response | The United Nations' global emergency response fund to deliver funding quickly to humanitarian responders. CERF's Rapid Response window allows country teams to kick-start relief efforts immediately. CERF's window for underfunded emergencies helps scale up and sustain protracted relief operations to avoid critical gaps when no other funding is available. | Emergency declaration through the top United Nations official of the country. The CERF Advisory Group provides policy guidance to the Secretary-General on the use and impact of the fund. | Varies per case. |
| UNICEF | Vaccine Independence Initiative | Pre-financing | Response | Prefinancing tool managed by UNICEF, offering a support mechanism for countries using their own domestic resources for procurement of health-related supplies. The tool helps countries bridge temporary short-term funding gaps, which might otherwise lead to supply shortages and stock-outs. | Any country that has a Programme Cooperation Agreement or Basic Cooperation Agreement with UNICEF. Governments must also have sufficient budgetary resources to purchase the vaccines and injection supplies and/or cold chain equipment | Flexible credit terms, allowing governments to pay after delivery. |
| Gavi | COVAX (No longer active) | Advance market commitment | Response | Financial mechanism within Gavi designed to secure funding for the equitable production and distribution of COVID-19 vaccines. The appeal sought contributions from donor countries and organizations to subsidize vaccine costs for low-income countries. | Economies approved by the Gavi Board based on income level and crisis management | Does not apply. |

*table continues next page*

**Table 13.2** Pandemic Financing Instruments Matched to Pandemic Phases (continued)

| Source | Facility | Instrument type | Pandemic phase(s) | Purpose | Trigger/Eligibility | Repayment terms |
|---|---|---|---|---|---|---|
| IMF | Extended Fund & Credit Facility (ECF) | Concessional loan | Recovery | Designed for medium- to long-term financial assistance and structural reforms. Although not tailored specifically for pandemics, the ECF becomes relevant in the postpandemic recovery phase because it offers an extended engagement period, enabling countries to implement comprehensive reforms that contribute to rebuilding and strengthening the economy after the crisis. | All LICs under the Poverty Reduction and Growth Trust facing a protracted balance of payments problem. | Grace period of 5½ years and a final maturity of 10 years. |
| ADB | Sustainable Economic Recovery Program | Concessional loan | Recovery | Designed to support post-COVID-19 economic recovery. These loans fund projects for rebuilding infrastructure, restoring essential services, and promoting overall economic rejuvenation. | Low- and lower-middle income country members (Bangladesh, to date). Implement urgent reforms for rapid economic recovery | Depending on group categorization: A, B, and C. |
| EBRD | Strategic and Capital Framework | Grant, concessional loan, and market-based loan | Recovery | Accelerates transition in the countries as they work through the crisis and recovery phases in response to the COVID-19 crisis. | Responsive to market and reform conditions with a special focus on the transition to a green, low-carbon economy. | Varies per case. |
| IMF | Catastrophe Containment and Relief Trust (CCRT) | Debt relief grant | Response, Recovery | Provides grants for debt relief for the poorest and most vulnerable countries hit by catastrophic natural disasters or public health disasters. The relief on debt service payments to IMF frees up resources to help countries meet exceptional balance of payments needs created by the disaster and to pay for containment and recovery. | IMF members qualify for CCRT relief if a life-threatening epidemic has affected several areas of their country. Significant economic disruption is defined as a cumulative loss of the country's real GDP of 10 percent or greater, or a cumulative loss of revenue and increase of expenditures equivalent to at least 10 percent of GDP. | Debt relief grants will be used to immediately cancel debt service coming due to the IMF equivalent to approximately 20 percent of a country's quota. |
| EBRD | Coronavirus Solidarity Package | Grant, concessional loan, and market-based loan | Response, Recovery | Includes a set of financial instruments tailored to address the immediate and long-term challenges posed by the pandemic. | The EBRD is responsive to market and reform conditions with a special focus on the transition to a green, low-carbon economy. | Varies per case. |
| Global Fund | COVID-19 Response Mechanism (C19RM) Appeal | Grant | Response, Recovery | The Global Fund's main avenue for providing grant support to LMICs for COVID-19 is through the C19RM, which extends beyond the emergency phase to support long-term programs and reinvestments. Although C19RM investments were available until December 31, 2023, countries can continue implementing interventions until December 2025. | Countries that received funding in Waves 1 and 2 need to demonstrate optimal use of their approved C19RM funds, including reinvestment where appropriate. | Does not apply. |

*table continues next page*

**Table 13.2** Pandemic Financing Instruments Matched to Pandemic Phases (continued)

| Source | Facility | Instrument type | Pandemic phase(s) | Purpose | Trigger/Eligibility | Repayment terms |
|---|---|---|---|---|---|---|
| Donor countries | Bilateral aid | Grant and concessional loan | Prevention, Preparedness, Response, Recovery | Support the recipient country's health care infrastructure, provide emergency relief, enhance disease surveillance, facilitate access to medical supplies and vaccines, and bolster recovery. | Low- or middle-income country facing significant public health challenges. Agreements are based on diplomatic and developmental priorities. | Varies per case. |
| Gates Foundation | Philanthropic funding | Grant | Prevention, Preparedness, Response, Recovery | Comprehensive funding encompassing research, development, and equitable distribution of vaccines, treatments, and diagnostics. Supports strengthening health systems and enhancing global disease surveillance and response capabilities. | Initiatives that address public health needs with innovative, scalable solutions, particularly in LMICs. Priority is given to proposals demonstrating potential for broad, global impact. | Does not apply. |

*Source:* Original table created for this publication.

*Note:* Green refers to prevention and preparedness, red to response, blue to recovery and reconstruction, and purple to multiple pandemic phases. ADB = Asian Development Bank; AfDB = African Development Bank; COVAX = COVID-19 Vaccines Global Access; EBRD = European Bank for Reconstruction and Development; GDP = gross domestic product; GNI = gross national income; IBRD = International Bank for Reconstruction and Development; IDA = International Development Association; IDB = Inter-American Development Bank; IMF = International Monetary Fund; IsDB = Islamic Development Bank; LICs = low-income countries; LMICs = low- and middle-income countries; PAHO = Pan American Health Organization; UNICEF = United Nations Children's Fund; UNOCHA = United Nations Office for the Coordination of Humanitarian Affairs; WHO = World Health Organization.

## Organizational Stakeholders in External Pandemic Financing

**International financial institutions** are multilateral development banks (and associated institutions) established by more than one country with the main purpose of providing financial support and advice to achieve development goals. The best-known international financial institutions were established after World War II to provide mechanisms for international cooperation in managing the global financial system. They include the World Bank, the International Monetary Fund (IMF), and regional development banks.

The World Bank is the largest development bank and plays a central role in providing grants and concessional loans through the International Development Agency to the poorest countries and concessional and nonconcessional loans through the International Bank for Reconstruction and Development to middle-income countries. The World Bank also provides other financial instruments such as insurance mechanisms and guarantees.

IMF serves as the international safeguard for economic stability, offering last-resort financing and expert guidance to countries for crisis management and prevention. It provides emergency loans and debt relief during fiscal emergencies that can have many causes, including epidemics and pandemics. IMF also helps countries tackle acute payment imbalances.

**Regional development banks** complement IMF and World Bank lending efforts, providing an array of financial instruments and playing a vital role in their respective regions thanks to their deep cultural understanding and networks. They include the African Development Bank, the Asian Development Bank, the Asian Infrastructure Investment Bank, the European Bank for Reconstruction and Development, the Inter-American Development Bank, the Islamic Development Bank, and the New Development Bank.

**Bilateral aid** refers to the direct transfer of financial, technical, or material (in-kind) assistance from one country to another. Funds can come in the form of grants or loans, often as part of a broader foreign policy strategy. Compared to multilateral aid, bilateral aid can be more flexible and quicker to mobilize because it involves direct country-to-country support.

**Global health initiatives (GHIs)** are collaborative international efforts that focus on particular health issues or diseases, as well as on strengthening health systems more generally—particularly in low- and middle-income countries. They function as public-private partnerships, and some are incorporated as a nonprofit organization in Switzerland. The strength of GHIs lies in their ability to pool resources, expertise, and efforts across multiple stakeholders, including governments, international organizations, the private sector, and civil society. High-profile, independently governed examples of GHIs include Gavi, the Vaccine Alliance; the Global Fund to Fight AIDS, Tuberculosis and Malaria; and Unitaid. GHIs differ from nongovernmental organizations because of the presence of government or United Nations agency representatives in their governance as primary financiers.

**Philanthropy** involves the use of private funds, often from individuals, foundations, or corporations. Philanthropic organizations can fill gaps in funding and often have more flexibility and can act more quickly than multilateral or bilateral funding bodies. The flexibility contributes to their ability to work more easily with both private, for-profit companies and nonprofit, nongovernmental entities than is often the case for multilateral and bilateral funders.

The exercise also found significant imbalance in the presence of instruments over the pandemic cycle, with only four dedicated to recovery. This finding highlights a notable deficiency in the pandemic financial architecture, which could lead to protracted and suboptimal recovery, particularly for countries experiencing high inflation and debt service payments in the aftermath of a pandemic such as COVID-19. Such an imbalance disproportionately affects lower-income countries reliant on external financing, exacerbating global health inequities and undermining the capacity to prepare for future pandemics.

The instruments can be classified across the pandemic cycle. For this exercise, selected instruments or mechanisms were curated and featured into four key areas, including instruments used during the COVID-19 pandemic as well as newer instruments or mechanisms developed afterward. Boxes 13.3–13.6 highlight the instruments selected to illustrate a range of financing approaches that have been actively used or newly introduced in pandemic preparedness and response. The selection was guided by two key criteria: (1) relevance to different phases of the pandemic cycle and (2) diversity in financial mechanisms, including grants, loans, insurance, and market-shaping instruments. Although not necessarily the only or best options available, the selected instruments represent notable examples of how different financing tools have been designed and deployed in real-world settings. Some, like the Pandemic Fund, reflect new efforts to address financing gaps in preparedness; others, like COVAX (COVID-19 Vaccines Global Access), demonstrate lessons learned from pandemic response financing. Readers should interpret these selections as illustrative rather than prescriptive, offering insights into the strengths, limitations, and design considerations of pandemic financing tools.

**Box 13.3**

## The New Mechanism for Pandemic Prevention and Preparedness: The Pandemic Fund

The Pandemic Fund, established in 2022 and hosted by the World Bank, with the World Health Organization as the technical lead, provides long-term grants to countries for pandemic prevention, preparedness, response, and recovery. In its first funding round in August 2023, the Pandemic Fund disbursed US$338 million to 37 countries for activities like enhancing surveillance, improving laboratory capacity, and training health care workers—almost entirely for prevention and preparedness. A second round of US$500 million has been approved. The Pandemic Fund aims to offer predictable, multiyear financing, with a focus on both national and regional health system strengthening, and will require ongoing monitoring to ensure its effectiveness. It does not yet have contingent financing mechanisms that would be activated in response to an outbreak, epidemic, or pandemic.

Box 13.4

## Financial Instruments for Emergency Response to Outbreaks and Epidemics

**World Health Organization (WHO) Contingency Fund for Emergencies (CFE).** This fund enables WHO to respond rapidly to disease outbreaks and health emergencies, often within 24 hours. CFE's flexibility allows WHO to allocate resources quickly where they are most needed, without being tied to specific purposes. In 2024, through July 23, seven countries contributed approximately US$15.4 million. These funds have been allocated across various crises, with US$7.3 million going to the Sudan conflict, US$6.5 million to the global dengue outbreak, and additional disbursements for emergencies in Ethiopia and the occupied Palestinian territories. In total, approximately US$32.5 million—drawing on both the US$15.4 million contributed in 2024 and existing funds—was disbursed to address global health crises through July 23. Since its inception in 2015, CFE has received approximately US$335 million from a relatively small number of countries, with Germany being the largest donor by far. CFE seems to be intended for WHO response to urgent, unplanned, and unbudgeted needs, but is apparently not a prenegotiated, triggerable mechanism for responding at the required scale to contain a large epidemic nor is it designed to fund associated nonhealth costs, such as those associated with suspending air travel, which response to an outbreak or epidemic can trigger.

**The World Bank Group's latest Crisis Preparedness and Response Toolkit.** Launched in 2023–24, this toolkit provides developing countries with tools to better respond to and prepare for crises. It includes the following:

- *Rapid response option.* Countries can quickly reallocate up to 10 percent of undisbursed World Bank financing to address immediate crisis needs, such as repurposing funds from infrastructure projects to provide emergency aid.
- *Prearranged financing.* Countries can access new budget support quickly when disasters strike, helping manage immediate impacts without compromising long-term development goals. This financing includes expanded options like the Development Policy Financing Catastrophe Deferred Drawdown Option and Investment Policy Financing with a Deferred Drawdown Option.
- *Catastrophe insurance.* Governments can embed catastrophe bonds and insurance in their financing operations, allowing them to receive payouts during crises without incurring additional debt. This insurance is supported by international reinsurance markets and private capital.
- *Climate resilient debt clauses.* Eligible countries can defer interest and fee payments on existing loans during disasters, enabling them to prioritize disaster recovery over debt repayment.

These tools aim to provide fast access to emergency funds, insurance payouts, and flexible financing options, helping countries manage crises more effectively while building long-term resilience

Box 13.5

## Insurance-Like Prepaid Mechanisms

**Pandemic Emergency Financing Facility (PEF).** Launched by the World Bank in July 2017, following the Ebola outbreak in West Africa, PEF aimed to improve funding and coordination during severe disease outbreaks. PEF had two funding channels, an insurance window and a cash window:

- *Insurance window.* This window targeted large, multicountry infectious disease outbreaks in countries eligible for assistance from the International Development Association and was backed by reinsurance markets and a Pandemic Bond. However, strict activation criteria delayed payouts, limiting its effectiveness.

*box continues next page*

Box 13.5 **Insurance-Like Prepaid Mechanisms** (continued)

- *Cash window.* Intended to function like a traditional trust fund and covering a broader range of diseases, the cash window disbursed immediate funds based on expert advice and PEF steering body approval. This functioning enabled quick response to outbreaks and was conceptually similar to the World Health Organization's Contingency Fund for Emergencies (refer to box 13.4).

Despite its aim to provide quick funding for outbreaks, PEF faced criticism for delayed payouts and limited scope, making its total disbursement of US$257.24 million insufficient to handle major health crises like COVID-19. PEF suffered from overly restrictive trigger conditions, which meant that funds were often not released until outbreaks had already escalated. Additionally, the total payout amounts were too small relative to the scale of actual pandemic response needs, and the structure of the insurance mechanism prioritized protecting investors over ensuring rapid response financing. These design flaws contributed to the lack of confidence in PEF, ultimately leading to its discontinuation.

The complete elimination rather than revision and adaptation of PEF amid the face of extensive criticism resulted in the loss of a useful mechanism that could have been improved. PEF's shortcomings highlight the need for a faster, more flexible, and better-funded mechanism for future global health emergencies.

**African Risk Capacity Group's parametric insurance.** African Risk Capacity Group, a specialized agency of the African Union, has launched a parametric insurance product to cover high-impact epidemic risks, with Senegal as the first African country to join. Developed in response to a 2015 request by African Finance Ministers, this insurance will provide rapid funding for outbreaks of Ebola, Marburg virus, and meningitis. The new product, supported by partners like AON, Ginkgo Bioworks, and Munich Re, and subsidized by the Swiss Agency for Development and Cooperation, aims to strengthen African Union Member States' capacity to respond to public health emergencies.

**Pandemic debt suspension clauses.** Barbados has completed a sovereign debt conversion focused on marine conservation, introducing the world's first "pandemic clause" in a bond issuance. This clause allows Barbados to defer interest payments for up to two years during a pandemic, as declared by the World Health Organization, giving the country fiscal space to address health emergencies. The bond, repayable over 15 years, also includes provisions for deferral during natural disasters like hurricanes and earthquakes. Supported by guarantees from the Inter-American Development Bank and The Nature Conservancy, the bond saves Barbados US$40 million to US$50 million, which will be used for marine conservation. This innovative financial tool is seen as a model for other countries to manage debt while investing in health and environmental sustainability.

Box 13.6

## Instruments for Product Development, Manufacturing, Purchasing, and Distribution

**COVAX.** COVID-19 Vaccines Global Access—abbreviated as COVAX and launched in April 2020 by the Coalition for Epidemic Preparedness Innovations; Gavi, the Vaccine Alliance; and the World Health Organization—aimed to ensure more equitable global access to COVID-19 vaccines, especially for low- and middle-income countries. It operated through two funding streams: self-financing high-income countries paid up front to secure vaccines, whereas lower-income countries received vaccines funded by donor grants through an advance market commitment. COVAX struggled, however, because many wealthy countries bypassed the initiative by making bilateral deals, leaving COVAX at a disadvantage in securing vaccine doses, delaying

*box continues next page*

vaccine distribution and undermining its equitable access goals. By the end of 2020, only US$400 million of the US$2.4 billion pledged had been disbursed. The initiative's challenges highlighted the importance of early pandemic financing and the need for stronger global cooperation and incentives to ensure timely and fair vaccine distribution in future pandemics.

**Gavi's First Response Fund.** Approved with a budget of US$500 million in June 2024, the First Response Fund is designed to secure early access to vaccines and maintain routine immunization programs during major public health emergencies. It is part of Gavi's Day Zero Financing Facility for Pandemics, which aims to provide up to US$2.5 billion in surge financing for rapid vaccine responses. As the fastest instrument in the financing facility, its purpose is to address urgent funding requirements until additional resources become available. It has three key objectives: to ensure swift vaccine access for Gavi-eligible countries, support vaccine delivery systems in those countries, and maintain routine immunization programs.

**African Vaccine Manufacturing Accelerator (AVMA).** A new financing mechanism launched in June 2024 to provide up to US$1 billion over a 10-year period, AVMA aims to expand the development of a sustainable vaccine manufacturing sector in Africa. AVMA operates through a pull financing mechanism, offering incentives to vaccine manufacturers to help cover the initial costs of development and production. This initiative, approved by the Gavi board in December 2023, was developed after nearly two years of collaboration among the Africa Centres for Disease Control and Prevention, the African Union, and Gavi, with input from a broad range of stakeholders, including partners, donors, industry representatives, and civil society. AVMA has two types of incentives:

- *Milestone payments.* Awarded when manufacturers obtain World Health Organization prequalification for designated priority vaccines, with payments ranging from US$10 million to US$25 million, depending on the technology used.
- *Accelerator payments.* Additional per-dose payments provided on top of standard market rates for vaccines produced under Gavi–United Nations Children's Fund tenders, with higher payments offered for comprehensive manufacturing processes of priority vaccines.

The goal of AVMA is to foster a robust vaccine manufacturing ecosystem in Africa, supporting at least four manufacturers over the next decade, thereby enhancing both the global vaccine market and Africa's capacity for pandemic preparedness. Questions remain about the adequacy of this fund to grow African manufacturing, and additional resources are expected to be required (Adeyi et al. 2024).

**International Finance Facility for Immunisation (IFFIm).** IFFIm is a multilateral development institution that leverages financial markets to accelerate the availability of funds for immunization programs. Established in 2006, IFFIm raises capital by issuing bonds backed by long-term donor pledges. The funds generated are then rapidly deployed through Gavi, to support vaccination initiatives in low- and middle-income countries. This innovative financing mechanism helps bridge the gap between the immediate need for vaccines and the timing of donor contributions, enhancing the impact of global immunization efforts.

IFFIm's bonds, known as Vaccine Bonds, are sold to institutional and individual investors globally, providing an attractive investment option with the added benefit of social impact. The long-term donor pledges, primarily from governments, provide robust security for these bonds, making them highly creditworthy and allowing IFFIm to secure favorable interest rates, maximizing the funds available for immunization programs. This funding model also offers flexibility in responding to health emergencies and supporting innovative vaccine delivery strategies. The quick availability of funds ensures that Gavi can act swiftly in rolling out vaccination campaigns, ultimately saving more lives and improving health outcomes.

## HOW MUCH PANDEMIC FINANCING IS NEEDED?

How does the investment needed to potentially avert a pandemic compare to the pandemic's losses or impacts? Past research has concluded that a small investment is needed to potentially avert a pandemic, compared to the tremendous losses of pandemics.

### The Large Economic Impact of Pandemics and Epidemics

Outbreaks, epidemics, and pandemics have had large economic impacts. Past studies have examined the tremendous losses of pandemics on an annualized or ongoing basis (Fan, Jamison, and Summers 2018; Glennerster, Snyder, and Tan 2022). Numerous studies have estimated the economic losses of recent pandemics and epidemics such as SARS (severe acute respiratory syndrome), Ebola, and COVID-19. SARS had significant impacts on the hardest hit locations—Canada; China; and Hong Kong SAR, China—with negative impacts on gross domestic product of US$3.2 billion to US$6.4 billion in Canada and US$3.7 billion in Hong Kong SAR, China (Keogh-Brown and Smith 2008). The estimated economic impact of the 2014 Ebola outbreaks in Guinea, Liberia, and Sierra Leone ranged from US$30 billion to US$50 billion (Obeng-Kusi, Martin, and Abraham 2024).

In contrast to SARS and Ebola, which had a geographically contained spread, COVID-19 had global impact. An early 2020 estimate of the economic cost of the COVID-19 pandemic suggested a cost of more than US$16 trillion globally (Cutler and Summers 2020). Gopinath (2020) called it the worst economic downturn since the Great Depression, estimating cumulative output loss over 2020–21 of about US$9 trillion. Further, countries continued to experience the economic impacts after the acute phase through the debt crises precipitated by the pandemic (Rogoff 2022).

### The Small Investment Required to Address Pandemics

By comparison, the amount of investment required to address pandemics is small. There is broad agreement about the need for more financing for pandemic preparedness and response, including by other researchers in this volume (Sureka et al. 2023). Questions about what to invest in and how much to invest for pandemic preparedness and response are joint questions, and researchers have examined the financing requirements in different ways. Table 13.3 provides a crude range of different estimates, each of which uses different methodologies (Fan, Smitham, et al. 2023). Estimates range from US$1.6 billion annually to US$65 billion needed in the first year, with similarly high levels expected in the second year.

**Table 13.3** Cost Estimates for Pandemic Preparedness and Response Using Different Definitions and Methodologies

| Source | Estimate |
|---|---|
| G20 High-Level Independent Panel on Financing the Global Commons for Pandemic Preparedness and Response (G20 HLIP 2021) | US$10 billion annually, plus US$5 billion to strengthen WHO and other existing institutions |
| World Bank and WHO for the G20 Joint Finance and Health Task Force (WHO and World Bank 2022) | US$10.5 billion annually in international financing for minimum priority PPR financing gap |
| McKinsey & Company (Craven et al. 2021) | US$20 billion to US$50 billion annually, after initial global investment of US$85 billion to US$130 billion over two years |
| Becker Friedman Institute, University of Chicago (Glennerster, Snyder, and Tan 2022) | US$5 billion annually, after US$60 billion up-front investment for vaccine production capacity and supply chain inputs |
| Center for Global Health Science & Security, Georgetown University (Eaneff et al. 2022) | US$124 billion over five years toward "demonstrated capacity" on JEE indicators |
| WHO (Clarke et al. 2022) | From US$1.6 billion per year for 139 LMICs to improve capacities to US$43 billion per year including for R&D |

*Source:* Fan, Smitham, et al. 2023.

*Note:* G20 = Group of Twenty; JEE = Joint External Evaluation; LMICs = low- and middle-income countries; PPR = pandemic preparedness and response; R&D = research and development; WHO = World Health Organization.

**Table 13.4** Health Expenditure, by Country Income Group, 2019

| Country income group | Number of countries | Population (million) | Health expenditure per capita | | Total health expenditure (billion) |
|---|---|---|---|---|---|
| | | | **Mean** | **Standard deviation** | |
| Low | 25 | 587 | 39.4 | 16.4 | 20.7 |
| Lower-middle | 53 | 3,308 | 141.9 | 127.5 | 306 |
| Upper-middle | 52 | 2,521 | 515.0 | 320.8 | 1,384 |
| High | 60 | 1,203 | 3,093.6 | 2,345.2 | 6,745 |

*Source:* Original table compiled using World Health Organization Global Health Expenditure Database.

*Note:* Total health expenditure is in current US dollars. The table does not show more recent data on health expenditure because they reflect expenditures during the pandemic, which were much higher than normal and are unlikely to be maintained in the intrapandemic period.

### Unequal Distribution of Financial Resources as Measured by Health Expenditures

The amounts required to invest in pandemics represent a fraction of available resources in high-income countries, which collectively spent US$6.7 trillion on health care in 2019 (table 13.4). By contrast, the needed funds would greatly exceed the available resources of low- and lower-middle-income countries. Health expenditure in low-income countries averaged US$39 per person and collectively, for 24 countries, totaled US$20.7 billion in 2019.

## CASE STUDY OF COVID-19 PANDEMIC FINANCING

This section explores pandemic financing using the COVID-19 pandemic as a case study and examines primarily development assistance for health and specifically for pandemics. This analysis uses data from the Institute for Health Metrics and Evaluation's Development Assistance for Health on COVID-19 Database (2020–2023) to assess the total volume of resources.[4] Table 13.5 provides an overview of the financial contributions made by various organizations and entities in response to the pandemic. It segments the data by year, detailing the annual funding amounts from 2020 to 2023, and shows the total for each contributor.

**Table 13.5** Development Assistance for Health (COVID-19) during the Pandemic, 2020–23

| | | 2020 | 2021 | 2022 | 2023 | Total |
|---|---|---|---|---|---|---|
| **UN agencies** | PAHO | 122,292 | 250,044 | 74,694 | 0 | 447,030 |
| | UNAIDS | 9,711 | 0 | 0 | 0 | 9,711 |
| | UNFPA | 109,282 | 28,181 | 7,541 | 0 | 145,004 |
| | UNICEF | 662,194 | 199,996 | 156,136 | 0 | 1,018,326 |
| | WHO | 1,318,499 | 1,265,464 | 861,201 | 135,505 | 3,580,669 |
| **MDBs** | ADB | 2,023,172 | 2,330,388 | 955,787 | 903,588 | 6,212,935 |
| | AfDB | 711,222 | 74,162 | 32,630 | 69,918 | 887,932 |
| | IDB | 406,835 | 222,430 | 221,032 | 203,397 | 1,053,694 |
| | WB_IBRD | 2,175,341 | 4,278,387 | 1,069,294 | 478,631 | 8,001,653 |
| | WB_IDA | 924,215 | 2,234,265 | 465,515 | 0 | 3,623,995 |
| **GHIs** | CEPI | 317,634 | 530,147 | 143,343 | 25,561 | 1,016,685 |
| | Gavi | 770,927 | 8,038,491 | 2,280,597 | 0 | 11,090,015 |
| | Global Fund | 975,089 | 5,461,119 | 504,618 | 698,399 | 7,639,225 |
| | Unitaid | 50,400 | 56,128 | 5,055 | 1,918 | 113,501 |
| **Foundations** | Gates Foundation | 325,511 | 270,047 | 93,032 | 75,354 | 763,944 |
| | Other | 646,643 | 632,243 | 40,077 | 0 | 1,318,963 |
| **Bilateral** | Bilateral | 7,174,648 | 13,647,397 | 14,000,446 | 9,835,250 | 44,657,741 |
| **Total (US$, thousand)** | | 18,723,615 | 39,518,889 | 20,910,998 | 12,427,521 | 91,581,023 |

*Source:* Original table compiled using the Institute for Health Metrics and Evaluation's Development Assistance for Health on COVID-19 Database 2020–2023. ADB = Asian Development Bank; AfDB = African Development Bank; CEPI = Coalition for Epidemic Preparedness Innovations; Gavi = Gavi, the Vaccine Alliance; GHIs = global health initiatives; IDB = Inter-American Development Bank; MDBs = multilateral development banks; PAHO = Pan American Health Organization; UN = United Nations; UNAIDS = Joint United Nations Programme on HIV/AIDS; UNFPA = United Nations Population Fund; UNICEF = United Nations Children's Fund; WB_IBRD = World Bank, International Bank for Reconstruction and Development; WB_IDA = World Bank, International Development Association; WHO = World Health Organization.

Over the period 2020–23, the grand total of development assistance for health for COVID-19 reached nearly US$91.6 billion. Annual contributions varied, with the highest funding in 2021 at US$39.5 billion, reflecting the global surge in response efforts during the peak of the pandemic. Bilateral contributions were the largest source of funding overall, followed by the World Bank (both the International Bank for Reconstruction and Development and the International Development Association), Gavi, the Global Fund, and WHO. Figure 13.4 shows the changes in contributions over time for each category of contributors. Overall, the substantial peak in funding in 2021 corresponds with the intensified global response efforts, including vaccine distribution and health care system support. The subsequent decrease in funding in 2022 and 2023 indicates a shift to long-term recovery efforts, which appear to be insufficient.

**Figure 13.4** Development Assistance for Health (COVID-19), 2020–23

(US$, billion)

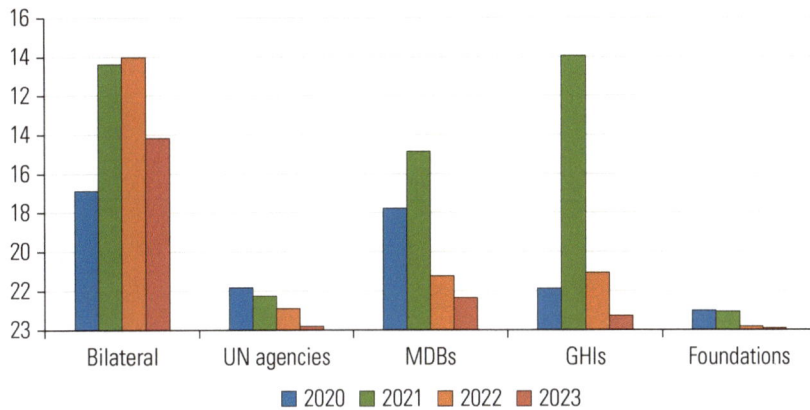

Source: Original figure created using the Institute for Health Metrics and Evaluation's Development Assistance for Health on COVID-19 Database 2020–2023.

Note: GHIs = global health initiatives; MDBs = multilateral development banks; UN = United Nations.

Specifically, whereas bilateral contributions remained steady but declined after 2022, financial assistance from most other agencies dropped to less than half of the 2021 disbursement levels in 2022, with a similar trend observed in 2023. Additional significant funding sources not incorporated in this analysis include the Asian Infrastructure Investment Bank's COVID-19 Crisis Recovery Facility, the International Monetary Fund's Rapid Credit Facility and Rapid Financing Instrument, and the New Development Bank's COVID-19 Emergency Program Loans. Primarily allocated for broader social and economic responses and recovery efforts, these funds did not appear in the Institute for Health Metrics and Evaluation health data.

Although figure 13.4 illustrates the year of funding distribution, it does not specify the precise timing of financial assistance. Past research has found that the timing of pandemic financing mattered greatly but that financing was delayed. Despite the size of resources available from multilateral development funds, their disbursement was slow (figure 13.5). Nevertheless, as noted by the World Bank (2022), the timing of the release of these resources was still faster than usual timescales (figure 13.6). Lagged financing has been found to be a major determinant of lagged purchase and thus lagged delivery of financing (Agarwal and Reed 2022).

**Figure 13.5** Multilateral Funding for the COVID-19 Response, March 2020 to March 2021

Funding committed (nominal US$, billions)                      Running total of aid flows (nominal US$, billiions)

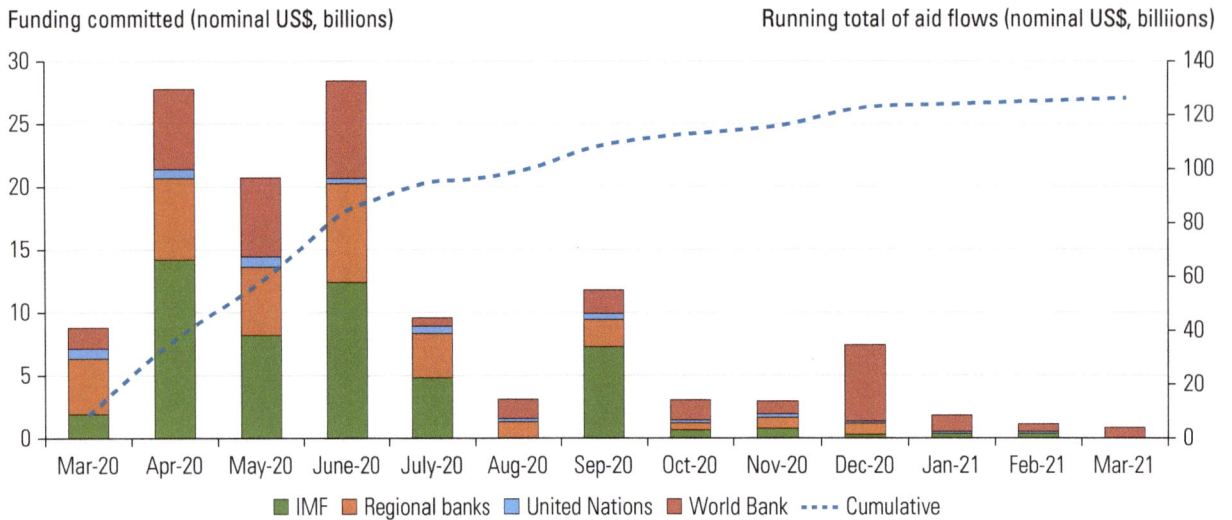

*Source:* Based on Hill et al. 2024.

*Note:* This figure is not limited to development assistance for health. IMF = International Monetary Fund.

**Figure 13.6** Cumulative World Bank Disbursements for COVID-19 Health and Social Response, by Financing Instrument, March 2020 to May 2021

Cumulative disbursements (US$, million)

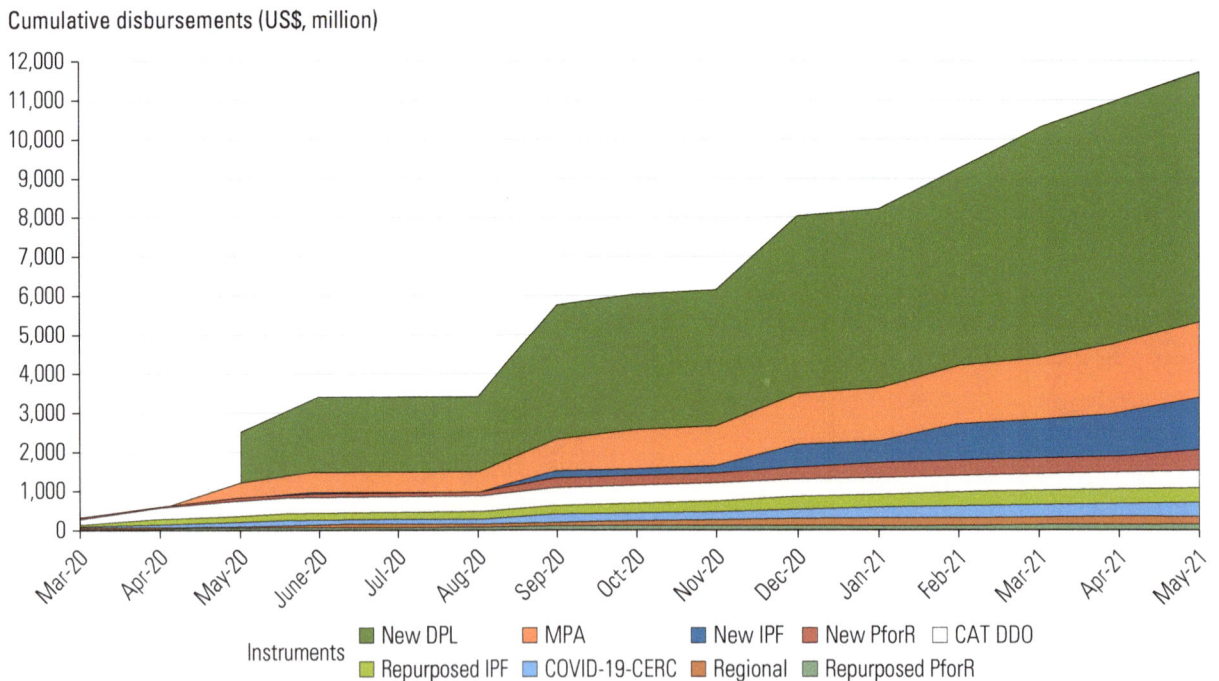

*Source:* World Bank 2022.

*Note:* This figure includes assistance for both health and social response. CAT DDO = Catastrophic Deferred Drawdown Option; CERC = Contingent Emergency Response Component; DPL = Development Policy Loan; IPF = Investment Project Financing; MPA = Multiphase Programmatic Approach; PforR = Program-for-Results.

## PANDEMIC FINANCING CONSIDERATIONS

Similar to the challenge posed by climate change, effectively combatting the threat of pandemics demands a strategic and coordinated financial approach. Addressing a global health crisis necessitates more than just good intentions; it requires substantial financial resources allocated throughout the pandemic cycle. This section outlines the kind of financing needed to address the distinct needs of each phase of the pandemic cycle: prevention, preparedness, response (early and late), and recovery and reconstruction.

Further, this chapter has primarily focused on, and has mostly limited its scope to, financing the health-related aspects of the pandemic cycle while acknowledging the broader economic and social financing needs that arise during pandemics—such as social protection measures, business support programs, and economic stimulus packages. Future work would benefit from considering how health financing is weighed and prioritized relative to economic and social support mechanisms from a policy perspective, as well as how pandemic financing strategies for health can be better integrated with broader economic resilience measures to create a more comprehensive and sustainable pandemic financing architecture.

### Prevention and Preparedness

The funding approach for pandemic prevention and preparedness is grounded in the recognition that such efforts constitute a public good, at least regional (in the case of viral hemorrhagic fevers) if not global (in the case of highly transmissible pathogens, particularly respiratory pathogens). Pandemics transcend borders, and investments in one country's preparedness efforts can yield benefits for global health security. However, disparities exist in the benefits and costs of pandemic preparedness across countries, influenced by factors such as outbreak likelihood, development level, infrastructure use, and variations in input costs, particularly labor.

Prevention and preparedness (P&P) are not candidates for contingent financing instruments because their costs, based on current capacity and needed capacity, are largely predictable. Instead of requiring funds to respond to a pandemic, P&P funds are needed to (1) create capacity to prevent and respond according to the level of pandemic risk and (2) maintain such capacity. These funds can be thought of as an initial fixed cost to create capacity (that could be credit-financed, spreading the cost over a number of years) combined with an annual maintenance cost (that would normally not be credit-financed other than to cover a short-term financing shortfall).

The cost of creating P&P capacity should be funded with a mixture of national funding, grants, and concessional or nonconcessional credits. As countries become richer, the funding mix should be decreasingly concessional, from pure grants and highly concessional financing for low-income countries to nonconcessional funding or less concessional funding for middle-income countries. Concessional and nonconcessional financing have as an important feature the role of government financing for repayment, ensuring that governments have "skin in the game" by co-investing external resources alongside external financing.

A fair global P&P financing system would consider both countries' funding of their own P&P efforts and their obligation to contribute to efforts regionally, globally, and in other countries. In some sense, the existing proportional contribution system (namely, the assessed member contributions to WHO) should support response to the pandemic cycle. This contribution system is based mainly on country gross domestic product, along with other factors. In practice, however, most of WHO's budget comes from discretionary sources rather than assessed member contributions; moreover, WHO played a smaller role in financing the pandemic cycle relative to other agencies. The Pandemic Fund considers whether the grant leverages other resources such as cofinancing from other donors and what it calls co-investment from the government itself, either in cash or in kind. A key objective for the Pandemic Fund is for its resources to expand overall health expenditures by even more than the size of its grant (and certainly not substitute for national P&P funding).

What proportion of its national P&P funding needs (as well as regional and global P&P funding needs, including subsidies to other countries) a particular country should pay is not simple, because a fair funding formula or allocation framework would consider a number of factors. The use of allocation frameworks or formulas is common among multilateral development banks and global health initiatives such as the Global Environment Facility; the Global Fund to Fight Aids, Tuberculosis and Malaria; and the International Development Association (Fan 2023; Fan, Glassman, and Silverman 2014).

Many have argued that the allocation framework should necessarily incorporate indexes based on pandemic preparedness, such as the International Health Regulations Joint External Evaluation Tool; however, this chapter eschews that approach because, among reasons explained elsewhere, preparedness indexes are not predictive of pandemic risk (Fan and Smitham 2023). Nevertheless, a lack of predictive power does not mean that these capacities are irrelevant or that they should not be invested in. Rather, these capacities may need to be improved or supplemented with more actionable indicators.

There will be reasonable disagreement about how the exact formula should be designed and which factors should be incorporated. Some of the factors to consider include the following:

- *Level of pandemic risk*, as measured in average annual loss or spark index (Fan 2023). It can incorporate or reflect other related aspects of pandemic risk, such as the likelihood of pathogen spillover, regional transmission patterns, and the potential for cross-border spread.
- *Ability to pay*, whether by income classification or per capita gross national income, adjusted by size of the population, and similar to the formulas used to calculate assessed contributions to the United Nations System.
- *Ability to benefit from P&P efforts*. Larger countries like China or the United States may derive more benefits themselves from localized outbreak containment, thereby limiting its impact to a specific state or province. In contrast, smaller

nations like Guatemala or Liberia could face nationwide repercussions even from minor outbreaks with a larger proportion of the total benefits of containment accruing to other countries. The return on investment and thus the ability of a country to benefit from P&P efforts and investment undoubtedly vary with significant implications for equity.

- *Need for P&P efforts.* The appropriate level of effort for P&P is related to the probability that a spillover event will occur and that an outbreak will need to be contained. Belize and Iceland have similar population sizes and both are small countries, but Belize has a much greater probability of zoonotic spillover events. Other measures of need could be need for surveillance capacity as measured by data capacity (for example, birth registration coverage), health worker capacity (for example, nurse availability per capita), and network capacity and connectivity (for example, mobile subscribers per capita) (Fan 2023), without which conducting surveillance will be very challenging.

- *Cost of P&P efforts.* Ability to pay (noted earlier) is strongly correlated with the cost of implementing P&P efforts in a country primarily because labor costs are strongly correlated with per capita gross national income and are the largest cost category. However, other differences between countries affect the difference in cost. One obvious factor is the previous category (need), which will determine the level of required effort. Another is the difference in the cost of implementation. For example, the population of Rwanda is more than four times that of Namibia but Namibia's land area is more than 30 times that of Rwanda, suggesting substantial per capita differences in the cost of a surveillance system. Using a cost-based approach on specific P&P functions (such as surveillance, laboratory networks, and workforce training) is one of multiple factors to determine the level of investments, but it differs from the notion of capacities as measured by aggregate scores.

The lack of annual and comprehensive data collected for all countries means that not all these factors can be included (Fan 2023). One challenge of the Joint External Evaluation data is that collection takes place only every five years at best. Thus, the use of a simple and objective indicator for which there are widely available and regularly reported data is preferred over aggregated, subjective indicators or indicators that are unavailable or unmeasurable.

This financing formula would create a set of countries that would be net recipients because their expected contribution is less than their domestic estimated cost, and a set of net contributors because their expected contribution is greater than their estimated domestic cost (for example, using work by Eaneff et al. 2022 as the basis for estimates of global needs and countries' obligations). These estimates will need to be regularly revised with better data on the cost of implementing P&P in different settings and should be formally adopted by WHO as the standard for estimating costs for pandemic P&P.

Achieving a global mechanism to ensure proportional contributions for pandemic preparedness involves several practical challenges. First, pandemic preparedness investments yield highly asymmetrical benefits. Wealthier nations, which tend to have stronger health and surveillance systems, have both the capacity and the incentive to invest in P&P for their own national security, even without external enforcement or creation of a separate proportional contribution mechanism. Second, the diversity of national interests, governance structures, and fiscal capacities makes it difficult to establish and enforce a universally accepted burden-sharing framework for pandemic financing, although the same could have been said for the original creation of United Nations agencies such as WHO or even of the multilateral development banks. The core challenge of pandemic financing is a lack of agreement on which mechanism to use as much as on the amount to be contributed.

Because some countries will not achieve acceptable P&P without major investment in basic health system infrastructure, the financing agreement could include the cost of upgrading infrastructure where possible. In some settings, such as conflict zones, resources may not be the binding constraint, or the level of acceptable P&P will need to consider what is possible with existing infrastructure.

Financing should also consider the time horizon of investments, such as whether the investments provide short-term capacity creation or long-term maintenance. The Pandemic Fund, with its project-based approach to funding, is arguably better placed to provide shorter-term, capacity-development resources, given the small amount of funding available globally as well as the short time horizon. The long-run horizon for maintenance or expansion of capacity requires ongoing, predictable funds as well as third-party independent evaluation using clear metrics to assess progress toward both improved capacity and sustainability.

Trust (and therefore participation) in a global P&P financing scheme will be achieved only if countries are confident not just that other countries are making the required investments but also that those investments are being translated into the desired P&P capacity. Funds that leave a country to fund regional or global capacity, or that fund P&P efforts in other countries, are relatively easy to track, at least from the perspective of donors. More difficult is tracking domestic expenditures on health, and specifically across the pandemic cycle (Fan and Smitham 2023).

Additionality of domestic resources can be assessed ex ante and ex post. Ex ante, additionality could be assessed by looking at project design—explicit arrangement for domestic finance has been set out in the assessment criteria of the Pandemic Fund's Technical Advisory Panel or auditable records through the public financial management and budgeting stage. Ex post, the use of WHO's Global Health Expenditure Database offers the possibility of detecting additional increases in government spending on health, despite a risk that conditionality on this metric may alter the unbiased nature of this data source, especially because the database is the benchmark methodology and tool for measuring government spending in comparison to external assistance on health. However, using the Global Health Expenditure Database to track whether government spending on pandemic preparedness has specifically increased will be very challenging. A third mechanism is a costing methodology employed by Eaneff et al. (2022) in estimating the amounts required for pandemic prevention and preparedness (refer to table 13.3). Thus, the alternative is to require financial control and clear accounting of spending, which returns to the core question of public capacity and governance, particularly in the area of public financial management and budget execution and implementation rates (Fan and Gupta 2024).

This chapter argues that the main kind of additionality to be assessed should relate to improved performance on preparedness (surveillance, laboratories, or human resources), rather than simply financial additionality. It is more important to track the capacity of P&P built and sustained by investments than to track domestic financial flows, if tracking only one of these is possible. Importantly, however, the limitations of existing metrics, such as the Joint External Evaluation and the States Parties Self-Assessment Annual Report, necessitate a broader approach. Their limited predictive power during COVID-19 suggests the need to supplement them with measures focused on functions or outcomes. Such measures could include real-time response capabilities, such as the speed of outbreak detection and containment; simulation-based evaluations, through which countries undergo regular stress tests of their pandemic preparedness systems; surge capacity readiness, measuring the ability to mobilize medical countermeasures, health workers, and emergency funding on short notice; and cross-border collaboration metrics—such as the timeliness and transparency of data sharing—to help assess whether countries are contributing to global health security.

The emphasis on inclusivity and solidarity as fundamental principles for pandemic P&P, although perhaps appearing idealistic, aligns with the pragmatic understanding that pandemics do not respect borders. COVID-19 underscored the interconnectedness of our global community, revealing that the virus's spread in one region could eventually affect all nations, regardless of their initial success in containment. This interconnectedness suggests that investing in universal pandemic P&P is a matter of enlightened self-interest. That it also respects the values of altruism and humanitarianism is an added benefit.

An efficient global preparedness system does not require every country to be fully prepared for all eventualities. Instead, it relies on the ability of countries to support one another, and on the flexibility of regional and global institutions to respond to acute needs in countries with less capacity. Global preparedness requires a well-articulated network of institutions that can work together to provide such cross-national, regional, or global technical and material support. The promising emergence in some countries of national institutes of public health that concentrate technical capacity independent of political cycles combined with regional institutions like the Africa Centres for Disease Control and Prevention (or perhaps enhanced capacity in regional WHO offices) should be further developed and included in P&P budgets at the national and regional levels. Networks, however, require institutional relationships built over time, transcending interpersonal relationships, and activities in the network that maintain those relationships.

Finally, investing in P&P does not occur in a vacuum, independent of other investments in health and social welfare. As examples, countries with generous national sick-leave policies can more easily detect outbreaks and more easily prevent workers from going to work when sick and spreading an infection. Countries with well-developed primary health care systems can use that infrastructure for surveillance of fevers of unknown origin. Countries with generous unemployment insurance can impose lockdowns with less impact on poverty. Countries with ubiquitous household internet access can more easily teach remotely, and so on. Although it is unreasonable to expect pandemic P&P financing streams to broadly develop a country's health and social services, a country with rudimentary services would need significantly more funding to achieve comparable levels of P&P, which can be unrealistic. No country experiencing famine or war could be expected to continue to prioritize P&P for its own human and financial resources, as demonstrated by the polio outbreak in Gaza in 2024. Thus, a universal P&P formula may have advantages of objectivity and fairness, but may miss out on the subjective characteristics for which country-specific adjustments would be merited in order to be fair.

### Response: Early and Late

In the response phase of a pandemic, urgency and timeliness are paramount and require defining and establishing a clear trigger. The trigger specifies when the response should be activated and should be defined in national and global pandemic preparedness and response plans. In theory, the world has an existing mechanism for reporting potential pathogens of pandemic potential through the International Health Regulations; however, in practice, significant gaps remain in the definition of a tiered system for communication about different tiers of responses (Fan, Cash, et al. 2023).

Financing and triggers both need to be designed in ways that account for reticence to report potential outbreaks, due to the negative economic consequences, as well as lack of capacity to adequately identify potential outbreaks. Delays in international reporting put other countries at risk because those countries cannot initiate appropriate complementary containment efforts. Thus, financing mechanisms may need to build in additional incentives (such as the liability for the costs incurred by other countries or a sanction mechanism similar to those imposed by the World Trade Organization for violations of trade agreements).

Day-zero financing or surge financing is crucial in this context, providing funds at the onset of a deadly outbreak to quickly purchase necessary resources, including products still in development through at-risk financing (Fan et al. 2024). The early and swift release of these funds is vital because delays can undermine intervention effectiveness and exacerbate the outbreak. Such resources should be allocated both to immediate containment efforts and to mitigate the economic and social impacts of these measures, ensuring that countries are not discouraged from early reporting.

Outbreaks tend to grow exponentially, and their containment becomes increasingly challenging with time. Unlike the fixed and recurrent expenditures necessary for

P&P, releasing financing for mounting a response is contingent upon the occurrence of an outbreak or epidemic. At the local level, such funding might come from a reserve fund within the ministry of health or finance, or from staff being diverted from their usual jobs to contain an outbreak, generating opportunity costs rather than a need for additional budget, or approvals from funders to reallocate resources for a given budget line or service area to the response. Response expenditures occur in addition to normal annual expenditures for P&P and do not occur except in response to an event.

The response phase comprises two critical stages: early and late. Early response focuses on containing the outbreak or epidemic, striving to prevent it from escalating into a pandemic. This stage mirrors the containment strategies employed during outbreaks like MERS (Middle East respiratory syndrome) and SARS. Rapid mobilization of resources is imperative to control the spread, reflecting a globally shared interest in averting a wider crisis.

Given the global benefit of early, effective response, funding should not be contingent upon a country's history of cooperation or prior investment in pandemic P&P. Although perhaps understandable, reluctance to assist nonparticipating countries is imprudent policy. Reserving fire brigades for houses that have paid a fire insurance premium is foolish because fires in uninsured houses will lead to fires in neighboring houses. Similarly, the rapid control of an outbreak benefits the world, regardless of individual countries' past actions or readiness levels. By dissociating funding from past behaviors and investments, the early response phase maximizes global welfare, recognizing that containing an outbreak anywhere benefits the world at large. In other words, withholding early response funding is not an effective means to incentivize the achievement of appropriate levels of P&P.

Several other mechanisms could be considered to incentivize better performance or good behavior in terms of P&P. Subsidies of pandemic insurance premiums could be made conditional on improvements to P&P capacity (to reward good behavior) while also giving higher subsidy for lower P&P capacity and higher P&P need (because rewarding need can also be interpreted as rewarding low performance or achievement). Donors could also condition other forms of assistance on P&P capacity, such as increasing a country's borrowing rates or insurance premiums as a penalty for having increased pandemic risk or failing to transparently report pandemic information in a timely manner. Taxes on international flights as well as taxes on the factors associated with spark risk, such as presence and size of wildlife markets, could also be used to account for the increased risk of pathogen spread, and so on.

Moreover, early response efforts should incentivize prompt reporting of cases by providing financial resources not just to curb the virus's spread but also to mitigate the social and economic repercussions of early reporting and early response. Measures such as airport closures and lockdowns, although crucial for public health, can significantly affect communities and businesses. Therefore, part of the funding could be allocated to compensate for such losses, although it may not be necessarily counted as part of the official development financing for health and pandemics. This approach not only alleviates the economic strain on affected areas but incentivizes early reporting good practices. Such funding should be very rapidly available, although it could come with riders that specify that countries not meeting certain conditions must return portions of it (for example, a country cannot retain funding to compensate for closure of airports if it never closed them).

Because of limited health personnel, especially in the short term before regional assistance can arrive, plans should be in place to provide appropriate additional funding to workers assuming additional risk and those working overtime. These efforts can be complemented with plans to pull in currently inactive workers, much as the military does with reserve troops. The rapidly available financing will not be useful if the mechanisms do not exist to channel the funds to workers, specifically through digital payment and banking. Similarly, and only somewhat less urgent, predesigned mechanisms need to exist to channel sick leave and unemployment compensation to recipients to enable local isolation and quarantine to contain an epidemic. Finally, commandeering resources to enable an effective early response will require predesigned compensation mechanisms. They can include prearranging hotel rooms for isolation and quarantine, or diverting oxygen supplies from commercial to health use, or using existing infrastructure such as call centers for expanded pandemic functions, before surges occur (Fan et al. 2021; Fan et al. 2022). Although properly considered P&P, these predesigned mechanisms are mentioned here because of their relationship with response instruments. Many questions persist about whether the investments made from response financing during the COVID-19 pandemic were durable and carried over to the future.

Late response occurs when containment efforts prove futile and the inevitability of a pandemic becomes apparent. Modeling can support an understanding of the unbiased forecast of the epidemic situation as well as trade-offs of different policy scenarios (Lee et al. 2022; Patouillard et al. 2024). At this stage, the primary focus shifts to minimizing the broader impacts—ranging from loss of life to economic repercussions—associated with the pandemic. Strategies and resource allocations in this phase pivot from containment to mitigation and the effective management of the pandemic's effects.

Early and late responses are not always easily distinguished, but modeling can assist. A country with a large epidemic may already be focused on mitigating the health impact of infections and the economic impact of the epidemic. Most other countries may still be focused almost entirely on preventing entry of the pathogen and rapidly extinguishing any outbreaks, with the goal of ultimately preventing a pandemic.

The most significant economic divergence between early and late response lies in the transition from actions serving as almost pure global public goods to those primarily benefiting domestic interests. Consequently, the economic rationale for global investment in national response differs. Although humanitarian considerations may still warrant assistance to countries that did not contribute to global preparedness, the argument for collective self-interest is less compelling in late-stage responses.

To extend the fire analogy, all countries should have immediate, unconditional access to the financial, human, and physical resources to put out a fire or contain an outbreak or epidemic, including the resources to compensate countries for the economic impact of reporting and containment efforts. However, the fire department is not responsible for securing an individual's property, finding them alternative housing, or paying the cost of rebuilding and refurnishing the house. For that, the individual must have purchased insurance. In the case of late response, this requirement could take the form of purchasing (at market or concessional rates) pandemic insurance, or prenegotiating contingent loans or grants, or accessing reserves or issuing bonds.

Pandemic financing for response may need to be linked to some other globalized sectors, such as trade and transportation, to create incentives for participation in prevention, preparedness, response, and recovery mechanisms.

This chapter has adopted mostly economic arguments for investing in pandemic preparedness and response. However, it does not discount the role of political arguments made for investment throughout the pandemic cycle, particularly from the lens of geopolitics and vaccine diplomacy, which unfolded during the COVID-19 pandemic when high-income countries were slow in sharing or selling vaccines to LMICs and China and Russia stepped in to offer their own domestically developed vaccines (Suzuki and Yang 2023).

Pandemic insurance mechanisms can also be intended for early response; however, in the case of the Pandemic Emergency Financing Facility, its failure to rapidly disburse on the order of days rather than months was its downfall (Boyce, Sorrell, and Standley 2023; Buckley and Pittluck 2016). Nonetheless, the potential of insurance-based mechanisms should not be dismissed entirely. Innovative models, such as parametric insurance, regional epidemic risk pools, and catastrophe bonds, offer ways to provide rapid payouts based on preagreed triggers. Although insurance alone cannot replace core preparedness investments, prefinanced, trigger-based mechanisms could complement existing pandemic financing tools by ensuring immediate release of funds when an outbreak crosses a predefined threshold. The limited adoption of pandemic insurance to date reflects both technical and political challenges—such as moral hazard, determining appropriate premiums, and setting effective triggers—rather than a fundamental lack of viability. Future designs should address these constraints while learning from past experiences to ensure that insurance plays a meaningful role in pandemic financing. Insurance mechanisms for pandemic response and reconstruction remain uncommon (refer to box 13.5). Development of such mechanisms at scale could harness private capital markets and still offer opportunities for donor financing to reduce effective premiums. Similarly, multilateral mechanisms (such as through the International Monetary Fund) exist for contingent responses to financial crises and could be adapted for responses to health crises.

Finally, late response can also be divided into subphases with different needs for financing. First, in the event of a pandemic with serious morbidity and mortality, countries will likely recognize the importance of attempting to minimize the number of infections until an effective vaccine or treatment is available. This phase is the most disruptive because personal protective equipment, physical distancing, isolation, and quarantine are the only available tools. Depending on the severity of the pathogen, countries may be willing to impose progressively stricter lockdown restrictions that have serious economic, social, and educational consequences of their own. Trade-offs between measures should consider multiple outcomes and considerations, not only health impacts, and can be illustrated through integrated modeling (Patouillard et al. 2024). Some interventions are less socially restrictive than others—for example, masks and hand washing are less invasive and draconian than individual home quarantine and border control, which are less draconian than mandatory mass lockdowns. The more draconian the measures, the greater the need to alleviate their impact.

Second, once vaccines or treatments are available, countries will seek to scale up coverage as quickly as possible in order to relax the restrictive measures imposed to reduce infections. In the event of partial effectiveness of the vaccine or treatment (whether because of limited efficacy or limited uptake), countries will seek to keep the incidence below the threshold that would saturate health services and cause the needless deaths of infected people. Dose optimization to maximize population-level benefits when vaccines are in short supply, with a transition to dose optimization to maximize individual benefit as supply constraints are relaxed, is an example of areas that require creative (public) financing of product development because such trials do not generate returns for vaccine companies (Więcek et al. 2022). Although research and development is a form of P&P, this chapter does not include it.

This section has discussed considerations for pandemic financing along the pandemic cycle, but detailed analyses for each remain necessary as part of any national preparedness planning process, particularly of pandemic insurance or contingent financing for late response actions, which were arguably underused during the COVID-19 pandemic. Such financing mechanisms will likely focus on ensuring effective medical care (for example, access to oxygen) for those infected across all of the subphases. Before the development of effective vaccines and therapies, enabling people to reduce contact and protect themselves will require financing. Once vaccines and therapies become available, they will need to be purchased, distributed, and delivered. Contingent financing could also fund massive scale-up (or repurposing) of production capacity for the vaccines or therapies.

## Recovery and Reconstruction

The recovery and reconstruction phase occurs in the aftermath of a pandemic. It involves facilitating comprehensive rebuilding and recovery from the multifaceted damage inflicted by the pandemic, such as restoring health care systems, addressing economic disruptions, compensating from disruptions in education, and supporting societal and behavioral rehabilitation. The international financial institutions of the World Bank, established as a means to provide financial assistance earmarked for recovery and reconstruction from war, could be applied to any major shock (war, natural disaster, or pandemic), with the notion that countries responsible for a war should not be penalized during the recovery process, lest such penalties reinvigorate chances of future war. Unlike financing for early response, however, this assistance could be highly conditional upon a country's level of preparedness and the effectiveness of its response efforts during the pandemic.

To continue the firefighting analogy, communities expect to put out fires without consideration of whether the property owner has insurance. If the owner lacks insurance, there is no expectation that the government or community will rebuild their house for them; however, the pandemic situation has an important difference. National leadership that did not buy insurance or appropriately prepare for a pandemic may well no longer be in power when the consequences of a pandemic occur. Furthermore, those who suffer most from the lack of foresight by leadership likely had no role in the decision to be unprepared. Thus, the threat of future refusal to provide assistance is likely less effective in this case than with homeowner's insurance. Using the firefighting analogy in this case may thus lend to extreme or impractical conclusions.

More immediate incentives that affect the leadership currently in power will be needed. To return to the homeowner's analogy (some of whom also may postpone paying for insurance), a highly effective incentive is that banks will refuse to provide a mortgage for an uninsured property. Similarly, countries could face restrictions on their ability to access global financial markets in the present if they do not participate to reduce future risk. Institutions such as the International Monetary Fund already offer, or even demand, a range of conditionalities for participation in the international financial system but currently lack any consideration of performance throughout the pandemic cycle.

By anchoring financial support to a country's readiness, or at least to improvements in these measures, policy makers not only incentivize investments in resilient health systems but also ensure that recovery efforts align with long-term resilience goals. As noted earlier in the allocation formula section, these incentives also need to be balanced with considerations of need, which can create perverse incentives to be unprepared, have greater need, and require greater external funding.

Prenegotiated financing mechanisms, such as cofinanced insurance, offer a range of advantages, particularly in their capacity to tailor premiums or fees according to a country's level of preparedness and preventative measures. This mechanism would be analogous to paying a lower homeowner's premium for homes with a fire-resistant roof and a sprinkler system. Even if preparedness cannot prevent a pandemic, it will reduce the impact of the pandemic and thus the need for recovery financing, in turn fostering incentives for investing in resilient health care systems and reducing overall risk exposure. Moreover, such mechanisms empower countries with autonomy over their recovery priorities, akin to receiving an insurance payout to rebuild after a disaster, as opposed to the negotiation process inherent in seeking a bank loan to finance reconstruction efforts.

A fundamental aspect of prenegotiated financing whether through insurance or contingent loans, is the principle of risk sharing. By engaging in these mechanisms, countries can distribute the financial burden among all participating nations at risk, fostering a collective responsibility for managing pandemic aftermaths. In contrast, postdisaster negotiations may lack this shared accountability from sharing burden, analogous to the difference between accessing insurance funds ahead of time and applying for a bank loan after a disaster.

## LESSONS, RECOMMENDATIONS, AND CONCLUSIONS

This review of pandemic financing has defined essential concepts in epidemiology and economics for informing pandemic financing throughout the pandemic cycle, framed pandemic financing in the context of health financing and its notable features of different financing instruments as well as the relevant organizations, emphasized the small amounts of financing needed relative to the costs and losses that pandemics impose, examined the flows of pandemic financing during the COVID-19 pandemic by key agencies and reviewed the key financial instruments used as well as those not used, and analyzed key pandemic financing considerations as policy makers plan for the pandemic cycle.

This review of the essential epidemiologic and economic concepts for the pandemic cycle also informs the selection of the following key principles for designing effective pandemic financing:

- *Timely (and therefore prearranged) financing*
  - Because the next pandemic could happen anytime, countries should make the needed investments in prevention and preparedness to get ready now, even if they need to borrow to create the capacity. Maintaining capacity will be much more affordable and will pay for itself in reduced risk of pandemics.
  - Given that outbreaks grow exponentially, time is of the essence in addressing an outbreak or epidemic, because these emergencies get worse and harder to contain by the hour. Prearranged financing is essential to eliminate delays in mounting an effective containment response.
  - If containment is not possible, avoidable delays in developing and deploying drugs and vaccines at scale can translate into some combination of trillions of dollars in economic costs and avertable death and disability.

Eliminating financing-caused delays can speed development, manufacturing, procurement, and distribution.

- *Public goods, market failures, and incentives.* Like the other public good–defined global challenge such as climate change, failure to act harms us all but also comes with incentives to free ride on others: Why should we pay if others will? Financing mechanisms for any investments in public goods (or preventing public harms) need to account for these problems and design accountability mechanisms that help to counteract incentives to free ride.

### Lessons from COVID-19

Amid the large array of pandemic financing tools available during the COVID-19 pandemic, the vast majority focused on response. Analysis of the strengths and weaknesses of the financing system and architecture during the COVID-19 pandemic results in the following five key messages.

First, the pattern of global financial assistance for COVID-19 was broadly similar to that for health official development assistance. Bilateral development agencies provided the largest share of resources, followed by the multilateral development banks, Gavi, and the Global Fund. WHO and other United Nations agencies provided miniscule financial contributions relative to the total resources made available.

Second, the lack of an existing dedicated facility for pandemic preparedness and response was notable and justified the creation of the Pandemic Fund. The current design of this facility focuses primarily on financing country-by-country, project-based, preparedness efforts. Other existing mechanisms, from bilateral official development assistance to multilateral development banks, could also fund these efforts. Questions remain about the additionality of the Pandemic Fund as well as whether it should develop contingent financing mechanisms to fund response efforts (early or late) in the future.

Third, the pandemic financing architecture is fragmented in terms of both number of organizations and number of financing tools, with significant implications for burden on receiving countries during a pandemic. The role of governance and coordination in reducing unnecessary delays and accessing funding cannot be underestimated. Similar problems became apparent with respect to the logistics of procurement and distribution of commodities, with both developed in the moment, creating considerable delays. Newly created mechanisms, such as COVAX, were too little, too late, and largely superseded by individual and bilateral efforts by countries (refer to box 13.6).

Fourth, concessional financing (primarily bilateral official development assistance, concessional loans, Gavi, the Global Fund, and philanthropy) represented the largest share of financing, followed by market rate loans. The analysis for this chapter did not measure the role of tools designed to respond to crises, such as contingent financing, debt service suspension, and insurance mechanisms, but their role is believed to be negligible. Contingent financing and prearranged agreements offer the potential to eliminate the delay in the flow of funds that marked most of the COVID-19 response. Promising examples that have emerged include the African Risk Capacity group, the new pandemic bond in Barbados, the Pandemic Emergency Financing Facility (improving its insurance mechanisms and triggers), and the World Bank's new Crisis Preparedness and Response Toolkit.

Finally, the response was too slow not only during the early response, when ultimately unsuccessful efforts to contain the virus were under way, but also during the late response as countries attempted to reduce its morbidity and mortality. This insufficient speed was most visibly apparent in lack of access to vaccines, but unnecessary delays due to lack of timely financing were apparent for diagnostics, monoclonal antibodies, ventilators, oxygen, drugs, and other supplies and equipment. These delays, resulting from the need to negotiate and execute financing instruments, were compounded by delays in comparative product evaluation (especially for diagnostics and vaccines), which hampered decision-making about product selection, and procurement delays caused by the lack of prenegotiated agreements. Delays also resulted from the free-for all in which the largest, wealthiest countries hoarded supplies because they could negotiate purchase agreements more quickly. There remains a need for a new at-risk response or surge financing mechanism that ensures equitable access to medical countermeasures. Negotiations for the Pandemic Accord, particularly on the pandemic access and benefits-sharing system, reflect the high priority and urgency of addressing this fatal weakness in the COVID-19 response.

Pandemic prevention, preparedness, response, and recovery and reconstruction will be effective only with the development of effective mechanisms to finance the required actions—and through the necessary organizational and governance mechanisms, the latter of which this chapter has not discussed at length. Although this chapter has outlined key principles and recommendations for future pandemic financing, translating them into actionable funding strategies requires further assessment of how existing instruments can be improved and where new mechanisms are needed. Some financing tools, such as contingent credit lines, emergency response grants, and pooled procurement mechanisms, already exist and could be scaled up or modified to better align with future pandemic needs. Others, such as prefinanced insurance mechanisms and at-risk financing for medical countermeasures, remain underused or largely undeveloped. Figure 13.7 provides a framework for future financing instruments, but an important next step will involve more detailed mapping—that is, distinguishing between what already exists, what can be adapted, and what must be newly created. Given the technical and political complexities involved in restructuring global pandemic financing, this chapter does not prescribe a definitive path forward. Nevertheless, future research and policy discussions should critically assess which existing instruments can be optimized and which gaps require entirely new solutions, ensuring that pandemic financing mechanisms are both practical and politically feasible.

**Figure 13.7** Instruments and Financing Mechanisms for Pandemic Phases

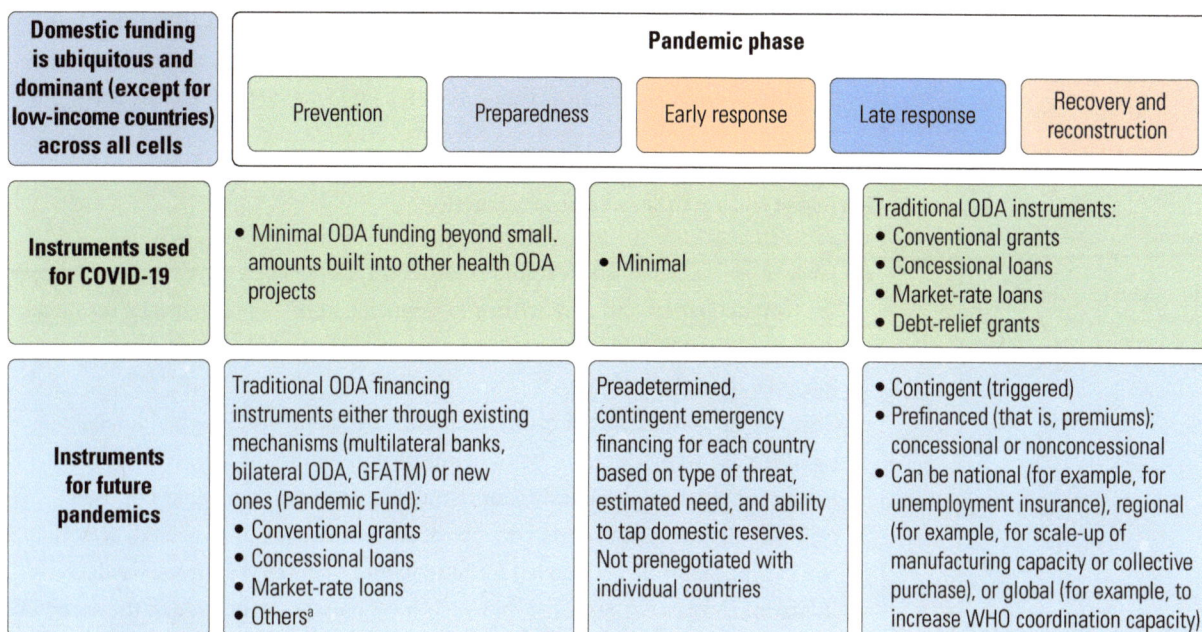

| Domestic funding is ubiquitous and dominant (except for low-income countries) across all cells | Pandemic phase | | | | |
|---|---|---|---|---|---|
| | Prevention | Preparedness | Early response | Late response | Recovery and reconstruction |
| **Instruments used for COVID-19** | • Minimal ODA funding beyond small amounts built into other health ODA projects | | • Minimal | Traditional ODA instruments: <br>• Conventional grants <br>• Concessional loans <br>• Market-rate loans <br>• Debt-relief grants | |
| **Instruments for future pandemics** | Traditional ODA financing instruments either through existing mechanisms (multilateral banks, bilateral ODA, GFATM) or new ones (Pandemic Fund): <br>• Conventional grants <br>• Concessional loans <br>• Market-rate loans <br>• Others[a] | | Preadetermined, contingent emergency financing for each country based on type of threat, estimated need, and ability to tap domestic reserves. Not prenegotiated with individual countries | • Contingent (triggered) <br>• Prefinanced (that is, premiums); concessional or nonconcessional <br>• Can be national (for example, for unemployment insurance), regional (for example, for scale-up of manufacturing capacity or collective purchase), or global (for example, to increase WHO coordination capacity) | |

*Source:* Original figure created for this publication.

*Note:* GFATM = Global Fund to Fight AIDS, Tuberculosis and Malaria; ODA = official development assistance; WHO = World Health Organization.

a. Loans appropriate for start-up costs or if the country is in short-term crisis; maintenance costs should incorporate a mix of grants and domestic financing.

## Recommendations

Drawing from those key messages, the chapter offers the following recommendations.

### Prevention and preparedness

- To ensure adequate financing of prevention and preparedness, establish clear and transparent indicators that define a minimum acceptable level of pandemic prevention and preparedness that can be improved by financing. Indicators should be simple, measurable, achievable, relevant to pandemic financing, and time-bound. Although this chapter does not discuss the existing array of international regulations and rules—such as the International Health Regulations, the negotiations under way on the Pandemic Accords, or prevailing tools like the Joint External Evaluation tool and others—its key message is that financing needs to be linked to progress that is independently and rigorously evaluated by a third party.
- Establish principles for how to distribute a global pandemic financing resource such as the Pandemic Fund across countries, on the presumption

that prevention and preparedness are global public goods. On the basis of those principles, define and use an allocation formula that can incorporate expected country costs for financing pandemic prevention and preparedness as well as standards for how much country and international sources should be expected to finance.

**Response and recovery and reconstruction**

- *Early response.* Establish clear and transparent triggers or a tiered scale of triggers for swift activation and deployment of financial, human, and material resources in response to an outbreak or epidemic of a new or reemerging pathogen (chapter 14 in this volume).
- Ensure that funding mechanisms are prearranged and are designed to enable rapid release when different types of outbreak or epidemic triggers occur. Financing must be much faster, more transparent, reimbursable if not used or justified, and used to fund actions within and outside of the health sector. Similar mechanisms are needed for human and material resources, particularly in planning for surge response, but such mechanisms are outside of the scope of this review.
- *Late response and recovery and reconstruction.* Develop a suite of contingent financing mechanisms to enable countries to cope with the late response to and recovery from large epidemics and pandemics. Mechanisms can include contingent grants, contingent loans, and insurance (refer to figure 13.7). These tools can be adapted to a country's ability to pay, with different levels of subsidy from the global community, comparable to other global development efforts. These mechanisms can be similar to those developed for response to and recovery from other major shocks. They differ from traditional grant and credit-based development assistance for health because, unlike much current development assistance for health, they are prenegotiated and contingent upon the occurrence of an epidemic or pandemic.

**Governance and continuous learning**

- Although extensive review of governance options for prevention, preparedness, response, and recovery was beyond the scope of this chapter, the public good nature of pandemics needs to be considered with respect to governance of financing mechanisms for global public goods.
- Pandemics are subject to the cycle of panic and neglect for many reasons, including the low frequency and high impact of such events, as well as the short time horizons of politicians. Leadership and governance, however, can ensure that lessons are learned and that pandemic preparedness and response plans evolve in response to those lessons. Learning can occur using real-world scenarios or simulation exercises of new potential pandemics to test and enhance preparedness plans, at hospital, local, national, and international levels. Review of best practices and lessons should be periodic and routine.

By exploring these strategies, the international community can create a resilient and equitable framework for pandemic preparedness, ultimately leading to stronger global health security.

## Conclusions

Global health financing mechanisms have historically not been designed to provide immediate or timely financial, material, and human support at the scale required to adequately respond to outbreaks and epidemics and prevent pandemics. Development assistance for health is designed to address ongoing health challenges, but pandemics require financing mechanisms that are triggered by an event or a set of conditions. This situation is much more akin to public and private insurance mechanisms than to traditional project-based or sectorwide development assistance. Such contingent mechanisms need to be implemented at the required scale and speed.

Reducing the risk of pandemics requires global cooperation with an effective system of rules and regulations that include positive and negative incentives. Just as homeowners in high-risk areas are required to clear flammable brush from around their houses, with inspectors verifying compliance, so too are transparency, verifiability, and accountability key to global financing mechanisms for pandemic prevention, preparedness, response, and recovery and reconstruction.

## NOTES

1. For more on the International Monetary Fund's tracker, refer to its "Policy Responses to COVID-19" web page, https://www.imf.org/en/Topics/imf-and-covid19/Policy-Responses -to-COVID-19.
2. *Non-flow financial instruments* refer to financial mechanisms that do not involve the continuous flow of funds from one entity to another over time. Unlike traditional grants or loans, which typically entail ongoing financial transactions, non-flow instruments may include options, swaps, guarantees, insurance contracts, or other derivative instruments that provide contingent coverage or protection against specific risks without necessitating regular payment streams. These instruments are often used in the context of risk management and financial hedging strategies, offering flexibility and tailored solutions to mitigate various types of financial risks.
3. This chapter mainly emphasizes the former functions of revenue mobilization and pooling, whereas it emphasizes less the function of payment and purchasing, recognizing that many incentives, particularly between international and national stakeholders, occur in the context of the latter function (that is, in the context of a contractual agreement involving payment). A third financing framework by Fan, Sharma, and Hou (2023) labeled the categories of the Roberts et al. (2008) framework as the means of financing, but emphasized two other aspects shared by both financing and purchasing, which pertains to the benefit package of services offered and the population eligibility or who is covered under such financing (Fan, Smitham, et al. 2023). This framework emphasis recognizes that the payment and purchasing function cannot be separated from the what and the who, and is consistent with the framework in this chapter, which emphasizes the list of pandemic actions—that is, the what.
4. Institute for Health Metrics and Evaluation, "Development Assistance for Health on COVID-19 Database 2020–2023," https://ghdx.healthdata.org/record/ihme-data /development-assistance-health-covid-2020-2023.

## REFERENCES

Adeyi, O., P. Yadav, R. Panjabi, and W. Mbacham. 2024. "The R21 Malaria Vaccine: Spotlight on Policy Goals and Pathways to African Vaccine Manufacturing." *PLOS Global Public Health* 4 (7): e0003412. https://doi.org/10.1371/journal.pgph.0003412.

Agarwal, R., and T. Reed. 2022. "Financing Vaccine Equity: Funding for Day-Zero of the Next Pandemic." *Oxford Review of Economic Policy* 38 (4): 833–50. https://doi.org/10.1093/oxrep/grac032.

Boyce, M. R., E. M. Sorrell, and C. J. Standley. 2023. "An Early Analysis of the World Bank's Pandemic Fund: A New Fund for Pandemic Prevention, Preparedness and Response." *BMJ Global Health* 8 (1): e011172. https://doi.org/10.1136/bmjgh-2022-011172.

Buckley, G. J., and R. E. Pittluck, eds. 2016. *Global Health Risk Framework: Pandemic Financing: Workshop Summary.* National Academies Press. https://doi.org/10.17226/21855.

Clarke, L., E. Patouillard, A. J. Mirelman, Z. J. M. Ho, T. T.-T. Edejer, and N. Kandel. 2022. "The Costs of Improving Health Emergency Preparedness: A Systematic Review and Analysis of Multi-country Studies." *eClinicalMedicine* 44. https://doi.org/10.1016/j.eclinm.2021.101269.

Craven, M., A. Sabow, L. Van der Veken, and M. Wilson. 2021. "Not the Last Pandemic: Investing Now to Reimagine Public-Health Systems." McKinsey & Company. https://www.mckinsey.com/industries/public-sector/our-insights/not-the-last-pandemic-investing-now-to-reimagine-public-health-systems.

Cutler, D. M., and L. H. Summers. 2020. "The COVID-19 Pandemic and the $16 Trillion Virus." *JAMA* 324 (15): 1495–96. https://doi.org/10.1001/jama.2020.19759.

Das Gupta, M., B. R. Desikachari, T. V. Somanathan, and P. Padmanaban. 2009. "How to Improve Public Health Systems: Lessons from Tamil Nadu." Policy Research Working Paper 5073, World Bank, Washington, DC. https://ideas.repec.org//p/wbk/wbrwps/5073.html.

Dieleman, J. L., C. M. Graves, and M. Hanlon. 2013. "The Fungibility of Health Aid: Reconsidering the Reconsidered." *Journal of Development Studies* 49 (12): 1755–62. https://doi.org/10.1080/00220388.2013.844921.

Dissanayake, R., and B. Camps Adrogué. 2022. "Building a Portfolio of Pull Financing Mechanisms for Climate and Development." CGD Policy Paper 273, Center for Global Development, Washington, DC. https://www.cgdev.org/publication/building-portfolio-pull-financing-mechanisms-climate-and-development.

Dissanayake, R., and B. Camps Adrogué. 2023. "The Case for More Pull Financing." CGD Brief, Center for Global Development, Washington, DC. https://www.cgdev.org/publication/case-more-pull-financing.

Dubois, P., Y. Lefouili, and S. Straub. 2021. "Pooled Procurement of Drugs in Low and Middle Income Countries." *European Economic Review* 132: 103655. https://doi.org/10.1016/j.euroecorev.2021.103655.

Eaneff, S., E. Graeden, A. McClelland, and R. Katz. 2022. "Investing in Global Health Security: Estimating Cost Requirements for Country-Level Capacity Building." *PLOS Global Public Health* 2 (12): e0000880. https://doi.org/10.1371/journal.pgph.0000880.

Fan, V. 2022. "Does Our State Government Have Too Many Boxes?" *Honolulu Civil Beat*, July 15, 2022. https://www.civilbeat.org/2022/07/does-our-state-government-have-too-many-boxes/.

Fan, V. 2023. "Resource Allocation Framework for Pandemic Risk and Surveillance: Version 1.0." CGD Note, Center for Global Development, Washington, DC. https://www.cgdev.org/publication/resource-allocation-framework-pandemic-risk-and-surveillance-version-10.

Fan, V., R. Agarwal, N. Madhav, C. Stefan, and C. Reynolds. 2024. "World Leaders' Must-Do List in 2024: Next Steps to Secure Pandemic Financing." *Center for Global Development* (blog), February 26, 2024. https://www.cgdev.org/blog/world-leaders-must-do-list-2024-next-steps-secure-pandemic-financing.

Fan, V., and S. Gupta. 2024. "Five Ideas for the Future of Global Health Financing: The Road Not Yet Taken." *Center for Global Development* (blog), June 5, 2024. https://www.cgdev.org /blog/five-ideas-future-global-health-financing-road-not-yet-taken.

Fan, V., and E. Smitham. 2023. "The Pandemic Fund's Results Framework: Early Reflections and Recommendations." *Center for Global Development* (blog), April 28, 2023. https:// www.cgdev.org/blog/pandemic-funds-results-framework-early-reflections-and -recommendations.

Fan, V., E. Smitham, L. Regan, P. Gautam, O. Norheim, J. Guzman, and A. Glassman. 2023. "Strategic Investment in Surveillance for Pandemic Preparedness: Rapid Review and Roundtable Discussion." CGD Policy Paper 298, Center for Global Development, Washington, DC. https://www.cgdev.org/publication/strategic-investment-surveillance -pandemic-preparedness-rapid-review-and-roundtable.

Fan, V. Y., R. Cash, S. Bertozzi, and M. Pate. 2023. "The When Is Less Important than the What: An Epidemic Scale as an Alternative to the WHO's Public Health Emergency of International Concern." *The Lancet Global Health* 11 (10): e1499–e1500. https://doi .org/10.1016/S2214-109X(23)00314-5.

Fan, V. Y., T. M. Fontanilla, C. T. Yamaguchi, S. M. Geib, J. R. Holmes, S. Kim, B. Do, et al. 2021. "Experience of Isolation and Quarantine hotels for COVID-19 in Hawaii." *Journal of Travel Medicine* 28 (7): taab096. https://doi.org/10.1093/jtm/taab096.

Fan, V. Y., A. Glassman, and R. L. Silverman. 2014. "How a New Funding Model Will Shift Allocations from the Global Fund to Fight AIDS, Tuberculosis, and Malaria." *Health Affairs (Project Hope)* 33 (12): 2238–46. https://doi.org/10.1377/hlthaff.2014.0240.

Fan, V. Y., D. T. Jamison, and L. H. Summers. 2018. "Pandemic Risk: How Large Are the Expected Losses?" *Bulletin of the World Health Organization* 96 (2): 129–34. https://doi .org/10.2471/BLT.17.199588.

Fan, V. Y., J. Sharma, and X. Hou. 2023. "Financing Primary Health Care for Older Adults: Framework and Applications." In *Silver Opportunity: Building Integrated Services for Older Adults around Primary Health Care*. Washington, DC: World Bank. 47–74. https://doi .org/10.1596/978-1-4648-1958-2.

Fan, V. Y., C. T. Yamaguchi, K. Pal, S. M. Geib, L. Conlon, J. R. Holmes, Y. Sutton, et al. 2022. "Planning and Implementation of COVID-19 Isolation and Quarantine Facilities in Hawaii: A Public Health Case Report." *International Journal of Environmental Research and Public Health* 19 (15): 9368. https://doi.org/10.3390/ijerph19159368.

G20 HLIP (Group of Twenty High Level Independent Panel). 2021. *A Global Deal for Our Pandemic Age: Report of the G20 High Level Independent Panel on Financing the Global Commons for Pandemic Preparedness and Response*. G20. https://pandemic-financing.org /report/foreword/.

Glennerster, R., C. M. Snyder, and B. J. Tan. 2022. "Calculating the Costs and Benefits of Advance Preparations for Future Pandemics." NBER Working Paper 30565, National Bureau of Economic Research, Cambridge, MA. https://doi.org/10.3386/w30565.

Gopinath, G. 2020. "The Great Lockdown: Worst Economic Downturn Since the Great Depression." *IMF Blog*, April 14, 2020. https://www.imf.org/en/Blogs/Articles/2020/04/14 /blog-weo-the-great-lockdown-worst-economic-downturn-since-the-great-depression.

Hale, T., N. Angrist, R. Goldszmidt, B. Kira, A. Petherick, T. Phillips, S. Webster, et al. 2021. "A Global Panel Database of Pandemic Policies (Oxford COVID-19 Government Response Tracker)." *Nature Human Behaviour* 5 (4): 529–38. https://doi.org/10.1038/s41562-021 -01079-8.

Hill, R., D. Patel, Y. Yang, and J. Gascoigne. 2024. "Funding COVID-19 Response: Tracking Global Humanitarian and Development Flows to Meet Crisis Needs." *Centre for Disaster Protection* (blog), June 25, 2024. https://www.disasterprotection.org/blogs/funding-covid -19-response-tracking-global-humanitarian-and-development-flows-to-meet-crisis-needs.

Keogh-Brown, M. R., and R. D. Smith. 2008. "The Economic Impact of SARS: How Does the Reality Match the Predictions?" *Health Policy* 88 (1): 110–20. https://doi.org/10.1016/j .healthpol.2008.03.003.

Kremer, M., J. Levin, and C. M. Snyder. 2020. "Advance Market Commitments: Insights from Theory and Experience." *AEA Papers and Proceedings* 110 (May): 269–73. https://doi .org/10.1257/pandp.20201017.

Laffont, J.-J. 1993. *A Theory of Incentives in Procurement and Regulation*. Cambridge: MIT Press. http://archive.org/details/theoryo_laf_1993_00_9636.

Laffont, J.-J., and D. Martimort. 2002. *The Theory of Incentives: The Principal-Agent Model*. Princeton University Press. https://doi.org/10.2307/j.ctv7h0rwr.

Lee, T. H., B. Do, L. Dantzinger, J. Holmes, M. Chyba, S. Hankins, E. Mersereau, K. Hara, K., and V. Y. Fan. 2022. "Mitigation Planning and Policies Informed by COVID-19 Modeling: A Framework and Case Study of the State of Hawaii." *International Journal of Environmental Research and Public Health* 19 (10): 6119. https://doi.org/10.3390 /ijerph19106119.

Obeng-Kusi, M., J. Martin, and I. Abraham. 2024. "The Economic Burden of Ebola Virus Disease: A Review and Recommendations for Analysis." *Journal of Medical Economics* 27 (1): 309–23. https://doi.org/10.1080/13696998.2024.2313358.

Pablos-Méndez, A., S. Villa, M. C. Monti, M. C. Raviglione, H. B. Tabish, T. G. Evans, and R. A. Cash. 2022. "Global Ecological Analysis of COVID-19 Mortality and Comparison between 'the East' and 'the West.'" *Scientific Reports* 12 (1): 5272. https://doi.org/10.1038/s41598-022 -09286-7.

Patouillard, E., V. Fan, E. Ozcelik, S. Alkenbrack, M. Cecchini, T. T. Torres Edejer, and A. Burns. 2024. "Navigating Pandemic Uncertainty: The Role of Integrated Modeling in Policymaking." *Center for Global Development* (blog), May 8, 2024. https://www.cgdev.org /blog/navigating-pandemic-uncertainty-role-integrated-modeling-policymaking.

Roberts, M., W. Hsiao, P. Berman, and M. Reich. 2008. *Getting Health Reform Right: A Guide to Improving Performance and Equity*. Oxford University Press. https://doi.org/10.1093/acp rof:oso/9780195371505.001.0001.

Rogoff, K. 2022. "Emerging Market Sovereign Debt in the Aftermath of the Pandemic." *Journal of Economic Perspectives* 36 (4): 147–66.

Sachs, J. D., S. S. A. Karim, L. Aknin, J. Allen, K. Brosbøl, F. Colombo, G. C. Barron, et al. 2022. "The *Lancet* Commission on Lessons for the Future from the COVID-19 Pandemic." *The Lancet* 400 (10359): 1224–80. https://doi.org/10.1016/S0140-6736(22)01585-9.

Schäferhoff, M., P. Chodavadia, S. Martinez, K. K. McDade, S. Fewer, S. Silva, D. Jamison, and G. Yamey. 2019. "International Funding for Global Common Goods for Health: An Analysis Using the Creditor Reporting System and G-FINDER Databases." *Health Systems and Reform* 5 (4): 350–65. https://doi.org/10.1080/23288604.2019.1663646.

Sureka, S., N. Madhav, B. Oppenheim, and V. Fan. 2023. "How Big Is the Risk of Epidemics, Really?" *Center for Global Development* (blog), November 13, 2023. https://www.cgdev .org/blog/how-big-risk-epidemics-really.

Suzuki, M., and S. Yang. 2023. "Political Economy of Vaccine Diplomacy: Explaining Varying Strategies of China, India, and Russia's COVID-19 Vaccine Diplomacy." *Review of International Political Economy* 30 (3): 865–90. https://doi.org/10.1080/09692290.2022 .2074514.

United Nations Brundtland Commission. 1987. *Report of the World Commission on Environment and Development: Our Common Future*. United Nations. http://www.un-documents.net/our -common-future.pdf.

Wagner, C. E., C. M. Saad-Roy, S. E. Morris, R. E. Baker, M. J. Mina, J. Farrar, E. Holmes, et al. 2021. "Vaccine Nationalism and the Dynamics and Control of SARS-CoV-2." *Science* 373 (6562): eabj7364. https://doi.org/10.1126/science.abj7364.

WHO (World Health Organization). 2022. *Joint External Evaluation Tool: International Health Regulations (2005), Third Edition*. Geneva: WHO. https://www.who.int/publications/i/item /9789240051980.

WHO (World Health Organization). 2023. "Strengthening the Global Architecture for Health Emergency Prevention, Preparedness, Response and Resilience (HEPR)." WHO, Geneva. https://www.who.int/publications/m/item/strengthening-the-global-architecture-for -health-emergency-prevention--preparedness--response-and-resilience.

WHO (World Health Organization). 2024. *Pandemic Influenza Preparedness Framework: Partnership Contribution High-Level Implementation Plan III 2024–2030.* Geneva: WHO. https://www.who.int/publications/i/item/9789240070141.

WHO (World Health Organization) and World Bank. 2022. "Analysis of Pandemic Preparedness and Response (PPR) Architecture, Financing Needs, Gaps and Mechanisms. G20 Joint Finance & Health Task Force." WHO and World Bank, Geneva and Washington, DC. https://thedocs.worldbank.org/en/doc /5760109c4db174ff90a8dfa7d025644a-0290032022/original/G20-Gaps-in-PPR-Financing -Mechanisms-WHO-and-WB-pdf.pdf.

Więcek, W., A. Ahuja, E. Chaudhuri, M. Kremer, A. Simoes Gomes, C. M. Snyder, A. Tabarrok, and B. J. Tan. 2022. "Testing Fractional Doses of COVID-19 Vaccines." *Proceedings of the National Academy of Sciences of the United States of America* 119 (8): e2116932119. https:// doi.org/10.1073/pnas.2116932119.

World Bank. 2022. *The World Bank's Early Support to Addressing Coronavirus (COVID-19) Health and Social Response: An Early-Stage Evaluation.* Independent Evaluation Group. Washington, DC: World Bank. https://ieg.worldbankgroup.org/evaluations/world-banks -early-support-addressing-covid-19.

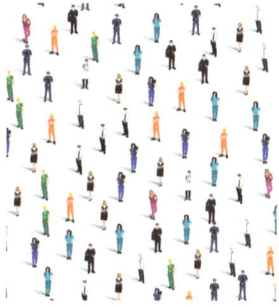

# 14

# Designing Trigger Mechanisms for Epidemic and Pandemic Financing and Response

Nita K. Madhav, Ben Oppenheim, and Cristina Stefan

## ABSTRACT

Nearly every consequential choice in epidemic and pandemic response requires a trigger of some kind: a set of criteria—often, but not always, quantitative—that determines whether alerts or public health declarations are issued, financing for outbreak containment and response is released, personnel and medical countermeasure deployments are surged, and so on. Triggers are sometimes implicit or internally facing, nested within expert guidance and decision-support processes, but are increasingly public facing to help stakeholders and citizens make sense of public health guidelines and decisions. Consequently, triggers are both increasingly used and increasingly visible, and are the subject of continuous innovation and debate. However, no established frameworks or standards exist to guide the development and integration of triggers into public health decision-making generally, or epidemic and pandemic financing and response specifically. This chapter presents a framework for high-quality trigger design with specific application to pandemic financing and response, with the goals of improving triggers' effectiveness and reliability, and providing clearer communication of their attributes and intended performance to stakeholders, including the public. It also includes a brief case study on the World Bank's Pandemic Emergency Financing Facility.

## INTRODUCTION

Nearly every consequential choice in epidemic and pandemic response requires a trigger of some kind: a set of criteria—often, but not always, quantitative—that determines whether alerts or public health declarations are issued, financing for outbreak containment and response is released, personnel and medical countermeasure deployments are surged, and so on. This chapter focuses mainly on the design and development of triggers for prearranged financing mechanisms. It also briefly discusses additional applications for triggers in epidemic and pandemic preparedness and response. The primary focus of this chapter is to explore the trigger design process and propose criteria that can be used to assess the quality of trigger designs, with the goal of supporting technical improvements to trigger designs in public health, especially for financing response activities. This chapter is not an argument to incorporate quantitative triggers into all financing mechanisms or decision processes; the suitability and feasibility of triggers (and of specific trigger designs) vary with different objectives, applications, scenarios, and risks.

A *trigger* is a prearranged mechanism or set of conditions that determines whether (or when) to activate a financial or operational response because an event has occurred or is predicted to occur. Triggers are perhaps best known for their use in insurance contracts, both private market contracts and sovereign disaster risk financing mechanisms that provide capital (typically from multilateral organizations or specialized capital pools) to governments. In the context of insurance, triggers represent a critical element of a contract that binds one party to release capital to another under preagreed conditions; of note, the trigger criteria are designed to correlate with the economic loss that the beneficiary of the financing would incur. The process of trigger design described in this chapter is intended to identify, address, and propose options to reduce information asymmetries that present a fundamental barrier to the quantification (including pricing) of risk and successful contracting to transfer it. However, triggers also have broad application to noncontractual settings, including in the design and implementation of decision processes. In the context of supporting decision-making, triggers can provide a structure to guide policy makers in making difficult choices (for example, whether and when to implement and relax public health restrictions).

Triggers have varying degrees of complexity. For example, a simple trigger could be designed to activate upon an emergency declaration by a ministry of health. A more complex trigger could incorporate multiple parameters that need to meet specific joint thresholds to activate.

The term "parametric trigger" comes from the use of a parameter or combination of parameters—quantitative in nature—that prompts the release of funds; each parameter has a threshold or required value that, if reached (or, in the case of multiparameter designs, collectively reached), triggers the release of funds. A parametric trigger can also take the form of an index, which involves the combination or calculation of a value or values based on measured parameters; data sources can vary greatly, from reported epidemiological data to meteorological data, to remote sensing or satellite data. Triggers can also be based on modeled results, which would be simulated by a model that takes the estimated parameter values as inputs.

Trigger design is currently the focus of technical and creative energy for a broad range of use cases, ranging from the insurance industry, risk modeling, and climate science to humanitarian and development applications. Designing triggers that work well, however, is challenging.

Disaster risk financing has numerous examples of trigger mechanisms—particularly parametric trigger mechanisms. This is especially so for natural hazards such as tropical cyclones, earthquakes, floods, and droughts (Cissé 2021). Despite standing to benefit substantially from preagreed funding mechanisms, the health sector has arguably been slow to consider and adopt these types of constructs.

## TRIGGERS FOR EPIDEMIC RISK FINANCING

In the late 2010s and early 2020s, financing mechanisms designed to mitigate risk from epidemics and pandemics began incorporating parametric triggers (refer to table 14.1 for selected examples).[1] In these financing mechanisms, a parametric trigger defines the necessary quantitative criteria for the release of capital during or following the occurrence of an epidemic. In the case of epidemics, the total loss includes the number of lives and livelihoods affected, along with budgetary expenses incurred during epidemic response activities such as contact tracing, vaccination, and clinical case management.

**Table 14.1** Attributes of Selected Epidemic and Pandemic Financing Instruments, Including Trigger Elements

| Instrument | Objective | Covered perils | Covered geographies | Trigger elements | Potential design challenge(s) |
|---|---|---|---|---|---|
| Pandemic Emergency Financing Facility (IBRD 2017) | To provide financing for multicountry epidemics and pandemics (rather than single-country outbreaks) | • Pandemic influenza<br>• Novel coronaviruses<br>• Filoviruses<br>• Lassa Fever<br>• Rift Valley Fever<br>• Crimean-Congo Hemorrhagic Fever<br><br>Other perils were covered in the cash (contingency) window | • IDA countries (World Bank 2021b) | Triggers were specific to bond class and pathogen group, and included the following:<br>• Cumulative cases<br>• Eligible event period<br>• Total confirmed deaths<br>• Geographic spread<br>• Growth rate<br>• Confirmation ratio for certain pathogens | • Received criticisms due to complex trigger design and timing of payouts for COVID-19<br>• Did not pay out during Ebola epidemics from the insurance window, but did pay from the cash (contingency) window |
| African Risk Capacity Outbreaks & Epidemics policy (Böhm 2023) | To provide rapid financing in the earliest stages of an epidemic | • Filoviruses<br>• Meningitis | • Senegal | • Total laboratory-confirmed cases (filoviruses)<br>• Districts in alert and epidemic phase (meningitis) | • Uncertainty about case counts very early in an outbreak |

*table continues next page*

| Instrument | Objective | Covered perils | Covered geographies | Trigger elements | Potential design challenge(s) |
|---|---|---|---|---|---|
| Pathogen Rx (ADB 2022) | To provide liquidity for private sector firms facing cash flow and/or operational disruption during an epidemic | "Infectious disease outbreaks"[a] | • Worldwide and regional | • Confirmed outbreak<br>• Infections<br>• Deaths<br>• Sentiment Index (Oppenheim et al. 2019)<br>• Proof of loss | • Coverage limited depending on geographic characteristics of the event<br>• Hybrid trigger, including indemnity component: proof of loss required (Wright and Lacovara 2020) |
| Munich RE Epidemic Risk Transfer Solutions[a] | To efficiently reallocate epidemic and pandemic risk across various stakeholders | • "Viral epidemic and pandemic outbreaks"[a] | • Worldwide and regional | • PHEIC<br>• Civil authority restriction<br>• Proof of loss | • Reliance on subjective triggers (for example, PHEIC)<br>• Proof of loss required from the insured (long time to assess the claim) |
| Gavi's First Response Fund (Gavi 2024) | To secure early access to vaccines and to protect existing immunization programs | • Pathogens with PHEIC potential<br>• Pathogens qualified as Grade 2 or 3 by WHO | • Gavi-eligible countries | • Pandemic or PHEIC declaration | • Reliance on subjective triggers (for example, PHEIC)<br>• Lack of predictability and transparency |

*Source:* Original table compiled for this publication.

*Note:* Pathogen Rx and Munich RE Epidemic Risk Transfer Solutions are private sector insurance structures. IDA = International Development Association; PHEIC = public health emergency of international concern; WHO = World Health Organization.

a. Munich Reinsurance, "Epidemic and Pandemic Risk Solutions," https://www.munichre.com/en/solutions/for-industry-clients/epidemic-risk-solutions.html.

Parametric triggers can be used to develop coverage through parametric insurance, which disburses funding without waiting for a claim assessment on the ground to determine the exact loss suffered by each insured party. This practice contrasts with indemnity insurance, which is defined by post facto reimbursement of actual losses incurred and typically requires proof of loss, such as (in the case of epidemics) evidence of fiscal outlays for containment and response activities. This same logic applies to noninsurance financing mechanisms: formal incorporation of a parametric trigger can release funding rapidly, without the need for expert assessments or ex post humanitarian appeals and response cost estimates from governments affected by disasters. Financing mechanisms may also use a hybrid trigger that combines both parametric and indemnity-based trigger criteria, though hybrid triggers are typically less common because of their complexity. Trigger mechanisms are often progressive or scaled, with additional triggers releasing more funding as an event progresses and more losses and operational costs are incurred.

The main rationale for using a parametric trigger is the predictability and speed at which a payout can be released. Because the payout can occur as soon as the trigger is reached, funds can be disbursed far more rapidly than in the case of an indemnity trigger, which typically requires a lengthy process: waiting until the damage occurs, proof of loss is submitted, the loss is independently assessed, an insurance adjustment is performed, and payment is eventually released. Financing mechanisms based on parametric triggers can pay out in days or weeks, whereas those incorporating indemnity-based triggers would more typically pay out in months or even years after an event has occurred. Some parametric trigger–based financing mechanisms have even been designed to release funds in advance of an event—for example, a novel African Risk Capacity drought insurance instrument (Maslo 2022).

A growing body of evidence confirms the significant welfare benefits of early response to catastrophes (Pople et al. 2021). Those benefits apply to a wide variety of crises, but especially to infectious disease events. Rapid financing can significantly reduce the financial and health impacts caused by epidemics. For epidemics, rapid access to capital can enable more timely and effective reduction and potential containment of disease transmission—for example, by supporting contact tracing; public education and risk-reduction campaigns; and diagnostic, drug, and vaccine distribution. Rapid containment can, in turn, reduce the severity and duration of an epidemic, leading to significant reductions in human and economic losses and, ultimately, preventing events from reaching their full potential magnitude. The effects of early mitigation can be especially significant for epidemics and pandemics, because (unlike other acute natural hazards such as earthquakes or hurricanes) some infectious disease events may last years (for example, the 1918 influenza pandemic and COVID-19 [coronavirus]) and others may last decades (for example, the human immunodeficiency virus and acquired immune deficiency syndrome [HIV/AIDS] pandemic).

The timeliness and predictability of funding can also provide incentives for all actors involved in outbreak detection and epidemic response: to detect and report potential threats to public health quickly, and to develop and maintain operational plans that will guide response activities. Prearranged, predictable financing can provide greater confidence that funding will be available, allowing agencies and leaders to focus on managing response activities rather than fundraising.

Although this discussion has focused primarily on disaster risk financing mechanisms for rapid response and mitigation of biological hazards, these financing mechanisms can serve other functions—for example, containment to reduce the risk of disease spread beyond the initially affected country. Optimal trigger design depends entirely upon the problem that the financing instrument is designed to solve. The following section discusses this issue further.

## BEYOND FINANCING: TRIGGERS FOR DECISION-MAKING

Triggers have a wide range of applications beyond financing mechanisms, including providing quantitative, objective criteria for implementing, altering, or ending containment policies, programs, or public declarations of health emergencies.

A key virtue of triggers is that they support the rapid implementation of decisions that have effectively been made in advance; triggers therefore provide both speed and insulation from political pressures that may quickly build up once a crisis occurs. Not all decisions require or necessarily benefit from being implemented via a trigger mechanism. A surprisingly wide range of decision processes are suitable, however, and many if not all policy and decision processes can benefit from the logical process of working through how they might be implemented using a trigger-like mechanism. The following subsections discuss a selection of illustrative, nonexhaustive examples of situations and decision points for which having a trigger mechanism in place could be beneficial during an epidemic or pandemic.

### Health Notifications, Alerts, and Emergency Declarations

One important category of decision-making during an outbreak or epidemic is whether to issue health notifications, alerts, or emergency declarations. Notable examples include the issuance of a notification by a health authority (for example, Disease Outbreak News from the World Health Organization [WHO]),[2] the dissemination of an alert (for example, the US Centers for Disease Control and Prevention's Health Alert Network Health Advisory),[3] the declaration of a public health emergency (for example, declaration by WHO of a public health emergency of international concern [PHEIC]),[4] and WHO's declaration of meningitis districts in alert or epidemic based on different disease thresholds (WHO 2014). The process for determining whether to issue a PHEIC has, in particular, been criticized for being complex and nontransparent; an empirical analysis of emergency committee deliberations found inconsistent application of criteria for determining whether to issue a PHEIC declaration (Fan et al. 2023; Mullen et al. 2020).

Public health emergency declaration processes often provide for substantial decision-making flexibility: this flexibility can be a virtue because there may be substantial uncertainty about the characteristics and severity of the potential threat, the speed of its development, and its potential impacts. The virtue of flexibility is that it can allow for scientific judgment to address these points of uncertainty; a vice is that it also allows for political factors—electoral costs, reputational risks, and fears of economic damages—to cloud judgment. Here, incorporation of quantitative triggers can help provide both expert guidance and political insulation, because some potentially "costly" aspects of the emergency declaration process can be addressed through preagreed mechanisms.

### Early-Stage Containment Measures

Very early in an outbreak, it may be possible to limit spread and contain the event while it is still relatively small and manageable. A key challenge is that data are often sparse and incomplete at this early stage, so substantial uncertainty can raise the political cost and risk associated with taking potentially costly steps to contain transmission. Data sparsity and uncertainty can also make it difficult to design an appropriate trigger to activate rapid response and containment measures; especially in this early stage of an outbreak, quantitative information may not yet be available or even known, and modeled estimates may have high levels of uncertainty. Therefore, binary parametric triggers or qualitative triggers may play a more important role than during other stages of an epidemic or pandemic. For example, a rapid risk assessment of a new respiratory virus may consider the presence or absence of sustained human-to-human transmission, among other relevant factors (FAO, WHO, and WOAH 2025; Ferguson et al. 2005; Longini et al. 2005), because it could potentially indicate elevated epidemic or pandemic risk. A critical priority during this early stage of an outbreak is to obtain as much relevant data as possible, which is much easier to do when persistent pathogen monitoring systems are already in place before an event.

## Epidemic Response and Mitigation If Initial Containment Is Unsuccessful

Once an outbreak has evaded containment and epidemic spread is under way, or seemingly inevitable, authorities—including national governments as well as international and multilateral agencies—need to make critical decisions about how to mitigate spread using a variety of tools.

### Targeted and Populationwide Interventions

Once the initial containment has failed, or is at high risk of failure, authorities may consider implementing targeted and populationwide interventions to curtail disease transmission. These measures may be taken with the goal of reducing pressure on health care systems ("flattening the epidemic curve"); protecting specific, vulnerable demographic groups; or limiting further geographic spread. They include the following:

- Implementation (and ending) of populationwide measures to reduce transmission, such as social distancing and mask mandates (refer to chapter 6 in this volume).
- Implementation (and ending) of targeted measures to reduce disease transmission (refer to chapter 7 in this volume), such as school closures (refer to chapter 8 in this volume). For example, a school might close in response to an outbreak or sharp increase in incidence in neighboring schools (Cauchemez et al. 2009). Alternatively, a pooled testing strategy could be used for decision-making based on positivity trends in schools (McKnight and Sureka 2024).
- Implementation of politically sensitive policy measures, such as travel restrictions, border closures, or trade restrictions. Having a predefined trigger in place could reduce the potential for a "knee-jerk" and effectively punitive reaction to a country's early detection and reporting of an outbreak, when such surveillance capability and behavior are precisely what should be incentivized. For example, South Africa suffered adverse consequences during the COVID-19 pandemic for being the first to detect and report the SARS-CoV-2 Omicron variant (Gudina and Gidi 2025).

### Medical Countermeasures

The applicability and set of choices regarding the deployment of medical countermeasures vary by pathogen, and by context. In the case of novel pathogens, diagnostics and vaccines need to be developed, tested, and deployed, and therapeutics either developed or identified from existing products. Known pathogens may also mutate, potentially compromising existing countermeasures and altering policy makers' choice sets. Last, countries may have vastly differing levels (and timing) of access to countermeasures, which can greatly influence decisions about deployment. Bearing these factors and constraints in mind, policy makers need to make decisions regarding

- Release of a government stockpile (for example of diagnostics, treatments, vaccines, or personal protective equipment);[5]
- Initiating a 100-day countdown for vaccine development (Pandemic Preparedness Partnership 2021);
- Government interventions to encourage or compel manufacturing of critical materials (masks, ventilators, vaccines, and so on), such as the US Defense Production Act (Hart 2024) and Operation Warp Speed during the COVID-19 pandemic (Lopez 2020); and
- Rapidly expanding clinical capacity, such as the activation of "surge" clinical facilities, emergency conversion of nonmedical facilities to provide care—for example, the Fangcang shelter hospitals built in China during the COVID-19 pandemic (Chen et al. 2020)—or construction of new hospital facilities.

## FRAMEWORK FOR HIGH-QUALITY TRIGGER DESIGN

An effective or high-quality trigger must possess the following qualities to be accepted by the involved parties in a financing transaction (the insured, the insurer, the reinsurer, donors, multilateral agencies, and so on) or policy process:

- *Simple.* Complicated triggers make it difficult to have an intuitive sense about whether and under what conditions a policy will trigger, potentially leading to misaligned expectations between counterparties (such as insurers and the insured). If a payout does not occur, does not occur rapidly enough, or does not occur at sufficient scale, it can lead to mistrust and a perception that the trigger and the underlying financial contract have been poorly designed, or even worse, made deliberately complicated to avoid making a payout.
- *Transparent.* So that anyone assessing whether the trigger threshold has been met possesses all the necessary information to perform the required calculations, all the involved parties in the transaction or the decision process must have access to the same underlying data used for calculation, as well as to the trigger calculations themselves.
- *Objective.* The trigger must be based on factors that can be reliably and consistently measured.

- *Verifiable.* It must be possible to independently and objectively corroborate that trigger conditions have been met (or not).
- *Preagreed.* Agreeing ahead of time ensures that the trigger has all the previously listed qualities and avoids confusion and delays during the assessment of whether trigger criteria have been met.

Appropriate trigger design is critical to ensure rapid disbursement of funds and to minimize the likelihood of inordinate and unpredictable payouts. Effective triggers can be developed by first establishing clear criteria for the context (when and for what) in which activation should occur. Crafting good triggers involves balancing the preferences and demands of the stakeholders, technical feasibility, and practical considerations (calculation processes, sources of data for the trigger and their reliability over time, failsafe procedures, and so on).

The trigger design process (part of a larger structuring process) is generally complex and involves the iterative exploration, development, testing, and calibration of various trigger concepts, in an effort to balance multiple design criteria and ensure that stakeholders are aware and aligned on what the instrument is designed to do (and what it is not designed to do). A thorough design process identifies requirements regarding the needs of responders at that specific moment, examines technical possibilities, and addresses potential failure points in advance. For whatever purpose the trigger is being designed, it behooves the developers of the trigger mechanism to follow an analytically sound design process that is transparent and inclusive of all stakeholder viewpoints. Ideally, a collaborative process of trigger design can help build trust and confidence between all the key stakeholders. The following subsections discuss key elements and considerations of the trigger design process.

### Event Definition

The foundational element of a trigger is an *event definition*, which clearly defines the types of adverse shocks to which the trigger applies. In the case of epidemic risk, a financing instrument may provide funding only for specific pathogens (for example, viral hemorrhagic fevers such as Ebola, Marburg, or Nipah viruses, which are capable of rapid, sustained transmission and have the potential to cause substantial societal and economic disruption) or only for epidemics of a magnitude that cannot be managed through routine health system functions and health budgets.

An event definition for an epidemic or pandemic may rely on a declaration by a health authority, such as a ministry of health or multilateral body (for example, Africa Centers for Disease Control or WHO). The authority may define the event on the basis of pathogen-specific criteria linked to the epidemiology of the disease and historical patterns in outbreak control. For example, an Ebola virus disease outbreak is declared once there is a single confirmed case based on laboratory testing.[6] Likewise, there may be specific criteria for declaring the end of the outbreak. For Ebola virus disease, the criterion is typically the end of 42 days with no new, epidemiologically linked cases (Djaafara et al. 2021). For other types of diseases, especially more routine occurrences such as meningitis, event definitions may be based on how far incidence has spiked above an established baseline of historical disease levels.

An event definition can also determine whether a series of losses is considered a single event or multiple occurrences. For example, substantial litigation took place over whether the two plane impacts on the World Trade Center in the 9/11 terrorist attacks should be considered separate events or a single attack, with substantial sums of money at stake (Johnson 2010). Similarly, an event definition for an epidemic or pandemic trigger could specify whether a mutation—for example, the emergence of a new variant or strain capable of more efficient transmission or immune evasion—is considered part of an ongoing outbreak or is a distinct event that could trigger a financing mechanism or policy response.

In addition to defining which events are covered, it is also important to define which events are not covered (that is, exclusions). Familiar insurance exclusions include "acts of God," terrorism, and war. In this case of epidemics, exclusions may include ongoing or foreseen events, such as epidemics already under way, as well as infectious disease hazards whose characteristics have not been accounted for in trigger design or pricing. For example, pandemic influenza is sometimes excluded because of its potential to be a systemic risk that could lead to correlated, catastrophic losses across far-flung geographical locations. Also sometimes excluded are biowarfare and bioterrorism, because they would fall more broadly under war or terrorism exclusions, and the accidental release of human-made or manipulated infectious agents, sometimes referred to as "bio-error" (refer to chapter 4 in this volume).

Another aspect of the coverage definition includes the covered geographic area—that is, the area within the geographic scope of the financing mechanism. This area can be defined by country or territorial boundaries, or even could be defined by a polygon (for example, "cat in a box"; refer to Franco et al. 2024). For epidemic or pandemic applications, such a polygon could be applied to a spark risk map and could be used as the basis for triggers following the progressive geographic spread of an epidemic beyond known hot spots.

As a general principle, the event definition should be developed drawing upon knowledge from all parties involved in epidemic preparedness and response, not just the health and finance sectors. Parties should include scientists and technical experts, community-based organizations, civil society, and government officials from the wide range of ministries whose missions and constituents are affected by epidemics (such as the education, labor, and security sectors). Their inclusion allows for incorporation of local context and local knowledge at the most fundamental level of design, ensuring that the trigger solves for real-world scenarios and problems.

## Quantitative Triggers

Quantitative triggers rely on measurable data and parameters. Several factors should be considered in determining which data and parameters to include. First and foremost, it must be determined which parameters are correlated to the outcome of interest, such as the loss to the insured. Second, the parameters should be easily measured. Third, the parameter values should be transparent, meaning they should be reported by an official, unbiased source, so that everyone has equal access to the information. Fourth, the source data should be reliable and updated in a timely fashion. Fifth, to ensure appropriate trigger calibration, there should be sufficient historical information to establish baseline levels or normal levels of risk. Sixth, if, for the purpose of designing a trigger, input data are transformed, the transformation methods should be well documented, including any relevant formulas and source code to perform the calculation. Finally, any methods used to fill data gaps (such as imputation), or reliance on alternative data sources, should be transparently described and well-documented.

In the case of epidemics and pandemics, quantitative triggers can be based on a number of parameter values, including reported measures of event severity (for example, laboratory-confirmed deaths or reduction in foot traffic) or reported government policy responses and actions for containment (closing borders, limiting social contact, establishing curfews, and so on) that can be measured categorically or via an index (Hale et al. 2021).

A range of data types and sources may be considered for incorporation into a trigger. The first is one based on independently reported (typically epidemiological) data. This data type is typically considered the most objective, because it comes from a third party (usually official) reporting source that would supply the information independent of any financing considerations. However, epidemiological data reported by a national government can pose potential challenges, most notably when a country that is covered by a disaster risk financing mechanism reports information that could activate a trigger (such as number of cases) and the national government itself is a beneficiary. In such situations, national statistical systems need to be independent, receive adequate financing, and produce high-quality data so that information is considered valid and trustworthy. One solution is to rely on data from other sources such as multilateral agencies. Of course, multilateral agencies, which generally rely on governments to provide data in the first place, can provide quality control and standards but not necessarily independence (World Bank 2021d).

A second type of data used to underpin a quantitative (and specifically parametric) trigger is an index, which is based on a calculated formula from reported data. For example, the Vita series of mortality bonds (Klein 2006) includes a mortality index that weights general population reported mortality to an insurance portfolio, thus building the correlation between the reported data on mortality rates and the estimated losses. Relatedly, a trigger can also incorporate parameters estimated from empirical data: for example $R_0$ can be calculated from reported epidemiological data and could (in theory) serve as a parameter in a trigger design. A third potential type of data used for a trigger is model output, often from a mechanistic model. In this kind of trigger, certain measured or reported parameter values are entered into a model and generate a modeled outcome, whether a loss estimate or index value, which ultimately will be compared against a trigger criterion.

Among these different types of trigger formulations, it is also important to consider the sources of error and uncertainty that may be present in the selected data and parameters (Mari and Giordani 2015). For example, confirmatory testing in a laboratory will be subject to measurement errors related to the sensitivity and specificity of the test; therefore, in some cases, corroborating the findings of an initial test may require a secondary test. Measurement error for empirical data can be highly variable across events and within events both over space (for example, because different countries have varying capacity or willingness to report accurate epidemiological data) and over time (for example, because of the intensification of surveillance during the course of an epidemic, the development and deployment of new diagnostic tests, or the failure of existing tests). For calculated parameters, these errors may have a complex interplay. For example, the case-fatality ratio (a measure of deaths divided by cases) could have ascertainment errors and biases in both the numerator and denominator (Lipsitch et al. 2015). However, this challenge could be partially mitigated for larger data sets of modeled or calculated parameter values, which could include point estimates and metrics of the uncertainty, such as a 95 percent confidence interval.

Trigger design frequently considers counts of confirmed or probable infections and deaths (refer to table 14.1). Verifying these parameters, however, may prove to be challenging during an epidemic. For example, case counts are often subject to underreporting (Meadows et al. 2022) or may not meet the condition of being verifiable, unless there is a laboratory confirmation. In a cruel irony, capacity for lab confirmation (and thus to meet trigger criteria) may be limited in those very settings, such as low-income and fragile states, that may benefit substantially from a disaster risk financing mechanism to cover response costs and economic losses. Design must also take into account stakeholder needs. For example, it may be difficult to get buy-in from public health stakeholders for a trigger based solely on counts of deaths—which are undesirable metrics from a public health standpoint and potentially present the risk of adverse media coverage (for example, McVeigh 2020)—whereas this may not be an obvious concern for financial stakeholders.

Emerging infectious disease surveillance approaches such as environmental monitoring can potentially unlock novel approaches to trigger design by generating data that could overcome some of the challenges of verifiability and underreporting described earlier. For example, wastewater testing for pathogens of interest could allow for triggers based on the detection of an emerging pathogen with epidemic potential (such as Nipah or Marburg viruses) in municipal sanitation (Grassly, Shaw, and Owusu 2024; Kilaru et al. 2023). However, more sophisticated trigger concepts, such as triggering based on a spike in concentration well in excess of typical levels, would require more established analytical methods for estimating epidemiological metrics of interest (cases, infection rates, and so on) from wastewater epidemiology metrics, along with a sufficiently long time series of data that would allow the establishment of baselines.

In deciding which parameters to include in the trigger design, decision-makers can employ certain methods to evaluate the importance of different components in the trigger calculation. For example, sensitivity testing is often an important step, used to understand which components of the trigger calculation are most influential. Additionally, it is critical to consider the correlation of the parameters and variables with the actual loss; this comparison is often achieved using historical data.

## Qualitative Triggers

Qualitative triggers—those based on subjective criteria such as declarations of a PHEIC, the issuance of Disease Outbreak News reports, or an emergency declaration by state actors—have been previously incorporated into trigger designs, including in Gavi's First Response Fund (box 14.1). As noted earlier, because such declarations are based upon expert judgment, political and economic considerations, and other subjective criteria, qualitative triggers can be problematic and thus must be designed with great care. The arbitrary nature of these factors suggests that triggers based on such criteria would not meet the qualities of being transparent and objective (Fan et al. 2023).

### Box 14.1

### Applying Qualitative Triggers to Vaccine Procurement for Epidemic Response

Qualitative triggers figure prominently in Gavi's First Response Fund. In June 2024, Gavi, the Vaccine Alliance launched the first "day zero" financing mechanism of "US$ 500 million designed to secure early access to vaccines and to protect existing immunization programmes within days of a pandemic or a public health emergency of international concern being declared" (Gavi 2024). The trigger is made such that 80 percent of funding will be disbursed for at-risk procurement of vaccines for pathogens with public health emergency of international concern potential when Gavi has no existing vaccine or outbreak response program. The remaining 20 percent of funds can be deployed for pathogens qualified as Grade 2 or 3 by the World Health Organization (WHO) but for which a vaccination response is needed, or in case routine immunization is at risk given the outbreak (as was the case in the 10th Ebola outbreak in the Democratic Republic of Congo, when routine measles immunizations dropped significantly). The final decision is made by a committee at Gavi using input from technical partners and WHO. What is unclear is whether a formal request from a given country is necessary to activate the discussions of the committee or if this committee meets regardless as long as the WHO classifications are communicated.

*box continues next page*

This trigger framework is unusual in that it relies on preagreed, albeit "soft," qualitative triggers that include WHO assessments and a public health emergency of international concern declaration as well as information gathering from other partners for a committee to launch the decision process. Although it is a quite flexible and all-encompassing mechanism—that is, it does not apply to a single pathogen and does not restrict disbursements to any country—it also has no participation cost from countries. Consequently, it retains significant discretion in how the funds are spent. The potential risk is that flexibility may create ambiguity, such that countries may not be able to easily anticipate which events will qualify and which will not, as well as the potential for such a mechanism to be perceived as arbitrary. These potential risks can be best mitigated through transparency, and active communication to countries and other stakeholders that might rely on the mechanism.

Without these types of efforts, such a flexible mechanism might fall short of ensuring the much needed predictability of funding and transparency that would empower countries to make the right decisions during the next epidemic or pandemic.

Moreover, subjectivity presents challenges for modeling, which is often used to inform trigger design in a financing mechanism. Subjectivity in trigger design makes it difficult to use modeling to estimate whether a trigger structure will pay out under the right conditions and whether the risk has been appropriately estimated and priced, leading to potentially higher than necessary risk premiums that incorporate an extra buffer for underestimated activation probability. It could also potentially bias the declaration process itself: decision-makers may become more (or less) likely to declare an emergency if such a declaration will trigger a payout. This bias—or political risk from the potential perception of bias—becomes even more problematic if the agency making the declaration also receives funding from the financial instrument.

**Trigger Timing**

The timing of the trigger, with respect to the epidemic curve and the pandemic financing cycle (Fan et al. 2024), is a crucial consideration. Early in an outbreak, while it is still small, disease control and response measures have a much greater chance for outbreak containment (refer to chapter 7 in this volume). Consequently, financing provided at this stage is likely to be highly cost-effective. At this early stage, there is also greater uncertainty about the number of cases or the presence of sustained human-to-human transmission: limited information and sometimes incomplete and fragmentary surveillance data can make it difficult to establish the expected trajectory of an outbreak. The African Risk Capacity structure is a notable example of a mechanism designed to trigger very early in an outbreak (refer to table 14.1).

Some triggers, however, may require data stability and a higher level of certainty about the magnitude of outbreak before activation. By the time these necessary criteria are met, several weeks or months might have passed and full containment may not be possible, but the financing could support public health and social measures to flatten the curve—including active case identification, case isolation, and contact tracing—and reduce the burden on the health system and overall impact of the event (refer to chapter 6 in this volume). This approach is probably most similar to the financing mechanism incorporated into the World Bank's Pandemic Emergency Financing Facility, or PEF (refer to table 14.1).

A third potential timepoint around which to build a trigger that is not often implemented is before an outbreak even reaches a country. For example, if an event affects one country, then a neighboring country could be the beneficiary of seed financing that would help support surveillance and containment measures designed to prevent introduction of the pathogen and spread of the epidemic. A potential design for such a concept was discussed previously in an Asian Development Bank report (ADB 2022). Although an anticipatory/containment design of this kind could potentially be effective and worth exploring, a key challenge is that it may be politically difficult to justify allocating response funds to a country that is not (yet) directly affected by a health emergency, especially if funds are limited and response activities in the directly affected country are underfinanced.

## Avoiding Recency Bias

A common pitfall in trigger design is to build a trigger for the event that occurred most recently—a behavior analogous to preparing to fight the last war. In the context of epidemic risk, this tendency could, for example, entail limiting the event definition to only those pathogens that have recently caused epidemics, or setting parameter combinations and thresholds based solely on observed data from recent outbreaks rather than modeled risk estimates that consider broader probability distributions (Madhav et al. 2023). Some mechanisms—notably the World Bank's PEF insurance window—have incorporated emerging pathogens (such as Rift Valley Fever virus) with known epidemic and potentially pandemic potential, but that have not caused large-scale public health emergencies to date. Incorporating wholly novel pathogens into a trigger structure is also possible, but doing so introduces challenges to risk modeling because of data sparsity.

Future epidemic and pandemic scenarios may look very different from the most recent events. As such, it is critical to consider the widest relevant range of scenarios that could occur and fit within the conceptual and policy objectives of the financing mechanism or policy process. Scenario planning processes as well as the use of simulation-derived event catalogs can provide structured ways to address and mitigate recency bias (Madhav, Stephenson, and Oppenheim 2021; Schwartz 1997).

## Flexibility

Flexibility in trigger design, such as incorporating technical and operational experts into consultation processes, can be advantageous, allowing for local context and local stakeholders' knowledge to be factored in, to "correct" mismatches between a predefined trigger and the reality on the ground. In this sense, a level of flexibility (as opposed to full discretion over the activation of funds for response) can sometimes enhance a mechanism's overall effectiveness.

Trigger mechanisms, especially for nonfinancial applications, could be built into a playbook or tiered response system that would allow some flexibility and adaptability during a crisis. An overly rigid system may be difficult to adhere to during a crisis—and the next crisis may look very different from the previous crises upon which design of the trigger criteria may have been based. It is important to think beyond previous events and to avoid recency bias—that is, over indexing on the most recent event to have occurred. For example, some financing mechanisms have a contingency fund component, which may relax some of the more rigid criteria and design principles that would underpin triggers for insurance-backed financing mechanisms that can come in later, at higher levels of severity of the outbreak.

Adding an element of flexibility can also diminish basis risk (that is, the chance of a false positive or false negative) and ensures that decision-makers have some ownership. To date, notable structures for epidemic risk financing have included asymmetric mechanisms to address basis risk, including cash windows that can (with some parameters and rules) release financing for events that would not otherwise qualify; however, no mechanisms appear to exist that address false positives, though these mechanisms are theoretically possible. The risk is that stakeholders who are unhappy with a specific decision may view flexibility as arbitrariness; this risk should be mitigated to the greatest extent possible with transparency, broad involvement of stakeholder groups in the development of decision-making rules and guidelines, and active communication once a potentially qualifying event has occurred.

### Testing, Refinement, and Calibration

During the process of designing the trigger, an important step is to test whether or not it performs as anticipated and desired—for example, whether it correctly activates under scenarios that the financing mechanism (or other policy intervention) is being designed to respond to. This step requires clarity and alignment regarding the types of scenarios that the mechanism is meant to address. Trigger designers should, in close conversation with stakeholders, define the types and severities of events that should trigger the mechanism; it is likely critical that they clearly define the types of scenarios that should not trigger it. In testing, the draft trigger concept would be calculated against historical epidemic events to determine which events would have set off the trigger and which ones would have not. If the results do not lead to the desired outcomes, then it is determined which parameters and thresholds led to the failure. The trigger will then be reformulated to ameliorate the issue and tested again. This iterative process typically entails multiple rounds of testing and refinement—with care given to understand the implications of design changes and ensure that a change to address one apparent failure does not cause other problems (such as causing the mechanism to trigger under undesirable circumstances; refer to the section "Trigger Failure" later in this chapter).

If the occurrence being tested against is a rare event, the trigger is also often tested against modeled or hypothetical scenarios, again to see under which scenarios the trigger conditions are met. When a full range of hypothetical, plausible scenarios is available, such as in a stochastic catalog (Madhav et al. 2023), then additional statistics may be calculated, such as the overall probability of the trigger conditions being met.

Upon completion of the iterative process, there should be agreement by all involved parties that the trigger is measurable, that the payout occurs with appropriate timing and predictability, and that stakeholder incentives and expectations are aligned—keeping in mind that, for triggers incorporated into disaster risk financing instruments, the stakeholders involved often span the public and private sectors (Schanz 2021).

## CASE STUDY: THE WORLD BANK PANDEMIC EMERGENCY FINANCING FACILITY

PEF, the first sovereign insurance mechanism for epidemic and pandemic risk, was issued in 2017, in reaction to the slow and initially inadequate donor financing response to the 2014 West Africa Ebola epidemic. It was designed to provide financing for several types of infectious disease risks and was organized into two classes. Class A was configured to release funding in the event of a large, multicountry outbreak of a respiratory pathogen (that is, an influenza virus or a novel coronavirus) that could develop into a pandemic. Class B was designed to provide funding to contain a multicountry epidemic, similar to the 2014 West Africa Ebola epidemic, caused by pathogens including filoviruses, novel coronaviruses, Lassa virus, Rift Valley Fever phlebovirus, or Nairovirus (the causative agent of Crimean-Congo Hemorrhagic Fever).

PEF was explicitly designed to provide financing for multicountry epidemics, rather than sustained epidemics within a single country. This design criterion would later lead to substantial criticism during the 2018–20 North Kivu Ebola epidemic (also known as the 10th Ebola outbreak in the Democratic Republic of Congo), which remained almost entirely contained within the Democratic Republic of the Congo and for which no payout from the insurance window was released (Jonas 2019).[7] However, PEF also included a *cash window*, a funding pool that could be flexibly deployed to support response activities for events that did not meet trigger criteria for either class. The cash window ultimately released funds to support the response to the North Kivu epidemic (World Bank 2019).

PEF had several other notable design characteristics. First, the International Development Association (IDA) countries[8] that were potential recipients of PEF funds did not have to pay for coverage. The World Bank financed the development and implementation of the PEF disaster risk financing mechanism with IDA funds; international donor funding paid the entirety of the premium. The use of IDA funds to finance PEF generated debate, particularly because IDA money flowed to private insurance companies in the form of premium payments (Jonas 2019). Although that critique relates to the source of funds, rather than to the trigger design, it may have amplified later concern over the complexity of the triggers themselves.

Second, the complexity of the triggers led to criticisms about the lack of transparency or verifiability of the triggers. Especially controversial was the complex growth rate trigger criterion, which did not have easily accessible methodological documentation and data that would allow it to be quickly replicated. Trigger complexity, including the growth rate trigger criterion, likely resulted from the interplay between competing stakeholder demands and budget constraints in the design of the trigger. The design of the trigger encapsulates the push and pull between stakeholders: the beneficiaries want to receive the funding as much and as soon as possible and often with minimal criteria, whereas the capital providers (especially if they include insurers and investment professionals) may demand indisputable confirmation of an event and evidence that the funds are needed. In the case of PEF, the growth rate trigger criterion may have arisen as a way to provide evidence that an eligible epidemic event was continuing to worsen, and thus the funds would still be necessary by the time they were disbursed. Other relevant factors in the trigger design were likely misaligned incentives and an attempt to limit the perception of inordinate payout risk on the part of capital market participants who would be more skeptical about a novel financing mechanism.

The COVID-19 pandemic met the trigger criteria for PEF on April 17, 2020, about five weeks after the WHO PHEIC declaration on March 11, 2020. Consequently, by September 30, 2020, beneficiary countries had received a full payout from Class A of over US$195 million. PEF funds were used to support varying response activities, specific to the needs of each beneficiary country. Funding uses included, for example, procurement of diagnostics and personal protective equipment, increasing diagnostic testing capacity in national labs, expansion of hospital bed capacity, investments in oxygen generation and distribution, and funding to mobilize skilled medical personnel (World Bank 2020, 2021a, 2021c). To ensure that the payout amount remains relevant to the stage of the outbreak, this six-month lag from meeting the trigger criteria to the completion of fund disbursement should ideally be shortened in future financing mechanisms for infectious disease risks. For PEF, detractors primarily criticized the payment amount as "too little, too late" for a pandemic of such magnitude. Arguably, however, no financing mechanism in existence at that time could have covered the entire cost of the COVID-19 pandemic, so a more appropriate bar would be to assess if the PEF financing was accretive to the other financing available at the time.

As noted earlier, it is critical to clearly articulate the problem that the financing instrument is designed to solve, which scenarios would lead to a payout, and which would not. Another aspect to be improved in future iterations of such global disaster risk products is the transparency about the rules of distributing the funds between beneficiaries when an event occurs.

PEF provides numerous lessons. As discussed earlier, an effective trigger should be simple, transparent, objective, verifiable, and preagreed. Of these characteristics PEF arguably fell short mainly in the areas of having a simple, transparent, and easily verifiable trigger (Meenan 2020). The first lesson from the PEF experience pointed to the challenges that arise with a complex trigger, which can make it difficult to verify and potentially lead to a lack of trust in the financing instrument as a whole.

A second major lesson involves transparency, pointing to the need for very early, frequent, and informative communication to all stakeholders (including the public) to ensure a high degree of comfort and understanding of the trigger design, the scenarios in which it is expected to trigger (and not trigger), what technical choices were made in the trigger design process, and why those choices were made. As noted earlier, PEF did not trigger a payout from its insurance mechanism for the North Kivu Ebola epidemic of 2018–20, leading to substantial criticism of its complex trigger structure (table 14.1; refer also to Brim and Wenham 2019). Although important lessons can be learned from the practical implementation of the trigger, PEF was fundamentally designed to respond to multicountry epidemics, rather than to sustained events that remained (largely) contained within a single country. Consequently, debate about the North Kivu nontrigger should have focused on the fundamental design and event definition, rather than narrowly on the trigger design. This debate also shows why careful concept testing and discussion regarding the event definition among all stakeholders—beneficiaries, trigger designers, donors, and governments—is so critical.

A third lesson, going beyond the trigger, is that PEF's cash window provided an effective way to maintain flexibility for situations when an epidemic might require rapid financing but when trigger criteria are not met for the insurance window. Maintaining this level of flexibility, both in the circumstances under which funds can be disbursed and in what they can be used for, is critical to ensure that funds can go to unanticipated needs that arise.

A fourth lesson that emerged was the need to closely engage beneficiary countries. Doing so helps build awareness and tie the financing mechanism with the creation of incentives to actions that can prepare for and reduce overall epidemic risk, such as investing in diagnostic capacity and pathogen monitoring programs.

Arguably the final lesson from PEF is one already gained from hard experience in other risk financing domains, such as climate and natural catastrophe risk. That is, designing financing mechanisms for challenges where both the risk (Meadows et al. 2023) and the fundamental science are rapidly evolving is difficult and requires a commitment to ongoing learning and dialogue. Ultimately, a proper independent evaluation will provide the most thorough assessment of the successes, challenges, and lessons learned from PEF.

## TRIGGER FAILURE

Parametric triggers can fail in many ways, which often fall in one of two main categories: false positives and false negatives. A *false positive* in the context of a financing instrument is an event that meets the criteria for release of funds but for which the actual losses incurred are zero or less than the payout amount. In this case, the providers of the capital "suffer" from a loss of their capital. This situation also potentially sends a signal that the trigger has inadequate science or design rigor behind it, thus the financing mechanism could be perceived as a "lottery." A *false negative* occurs when the trigger criteria are not met even though substantial losses are incurred. In this case, the beneficiary or insured suffers, because they are affected by real losses and expenses that they expected to have covered by the financing mechanism. The goal during the trigger design and calibration phase of the structuring process is to minimize the probability of both types of errors, also described by practitioners as "basis risk." During this process, and to minimize basis risk, the trigger criteria will be tested and configured using historical data and model estimates so as to maximize correlation to actual loss.

Ambiguous situations also arise. Consider, for example, a scenario in which a trigger is designed to support early response and containment of Nipah virus disease epidemics in South Asia, and is configured to pay out when 20 deaths caused by Nipah virus occur. An outbreak subsequently occurs in Bangladesh: 40 people are infected, 20 people recover, and 19 people die within the first three weeks; the final infected person remains in the clinic for a week, then dies. The policy pays out, but the outbreak is over. Capital providers may view this event as a false positive, because the outbreak is no longer active. However, the policy could still be effective, because it could provide financing to the country for response and containment activities initiated earlier in the outbreak, and prospectively for any ongoing surveillance to ensure rapid detection of any additional cases. Capital providers and the recipient countries may have honestly diverging points of view over whether the financing mechanism and trigger structure were successfully designed. The converse problem could occur under a more complex trigger structure—for example, one that includes infections, deaths, and the growth rate (that is, trajectory of the epidemiological curve). In such a circumstance, case or death trigger criteria could be met slowly enough that the growth trigger is not reached, which could lead to complaints—as in the case of PEF—that the policy should nevertheless have triggered.

Triggers could potentially be manipulated or gamed, or the presence of a financing mechanism may create perverse incentive structures that alter the probability of a payout. First, having a financing mechanism in place may, in theory, create a *moral hazard*, an incentive to take riskier actions or forego risk-reducing actions

(Rowell and Connelly 2012). In the context of epidemics, moral hazard—that is, misaligned incentives—could conceivably include relaxing disease control measures until the trigger is met (a risk that could become more substantial as the proximity of breaching the trigger point increases). A perhaps more plausible version of this risk could be that a country applies tentative or inadequate populationwide measures to reduce disease transmission, knowing that such measures may be economically damaging and that additional financing support is more likely to be triggered if the partial measures are unsuccessful.

A more plausible—and, indeed, a positive externality—incentive created by a financing structure may be to intensify surveillance and case detection efforts. From the perspective of the insurer or capital provider, however, this incentive may be problematic, because trigger design or pricing efforts would not have taken more intensive surveillance (and, presumably, case identification) into account. These dynamics may vary by disease. For example, for endemic diseases with incomplete surveillance—such as Lassa Fever in portions of West Africa—the presence of a sufficiently large financing mechanism could lead to investments in surveillance that increase the probability of detecting baseline levels of endemic transmission and, therefore, of triggering a payout. In contrast, the investment case for a country to recoup surveillance expenses by detecting less frequent occurrences, such as a spillover of Nipah virus in Malaysia, may be more limited.

Importantly, the risk that surveillance improvements will lead to unanticipated increases in the likelihood of triggering a financing mechanism depends entirely on the size (and perceived probability) of the payout relative to the cost of surveillance, including potential negative consequences and disincentives for outbreak reporting, for example international trade restrictions. This situation is unlikely given the cost of sustained, high-quality surveillance relative to the typical, relatively modest payouts built into disaster risk financing mechanisms for epidemic risk.

The risk associated with false positive payout can be mitigated by various approaches, including by limiting the use of funds to preagreed uses that will not apply if an epidemic response is not warranted, by designing a policy that reimburses for already incurred expenses, or by requiring that the beneficiary provide proof of loss before the funds are released. These limitations, however, turn a relatively simple parametric mechanism into a more complicated, indemnity-like mechanism, potentially preserving the speed with which financing can be released but adding complexity and auditing requirements to the postdisaster recovery phase. Because false positives have effectively been priced into the mechanism design, another approach can be to roll unspent funds from false positives into a cash window, to be expended on other crisis response activities, including payment for false negatives. Although theoretically feasible, such mechanisms would be operationally and politically challenging, and could potentially increase the scope for miscommunication and misaligned expectations between stakeholders.

Mitigating the risk from false negatives—that is, payouts that should occur but do not—is perhaps more challenging. One option previously tested in disaster risk financing instruments is to include a cash window or contingency window—that is, a pool of capital that can be flexibly deployed for a variety of purposes, including supporting response costs for an event that meets the stated intent of the financing mechanism but that, because of some unforeseen complexity or challenges, does not meet the trigger criteria (World Bank 2021b). To build trust and predictability for the beneficiary, cash windows must also have a detailed operations playbook explaining what they are intended for and who makes the payout decision using either a set of criteria or parametric logic to channel and delimit the use of funds—for example, a cash window could require at least $N$ reported, laboratory-confirmed deaths caused by a viral pathogen.

## CONCLUSIONS

Well-defined triggers can provide clarity and speed to complex decision-making processes that often take place, unrehearsed, in the midst of an active crisis. Parametric triggers have been most frequently employed in insurance and natural hazards risk financing instruments. That said, many decision processes and financing mechanisms in the health sector resemble these instruments, in the sense that they formally incorporate variables; transparent, measurable thresholds; and other objective criteria to guide or even bind complex decision-making processes based on preagreed terms.

This chapter is not a call to blindly adopt triggers, parametric or otherwise, in epidemic financing and policy processes.[9] Rather, it urges readers to use and learn from sound design principles in the development of triggers, whether qualitative, quantitative, or a mixture of both. The most fundamental design principle is to design with care and incorporate diverse knowledge—especially practical, operational knowledge—about the risk context. Doing so means designing with broad participation, as well as transparency, to ensure that the purpose of the trigger is clear, understood, and accepted by all involved. All other design principles are, in an important sense, technical and can be addressed through careful and iterative analysis, testing, and refinement.

This chapter has focused primarily on the design of triggers for financing mechanisms. Importantly, no single comprehensive crisis financing structure will be applicable for all future threats, including biological threats (Centre for Disaster Protection and Airbel Impact Lab 2021). Instead, triggers should be designed to address specific, well-defined problems and risks, using a clear event definition and appropriate technical design. Triggers can also be designed to support policy decisions once an epidemic or pandemic has occurred, notably whether and how intensely to apply populationwide disease control measures, and when to relax or end such measures. A primary virtue of triggers is that they can be built into a range of playbooks tailored to specific scenarios and risks, helping guide policy makers to determine which decision frameworks are sound, and perhaps alerting them to scenarios in which prior guidance—and the factors and thresholds that it is rooted in—may not be fit for purpose.

Finally, if designed with care, triggers offer an efficient, objective, and predictable way to mobilize money to contain crises and save lives and livelihoods. Ultimately, what is needed is strong, credible, and consistent commitment from funders to provide adequate prearranged financing for epidemic preparedness and response in a predictable and timely way. Without that commitment, effective containment and response to epidemics and pandemics will remain impossible to achieve. With it, a more secure future is possible.

## ACKNOWLEDGMENTS

The authors thank Ruchir Agarwal, Stefano Bertozzi, Victoria Fan, Joseph Fridman, Dean Jamison, Magnus Lindelow, Serina Ng, Ole F. Norheim, Hitoshi Oshitani, Siddhanth Sharma, Simon Young, and several anonymous reviewers for their valuable technical and editorial contributions. The views expressed in this paper are those of the authors and should not be attributed to the authors' respective organizations.

## NOTES

The authors gratefully acknowledge the University of Bergen Centre for Ethics and Priority Setting in Health and the Norwegian Agency for Development Cooperation (NORAD) (RAF-18/0009) for providing funding support. Nita K. Madhav and Ben Oppenheim are employed by Ginkgo Bioworks. Cristina Stefan is an employee of the Centre for Disaster Protection.

1. Of note, mortality bonds incorporating index-based parametric triggers, such as Vita bonds, were introduced before this period (as discussed in the subsection "Quantitative Triggers").
2. WHO, "Disease Outbreak News (DONs)," https://www.who.int/emergencies/disease-outbreak-news.
3. US Centers for Disease Control and Prevention, "Health Alert Network (HAN)," https://www.cdc.gov/han/php/about/index.html.
4. WHO, "Emergencies: International Health Regulations and Emergency Committees," https://www.who.int/news-room/questions-and-answers/item/emergencies-international-health-regulations-and-emergency-committees.
5. Biomedical Advanced Research and Development Authority, "Influenza & Emerging Infectious Diseases Pandemic Vaccines and Adjuvants Program," https://medicalcountermeasures.gov/barda/influenza-and-emerging-infectious-diseases/pandemic-vaccines-adjuvants.
6. WHO, "Ebola and Marburg Virus Outbreak Toolbox," https://www.who.int/emergencies/outbreak-toolkit/disease-outbreak-toolboxes/ebola-and-marburg-virus-outbreak-toolbox.

7. Apart from four deaths in Uganda, which occurred when a family crossed the border from the Democratic Republic of Congo into Uganda to seek treatment.
8. Countries eligible for grants and concessional loans from IDA, which provides support to countries that cannot borrow funds at the market rate.
9. That is to say, it does not propose a hegemonic parametric agenda but, rather, thoughtful application of parametric approaches when appropriate.

## REFERENCES

ADB (Asian Development Bank). 2022. *Building Resilience to Future Outbreaks: Infectious Disease Risk Financing Solutions for the Central Asia Regional Economic Cooperation Regio.* Manila: ADB. http://dx.doi.org/10.22617/TCS220010-2.

Böhm, H. 2023. "Insuring Pandemics in Non-Life (Structuring and Modelling)." Presentation at Weiterbildungstag der DGVFM, University of Hannover, Germany, September 28. https://www.insurance.uni-hannover.de/fileadmin/house-of-insurance/Research_and _Events/Events/2023/Boehm_20230928_ERS_DGVFM.pdf.

Brim, B., and C. Wenham. 2019. "Pandemic Emergency Financing Facility: Struggling to Deliver on Its Innovative Promise." *BMJ* 367: l5719. https://doi.org/10.1136/bmj.l5719.

Cauchemez, S., N. M. Ferguson, C. Wachtel, A. Tegnell, G. Saour, B. Duncan, and A. Nicoll. 2009. "Closure of Schools during an Influenza Pandemic." *The Lancet Infectious Diseases* 9 (8): 473–81.

Centre for Disaster Protection and Airbel Impact Lab. 2021. "Exploring a Role for Triggers and Risk-Informed Financing in Complex Crises: COVID-19 as a Case Study." Centre for Disaster Protection and Airbel Impact Lab. https://static1.squarespace.com /static/61542ee0a87a394f7bc17b3a/t/61b9bac5ea9b8309d46070a1/1639561925573/airbel -risk-informed-financing%2B%281%29.pdf.

Chen, S., Z. Zhang, J. Yang, J. Wang, X. Zhai, T. Bärnighausen, and C. Wang. 2020. "Fangcang Shelter Hospitals: A Novel Concept for Responding to Public Health Emergencies." *The Lancet* 395 (10232): 1305–14.

Cissé, J. D. 2021. "Climate and Disaster Risk Financing Instruments: An Overview." United Nations University Institute for Environment and Human Security. https://climate -insurance.org/wp-content/uploads/2021/05/Climate-and-Disaster-Risk-Financing -Instruments.pdf.

Djaafara, B. A., N. Imai, E. Hamblion, B. Impouma, C. A. Donnelly, and A. Cori. 2021. "A Quantitative Framework for Defining the End of an Infectious Disease Outbreak: Application to Ebola Virus Disease." *American Journal of Epidemiology* 190 (4): 642–51.

Fan, V. Y., R. Cash, S. Bertozzi, and M. Pate. 2023. "The When Is Less Important than the What: An Epidemic Scale as an Alternative to the WHO's Public Health Emergency of International Concern." *The Lancet Global Health* 11 (10): e1499–e1500.

Fan, V. Y., S. Kim, D. Pineda, and S. M. Bertozzi. 2024. "Financing the Pandemic Cycle: Prevention, Preparedness, Response, and Recovery and Reconstruction." CGD Policy Paper 334, Center for Global Development, Washington, DC.

FAO (Food and Agriculture Organization of the United Nations), WHO (World Health Organization), and WOAH (World Organisation for Animal Health). 2025. "Updated Joint FAO/WHO/WOAH Public Health Assessment of Recent Influenza A(H5) Virus Events in Animals and People." WHO, Geneva. https://www.who.int/publications/m/item/updated -joint-fao-who-woah-public-health-assessment-of-recent-influenza-a(h5)-virus-events-in -animals-and-people_apr2025.

Ferguson, N. M., D. A. Cummings, S. Cauchemez, C. Fraser, S. Riley, A. Meeyai, S. Iamsirithaworn, and D. S. Burke. 2005. "Strategies for Containing an Emerging Influenza Pandemic in Southeast Asia." *Nature* 437 (7056): 209–14.

Franco, G., L. Lemke-Verderame, R. Guidotti, Y. Yuan, G. Bussi, D. Lohmann, and
P. Bazzurro. 2024. "Typology and Design of Parametric Cat-in-a-Box and Cat-in-a-Grid
Triggers for Tropical Cyclone Risk Transfer." *Mathematics* 12 (11): 1768.

Gavi. 2024. "How Day Zero Financing Could Help Protect the World during the Next
Pandemic." *Gavi Matters*, June 12, 2024. https://www.gavi.org/vaccineswork/how-day
-zero-financing-could-help-protect-world-during-next-pandemic.

Grassly, N. C., A. G. Shaw, and M. Owusu. 2024. "Global Wastewater Surveillance for
Pathogens with Pandemic Potential: Opportunities and Challenges." *The Lancet Microbe*
6 (1): 100939.

Gudina, E. K., and N. W. Gidi. 2025. "Travel Bans Did Not Contain Omicron: A Call for
Data-Driven Public Health Responses." *The Lancet Global Health* 13 (2): e179–80.

Hale, T., N. Angrist, R. Goldszmidt, B. Kira, A. Petherick, T. Phillips, S. Webster, et al. 2021.
"A Global Panel Database of Pandemic Policies (Oxford COVID-19 Government Response
Tracker)." *Nature Human Behaviour* 5 (4): 529–38.

Hart, D. M. 2024. "The Defense Production Act: National Security as a Potential Driver
of Domestic Manufacturing Investment." Bipartisan Policy Center, Washington, DC.
https://bipartisanpolicy.org/download/?file=/wp-content/uploads/2024/02/The-Defense
-Production-Act-National-Security-as-a-Potential-Driver-of-Domestic-Manufacturing
-Investment.pdf.

IBRD (International Bank for Reconstruction and Development). 2017. *Pandemic Emergency
Financing Facility Final Prospectus.* Washington, DC: World Bank. https://thedocs
.worldbank.org/en/doc/f355aa56988e258a350942240872e3c5-0240012017/original/PEF
-Final-Prospectus-PEF.pdf.

Johnson, S. G. 2010. "Ten Years after 9/11: Property Insurance Lessons Learns." *Tort Trial &
Ins. Prac. LJ* 46: 685.

Jonas, O. 2019. "Pandemic Bonds: Designed to Fail in Ebola." *Nature* 572 (7769): 285–86.

Kilaru, P., D. Hill, K. Anderson, M. B. Collins, H. Green, B. L. Kmush, and D. A. Larsen. 2023.
"Wastewater Surveillance for Infectious Disease: A Systematic Review." *American Journal
of Epidemiology* 192 (2): 305–22.

Klein, R. 2006. "Mortality Catastrophe Bonds as a Risk Mitigation Tool." *Reinsurance Section
News*, May 2006, Issue 57.

Lipsitch, M., C. A. Donnelly, C. Fraser, I. M. Blake, A. Cori, I. Dorigatti, N. M. Ferguson, et al.
2015. "Potential Biases in Estimating Absolute and Relative Case-Fatality Risks during
Outbreaks." *PLOS Neglected Tropical Diseases* 9 (7): e0003846.

Longini, I. M., A. Nizam, S. Xu, K. Ungchusak, W. Hanshaoworakul, D. A. Cummings, and
M. E. Halloran. 2005. "Containing Pandemic Influenza at the Source." *Science* 309 (5737):
1083–87.

Lopez, C. T. 2020. "Operation Warp Speed Accelerates COVID-19 Vaccine Development."
*DOD News*, June 16, 2020. https://www.defense.gov/News/News-Stories/Article/Article
/2222284/operation-warp-speed-accelerates-covid-19-vaccine-development/.

Madhav, N. K., B. Oppenheim, N. Stephenson, R. Badker, D. T. Jamison, C. Lam, and
A. Meadows. 2023. "Estimated Future Mortality from Pathogens of Epidemic and
Pandemic Potential." CGD Working Paper 665, Center for Global Development,
Washington, DC. https://www.cgdev.org/sites/default/files/estimated-future-mortality
-pathogens-epidemic-and-pandemic-potential.pdf.

Madhav, N., N. Stephenson, and B. Oppenheim. 2021. "Multipathogen Event Catalogs:
Technical Note." World Bank, Washington, DC. https://documents1.worldbank.org
/curated/en/181791625232959415/pdf/Multi-Pathogen-Event-Catalogs-Technical-Note.pdf.

Mari, L., and A. Giordani. 2015. "Modelling Measurement: Error and Uncertainty." In *Error
and Uncertainty in Scientific Practice*, edited by M. Boumans, G. Hon, and A. Petersen,
79–96. Routledge.

Maslo, D. 2022. "How Anticipatory Insurance Can Help Africa Better Prepare and Respond
to Natural Disasters." *Forum Stories*, November 1, 2022. https://www.weforum.org
/stories/2022/11/africaanticipatory-insurance-africa-natural-disasters-response/.

McKnight, M., and S. Sureka. 2024. "Deploying Biotechnology at Scale through Systems Integration to Combat COVID-19." In *The COVID-19 Pandemic: Science, Technology, and the Future of Healthcare Delivery*, edited by J. M. Rosen and R. R. Colwell, 361–68. Springer.

McVeigh, K. 2020. "World Bank's $500m Pandemic Scheme Accused of 'Waiting for People to Die.'" *Guardian*, February 28, 2020. https://www.theguardian.com/global -development/2020/feb/28/world-banks-500m-coronavirus-push-too-late-for-poor -countries-experts-say.

Meadows, A. J., B. Oppenheim, J. Guerrero, B. Ash, R. Badker, C. K. Lam, C. Pardee, et al. 2022. "Infectious Disease Underreporting Is Predicted by Country-Level Preparedness, Politics, and Pathogen Severity." *Health Security* 20 (4): 331–38. https://doi.org/10.1089/hs.2021.0197.

Meadows, A. J., N. Stephenson, N. K. Madhav, and B. Oppenheim. 2023. "Historical Trends Demonstrate a Pattern of Increasingly Frequent and Severe Spillover Events of High-Consequence Zoonotic Viruses." *BMJ Global Health* 8 (11): e012026. https://doi .org/10.1136/bmjgh-2023-012026.

Meenan, C. 2020. "The Future of Pandemic Financing: Trigger Design and 2020 Hindsight." *Centre for Disaster Protection* (blog), May 19, 2020. https://www .disasterprotection.org/blogs/the-future-of-pandemic-financing-trigger-design-and-2020 -hindsight?rq=conor%20meenan/.

Mullen, L., C. Potter, L. O. Gostin, A. Cicero, and J. B. Nuzzo. 2020. "An Analysis of International Health Regulations Emergency Committees and Public Health Emergency of International Concern Designations." *BMJ Global Health* 5(6).

Oppenheim, B., V. Serhiyenko, J. Guerrero, P. Ayscue, S. Cheeseman Barthel, N. Madhav, and C. Steffan. 2019. "System for Determining Public Sentiment towards Pathogens." US Patent Application Publication No. US 2019/370834 A1. https://patentimages.storage.googleapis .com/a2/26/bf/949e61ba5643cf/US20190370834A1.pdf.

Pandemic Preparedness Partnership. 2021. "100 Days Mission to Respond to Future Pandemic Threats: Reducing the Impact of Future Pandemics by Making Diagnostics, Therapeutics and Vaccines Available within 100 Days." A Report to the G7 by the Pandemic Preparedness Partnership. https://assets.publishing.service.gov.uk/government /uploads/system/uploads/attachment_data/file/992762/100_Days_Mission_to_respond _to_future_pandemic_threats__3_.pdf.

Pople, A., R. Hill, S. Dercon, Sand B. Brunckhorst. 2021. "Anticipatory Cash Transfers in Climate Disaster Response." CGD Working Paper 6, Centre for Disaster Protection, London. https://www.disasterprotection.org/publications-centre/anticipatory-cash -transfers-in-climate-disaster-response.

Rowell, D., and L. B. Connelly. 2012. "A History of the Term 'Moral Hazard.'" *Journal of Risk and Insurance* 79(4): 1051–75.

Schanz, K.-U. 2021. "Public-Private Solutions to Pandemic Risk: Opportunities, Challenges, Trade-Offs." The Geneva Association, Zürich. https://www.genevaassociation.org/sites /default/files/pandemic_risks_report_web.pdf.

Schwartz, P. 1997. *Art of the Long View: Planning for the Future in an Uncertain World*. John Wiley & Sons.

WHO (World Health Organization). 2014. "Meningitis Outbreak Response in Sub-Saharan Africa: WHO Guideline." WHO, Geneva. http://www.who.int/iris/handle/10665/144727.

World Bank. 2019. "The Pandemic Emergency Financing Facility (PEF) Released an Additional $10 Million for Ebola Response Activities in the Democratic Republic of Congo." News statement, May 9, 2019. https://www.worldbank.org/en/news /statement/2019/05/09/the-pandemic-emergency-financing-facility-pef-released-an -additional-10-million-for-ebola-response-activities-in-the-democratic-republic-of-congo.

World Bank. 2020. "Kosovo Pandemic Emergency Financing Recipient Executed Trust Fund." Preliminary Stakeholder Engagement Plan, World Bank, Washington, DC. https://documents1.worldbank.org/curated/en/213091596650826978/pdf/Stakeholder -Engagement-Plan-SEP-Kosovo-Pandemic-Emergency-Financing-RETF-P174452.pdf.

World Bank. 2021a. "Bangladesh—COVID-19 Emergency Response and Pandemic Preparedness Project: Restructuring and Additional Financing." Report No. PAD4281, World Bank, Washington, DC. http://documents.worldbank.org/curated /en/753391616378524213.

World Bank. 2021b. "Fact Sheet: Pandemic Emergency Financing Facility." Brief, April 27, 2021. https://www.worldbank.org/en/topic/pandemics/brief/fact-sheet-pandemic -emergency-financing-facility.

World Bank. 2021c. "Implementation Completion and Results Report (ICR) Document – COVID-19 Pandemic Emergency Financing Facility Project (P174366)." Report No. ICR00005541, World Bank, Washington, DC. http://documents.worldbank.org/curated /en/404431630803265286.

World Bank. 2021d. *World Development Report 2021: Data for Better Lives*. Washington, DC: World Bank.

Wright, C., and P. Lacovara. 2020. *PathogenRX: An Exclusive Analytics and Insurance Solution for Outbreaks, Epidemics, and Pandemics*. Marsh, LLC. https://www.marsh.com/content /dam/marsh/Documents/PDF/US-en/pathogenrx-fact-sheet.pdf.

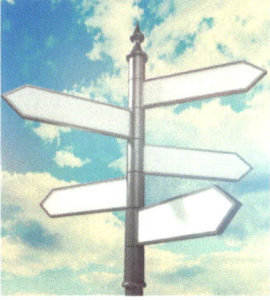

# 15

# Ethical Issues in Pandemic Prevention, Preparedness, and Response

Govind Persad

## ABSTRACT

Pandemic policies raise complex ethical challenges, as well as scientific and technical ones. This chapter examines four critical areas where ethical analysis is essential for effective pandemic prevention, preparedness, and response: spending decisions, clinical research, restrictions on rights and freedoms, and fair allocation of scarce medical resources.

Spending on pandemic prevention, preparedness, and response often involves trade-offs with other societal priorities, such as education, infrastructure, and environment. Navigating these trade-offs requires careful consideration of opportunity costs and distributional impacts.

Rights and freedoms can likewise present difficult trade-offs when pandemic policies restrict individual liberties, requiring clear goals and proportionate responses that consider differential impacts across populations.

Clinical research during pandemics must maintain ethical standards while addressing urgent public health needs. This chapter illustrates this imperative by exploring how ethical standards apply to challenge trials and to randomized studies of policy interventions.

Finally, scarce pandemic countermeasures like vaccines and therapeutics demand fair allocation frameworks that serve four core objectives: benefiting people, mitigating disadvantage, ensuring equal concern, and recognizing reciprocity.

## INTRODUCTION

Pandemics present important ethical challenges as well as scientific and technical ones. Other chapters in this volume raise questions with ethical dimensions:

- How much should we spend on pandemic prevention and preparedness compared to other societal priorities? (chapter 1)
- Should live animal markets be eliminated to prevent pandemics? (chapter 3)
- Should barriers to dual-use research on pathogens that present pandemic risk be heightened? (chapter 4)
- Which countries and people should be prioritized to receive scarce vaccines? (chapters 9, 10, and 11)
- What posttrial access to interventions should research participants receive? (chapter 11)
- When, if ever, should schools be closed in a pandemic? (chapter 8)
- How much should each country contribute to pandemic financing efforts? (chapter 13)

These questions have scientific and technical dimensions as well as ethical ones. For instance, determining how much to spend on pandemic prevention and preparedness should be informed by expected outcomes of spending, such as the number of deaths expected to be averted. By contrast, assigning relative importance to different types of outcomes—such as deaths earlier in life as opposed to later (chapter 2)—is an ethical question.

Ethical dimensions of pandemic decision-making are often signposted by explicit appeals to ethical concepts such as equity, need, and solidarity. At other times, ethical dimensions instead appear as tacit assumptions, such as that generating a larger total quantity of health or averting more deaths should be primary goals of pandemic policy.

Both explicit invocation of ethical concepts and tacit adoption of ethical commitments merit careful ethical analysis. It is widely accepted that pandemic response should be equitable, but equity is often left undefined. Defining equity more precisely in turn raises questions. For instance, some assert that it is inequitable for countries' ability to pay to affect their vaccine access (chapter 9). This concern stands in tension with allowing wealthier countries to spend more than others on other types of health technologies (Krohmal and Emanuel 2007). Others define equity as responsiveness to needs, but needs themselves require definition. For instance, chapter 13 sensibly asserts that "limited resources" should be "allocated where they are most needed"—a proposal that in turn requires a definition of need. Related to this concern, some deny that overall cost-effectiveness should be the primary basis for assessing policies. They argue that a policy that is not the most cost-effective might have preferable distributional consequences because it better advances the health of those who are worst off or have more severe disease. Last, ethics must be engaged with, but is not determined by, the socioeconomic and cultural landscape. Understanding public preferences, as well as the potential for influence by financially motivated firms and other actors, is important to ethical analysis and implementation of ethical frameworks, but those considerations do not determine the proper answer to ethical questions.

Pandemic response also raises challenging ethical questions because preventing pandemic harms is, and should be, just one among many societal priorities. As other chapters recognize, public spending on pandemic prevention, preparedness, and response can crowd out other spending priorities both inside and outside health systems, such as spending on chronic disease, environmental remediation, or infrastructure. The use of nonpharmaceutical interventions, like activity closures to reduce pandemic spread, can set back other important societal goals like education (chapter 8). Spending on pandemic prevention and preparedness must be balanced against other health system spending (chapter 12) and other needs more generally (chapter 2).

If preventing pandemic harms always took priority over other goals, the ethics of pandemic response would be simple. Any trade-offs with other societal aims could safely be ignored. Because averting pandemic harms is not all that matters, however, pandemic policies must always be considered against the backdrop of overall societal policies. Policies that would be appropriate to adopt if only pandemics mattered sometimes should not be adopted because other things matter as well. Moreover, pervasive trade-offs also exist among different pandemic policies—such as spending on some vaccines as opposed to others.

The pervasiveness of trade-offs and the relevance of other social objectives illustrate the ethical flaws of one popular slogan, "Nobody is safe until everyone is safe" (Takemi and Steiner 2020). Achieving complete and universal safety—"everyone is safe"—is impracticable because most pandemic pathogens cannot be eradicated.[1] Aiming at the mirage of making "everyone" safe will lead to the pursuit of increasingly burdensome measures despite diminishing returns. The ethical goal of pandemic policy must instead be to make people *safer* in a fair, equitable, and reasonable way. Fairness does not require identical or complete protection against infection for all populations. Rather, policy makers must identify which measures provide sufficient protection against pandemic harms at an acceptable level of cost and burden, and consider how to fairly distribute that protection. They must make these decisions responsively and transparently both during and outside of active health emergencies.

This chapter analyzes four illustrative contexts in which pandemic prevention, preparedness, and response present challenging ethical issues: (1) spending, (2) clinical research, (3) restrictions on rights and freedoms, and (4) fair allocation of scarce interventions. Table 15.1 explains each context's core ethical values, quantitative and implementation dimensions, and pitfalls to avoid. This chapter focuses on these four contexts because they cut across a variety of chapter topics, although it recognizes the relevance of other contexts such as health care provision. Each topic connects with others—greater spending, for instance, could ease clinical research, reduce the need to restrict rights, and mitigate scarcity. Each, however, implicates distinctive ethical values, making it useful to analyze each in depth while noting connections across them.

**Table 15.1** Ethical Issues in Pandemic Prevention, Preparedness, and Response

| Relevant ethical context | Ethical values | Quantitative operationalization | Implementation choices | Pitfalls to avoid |
|---|---|---|---|---|
| Spending | Maximizing net benefit<br><br>Mitigating relative disadvantage<br><br>Mitigating absolute disadvantage<br><br>Mitigating clustered disadvantage<br><br>Identifying values (if any) that are insulated from trade-offs | Cost-benefit analysis<br><br>Cost-effectiveness analysis<br><br>Extended cost-effectiveness analysis<br><br>Distributional cost-effectiveness analysis<br><br>Cost-consequence analysis<br><br>Social welfare function | Direct spending (for example, cash payments)<br><br>Implicit spending (for example, grants of IP rights) | Ignoring potential opportunity costs of pandemic spending<br><br>Assuming that an intervention having a good value somewhere makes it a good value everywhere |
| Clinical research | Social value<br><br>Scientific validity<br><br>Fair subject selection<br><br>Favorable risk-benefit ratio<br><br>Independent review<br><br>Informed consent<br><br>Respect for participants | Estimation of social value and risk-benefit ratio<br><br>Assessment of public trust effects<br><br>Assessment of fairness of subject selection | Permitting vs. prohibiting CHI trials<br><br>Permitting vs. prohibiting randomized trials of policies | Ignoring the ethical problems (for example, spending on ineffective treatments) presented by *not* conducting research<br><br>Applying exceptionalist standards to CHI trials |
| Rights and freedoms | Freedom of movement<br><br>Freedom of association<br><br>Education<br><br>Intellectual freedom | Defining threshold of allowable pandemic risk | Command-and-control regulation<br><br>Overall risk cap<br><br>Pricing risky activities | Equating differential treatment with discrimination<br><br>Failing to define goals and endpoints for rights-limiting policies |
| Fair allocation of scarce medical resources | Benefiting people and preventing harm<br><br>Mitigating disadvantage<br><br>Equal concern<br><br>Reciprocity | Measuring expected benefit (for example, averted deaths, averted years of life lost, or potential years of life lost)<br><br>Measuring mitigation of disadvantage | Points systems<br><br>Categorized priority systems<br><br>Levels for decision (individual, regional, country, global) | Focusing only on a single type of harm (for example, deaths)<br><br>Failure to create and implement an allocation framework |

*Source:* Original table prepared for this publication.

*Note:* CHI = controlled human infection; IP = intellectual property.

## SPENDING

Spending on pandemic prevention, preparedness, and response presents inevitable opportunity costs. Pandemic-oriented spending consumes resources that might instead be used to pursue other societal goals. For instance, some have proposed stockpiling pandemic response interventions such as ventilators. Amassing stockpiles, however, competes with other societal priorities that might be more important, such as funding health care for nonpandemic conditions, education, or environmental protection (Halpern and Miller 2020). Because of the inevitability of opportunity costs, different types of pandemic spending must be compared against one another, and the size of the pandemic budget compared against other budgets.

Trade-offs between pandemic spending and other aims diminish when pandemic investments also deliver value in nonpandemic times. A ventilator stockpile largely sits idle outside a pandemic. By contrast, growing the public health and medical workforce could provide available personnel to address nonpandemic problems— serving as a dual-use investment that both supports routine care and public health and is available to address outbreaks and emergencies (chapter 11). As noted in chapter 12, staff shortages rather than physical equipment tended to be the limiting factor during most COVID-19 pandemic surges. In addition to a stronger workforce, some pandemic response technologies also have co-benefits outside pandemics. For instance, reconfiguring physical spaces to reduce pandemic disease spread could potentially also mitigate nonpandemic conditions such as common respiratory infections or indoor particulate pollution.

Economic analyses could help elucidate the likely benefits and costs of pandemic investments, including benefits that come in nonpandemic times or address nonpandemic harms (Persad and Pandya 2022). For instance, biosafety measures' expected costs and benefits can be better understood via economic analysis (chapter 12).

In addition to learning from economic analyses, policy decisions must grapple with fundamental ethical questions about the fair distribution of benefits, as well as proposals that some rights should be insulated from economic and opportunity-cost analysis. Most accounts of fair distribution evaluate policies by considering factors beyond net benefit. One commonly considered factor is how badly the worst-off individuals will fare under a policy, either relative to others or in absolute terms. Another is whether a policy weakens the link between pandemic harms and social disadvantage: that is, whether a policy mitigates differential pandemic outcomes that constitute health disparities or inequities (Braveman 2006). Economic evaluations can consider these distributional factors through the use of distributional and extended cost-effectiveness analyses or social welfare functions. Understanding community values can help in making spending decisions, but the consideration of such values must be done carefully and with attention to the risk of overrepresenting particularly vocal groups (McCoy et al. 2019). The breadth of health emergencies' effects, for instance, makes efforts to focus primarily on those directly affected dubious.

By contrast to distributional factors that can be represented in economic analyses, a truly absolute right—one admitting no trade-offs—is difficult to represent in an economic evaluation. In a pandemic context, however, it is hard to envision a positive claim to medical assistance that is genuinely absolute, as opposed to particularly important.

Importantly, economic analyses must compare a given spending proposal to alternative uses of the same funds. For instance, the One Health chapter describes the cost of identifying all viruses of pandemic risk at about US$4 billion (chapter 3). When deciding whether to invest in identifying all viruses presenting pandemic risk, decision-makers should ask both (1) whether this investment is a *superior* use of limited funds compared to some alternative spending currently occurring, and (2) whether it is the *optimal* use of limited funds. A proposal whose benefits exceed its costs may nevertheless be suboptimal, because some alternative proposal provides even more benefit compared to its cost and both proposals cannot be simultaneously adopted.

The need to compare spending proposals becomes particularly urgent in countries that, before a pandemic, could deliver only a very limited package of health interventions. As chapter 12 notes, "local context, cost drivers, and epidemiology" can "greatly influence the overall value for money" that a given intervention provides. The merits of investing in advanced care at the level of intensive care units, for instance, depend on local health system conditions (chapter 12). Philanthropic funders, particularly from high-income countries, should not assume that, because an intervention represents a good buy domestically, it is appropriate to fund abroad (Persad 2015).

Biomedical innovations that support pandemic response, such as vaccines and antiviral medications, present distinctive spending questions. These interventions tend to be scarce at first, but scarcity could be mitigated by spending more in advance to encourage research, development, and manufacturing. Rather than up-front spending, however, governments often seek to encourage research, development, and manufacturing by granting innovators exclusive rights, such as patents, to market an innovation for some period of time.

Determining the optimal quantity and mechanism for spending to encourage innovation for pandemic response is an important and challenging task. Some have argued that access to interventions would be best promoted by suspending the enforcement of intellectual property (IP) rights or not granting them in the first place (Foss-Solbrekk 2021)—an appealing short-term solution for advocates and governments because it requires no up-front spending. But suspending IP rights without replacing them with alternative innovation incentives would be misguided. First, taken by itself, suspending the enforcement of IP rights in pandemic interventions would reduce the incentive to develop such interventions (Hemel and Ouellette 2023). As chapter 11 notes, the goal must be to "ensure market access for target populations without setting prices so low as to jeopardize incentives for pharmaceutical innovation or manufacturing." Chapter 10 likewise notes that "incentivizing socially valuable vaccine investments without 'giving away the store' to pharmaceutical manufacturers may require carefully designed policies." Second, suspending enforcement is not likely to promote manufacturing without some other form of spending to encourage knowledge transfer.

Rather than IP suspension alone, properly encouraging future innovation will require policies that reward and fund that innovation (Emanuel et al. 2021a). Such policies could employ alternatives to grants of IP rights. Prizes for pandemic response innovations, for instance, could encourage investment in the development of such innovations (Sampat and Shadlen 2021). So could patent buy-outs or "push" funding that supports research on specific interventions (refer to chapter 10).

## CLINICAL RESEARCH

Determining the best strategies for pandemic prevention and response often requires research on human subjects. When is such clinical research ethical? Research ethics does not disappear in pandemics (London and Kimmelman 2020). Rather, the same fundamental ethical requirements remain relevant. One prominent account of clinical research identifies seven ethical principles: (1) social value, (2) scientific validity, (3) fair subject selection, (4) favorable risk-benefit ratio, (5) independent review, (6) informed consent, and (7) respect for participants (Emanuel, Wendler, and Grady 2000).

This section will apply these principles to two debates that often arose during the COVID-19 pandemic and appear likely to arise in other pandemics. One centered on the ethics of controlled human infection (CHI) trials, often dubbed "challenge trials," which would have intentionally exposed consenting subjects to a pandemic pathogen in order to evaluate countermeasures such as vaccines. Another debate involved population-level research on nonpharmaceutical countermeasures such as mask policies or indoor ventilation. Although other research ethics problems, such as poorly designed trials, were even more widespread (refer to chapter 11), and other problems such as setting research priorities (Pierson and Millum 2018) remain crucial, CHI trials and population-level randomized trials raise particularly interesting and distinctive ethical questions in pandemic contexts.

### Challenge Trials

The primary ethical argument in favor of CHI trials emphasizes the first principle from Emanuel, Wendler, and Grady (2000): social value. At certain points in the COVID-19 pandemic, more than 10,000 people were dying worldwide per day. Accelerating the development of countermeasures by even a day could therefore have provided enormous benefits (Chappell 2022).

Most arguments against CHI trials charge that CHI trials would have violated some other ethical requirement. Consider fair subject selection. Some worried about the underrepresentation of groups facing a disproportionate burden of disease— for instance, that CHI trials in the United States during COVID-19 would enroll disproportionately fewer racial and ethnic minorities, who faced an outsized burden of disease. Others worried about overrepresentation of these groups—that efforts to recruit participants at high baseline risk of COVID-19 infection would lead to "targeted recruitment of minority groups," which would heighten distrust (Spinola et al. 2020, 1573). Despite the importance of fair subject selection, fairness does not require perfection, and CHI trials do not face distinctive selection problems. There is no evidence to suggest that underenrollment is a greater problem for CHI trials than for other trial designs. Nor does enrolling participants at high exposure risk require race-targeted recruitment.

Many arguments criticized CHI trials' risk-benefit ratio. Some claimed that CHI trials have no prospect of direct benefit to participants, only a prospect of harm. The risk-benefit requirements for ethical research, however, do not require a prospect of benefit to participants themselves. Rather, when risks to participants outweigh benefits to them, ethical evaluation requires considering whether "the societal benefits in terms of knowledge justify the excess risks to individual subjects" (Emanuel, Wendler, and Grady 2000, 2706). Given the great value of knowledge about potential pandemic interventions, CHI trials could potentially satisfy the risk-benefit requirement even if they present net risks to participants. Moreover, some CHI participants might benefit from better-quality care than available outside trials or from protection conferred by the study intervention. CHI trials of pandemic pathogens might thus in fact have a prospect of benefit.

Others charged that participants from lower- and middle-income countries would participate in CHI trials without their communities reaping the benefits of their participation (Moodley, Maasdorp, and Rennie 2021). Concerns about community benefits, however, do not distinctively apply to CHI trials and are a familiar topic in the ethics of international clinical research (Wendler and Shah 2017). Chapter 11, for instance, notes that clinical research in low- and middle-income countries raises questions about "the equitable distribution of research benefits and market access."

Some argue that there is an absolute upper limit on the expected severity of research-related harms that cannot be exceeded, irrespective of the social value of knowledge and even if participants consent (Resnik 2012). Belief in upper risk limits may have undergirded some commentators' belief that COVID-19 CHI trials were unacceptable in the absence of a "rescue therapy" that limits the severity of disease (Sulmasy 2021). Such an upper limit might proscribe, for instance, CHI trials of pathogens with very high infection fatality rates such as Ebola virus, even when the trials have high expected social value and even when participants have consented. Others, however, argue that no universal upper limit on risk exists (Steel 2020).

Informed consent to CHI trials has also been challenged: some argue that COVID-19's novel nature and unknown long-term risk profile would have precluded informed consent to COVID-19 CHI trials (Spinola et al. 2020). This argument is implausible. Individuals could and did informedly consent to other in-person activities, such as providing or receiving medical care, that would have exposed them to COVID-19. Additionally, participants can informedly consent to research that exposes them to risks that are not fully understood (Schaefer et al. 2020).

Others worried that payment would lead participants to consent to research they would have otherwise declined to join (Sulmasy 2021). However, a participant can elect to join a study because of payment, or even in order to be paid, while still informedly consenting. Payment vitiates informed consent only if it precludes appropriate consideration of research risks and benefits (Cryder et al. 2010).

The right to withdraw from research was also raised as a concern about CHI trials. If volunteers were infected during the study, critics claim they "would need to stay on the research unit, making the right to withdraw meaningless" (Spinola et al. 2020, 1573). Again, this concern is dubious. Participants in inpatient, non-CHI trials *unrelated* to a pandemic disease would also need to take isolation precautions if they contract the pandemic disease during those trials. The possibility that isolation precautions will be needed does not make inpatient trials ethically impermissible. Furthermore, infected volunteers would not necessarily need to stay on the research unit—they might allowably be discharged whenever any other individual with the pandemic disease could likewise be discharged.

Last, some charged that CHI trials do not produce scientifically valid results because they must exclude participants at high risk of complications (Moodley, Maasdorp, and Rennie 2021). Scientific validity and social value, although framed as distinct principles, are closely linked: presumably, scientific validity matters because scientifically valid results are more likely to enable socially valuable outcomes. Concerns about CHI trials' scientific validity could be addressed in two ways. One is to let CHI trials enroll consenting individuals even if those individuals face higher risk of severe outcomes, which would enable the participant population to mirror the population of ultimate recipients (Chappell 2022). The other is to exclude consenting participants on risk grounds and justify doing so on the basis that such exclusions are common outside CHI trials and consistent with scientific validity (Eyal and Gerhard 2022). For instance, long-term care facility residents were starkly underrepresented in the actual, non-CHI trials used to test COVID-19 vaccines, yet were among the first groups to receive vaccines (Branswell 2020). No trial design perfectly mirrors actual use. Trade-offs between scientific validity and individual risk are inevitable: enrolling participants at greater risk of serious outcomes will enhance validity but heighten risk.

Beyond these seven principles of ethical research, some have argued that researchers' professional duties prohibit them from intentionally infecting even consenting participants. These arguments often conceive of health professionals' role responsibilities as requiring nonmaleficence. Although nonmaleficence could justify professionals individually declining to conduct CHI trials, reasonable pluralism about health professionals' role responsibilities counsels against entrenching these conceptions as legal prohibitions on CHI trials.

Other objections, finally, contend that CHI trials—despite initial appearances—may lack net social value. This objection is the most promising but requires factual assessment rather than speculation. One social value objection contends that CHI trials would have led to public distrust in research if participants became severely ill or died. Others have argued that CHI trials "endanger ... our whole society (its moral fabric), by making it less likely that we will take the sort of relatively easy measures prescribed by experts to avoid future crises" (Bramble 2021). This claim, however, is a factual and empirically assessable one, not an ethical conjecture. Some studies suggest that public trust would have been preserved as long as the public understood that trial participants were voluntarily taking these risks in order to realize a socially valuable outcome (Broockman et al. 2021). Furthermore, any loss of public trust due to poor CHI trial outcomes would need to be weighed against dimensions of social value other than public trust.

Another objection contends that CHI trials might not have in fact accelerated access to countermeasures (Shah et al. 2020). During the COVID-19 pandemic, rampant viral spread made it tenable to conduct conventional, non-CHI trials. Additionally, regulators might not have approved vaccines on the basis of data from challenge trials alone. Whether CHI trials in fact could accelerate the development of certain types of countermeasures is, as objectors acknowledge, an empirically assessable question. The answers will likely depend on the type of countermeasure and the nature of the pandemic in question.

## Randomizing Nonpharmaceutical and Policy Interventions

Deciding whether to implement nonpharmaceutical interventions such as masking or school closures, or to make policy choices like pausing elective procedures during pandemic surges, also benefits from a high-quality evidence base. Perhaps chapter 8's most decisive takeaway is that we lack high-quality evidence regarding the effect of school closures on pandemic disease.

Strengthening the evidence base for nonpharmaceutical and policy interventions can be done through systematic research, including randomizing populations to different interventions. During the COVID-19 pandemic, however, prominent researchers and officials rejected randomized trials of mask policies as unethical because masks had proven beneficial on the basis of mechanistic plausibility or observational studies (Czypionka et al. 2021). Similar arguments could be leveled against randomized trials of other nonpharmaceutical interventions such as reducing the density of activities or improving ventilation (for example, Gilman et al. 2020).

Randomized trials of nonpharmaceutical interventions can be ethical even if other evidence already exists. Understanding *how much* benefit nonpharmaceutical interventions like masking or ventilation provide is crucial for deciding how much to invest in implementing these interventions. Another important argument for randomized trials is that the absence of high-quality evidence creates room for financially motivated actors to market unproven interventions to the public and to governments. High-quality evidence ensures that limited resources can be directed toward valuable treatments, and enables health care and allied professionals to act in accordance with their professional obligations to provide effective treatment.

The ethical starting point should be that, when evidence about the magnitude of multiple policies' benefits is of low enough quality that no policy is clearly best, it is acceptable to compare these policies in a formal randomized trial, rather than merely picking among them. Moreover, at the population level, it is neither practicable nor necessary to require more individualized consent for randomization between two acceptable policies than would be required in order to choose one of the policies for universal application. For instance, if it is acceptable for a community to require high-filtration masks, to require only cloth masks, or to require no masks at all, it should also be acceptable to rigorously compare these policies using randomization. The same is true for other interventions such as activity closures. Notably, randomized designs have been used to test some policies such as incentives for vaccination uptake (Milkman et al. 2022).

## RIGHTS AND FREEDOMS IN PANDEMIC POLICY

Many pandemic policies present trade-offs with individual rights and freedoms. Chapter 3, for instance, discusses how animal agriculture practices, trade, and human population movement can increase pandemic risk. Yet many risk-producing activities (such as long-distance travel or consuming farmed animals) are highly valued parts of people's lives (Barnhill and Bonotti 2022). Chapter 4, meanwhile, discusses biosecurity, including scientific research on pathogens that could cause pandemics. Limiting such research could reduce some pandemic risks but could impinge on an exercise of intellectual freedom that has value even beyond its potential to prevent future pandemics. Chapter 8 discusses education in the context of pandemic school closures—it emphasizes schools' role in generating human capital and meeting basic needs, but notes that education is also recognized as an important individual human right.

Addressing trade-offs between pandemic prevention, preparedness, and response and individual freedoms requires policy makers to identify which freedoms are most important and consider how to effectively prevent pandemics while securing those freedoms. One way to conceptualize this trade-off is to imagine a pandemic risk budget, in which each activity—such as keeping schools open—consumes a portion of the risk budget proportional to the risk it presents (Budish 2020). This risk budget should prioritize more important activities over less important ones, just as a household or national budget prioritizes more important over less important spending.

Identifying more important activities or freedoms, however, can be challenging. Optimistically, we might hope to identify a ranking of rights with which nobody can reasonably disagree. For instance, keeping in-person schools open seems more important than keeping live animal markets open. The COVID-19 pandemic indicated that primary and secondary education are highly beneficial and particularly difficult to conduct remotely (Levinson, Cevik, and Lipsitch 2020). The same is true of medical primary care services. In contrast, we learned that some other activities can be effectively carried out remotely: the difference between watching a movie in person or attending a workplace meeting in person versus conducting these same activities remotely is much smaller than the difference between in-person and remote primary education.

However, some might object that education is easier to conduct remotely than live animal markets, or that live animal markets or in-person workplace meetings are necessary to cultural or religious practices. Ultimately, such choices may require recourse to voting processes or elected decision-makers.

Ethical trade-offs with individual freedom are particularly stark when the intervention must be or is implemented without allowing individuals to opt in or out—for example, with activity and travel restrictions, such as school and border closures, and density limits. Assessment of these trade-offs must recognize that restricting some freedoms (for instance, restricting animal markets) may enable others (for instance, continuing to practice animal agriculture).

A further issue is that the burdens and benefits of restrictions are often unevenly distributed. People at high risk of poor outcomes from a pandemic disease may benefit more from restrictions, whereas people who depend on restricted activities are more burdened. Border closures, for instance, may benefit people who do not travel and are at high medical risk if infected, but harm those who travel to visit loved ones or depend on employment activities that require crossing borders.

Pandemic policy should also recognize that closing one activity or space inevitably redirects people to other activities or spaces (Marcus 2020). For instance, closing outdoor playgrounds may increase risk if it leads people to gather indoors. Closing schools or workplaces may increase risk if people instead gather in higher-risk settings.

Border and school closures are two useful policies to analyze from an individual rights and freedoms perspective because both were widely adopted during the COVID-19 pandemic and both also stand in clear tension with important individual rights—the right to education and the right to travel. In addition, both border and school closures could be imposed in either universal or partial fashion. For instance, borders and schools could be open only to individuals who have received a vaccine or who take relevant nonpharmaceutical measures (Persad and Emanuel 2020).

In addition to partial closures based on vaccination status or taking nonpharmaceutical measures, it is also possible to target partial closures based on medical vulnerability. For instance, during COVID-19, older adults were often prioritized for vaccine access because they faced higher risk of severe outcomes if infected (Saadi et al. 2021). Analogously, older adults could also have been prioritized for mask requirements, particularly for high-quality masks that protect wearers, or for vaccine requirements (Williams 2022). Or they could have been distinctively excluded from certain spaces where infection was prevalent (Savulescu and Cameron 2020). In general, societies seemed more willing to target pure benefits, such as priority vaccine access, toward people at high risk than to similarly target interventions like vaccine or mask requirements that would both protect and burden people at high risk. Targeting burdensome interventions, however, can also be justifiable when it enables effective pandemic policy at less cost to individual freedom. Invidious discrimination treats people differently on the basis of irrelevant differences such as skin color; in contrast, risk of poor outcomes if infected is a relevant difference that could justify differential treatment.

Rights and freedoms are also implicated when interventions require uptake by individuals. Examples include vaccination, testing, and the use of nonpharmaceutical protective equipment such as masks. Policy makers have a variety of options to increase uptake, including educational programs, exhortations, financial incentives, and requirements (refer to chapter 7). When practicable, it is preferable to begin with voluntary programs before implementing requirements (Mello, Silverman, and Omer 2020). Requirements, however, can be acceptable when they promise sufficiently great benefits in comparison to their burdens.

Last, protecting rights and freedoms requires clearly defining the goal of pandemic response interventions. Even very restrictive interventions may be justifiable when hospitalizations threaten health system functioning, or when these interventions have good prospects of stalling disease spread. In contrast, deciding whether to continue the use of interventions—particularly burdensome ones—in less exigent circumstances is more challenging. For instance, some have argued that medical personnel should be required to wear masks upon request, or that coworkers of an employee at greater risk of severe COVID-19 outcomes should similarly be required to wear masks as an accommodation of that coworker (Raz and Dorfman 2021). Outside of a crisis that threatens health system functioning, it is harder to justify long-term mandatory masking even if it protects some individuals' health. Determining which measures are justified requires identifying and balancing the interests of health professionals, patients, and the broader public.

Precisely defining the goal of pandemic response, however, remains challenging. In other contexts, some have suggested using the harm of common diseases such as seasonal influenza as a baseline (Emanuel et al. 2021b). The "nobody is safe until everyone is safe" approach, meanwhile, suggests that zero deaths should be the goal. A zero-death goal, however, violates what this chapter stated at the outset: preventing pandemic harm is not all that matters, and pandemic prevention frequently presents trade-offs. It is unlikely that a universal threshold can be identified, but we can at least say that the criteria for phasing interventions in and out should be based on interventions' benefit, their cost, and their burden on freedoms and rights, with interventions that are cost-effective and minimally jeopardize freedoms implemented before more burdensome interventions like school closures (chapter 8).

## FAIRLY ALLOCATING SCARCE INTERVENTIONS

Some pandemic response interventions are expected to be initially or persistently scarce, such that not everyone who can benefit will be able to receive them. During the COVID-19 pandemic, scarcity existed for testing, vaccines, antiviral medications, and critical care interventions like intensive care unit beds and medical personnel. Vaccines and antivirals were also scarce during the mpox public health emergency. This scarcity creates the need for fair allocation of interventions among nations, subnational entities, medical facilities, and ultimately patients.

**Table 15.2** Ethical Objectives and Priority Groups for Allocation

| Ethical objective | Priority groups |
|---|---|
| Benefiting people and reducing harm | Those likely to suffer serious direct harms (death, loss of future life, loss of function) without the intervention |
| | Those (such as caregivers) whose subjection to direct harm will deprive others of crucial benefits |
| | For a communicable illness, those who are likely to transmit illness to others (refer to chapter 8 on indirect benefits of vaccination) |
| Mitigating disadvantage | Those whose lives will worsen overall if they do not receive the intervention |
| | Those who have been subject to systematic disadvantage |
| Affording equal concern | All groups |
| Reciprocity | Those who have taken steps that mitigated pandemic harms |

*Source:* Adapted from Emanual and Persad 2023.

The most central objective of fair allocation in a pandemic is to benefit people and reduce harms (Emanuel and Persad 2023). Importantly, this objective aligns with other aspects of pandemic response, which also usually emphasize benefiting people and preventing harm. Other important ethical objectives include mitigating disadvantage, equal concern for potential recipients, and reciprocity (table 15.2).

In allocation policy, harms beyond imminent loss of life should be considered. Some have argued that pandemic response should ignore differences in how much life patients stand to lose and consider only how likely patients are to die in the immediate term after contracting the pandemic disease (Gaurke et al. 2021; Rajczi et al. 2021). This approach is contrary both to harm prevention and to mitigating disadvantage. The COVID-19 pandemic, which disproportionately killed people later in their lives, was awful. Far worse, however, would be a pandemic disease with similar transmissibility and infection fatality rate to COVID-19, but age-neutral severity and death rates (Ruf and Knuf 2014) (figure 15.1). Such a disease would kill nearly 10 million people under the age of 40, including millions of children, rather than the few thousands of younger people who died of COVID-19. Tens of millions more years of life would be lost. Moreover, because of the life-shortening effects of social disadvantage (Chetty et al. 2016; Vyas, Hathi, and Gupta 2022), the people who die earlier in life from this disease would more likely have been disadvantaged in other respects as well, compared to the older adults who disproportionately died from COVID-19.

Focusing only on immediate death is likewise misguided for diseases with a lower fatality rate that may cause intense suffering, such as mpox, or may cause long-term loss of function, such as Zika. In addition, policies should account for the severe indirect harm to children and dependents when pandemic diseases kill parents and caregivers or render them unable to provide needed care (Gorin 2021). Widespread loss of crucial caregivers marked the worst parts of the human immunodeficiency virus (HIV) epidemic (De Wagt and Connolly 2005).

**Figure 15.1** Actual and Population-Proportional Excess Deaths from COVID-19, by Age Range, January 2020–December 2021

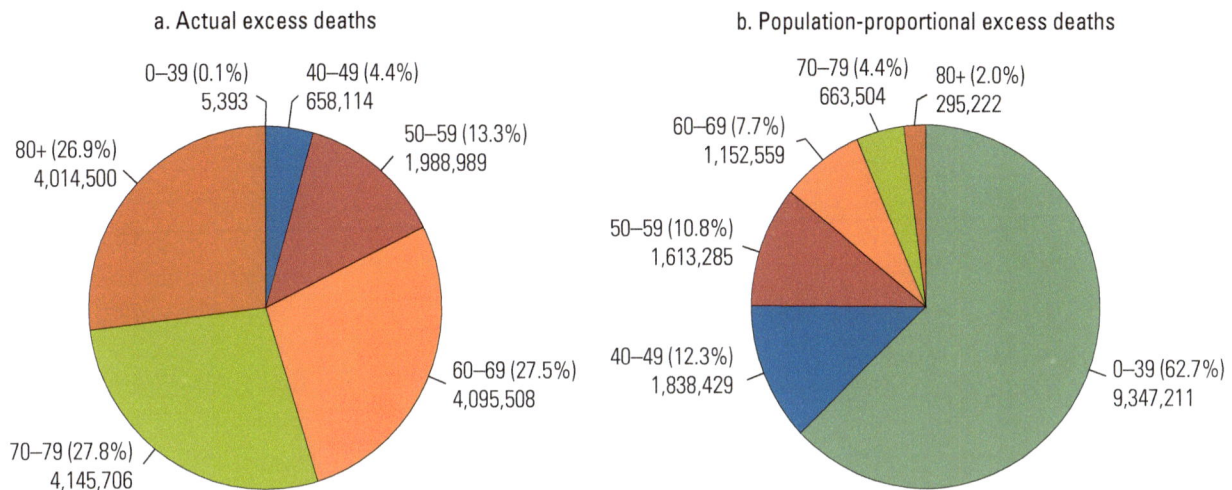

a. Actual excess deaths

0–39 (0.1%)
5,393

40–49 (4.4%)
658,114

50–59 (13.3%)
1,988,989

80+ (26.9%)
4,014,500

60–69 (27.5%)
4,095,508

70–79 (27.8%)
4,145,706

b. Population-proportional excess deaths

70–79 (4.4%)
663,504

80+ (2.0%)
295,222

60–69 (7.7%)
1,152,559

50–59 (10.8%)
1,613,285

40–49 (12.3%)
1,838,429

0–39 (62.7%)
9,347,211

*Sources:* Based on data from Wong et al. 2023 (panel a) and 2023 data from https://population.un.org/wpp/downloads?folder=Standard%20 Projections&group=Population (panel b)

For interventions like vaccines and antiviral medications that prevent pandemic exposure from resulting in severe disease, benefiting people and mitigating disadvantage generally align. In general, disadvantaged people are more exposed to pathogens and so stand to gain more from interventions that forestall pandemic harms among exposed individuals. This reality supports integrating indexes of disadvantage into decisions about who should be first to receive an antiviral medication or vaccine (Kaalund et al. 2022).

In contrast, for critical care interventions that treat patients who are already severely ill, benefiting people and mitigating disadvantage will more often—but not always—stand at odds. Sometimes, disadvantage may reduce prospect of benefit: a disadvantaged candidate for treatment may be less likely to survive even if they receive interventions, or may have a lower posttreatment lifespan. In these difficult situations, mitigating disadvantage must sometimes give way: it can be justified to greatly benefit a better-off person rather than to modestly benefit a worse-off person (Parfit 2012).

Reciprocity presents distinctive issues. Frontline medical personnel potentially have reciprocity-based claims to scarce pandemic interventions. So do others who have worked to reduce pandemic harms, such as participants in research on pandemic interventions (Rid, Lipsitch, and Miller 2021). Meanwhile, individuals whose conduct exacerbated pandemic harms may be subject to claims of negative reciprocity that justify prioritizing others above them for interventions (Persad and Largent 2022). Particularly if reciprocity-based prioritization would worsen outcomes or exacerbate disadvantage, however, reciprocity-based claims might instead be better addressed using nonmedical resources. Medical personnel's reciprocity claims could be recognized with hazard pay (Jølstad and Solberg 2023), or trial participants compensated with benefits other than priority access to scarce pandemic countermeasures.

Backward-looking principles other than reciprocity may likewise have little purchase in pandemic contexts (refer to Moodley et al. 2020). Even if a group has historically been unjustly denied access to medicines or otherwise unfairly disadvantaged, prioritizing its members for access to pandemic interventions may not be the ethically best way of addressing their claims. Financial compensation or access to nonpandemic interventions may be preferable.

Some have questioned whether these and other ethical principles for allocation are applicable across different cultural contexts (Moodley et al. 2020). Each principle's application should be sensitive to context. In particular, how to best benefit people and limit harm will depend on context. A pathogen may disproportionally affect different populations in different countries. For instance, during the 2022 mpox public health emergency, most cases and hospitalizations in Europe and North America involved men who have sex with men, differing from the historic distribution of cases and severe outcomes in the African countries where mpox had been endemic (Mitjà et al. 2023).

## CONCLUSIONS

Pandemic prevention, preparedness, and response require navigating complex ethical terrain across multiple domains. Success demands both rigorous quantitative analysis and careful consideration of ethical values. For spending decisions, cost-effectiveness and distributional analyses should inform priorities while avoiding the trap of ignoring opportunity costs. In clinical research, maintaining consistent ethical values in pandemic contexts remains crucial. Regarding rights and freedoms, policy makers must define clear thresholds for allowable pandemic risk and endpoints for restrictions, while recognizing that differential treatment based on different expected outcomes is not necessarily discriminatory. Frameworks for allocating scarce resources should seek to operationalize ethical objectives like benefiting people, mitigating disadvantage, and recognizing reciprocity.

Common pitfalls to avoid include focusing on single types of harm while ignoring others, assuming interventions that work in one context will work equally well elsewhere, failing to define clear goals and endpoints for rights-limiting policies, and not creating comprehensive frameworks. Success requires quantifying trade-offs when possible, while remaining attentive to ethical values that resist pure quantification. Implementation choices should favor evidence-based, contextually appropriate approaches that acknowledge both the urgency of pandemic response and the continuing importance of other societal priorities.

## ACKNOWLEDGMENTS

Thanks to Ole Norheim, Ezekiel Emanuel, Seema Shah, and Johan Dellgren for discussion, and to Liz Ignowski and Halli Berrebbi for research assistance.

## NOTE

1. Carter Center, "Diseases Considered as Candidates for Global Eradication by the International Task Force for Disease Eradication," https://www.cartercenter.org/resources /pdfs/news/health_publications/itfde/updated_disease_candidate_table.pdf.

## REFERENCES

Barnhill, A., and M. Bonotti. 2022. *Healthy Eating Policy and Political Philosophy: A Public Reason Approach*. Oxford University Press.

Bramble, B. 2021. "Challenge Trials Are a Poor Substitute for an Effective Pandemic Response." *Cato Unbound*, March 11, 2021. https://www.cato-unbound.org/2021/03/11 /ben-bramble/challenge-trials-are-poor-substitute-effective-pandemic-response/.

Branswell, H. 2020. "CDC Advisory Panel's Lone Dissenter on Why Long-Term Care Residents Shouldn't Receive Covid-19 Vaccine First." *STAT*, December 3, 2020. https:// www.statnews.com/2020/12/03/cdc-advisory-panels-lone-dissenter-on-why-long-term -care-residents-shouldnt-receive-covid-19-vaccine-first/.

Braveman, P. 2006. "Health Disparities and Health Equity: Concepts and Measurement." *Annual Review of Public Health* (27): 167–94. https://doi.org/10.1146/annurev .publhealth.27.021405.102103.

Broockman D., J. Kalla, A. Guerrero, M. Budolfson, N. Eyal, N. P. Jewell, M. Magalhaes, and J. S. Sekhon. 2021. "Broad Cross-National Public Support for Accelerated COVID-19 Vaccine Trial Designs." *Vaccine* 39 (2): 309–16. https://doi.org/10.1016/j.vaccine.2020.11.072.

Budish, E. 2020. "Maximize Utility Subject to $R \leq 1$: A Simple Price-Theory Approach to Covid-19 Lockdown and Reopening Policy." NBER Working Paper 28093, National Bureau of Economic Research, Cambridge, MA. https://doi.org/10.3386/w28093.

Chappell, R. Y. 2022. "Pandemic Ethics and Status Quo Risk." *Public Health Ethics* 15 (1): 64–73. https://doi.org/10.1093/phe/phab031.

Chetty, R., M. Stepner, S. Abraham, S. Lin, B. Scuderi, N. Turner, A. Bergeron, and D. Cutler. 2016. "The Association between Income and Life Expectancy in the United States, 2001–2014." *JAMA* 315 (16): 1750–66.

Cryder, C. E., A. J. London, K. G. Volpp, and G. Loewenstein. 2010. "Informative Inducement: Study Payment as a Signal of Risk." *Social Science & Medicine* 70 (3): 455–64. https://doi .org/10.1016/j.socscimed.2009.10.047.

Czypionka, T., T. Greenhalgh, D. Bassler, and M. B. Bryant. 2021. "Masks and Face Coverings for the Lay Public: A Narrative Update." *Annals of Internal Medicine* 174 (4). https://doi .org/10.7326/M20-6625.

De Wagt, A., and M. Connolly. 2005. "Orphans and the Impact of HIV/AIDS in Sub-Saharan Africa." *Food Nutrition and Agriculture* 34. https://www.researchgate.net /publication/266160962_Orphans_and_the_impact_of_HIVAIDS_in_sub-Saharan _Africa.

Emanuel, E. J., A. Buchanan, S. Y. Chan, C. Fabre, D. Halliday, J. Heath, L. Herzog, et al. 2021a. "What Are the Obligations of Pharmaceutical Companies in a Global Health Emergency?" *The Lancet* 398 (10304): 1015–20. https://doi.org/10.1016/s0140 -6736(21)01378-7.

Emanuel, E. J., A. Buchanan, S. Y. Chan, C. Fabre, D. Halliday, R. J. Leland, F. Luna, et al. 2021b. "On the Ethics of Vaccine Nationalism: The Case for the Fair Priority for Residents Framework." *Ethics and International Affairs* 35 (4): 543–62. https://doi.org/10.1017 /S0892679421000514.

Emanuel, E. J., and G. Persad. 2023. "The Shared Ethical Framework to Allocate Scarce Medical Resources: A Lesson from COVID-19." *The Lancet* 401 (10391): 1892–902.

Emanuel, E. J., D. Wendler, and C. Grady. 2000. "What Makes Clinical Research Ethical?" *JAMA* 283 (20). https://doi.org/10.1001/jama.283.20.2701.

Eyal, N., and T. Gerhard. 2022. "Do Coronavirus Vaccine Challenge Trials Have a Distinctive Generalisability Problem?" *Journal of Medical Ethics* 48 (9). https://doi.org/10.1136/medethics-2020-107109.

Foss-Solbrekk, K. 2021. "The IP Waiver and COVID-19: Reasons for Unwavering Support." *Journal of Intellectual Property Law & Practice* 16 (12): 1347–59. https://doi.org/10.1093/jiplp/jpab150.

Gaurke, M. K., B. Prusak, K. Y. Jeong, E. Scire, and D. P. Sulmasy. 2021. Life-Years & Rationing in the Covid-19 Pandemic: A Critical Analysis. *The Hastings Center Report* 51 (5): 18–29. https://doi.org/10.1002/hast.1283.

Gilman R. T., S. Mahroof-Shaffi, C. Harkensee, and A. T. Chamberlain. 2020. "Modelling Interventions to Control COVID-19 Outbreaks in a Refugee Camp." *BMJ Global Health* 5 (12). https://doi.org/10.1136/bmjgh-2020-003727.

Gorin, M. 2021. "Prioritizing Parents." *Journal of Practical Ethics* 9 (1). https://doi.org/10.3998/jpe.1183.

Halpern, S. D., and F. G. Miller. 2020. "The Urge to Build More Intensive Care Unit Beds and Ventilators: Intuitive but Errant." *Annals of Internal Medicine* 173 (4). https://doi.org/10.7326/m20-2071.

Hemel, D. J., and L. L. Ouellette. 2023. "Valuing Medical Innovation." *Stanford Law Review* 75 (3): 517. https://www.stanfordlawreview.org/print/article/valuing-medical-innovation/.

Jølstad, B., and C. T. Solberg. 2023. "Reciprocity as an Argument for Prioritizing Health Care Workers for the COVID-19 Vaccine." *De Ethica* 7 (2). https://doi.org/10.3384/de-ethica.2001-8819.237228.

Kaalund K., A. Thoumi, N. A. Bhavsar, A. Labrador, and R. Cholera. 2022. "Assessment of Population-Level Disadvantage Indices to Inform Equitable Health Policy." *The Milbank Quarterly* 100 (4): 1028–75. https://doi.org/10.1111/1468-0009.12588.

Krohmal, B. J., and E. J. Emanuel. 2007. "Access and Ability to Pay: The Ethics of a Tiered Health Care System." *Archives of Internal Medicine* 167 (5): 433–37. https://doi.org/10.1001/archinte.167.5.433.

Levinson M., M. Cevik, and M. Lipsitch. 2020. "Reopening Primary Schools during the Pandemic." *New England Journal of Medicine* 383 (10): 981–85. https://doi.org/10.1056/NEJMms2024920.

London, A. J., and J. Kimmelman. 2020. "Against Pandemic Research Exceptionalism." *Science* 368 (6490): 476–77. https://doi.org/10.1126/science.abc1731.

Marcus, J. 2020. "Quarantine Fatigue Is Real." *The Atlantic*, May 11, 2020. https://www.theatlantic.com/ideas/archive/2020/05/quarantine-fatigue-real-and-shaming-people-wont-help/611482/.

McCoy, M. S., J. Warsh, L. Rand, M. Parker, and M. Sheehan. 2019. "Patient and Public Involvement: Two Sides of the Same Coin or Different Coins Altogether?" *Bioethics* 33(6): 708–15. https://doi.org/10.1111/bioe.12584.

Mello, M. M., R. D. Silverman, and S. B. Omer. 2020. "Ensuring Uptake of Vaccines against SARS-CoV-2." *New England Journal of Medicine* 383 (14): 1296–99. https://doi.org/10.1056/NEJMp2020926.

Milkman, K. L., L. Gandhi, S. F. Ellis, H. N. Graci, D. M. Gromet, R. S. Mobarak, A. M. Buttenheim, et al. 2022. "A Citywide Experiment Testing the Impact of Geographically Targeted, High-Pay-Off Vaccine Lotteries." *Nature Human Behaviour* 6 (11): 1515–24. https://doi.org/10.1038/s41562-022-01437-0.

Mitjà, O., D. Ogoina, B. K. Titanji, C. Galvan, J.-J. Muyembe, M. Marks, and C. M. Orkin. 2023. "Monkeypox." *The Lancet* 401 (10370): 60–74. https://doi.org/10.1016/S0140-6736(22)02075-X.

Moodley, K., E. Maasdorp, and S. Rennie. 2021. "Could Human Challenge Studies for COVID-19 Vaccines Be Justified in South Africa?" *South African Medical Journal* 111 (6): 559–62. https://pubmed.ncbi.nlm.nih.gov/34382566/.

Moodley, K., L. Ravez, A. E. Obasa, A. Mwinga, W. Jaoko, D. Makindu, F. Behets, and S. Rennie. 2020. "What Could 'Fair Allocation' during the Covid-19 Crisis Possibly Mean in Sub-Saharan Africa?" *Hastings Center Report* 50 (3): 33–35. https://doi.org/10.1002 /hast.1129.

Parfit, D. 2012. "Another Defence of the Priority View." *Utilitas* 24 (3): 399–440. https://doi .org/10.1017/s095382081200009x.

Persad, G. 2015. "The Medical Cost Pandemic: Why Limiting Access to Cost-Effective Treatments Hurts the Global Poor." *Chicago Journal of International Law* 15 (2): Article 6. https://chicagounbound.uchicago.edu/cjil/vol15/iss2/6/.

Persad, G., and E. J. Emanuel. 2020. "The Ethics of COVID-19 Immunity-Based Licenses ('Immunity Passports')." *JAMA Network*, May 6, 2020. https://doi.org/10.1001/jama .2020.8102.

Persad, G., and E. A. Largent. 2022. "COVID-19 Vaccine Refusal and Fair Allocation of Scarce Medical Resources. *JAMA Health Forum* 3 (4): e220356. https://jamanetwork.com /journals/jama-health-forum/fullarticle/2790959.

Persad, G., and A. Pandya. 2022. "A Comprehensive Covid-19 Response—the Need for Economic Evaluation." *New England Journal of Medicine* 386 (26): 2449–51. https://doi .org/10.1056/nejmp2202828.

Pierson, L., and J. Millum. 2018. "Health Research Priority Setting: The Duties of Individual Funders." *American Journal of Bioethics* (18) 11: 6–17. https://doi.org/10.1080/15265161.2 018.1523490.

Rajczi, A., J. Daar, A. Kheriaty, and C. Dastur. 2021. "The University of California Crisis Standards of Care: Public Reasoning for Socially Responsible Medicine." *The Hastings Center Report* 51 (5): 30–41. https://doi.org/10.1002/hast.1284.

Raz, M., and D. Dorfman. 2021. "Bans on COVID-19 Mask Requirements vs Disability Accommodations: A New Conundrum. *JAMA Health Forum* 2 (8): e211912. https://doi .org/10.1001/jamahealthforum.2021.1912

Resnik, D. B. 2012. "Limits on Risks for Healthy Volunteers in Biomedical Research." *Theoretical Medicine and Bioethics* 33 (2): 137–49. https://doi.org/10.1007/s11017-011 -9201-1.

Rid, A., M. Lipsitch, and F. G. Miller. 2021. "The Ethics of Continuing Placebo in SARS-CoV-2 Vaccine Trials." *JAMA* 325 (3): 219–20. https://doi.org/10.1001/jama.2020.25053.

Ruf, B. R., and M. Knuf. 2014. "The Burden of Seasonal and Pandemic Influenza in Infants and Children." *European Journal of Pediatrics* 173 (3): 265–76. https://doi.org/10.1007 /s00431-013-2023-6.

Saadi, N., Y.-L. Chi, S. Ghosh, R. M. Eggo, C. V. McCarthy, M. Quaife, J. Dawa, et al. 2021. "Models of COVID-19 Vaccine Prioritisation: A Systematic Literature Search and Narrative Review." *BMC Medicine* 19: 318. https://doi.org/10.1186/s12916-021-02190-3.

Sampat, Bhaven N., and Kenneth C. Shadlen. 2021. "The COVID-19 Innovation System." *Health Affairs* 40 (3). https://doi.org/10.1377/hlthaff.2020.02097.

Savulescu J., and J. Cameron. 2020. "Why Lockdown of the Elderly Is Not Ageist and Why Levelling Down Equality Is Wrong." *Journal of Medical Ethics* 46 (11). https://doi .org/10.1136/medethics-2020-106336.

Schaefer, G. O., C. C. Tam, J. Savulescu, and T. C. Voo. 2020. "COVID-19 Vaccine Development: Time to Consider SARS-CoV-2 Challenge Studies?" *Vaccine* 38 (33): 5085–88. https://doi.org/10.1016/j.vaccine.2020.06.007.

Shah, Seema K., Franklin G. Miller, Thomas C. Darton, Devan Duenas, Claudia Emerson, Holly Fernandez Lynch, Euzebiusz Jamrozik, et al. 2020. "Ethics of Controlled Human Infection to Address COVID-19." *Science* 368 (649300): 832–34.

Spinola, S. M., G. D. Zimet, M. A. Ott, and B. P. Katz. 2020. "Human Challenge Studies Are Unlikely to Accelerate Coronavirus Vaccine Licensure due to Ethical and Practical Issues." *The Journal of Infectious Diseases* 222 (9): 1572–74. https://doi.org/10.1093/infdis/jiaa457.

Steel, R. 2020. "Reconceptualising Risk–Benefit Analyses: The Case of HIV Cure Research." *Journal of Medical Ethics* 46 (3). https://doi.org/10.1136/medethics-2019-105548.

Sulmasy, Daniel P. 2021. "Are SARS-CoV-2 Human Challenge Trials Ethical?" *JAMA Internal Medicine* 181 (8): 1031–32. https://doi.org/10.1001/jamainternmed.2021.2614.

Takemi, K., and C. Steiner. 2020. "COVID-19: Nobody Is Safe until Everyone Is Safe." *UNDP Asia and the Pacific* (blog), December 9, 2020. https://www.undp.org/asia-pacific/blog/covid-19-nobody-safe-until-everyone-safe.

Vyas, S., P. Hathi, and A. Gupta. 2022. "Social Disadvantage, Economic Inequality, and Life Expectancy in Nine Indian States." *Proceedings of the National Academy of Sciences.* 119 (10): e2109226119. https://doi.org/10.1073/pnas.2109226119.

Wendler, D., and S. K. Shah. 2017. "Fair Benefits and Its Critics: Who Is Right?" *Journal of Health Care Law & Policy* 20 (1). https://www.ncbi.nlm.nih.gov/pmc/articles/PMC10569338/pdf/nihms-1885492.pdf.

Williams, B. M. 2022. "The Ethics of Selective Mandatory Vaccination for COVID-19." *Public Health Ethics* 15 (1): 74–86. https://doi.org/10.1093/phe/phab028.

Wong, M. K., D. J. Brooks, J. Ikejezie, M. Gacic-Dobo, L. Dumolard, Y. Nedelec, C. Steulet, at al. 2023. "COVID-19 Mortality and Progress toward Vaccinating Older Adults—World Health Organization, Worldwide, 2020–2022." *MMWR Morbidity and Mortality Weekly Report* 72 (5): 113–18. https://doi.org/10.15585/mmwr.mm7205a1.

# Acknowledgments

The fourth edition of *Disease Control Priorities* (*DCP4*) draws on the global health knowledge of institutions and experts from around the world, including volume editors, chapter authors, peer reviewers, and research and staff assistants. The finalization of this second volume would not have been possible without the intellectual vision, enduring support, and invaluable contributions of these individuals.

We owe gratitude to the financial sponsors of this effort. We are indebted to the Gates Foundation for supporting and funding the DCP Country Translation projects that helped us stake out the direction for future work in DCP4. We acknowledge the Research Council of Norway that—through its Centre of Excellence grant to the Bergen Centre for Ethics and Priority Setting in Health (BCEPS) at the University of Bergen—has enabled us to set up and develop a core analytics team for evidence collection, mathematical modeling, and economic evaluations. A special thank you goes to the Norwegian Agency for Development Cooperation (Norad) and the Trond Mohn Foundation, which have co-funded much of the ongoing country engagement work, including local capacity strengthening and master's and PhD training in health economics, ethics, and priority setting.

We are grateful to the University of Bergen, the Department of Global Public Health and Primary Care, and BCEPS for supporting the training of numerous students and creating a home base for the DCP4 Secretariat, a base that provides intellectual collaboration, logistical coordination, and administrative and social support. We thank those who worked behind the scenes within the department to ensure this work ran smoothly, including Wafa Aftab, Austen Davis, Øystein Ariansen Haaland, Kjell Arne Johanson, Solomon Memirie, Omar Mwalim, Jan-Magnus Økland, Bjarne Robberstad, Guri Rørtveit, Ingvild Sandøy, Maria Sollohub, and Jana Wilbricht.

The World Bank provided exceptional guidance and support throughout the planning phase, the review process, and the demanding production and design process. Within the World Bank, we especially thank Jung-Hwan Choi, Victoria Y. Fan, Magnus Lindelow, Martin Mpungu Lutalo, Juan Pablo Uribe, Monique Vledder, and Feng Zhao who served as champions of DCP4; and we thank the numerous expert reviewers of all chapters (refer to the list of reviewers). Mary Fisk oversaw the editing and publication of the series with diligence and expertise, and we are pleased to have had designer Debra Naylor, who developed the beautiful and crisp design for this volume and the series as a whole. Additionally, we thank Acquisitions Editor Jewel McFadden of World Bank publications for providing professional counsel on contracts, communications, and marketing strategies.

# Volume and Series Editors

## VOLUME EDITORS

### Stefano M. Bertozzi

Stefano M. Bertozzi is former dean and professor of health policy at the University of California, Berkeley School of Public Health. He previously led HIV and tuberculosis programs at the Gates Foundation and directed Mexico's Instituto Nacional de Salud Pública (INSP) Center for Evaluation Research. He was the last director of the World Health Organization's Global Programme on AIDS and has worked with the Joint United Nations Programme on HIV/AIDS, the World Bank, and the government of the Democratic Republic of Congo.

He is founding editor in chief of *Rapid Reviews\Infectious Diseases*. A member of the National Academy of Medicine, Dr. Bertozzi holds a biology degree and a PhD in health policy from the Massachusetts Institute of Technology (MIT); he earned his MD at the University of California, San Diego, and trained in internal medicine at the University of California, San Francisco.

### Victoria Y. Fan

Victoria Y. Fan is a senior economist in health financing at the World Bank. She previously served at the Center for Global Development from 2022–24 and 2011–14. From 2014 to 2024, she was faculty at the University of Hawaii, including tenured associate professor and interim director of the Center on Aging. At the University of Hawaii, she founded the Pacific Health Analytics Collaborative, a laboratory with more than 120 employees that conducted policy research on social determinants of health and mental health. During the COVID-19 (coronavirus) pandemic, she established and chaired the Hawaii Pandemic Applied Modeling working group advising state leaders and served as executive director of Hawaii CARES, the state's integrated call center and managed care network for mental health and substance use. She has more than 200 publications, including 70 articles in peer-reviewed journals. She holds a doctorate in health systems from Harvard University and a bachelor's in mechanical engineering from MIT. She was born and raised in Hawaii.

### Dean T. Jamison

Dean T. Jamison is professor emeritus of health economics at the University of California, San Francisco. He has worked at the World Bank as manager of both its education policy division and its health, nutrition, and population division. His subsequent career was in academia, including eight years as director of UCLA's Center for Pacific Rim Studies. At the World Bank, he initiated the *Disease Control Priorities* series. Jamison studied at Stanford University and at Harvard University, where he received his PhD in economics under Kenneth Arrow. He is a member of the Academy of Medicine of the US National Academies of Science, Engineering, and Medicine.

### Hitoshi Oshitani

Hitoshi Oshitani is a professor for the Department of Virology at Tohoku University Graduate School of Medicine in Japan. Before joining Tohoku University, he was a regional adviser of the World Health Organization Western Pacific Regional Office in Manila from 1999 to 2005, where he was responsible for emerging diseases, including severe acute respiratory syndrome and avian and pandemic influenza. He worked as a technical expert for Japan International Cooperation in Zambia from 1991 to 1994. His main research interest is epidemiology and control of viral infections, particularly respiratory viruses such as influenza and respiratory syncytial viruses. His research group has been conducting research in Japan and other countries such as Mongolia, the Philippines, and Zambia. He was a member of the Advisory Board and the Subcommittee on COVID-19 for the government of Japan during the COVID-19 pandemic. He is also a member of the Strategic and Technical Advisory Group on Infectious Hazards with Pandemic and Epidemic Potential, and other technical groups of the World Health Organization.

### Siddhanth Sharma

Dr. Siddhanth Sharma is a public health physician at the Burnet Institute in Australia, where he leads research on developing and evaluating interventions to improve indoor air quality. Before joining Burnet, Dr. Sharma contributed to communicable disease control efforts and supported environmental health projects for the Western Australian Department of Health, including work on climate change and outdoor air quality. He holds a masters of public health degree from Harvard University and a medical degree from the University of Notre Dame Australia.

### Muhammad Ali Pate

Muhammad Ali Pate serves as Nigeria's coordinating Minister of Health and Social Welfare. He formerly served as the global director of the Health, Nutrition and Population Global Practice at the World Bank and was Julio Frenk Professor of the Practice of Public Health Leadership in the Department of Global Health and Population at the Harvard T. H. Chan School of Public Health.

Dr. Pate is an MD trained in both internal medicine and infectious diseases, with an MBA from Duke University. Previously, he studied at the University College London. He also holds a master's in health system management from the London School of Hygiene and Tropical Medicine.

### Ole F. Norheim

Ole F. Norheim is a physician and Mary B. Saltonstall Professor of Ethics and Population Health at the Department of Global Health and Population, Harvard T. H. Chan School of Public Health. He co-founded the Bergen Centre for Ethics and Priority Setting in Health at the University of Bergen, Norway, and is an adjunct researcher at the center.

His research interests include theories of distributive justice, inequality in health, priority setting in health systems, and how to achieve universal health coverage in low- and middle-income countries. He is the lead series editor of *Disease Control Priorities* (fourth edition) and a member of the *Lancet* Commission on Investing in Health and the *Lancet* Commission on Sustainable Healthcare. Dr. Norheim is an elected member of the Norwegian Academy of Science and Letters. He has served as head of the Norwegian Biotechnology Advisory Board (2019–23), as chair of the World Health Organization's Consultative Group on Equity and Universal Health Coverage (2012–14), and on the third Norwegian National Committee on Priority Setting in Health Care (2013–14).

## SERIES EDITORS

### Ole F. Norheim

Refer to the list of volume editors.

### David A. Watkins

David A. Watkins is an associate professor in the Division of General Internal Medicine and in the Department of Global Health at the University of Washington. He currently leads the University of Washington site for the Disease Control Priorities Project and is affiliated with the Implementation Science Program in the Department of Global Health. Additionally, he is the co-director of the Learning for Action in Policy Implementation and Health Systems initiative. He studies health system reform and policy challenges, with a particular emphasis on universal health coverage and the growing burden of noncommunicable diseases in low-income countries. His team works in three thematic areas: (1) population and economic modeling to support policy analysis, (2) integrated health care delivery, and (3) use of evidence in policy formulation. In addition to his scholarly work, Dr. Watkins teaches global noncommunicable diseases and quantitative research methods and practices as a hospitalist at Harborview Medical Center.

**Kalipso Chalkidou**

Kalipso Chalkidou is the director of the Department of Health Financing and Economics at the World Health Organization headquarters. Before that, she founded and ran the Department of Health Finance at the Global Fund to Fight AIDS, Tuberculosis and Malaria. She also served as director of global health policy and was a senior fellow at the Center for Global Development. She is a visiting professor of global health at the School of Public Health, Imperial College London.

Her past work has concentrated on helping governments build technical and institutional capacity for using evidence to inform health policy as they move toward universal health coverage. She is interested in how local information, local expertise, and local institutions can drive scientific and legitimate health care resource allocation decisions. She has been involved in the Chinese rural health reforms and in national health reform projects in Colombia, Ghana, India, South Africa, Türkiye, and the Middle East, working with the Inter-American Development Bank; the Pan American Health Organization; the UK Foreign, Commonwealth & Development Office; and the World Bank, as well as national governments.

**Victoria Y. Fan**

Refer to the list of volume editors.

**Muhammad Ali Pate**

Refer to the list of volume editors.

**Dean T. Jamison**

Refer to the list of volume editors.

# Contributors

**Olaolu M. Aderinola**

- Emergency Preparedness and Response Cluster, WHO Regional Office for Africa, Brazzaville, Republic of Congo

**Puspanjali Adhikari**

- Kathmandu University, Nepal

**David Agus**

- Ellison Medical Institute, Los Angeles, California, United States

**Megan Akodu**

- Ellison Institute of Technology, Oxford, United Kingdom

**Ahmad Al-Kasir**

- Ellison Medical Institute, Los Angeles, California, United States

**Patrick Amoth**

- Ministry of Health, Kenya

**Brett N. Archer**

- Health Emergencies Programme, World Health Organization, Geneva, Switzerland

**Rinette Badker**

- Ginkgo Bioworks, Emeryville, California, United States

**Valentina Baltag**

- World Health Organization, Geneva, Switzerland

**Till Bärnighausen**

- Heidelberg Institute of Global Health, Germany

**Biniam Bedasso**

- Center for Global Development, Washington, DC, United States

**John Bell**

- Ellison Institute of Technology, Oxford, United Kingdom

**Kirsten Bell**

- Ellison Institute of Technology, Oxford, United Kingdom

**Tamsin Berry**

- Ellison Institute of Technology, Oxford, United Kingdom

**Franck Berthe**

- World Bank, Washington, DC, United States

**Stefano M. Bertozzi**

- University of California, Berkeley, California, United States

**David E. Bloom**

- Harvard T. H. Chan School of Public Health, Boston, Massachusetts, United States

**Donald A. P. Bundy**

- London School of Hygiene and Tropical Medicine, United Kingdom

**Carmen Burbano**

- World Food Programme, Rome, Italy

**David Canning**

- Harvard T. H. Chan School of Public Health, Boston, Massachusetts, United States

**Bin Cao**

- Capital Medical University, Beijing, China

**Lúcia Chambal**

- Maputo Central Hospital, Maputo, Mozambique

**Catherine Che**

- Department of Economics, University of California, Berkeley, California, United States

**Simiao Chen**

- University of Heidelberg, Germany

**Wenjin Chen**

- University of Heidelberg, Germany

**Sarrin Chethik**

- Market Shaping Accelerator, University of Chicago, Illinois, United States

**Matchecane Cossa**

- Maputo Central Hospital, Maputo, Mozambique

**Greta Davis**

- University of California, San Francisco, California, United States

**Olivier le Polain de Waroux**

- Health Emergencies Programme, World Health Organization, Geneva, Switzerland

**W. John Edmunds**

- London School of Hygiene and Tropical Medicine, United Kingdom

**Victoria Y. Fan**

- World Bank, Washington, DC; formerly Center for Global Development, Washington, DC, United States

**Maddalena Ferranna**

- University of Southern California, Los Angeles, California, United States

**Jane Fieldhouse**

- University of California, Davis, California; formerly University of California, San Francisco, California, United States

**Ugo Gentilini**

- World Bank, Washington, DC, United States

**Rachel Glennerster**

- Department of Economics, University of Chicago, United States

**Tracey Goldstein**

- Colorado State University (contributed while at United States Agency for International Development), United States

**Kumeren Govender**

- Ellison Institute of Technology, Oxford, United Kingdom

**Lee M. Hampton**

- US Centers for Disease Control and Prevention, Atlanta, Georgia, United States

**Eric Hanushek**

- Stanford University, Stanford, California, United States

**Ines Hassan**

- Ellison Institute of Technology, Oxford, United Kingdom

**Karli Tyance Hassell**

- Central Council of the Tlingit and Haida Indian Tribes of Alaska

**Sean Hillier**

- York University, Toronto, Canada

**Chikwe Ihekweazu**

- Health Emergencies Programme, World Health Organization, Geneva, Switzerland; World Health Organization Hub for Pandemic and Epidemic Intelligence, Berlin, Germany

**Dean T. Jamison**

- University of California, San Francisco, California, United States

**Julian Jamison**

- Universities of Oxford and Exeter, United Kingdom

**Lirui Jiao**

- University of North Carolina, United States

**Sun Kim**

- Harvard T. H. Chan School of Public Health, Boston, Massachusetts, United States

**Rassin Lababidi**

- Chatham House, London, United Kingdom

**Cathine Lam**

- Ginkgo Bioworks, Emeryville, California, United States

**Christopher T. Lee**

- Resolve to Save Lives, New York, United States

**Greg Lewis**

- Future of Humanity Institute, University of Oxford, United Kingdom

**Henry Li**

- Tony Blair Institute for Global Change, London, United Kingdom

**Gabriel Assis Lopes do Carmo**

- Federal University of Minas Gerais, Brazil

**Catherine Machalaba**

- The Nature Conservancy, United States; formerly EcoHealth Alliance

**Nita K. Madhav**

- Ginkgo Bioworks, Emeryville, California, United States

**Sri Harshavardhan Malapati**

- Harvard University, Boston, Massachusetts, United States

**Romina Mariano**

- Africa Clinical Research Network, Harare, Zimbabwe

**Jonna Mazet**

- University of California, Davis, California, United States

**Claire T. McMahon**

- Market Shaping Accelerator, University of Chicago, Illinois, United States

**Amanda Meadows**

- Ginkgo Bioworks, Emeryville, California, United States

**Elizabeth Mumford**

- University of Surrey, United Kingdom

**Ole F. Norheim**

- Harvard T. H. Chan School of Public Health, Boston, Massachusetts, United States

**Ben Oppenheim**

- Ginkgo Bioworks, Emeryville, California; Center for Global Development, Washington, DC, United States

**Hitoshi Oshitani**

- Tohoku University, Japan

**Geoffrey Otim**

- SynBio Africa, Makerere University, Kampala, Uganda

**Qian Yi Pang**

- Ellison Institute of Technology, Oxford, United Kingdom

**Muhammad Ali Pate**

- Ministry of Health and Social Welfare of Nigeria

**Edith Patouillard**

- World Health Organization, Geneva, Switzerland

**Sharmila Paul**

- University of California, San Francisco, California, United States

**Alexandra Penn**

- University of Sussex, United Kingdom; formerly University of Surrey, United Kingdom

**Govind Persad**

- University of Denver, Colorado, United States

**Diego Pineda**

- University of California, Berkeley, California, United States

**Nistara Randhawa**

- University of California, Davis, California, United States

**John Rose**

- University of California, San Francisco, California, United States

**Sophie Rose**

- Centre for Long-Term Resilience, London, United Kingdom

**Jonathan Rushton**

- University of Liverpool, United Kingdom

**Linda Schultz**

- London School of Hygiene and Tropical Medicine, United Kingdom

**Gabriel Seidman**

- Ellison Institute of Technology, Oxford, United Kingdom

**Siddhanth Sharma**

- Burnet Institute, Melbourne, Australia

**Zara Shubber**

- World Bank, Washington, DC, United States

**Christopher M. Snyder**

- Department of Economics, Dartmouth College, Hanover, New Hampshire, United States

**Emily Stanger-Sfeile**

- Tony Blair Institute for Global Change, London, United Kingdom

**Cristina Stefan**

- Centre for Disaster Protection, London, United Kingdom

**Nicole Stephenson**

- Ginkgo Bioworks, Emeryville, California, United States

**Anna-Maria Tammi**

- Global Partnership for Education, Washington, DC, United States

**Dipesh Tamrakar**

- Kathmandu University, Nepal

**Eri Togami**

- Johns Hopkins University, Baltimore, Maryland, United States

**Helene-Mari van der Westhuizen**

- University of Oxford, United Kingdom

**Sabine L. van Elsland**

- MRC Centre for Global Infectious Disease Analysis, Imperial College London, United Kingdom

**Supaporn Wacharapluesadee**

- Thai Red Cross Emerging Infectious Diseases Clinical Center, King Chulalongkorn Memorial Hospital, Chulalongkorn University, Thailand

**Chen Wang**

- Chinese Academy of Medical Sciences, Beijing, China

**Darcy Ward**

- Tony Blair Institute for Global Change, London, United Kingdom

**Kathleen Warren**

- Health Emergencies Programme, World Health Organization, Geneva, Switzerland

**David A. Watkins**

- University of Washington, Seattle, Washington, United States

**Charles Whittaker**

- MRC Centre for Global Infectious Disease Analysis, Imperial College London, United Kingdom; Division of Infectious Diseases and Vaccinology, School of Public Health, University of California, Berkeley, California, United States

**Bridget Williams**

- Uehiro Centre for Practical Ethics, University of Oxford, United Kingdom

**Jiuyang Xu**

- China-Japan Friendship Hospital, Beijing, China

**Lan Xue**

- Tsinghua University, Beijing, China

**Jakob Zinsstag**

- Swiss Tropical and Public Health Institute, Allschwil, Switzerland

# Reviewers

**Shuchi Anand**

- Stanford University, Stanford, California, United States

**Sulzhan Bali**

- World Bank, Washington, DC, United States

**Stefano M. Bertozzi**

- University of California, Berkeley, California, United States

**Mark Blecher**

- National Treasury, South Africa

**Mukesh Chawla**

- World Bank, Washington, DC, United States

**Nejma Cheikh**

- World Bank, Washington, DC, United States

**Alex Cook**

- National University of Singapore, Singapore

**Benjamin Cowling**

- University of Hong Kong, Hong Kong SAR, China

**Nir Eyal**

- Rutgers University, New Brunswick, New Jersey, United States

**Clementine Fu**

- World Bank, Washington, DC, United States

**Ramesh Govindaraj**

- World Bank, Washington, DC, United States

**Moytrayee Guha**

- World Bank, Washington, DC, United States

**Nilofer Habibullah**

- World Bank, Washington, DC, United States

**Katharina Hauck**

- Imperial College London, United Kingdom

**Kathryn Jacobsen**

- University of Richmond, Richmond, Virginia, United States

**Dean T. Jamison**

- University of California, San Francisco, California, United States

**Magnus Lindelow**

- World Bank, Washington, DC, United States

**Joe Millum**

- University of St. Andrews, Scotland

**Linda Mobula**

- World Bank, Washington, DC, United States

**Suresh Kunhi Mohammed**

- World Bank, Washington, DC, United States

**Son Nam Nguyen**

- World Bank, Washington, DC, United States

**Ole F. Norheim**

- Harvard T. H. Chan School of Public Health, Boston, Massachusetts, United States; University of Bergen, Norway

**Ben Oppenheim**

- Ginkgo Bioworks, Emeryville, California, United States; Center for Global Development, Washington, DC, United States

**Hitoshi Oshitani**

- Tohoku University, Japan

**Joao Pires**

- World Bank, Washington, DC, United States

**Siddhanth Sharma**

- Burnet Institute, Melbourne, Australia

**Woutrina Smith**

- University of California, Davis, California, United States

**Karin Stenberg**

- World Health Organization, Geneva, Switzerland

**Jonathan Suk**

- European Centre for Disease Prevention and Control, Solna, Sweden

**Jeremy Veillard**

- World Bank, Washington, DC, United States

**Saul Walker**

- Foreign, Commonwealth & Development Office, London, United Kingdom

**David A. Watkins**

- University of Washington, Seattle, Washington, United States

**Martin Weber**

- World Health Organization Regional Office for Europe, Copenhagen, Denmark

**Paul Wilson**

- Columbia University, New York, United States

www.ingramcontent.com/pod-product-compliance
Lightning Source LLC
Chambersburg PA
CBHW050900210326

41597CB00002B/26